T0310731

Data Mining in Public and Private Sectors: Organizational and Government Applications

Antti Syväjärvi
University of Lapland, Finland

Jari Stenvall
Tampere University, Finland

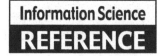

INFORMATION SCIENCE REFERENCE

Hershey · New York

Director of Editorial Content:	Kristin Klinger
Director of Book Publications:	Julia Mosemann
Acquisitions Editor:	Lindsay Johnston
Development Editor:	Joel Gamon
Publishing Assistant:	Keith Glazewski
Typesetter:	Michael Brehm
Production Editor:	Jamie Snavely
Cover Design:	Lisa Tosheff
Printed at:	Yurchak Printing Inc.

Published in the United States of America by
Information Science Reference (an imprint of IGI Global)
701 E. Chocolate Avenue
Hershey PA 17033
Tel: 717-533-8845
Fax: 717-533-8661
E-mail: cust@igi-global.com
Web site: http://www.igi-global.com/reference

Library of Congress Cataloging-in-Publication Data

Data mining in public and private sectors : organizational and government
applications / Antti Syvajarvi and Jari Stenvall, editors.
     p. cm.
  Includes bibliographical references and index.
  Summary: "This book, which explores the manifestation of data mining and how
it can be enhanced at various levels of management, provides relevant
theoretical frameworks and the latest empirical research findings"--Provided
by publisher.
  ISBN 978-1-60566-906-9 (hardcover) -- ISBN 978-1-60566-907-6 (ebook) 1.
Data mining. I. Syväjärvi, Antti. II. Stenvall, Jari.
  QA76.9.D343D38323 2010
  006.3'12--dc22
                        2010010160

British Cataloguing in Publication Data
A Cataloguing in Publication record for this book is available from the British Library.

All work contributed to this book is new, previously-unpublished material. The views expressed in this book are those of the authors, but not necessarily of the publisher.

Table of Contents

Section 2
Data Mining as Privacy, Security and Retention of Data and Knowledge

Section 3
Data Mining in Organizational Situations to Prepare and Forecast

Detailed Table of Contents

Section 1
Data Mining Studied in Management and Government

    Dries Verlet, Ghent University, Belgium
    Carl Devos, Ghent University, Belgium

In Chapter researchers have studied the performance measurement in public administration and focus on a few common difficulties that might occur when measuring performance in the public sector. They emphasize the growing attention for policy evaluation and especially for the evidence-based policy, and thus discuss the role of data mining in public knowledge discovery and its sensitive governmental position in the public sector.

    José Luis Zafra-Gómez, Granada University, Spain
    Antonio Manuel Cortés-Romero, Granada University, Spain

The Chapter is focused on local governments and those economic conditions. Data mining technique is used and related to local municipalities' financial dimensions like budgetary stability, solvency, flexibility and independence. Authors have examined a wide range of indicators in public accounts and thus they build up principal factors for dimensions. A model will be developed to measure and explain the financial conditions in local governments.

The Chapter show strategies employed by the public long-term care systems operated by each U.S. state
government. Researchers have employed data mining using fuzzy decision trees as a timely exposition
and with the employment of set-theoretic approaches to organizational configurations. The use of fuzzy
decision trees is seen relevant in organizational and government research as it assist to understand government attributes and positions in a general service strategy.

Chapter 4

In Chapter, the performance of local administrative regions is studied in order to recognize both factors
related to performance and their interactions. Through data mining researchers introduce the basic unit
concept for public services, which enables the measurement of local government performance. Authors
report a range of results and argue how current findings can be used to improve decision making and
management of administrative regions.

Chapter 5

In this Chapter researchers have studied public service productivity in the area of child day care. Accordingly there is not enough knowledge about productivity drivers in public organizations and thus the
data mining might be helpful. Some operational factors of public service productivity are studied. The
data mining is seen as a method, but it also emerges as a procedure for either organizational management or government use.

Section 2
Data Mining as Privacy, Security and Retention of Data and Knowledge

In current Chapter, the mobile computing technology and certain challenges of data mining are under scrutiny. The Chapter deals with issues like privacy and security. It indicates higher level of knowledge related to technology and less to knowledge about privacy, safety and security. The more important role of data mining and its sub themes are demanded by various means and an attempt to improve knowledge with mobile computing technology is introduced.

Chapter 7

In Chapter the privacy preserving data mining is introduced and discussed. The privacy is a growing and world wide concern with information and information exchange. This Chapter highlights the importance of privacy with data and information management issues that can be related to both public and private organizations. Finally it is provided some viewpoints for potential future research directions in the field of privacy-aware data mining.

Chapter 8

Information flows are huge in organizational and government surroundings. The aim of Chapter is to face some organizational data retention challenges for both internet service providers and government authorities. Modern organizations have to develop data and information security policies in order to act against unauthorized accesses or disclosures. Data warehouse architecture for retaining data is presented and a data warehouse schema following EU directive is elaborated.

Chapter 9

Knowledge is one of the most important resources for current and future organizational activities. This Chapter is focused on knowledge and data mining as it discuss how those are related to knowledge management. Validity of knowledge is analyzed in the respect of organizational studies. Following information and Penrose's steps, the security and knowledge become resources for standardization and those are further identified as being data mining based.

Section 3
Data Mining in Organizational Situations to Prepare and Forecast

    Jue Wang, Chinese Academy of Sciences, China
    Wei Xu, Renmin University, China
    Xun Zhang, Chinese Academy of Sciences, China
    Yejing Bao, Beijing University of Technology, China
    Ye Pang, The People's Insurance Company (Group) of China, China
    Shouyang Wang, Chinese Academy of Sciences, China

To perform and to forecast on the basis of data and information are challenging. Data mining based activities are studied in the case of oil markets as two separate mining models are implemented in order to analyze and forecast. According to Chapter, proposed models create improvements as well as the overall performance will get better. Thus, the data mining is taken as a promising approach for private organizations and governmental agencies to analyze and to predict.

    Vincent Lemaire, France Télécom, France
    Carine Hue, GFI Informatique, France
    Olivier Bernier, France Télécom, France

This Chapter offers a general, but simultaneously comprehensive way for organizations to deal with data mining opportunities and challenges. An important issue for any organization is to recognize the linkage between certain probabilities and relevant input values. More precisely the Chapter shows the predictive probability of specified class by exploring the possible values of input variables. All these are in relation to data mining and proposed processes show such findings that might be relevant for various organizational situations.

    Mirco Nanni, ISTI Institute of CNR, Italy
    Laura Spinsanti, Ecole Polytechnique Fédérale de Lausanne, Switzerland

Current Chapter debates about multifaceted challenge of forecasting in the private sector. Now in retail trade situations, the response of clients to product promotions and thus to certain business operations are studied. In the sense of data mining, the approach consists of multi-class classifiers and discretization of sales values. In addition, quality measures are provided in order to evaluate the accuracy of forecast for sales. Finally a scheme is drafted with forecast functionalities that are organized on the basis of business needs.

For any business it is important to prepare yourself according to changing situations. Changes may occur because of many reasons, but probably one of most vital is the competition feature. In Chapter, the data mining has both preparative and preventative role as development of an early caution system is described. This system might be a supportive element for business management and it may be used in the retail industry. Data mining is seen as a possibility to tackle competition.

Section 4
Data Mining as Applications and Approaches Related to Organizational Scene

This Chapter takes part to organizational studies by describing how potential the data mining might be to extract implicit, unknown and vital information. The data mining analysis is carried out with CaRBS and an application is considered by using data drawn from a large multipurpose public organization. The final aim is to study the argument that consensus on organization's strategic priorities is somehow determined by structures, processes and operational environment.

Networks and networked collaboration are progressively more essential research objectives in the organizational panorama. The Chapter deals with data mining and applies some new prospects into the field of inter-organizational business networks. A novel research framework for network-wide knowledge discovery is presented and by theoretical discussion a more multidisciplinary orientated research and information conceptualization is implemented. These viewpoints allow an approach to proceed with data mining, network knowledge and governance.

In many occasions both the evidence and the evidence-based practices are seen as factors of organizational success and advantage. In this Chapter, the clinical data mining is introduced as practice-based approach for organizational and government functions. Assorted exemplars from health and human service settings are under scrutiny. The clinical data management has gained recognition among social and health care sectors, and additionally other useful benefits are introduced. Above all, the importance of evidence-informed practice is finally highlighted.

Chapter 17

The project oriented environment is a reality for both private and public sectors. The Chapter presents the data mining concept together with rather dynamic organizational project management environment. Processes that control the information flow for generating data warehouses are identified and some key data warehouse contents are defined. Accordingly the data mining may be utilized successfully, but still some critical issues should be tackled in private and public sectors.

Chapter 18

The aim of Chapter is to explore data mining in terms of knowledge discovery in networked environment. Communicational and collaborative network activities are targeted as the author structuralizes not only explicit information contents but also valid information types in relation to knowledge and networks. It is shown how data and knowledge requirements vary according to situations and thus flexible data mining and knowledge discovery systems are needed.

Foreword

Data mining has developed rapidly and has become very popular in the past two decades, but actually has its origin in the early stages of IT, then being mostly limited to one-dimensional searching in databases. The statistical basis of what is now also referred to as data mining has often been laid centuries ago. In corporate environments data driven decisions have quickly become the standard, with the preparation of data for management becoming the focus of the fields of MIS (management information systems) and DSS (decision support systems) in the 1970's and 1980's. With even more advanced technology and approaches becoming available, such as data cubes, the field of business intelligence took off quickly in the 1990's and has since then played a core role in corporate data processing and data management in public administration.

Especially in public administration, the availability and the correct analysis of data have always been of major importance. Ample amounts of data collected for producing statistical analyses and forecasts on economic, social, health and education issues show how important data collection and data analysis have become for governments and international organisations. The resulting, periodically produced statistics on economic growth, the development of interest rates and inflation, household income, education standards, crime trends and climate change are a major input factor for governmental planning. The same holds true for customer behaviour analysis, production and sales statistics in business.

From a researchers point of view this leads to many interesting topics of a high practical relevance, such as how to assure the quality of the collected data, in which context to use the collected data, and the protection of privacy of employees, customers and citizens, when at the same time the appetite of businesses and public administration for data is growing exponentially. While in previous decades storage costs, narrow communications bandwidth and inadequate and expensive computational power limited the scope of data analysis, these limitations are starting to disappear, opening new dimensions such as the distribution and integration of data collections, in its most current version "in the cloud". Systems enabling almost unlimited ubiquitous access to data and allowing collaboration with hardly any technology-imposed time and location restrictions have dramatically changed the way in which we look at data, collect it, share it and use it.

Covering such central issues as the preparation of organisations for data mining, the role of data mining in crisis management, the application of new algorithmic approaches, a wide variety of examples of applications in business and public management, data mining in the context of location based services, privacy issues and legal obligations, the link to knowledge management, forecasting and traditional statistics, and the use of fuzzy systems, to summarize only the most important aspects of the contributions in this book, it provides the reader with a very interesting overview of the field from an application oriented perspective. That is why this book can be expected to be a valuable resource for practitioners and educators.

Gerald Quirchmayr, professor
University of Vienna, Austria
Department of Distributed and Multimedia Systems

Gerald Quirchmayr *holds doctors degrees in computer science and law from Johannes Kepler University in Linz (Austria) and currently he is Professor at the Department of Distributed and Multimedia Systems at the University of Vienna. His wide international experience ranges from the participation in international teaching and research projects, very often UN- and EU-based, several research stays at universities and research centers in the US and EU Member States to extensive teaching in EU staff exchange programs in the United Kingdom, Sweden, Finland, Germany, Spain, and Greece, as well as teaching stays in the Czech Republic and Poland. He has served as a member of program committees of many international conferences, chaired several of them, has contributed as reviewer to scientific journals and has also served on editorial boards. His major research focus is on information systems in business and government with a special interest in security, applications, formal representations of decision making and legal issues.*

Preface

Attempts to get organizational or corporate data under control began more profoundly in the late 1960s and early 1970s. Slightly later on, due to management studies and the development of information societies and organizations, the importance of data in administration and management became even more evident. Since then the data/information/knowledge based structures, processes and actors have been under scientific study. Data mining has originally involved research that is mainly composed of statistics, computer science, information science, engineering, etc. As stated and particularly due to knowledge discovery, knowledge management, information management and electronic government research, the data mining has been related more closely to both public and private sector organizations and governments. Many organizations in the public and private sector generate, collect and refine massive quantities of data and information. Thus data mining and its applications have been implemented, for example, in order to enhance the value of existing information, to highlight evidence-based practices in management and finally to deal with increasing complexities and future demands.

Indeed data mining might be a powerful application with great potential to help both public and private organizations focus on the most important information needs. Humans and organizations have been collecting and systematizing data for eternity. It has been clear that people, organizations, businesses and governments are increasingly acting like consumers of data and information. This is again due to the advancement in organizational computer technology and e-government, due to the information and communication technology (ICT), due to increasingly demanding work design, due to the organizational changes and complexities, and finally due to new applications and innovations in both public and private organizations (e.g. Tidd et al. 2005, Syväjärvi et al. 2005, Bauer et al. 2006, de Korvin et al. 2007, Burke 2008, Chowdhury 2009). All these studies authorize that data has an increasing impact for organizations and governance in public and private sectors.

Hence, the data mining has become an increasingly important factor to manage, with information in increasingly complex environments. Mining of data, information, and knowledge from various databases has been recognized by many researchers from various academic fields (e.g. Watson 2005). Data mining can be seen as a multidisciplinary research field, drawing work from areas like database technology, statistics, pattern recognition, information retrieval, learning and networks, knowledge-based systems, knowledge organizations, management, high-performance computing, data visualization, etc. Also in organizational and government context, the data mining can be understood as the use of sophisticated data analysis applications to discover previously unknown, valid patterns and relationships in large data sets. These objectives are apparent in various fields of the public and private sectors. All these approaches are apparent in various fields of both public and private sectors as will be shown by current chapters.

DATA MINING LINKED TO ORGANIZATIONAL AND GOVERNMENT CONDITIONS

The data mining seen as the extraction of unknown information and typically from large databases can be a powerful approach to help organizations to focus on the most essential information. Data mining may ease to predict future trends and behaviors allowing organizations to make information and evidence-based decisions. Organizations live with their history, present activities, but prospective analyses offered by data mining may also move beyond the analyses of past or present events. These are typically provided by tools of decision support systems (e.g. McNurlin & Sprague 2006) or possibilities offered either by information management or electronic government (e.g. Heeks 2006, de Korvin et al. 2007, Syväjärvi & Stenvall 2009). Also the data mining functionalities are in touch with organizational and government surroundings by traditional techniques or in terms of classification, clustering, regression and associations (e.g. Han & Kamber 2006). Thus again, the data needs to be classified, arranged and related according to certain situational demands.

It is fundamental to know how data mining can answer organizational information needs that otherwise might be too complex or unclear. The information that is needed, for example, should usually be more future-orientated and quite frequently somehow combined with possibilities offered by the information and communication technology. In many cases, the data mining may reveal such history, indicate present situation or even predict future trends and behaviors that allow either public policies or businesses to make proactive and information driven decisions. Data mining applications may possibly answer organizational and government questions that traditionally are too much resource consuming to resolve or otherwise difficult to learn and handle. These viewpoints are important in terms of sector and organization performance and productivity plus to facilitate learning and change management capabilities (Bouckaert & Halligan 2006, Burke 2008, Kesti & Syväjärvi 2010).

Data mining in both public and private sector is largely about collecting and utilizing the data, analyzing and forecasting on the basis of data, taking care of data qualities, and understanding implications of the data and information. Thus in organizational and government perspective, the data mining is related to mining itself, to applications, to data qualities (i.e. security, integrity, privacy, etc.), and to information management in order to be able to govern in public and private sectors. It is clear that organization and people collect and process massive quantities of data, but how they do that and how they proceed with information is not that simple. In addition to the qualities of data, the data mining is thus intensely related to management, organizational and government processes and structures, and thus to better information management, performance and overall policy (e.g. Rochet 2004, Bouckaert & Halligan 2006, Hamlin 2007, Heinrich 2007, Krone et al. 2009). For example, Hamlin (2007) concluded that in order to satisfy performance measurement requirements policy makers frequently have little choice but to consider and use a mix of different types of information. Krone et al. (2009) showed how organizational structures facilitate many challenges and possibilities for knowledge and information processes.

Data mining may confront organizational and governmental weaknesses or even threats. For example, in private sector competition, technological infrastructures, change dynamics and customer-centric approaches might be such that there is not always space for proper data mining. In the public sector, the data or information related to service delivery originates classically from various sources. Also public policy processes are complex in their nature and include, for example, multiplicity of actors, diversified interdependent actors, longer time spans and political power (e.g. Hill & Hupe 2003, Lamothe & Dufour 2007). Thus some of these organizational and government guidelines vigorously call for better quality data, more experimental evaluations and advanced applications. Finally because of the absence of high-quality data and easily available information, along with high-stakes pressures to demonstrate organizational improvements, the data for these purposes is still more likely to be misused or manipulated. However, it is evident that organizational and government activities confront requirements like predicting and forecasting, but also vital are topics like data security, privacy, retention, etc.

In relation to situational organization and government structures, processes and people, the data mining is especially connected to qualities, management, applications and approaches that are linked to data itself. In existing and future organizational and government surrounding, electronic-based views and information and communication technologies also have a significant place. In current approach of data mining in public and private sectors, we may thus summarize three main thematic dimensions that are data and knowledge, information management and situational elements. By data and knowledge we mean the epistemological character of data and demands that are linked to issues like security, privacy, nature, hierarchy and quality. The versatile information management refers here to administration of data, data warehouses, data-based processes, data actors and people, and applied information and communication technologies. Situational elements indicate operational and strategic environments (like networks, bureaucracies, and competitions, etc.), but also stabile or change-based situations and various timeframes (e.g. past-present-future). All these dimensions are revealed by present chapters.

THE BOOK STRUCTURE AND FINAL REMARKS

This book includes research on data mining in public and private sectors. Furthermore, both organizational and government applications are under scientific research. Totally eighteen chapters have been divided to four consecutive sections. Section 1 will handle data mining in relation to management and government, while Section 2 is about data mining that concentrates on privacy, security and retention of data and knowledge. Section 3 relates data mining to such organizational and government situations that require strategic views, future preparations and forecasts. The last section, Section 4, handles various data mining applications and approaches that are related to organizational scenes.

Hence, we can presuppose how managerial decision making situations are followed by both rational and tentative procedures. As data mining is typically associated with data warehouses (i.e. various volumes of data and various sources of data), we are able to clarify some key dimension of data mined decisions (e.g. Beynon-Davies 2002). These include information needs, seeks and usages in data and information management. As data mining is seen as the extraction of information from large databases, we still notice the management linkage in terms of traditional decision making phases (i.e. intelligence, design, choice and review) and managerial roles like informational roles (Minztberg 1973, Simon 1977). In relation to the management, it is obvious that organizations need tools, systems and procedures that might be useful in decision making. Management of information resources means that data has meaning and further it is such information demands of expanded information resources to where the job of managing has also expanded (e.g. McNurlin & Sprague 2006).

In organizational and government surroundings, it is valuable to notice that data mining is popularly referred to knowledge and knowledge discovery. Knowledge discovery is about combining information to find hidden knowledge (e.g. Papa et al. 2008). However, again it seems to be important to understand how "automated" or convenient is the extraction of information that represents stored knowledge or information to be discovered from large various clusters or data warehouses. For example, Moon (2002) has argued that information technology has given possibilities to handle information among governmental agencies, to enhance internal managerial efficiency and the quality of public service delivery, but simultaneously there are many barriers and legal issues that cause delays. Consequently one core factor here is the security of data and information. The information security in organizational and government context means typically protecting of information and information systems from unauthorized access, use, disclosure, modification and destruction (e.g. Karyda, Mitrou & Quirchmayr 2006, Brotby 2009). Organizations and governments accumulate a great deal of information and thus the information security is needed to study in terms of management, legal informatics, privacy, etc. Finally the latter has profound arguments as information security policy documents can describe organizational and government intentions with information.

Data mining is stressed by current and future situations that are changing and developing rather constantly both in public and private sectors. Situational awareness of past, present and future circumstances denote understanding of such aspects that are relevant for organizational and government life. In this context data mining is connected to both learning and forecasting capabilities, but also to organizational structures, processes and people that indeed may fluctuate. However, preparing and forecasting according to various organizational and government situations as well as structural choices like bureaucratic, functional, divisional, network, boundary-less, and virtual are all in close touch to data mining approaches. Especially in the era of digital government organizations simply need to seek, to receive, to transmit and finally to learn with information in various ways. As related to topics like organizational structures, government viewpoints and to the field of e-Government, thus it is probably due to fast development, continuous changes and familiarity with technology why situational factors are progressively more stressed (e.g. Fountain 2001, Moon 2002, Syväjärvi et al. 2005, Bauer et al. 2006, Brown 2007). In case of data mining, it is important to recognize that these changes deliver a number of challenges to citizens, businesses and public governments. As a consequence, the change effort for any organization is quite unique to that organization (rf. Burke 2008). For instance, Heeks (2006) assumes that we need to see how changing and developing governments are management information systems. Barrett et al. (2006) studied organizational change and concluded what is needed is such studies that draw on and combine both organizational studies and information system studies.

As final remarks we conclude that organizational and government situations are becoming increasingly complex as well as data has become more important. Some core demands like service needs and conditions, ubiquitous society, organizational structures, renewing work processes, quality of data and information, and finally continuous and discontinuous changes challenge both public and private sectors. Data volumes are still growing, changing very fast and increasing almost exponentially, and are not likely to stop. This book aims to provide some relevant frameworks and research in the area of organizational and government data mining. It will increase understanding how of data mining is used and applied in public and private sectors. Mining of data, information, and knowledge from various locations has been recognized here by researchers of multidisciplinary academic fields. In this book it is shown that data mining, as well as its links to information and knowledge, have become very valuable resources for societies, organizations, actors, businesses and governments of all kind.

Indeed both organizations and government agencies need to generate, to collect and to utilize data in public and private sector activities. Both organizational and government complexities are growing and simultaneously the potential of data mining is becoming more and more evident. However, the implications of data mining in organizations and government agencies remain still somewhat blurred or unrevealed. Now this uncertainty is at least partly reduced. Finally this book will be for researchers and professionals who are working in the field of data, information and knowledge. It involves advanced knowledge of data mining and from various disciplines like public administration, management, information science, organization science, education, sociology, computer science, and from applied information technology. We hope that this book will stimulate further data mining based research that is focused on organizations and governments.

Antti Syväjärvi
Jari Stenvall
Editors

REFERENCES

Barrett, M. Grant, D. & Weiles, N. (2006). ICT and Organizational Change. *The Journal of Applied Behavioral Change, 42*(1), 6–22.

Bauer, T.N., Truxillo, D.M., Tucker, J.S., Weathers, V., Bertolino, M., Erdogan, B. & Campion, M.A. (2006). Selection in the Information Age: The Impact of Privacy Concerns and Computer Experience on Applicant Reactions. *Journal of Management, 32*(5), 601–621.

Beynon-Davies, P. (2002). *Information Systems: an Introduction to Informatics in Organizations*. New York: Palgrave Publishers, Ltd. USA.

Bouckaert, G. & Halligan, J. (2006). Performance and Performance Management. In B.G. Peter, & J. Pierre (eds.), *Handbook of Public Policy,* (pp. 443–459). London: SAGE Publications.

Burke, W. (2008). *Organization Change – Theory and Practice,* (2nd Ed.). New York: SAGE Publication.

Brotby, K. (2009). *Information Security Governance*. New York: John Wiley & Sons.

Brown, M. (2007). Understanding e-Government Benefits. An Examination of Leading-Edge Local Governments. *The American Review of Public Administration, 37*(2), 178–197.

Chowdhury, S.I. (2009). *A Conceptual Framework for Data Mining and Knowledge Management*. In H. Rahman (ed.) *Social and Political Implications of Data Mining*. Hershey, PA: IGI Global.

Fountain, J. (2001). *Building the Virtual State: Information Technology and Institutional Change*. Washington, DC: Brookings Institution. USA.

de Korvin, A. Hashemi, S. & Quirchmayr, G. (2007). Information Preloading Strategies for e-Government Sites based on User's Stated Preference. *Journal of Enterprise Information Management, 20*(1), 119–131.

Hamlin, R.G. (2007). An Evidence-based Perspective on HRD. *Advances in Developing Human Resources, 9*(1), 42–57.

Han, J. & Kamber, M. (2006). *Data Mining: Concepts and Techniques,* (2nd Ed.). San Francisco: Morgan Kaufmann Publishers, Elsevier Inc.

Heeks, R. (2006). *Implementing and Managing e-Government*. London: SAGE Publications.

Hill, M.J. & Hupe, P.L. (2003). The Multi-Layer Problem in Implementation Research. *Public Management Review*, *5*(4), 469–488.

Heinrich, C.J. (2007). Evidence based Policy and Performance Management. *The American Review of Public Administration, 37*(3), 255–277.

Karyda, M., Mitrou, E. & Quirchmayr, G. (2006). A Framework for Outsourcing IS/IT Security Services. *Information Management & Computer Security, 14*(5), 402–415.

Kesti, M. & Syväjärvi, A. (2010). Human Tacit Signals at Organization Performance Development. *Industrial Management and Data Systems*, (In press).

Lamothe, L. & Dufour, Y. (2007). Systems of Interdependency and Core Orchestrating Themes at Health Care Unit Level – A Configurational Approach. *Public Management Review, 9*(1), 67–85.

Krone, O., Syväjärvi, A. & Stenvall, J. (2009). Knowledge Integration for Enterprise Resources Planning Application Design. *Knowledge and Process Management, 16*(1), 1–12.

McNurlin, B. & Sprague, R.H. (2006). *Information Systems Management in Practice*. New York: Prentice Hall, USA.

Minztberg, H. (1973). *The Nature of Managerial Work*. New York: Harper & Row.

Moon, M.J. (2002). The Evolution of E-Government among Municipalities – Rhetoric or Reality? *Public Administration Review, 62*(4), 424–433.

Papa, M.J., Daniels, T.D. & Spiker, B.K. (2008) *Organizational communication. Perspectives and Trends*. London: SAGE Publications.

Rochet, C. (2004). Rethinking the Management of Information in the Strategic Monitoring of Public Policies by Agencies. *Industrial Management & Data Systems, 104*(3), 201–208.

Simon, H. (1977). *A New Science of Management Decisions*. Upper Saddle River, NJ: Prentice Hall.

Syväjärvi, A. Stenvall, J. Harisalo, R. & Jurvansuu, H. (2005). The Impact of Information Technology on Human Capacity, Interprofessional Practice and Management. *Problems and Perspectives in Management, 1*(4), 82–95.

Syväjärvi, A. & Stenvall, J. (2009). *Core Governmental Perspectives of e-Health*. In J. Tan, (ed.), *Medical Informatics: Concepts, Methodologies, Tools, and Applications*. Hershey, PA: Medical Information Science Reference.

Tidd, J., Bessant, J. & Pavitt, K. (2005). *Managing Innovation: Integrating Technological, Market and Organizational Change,* (3rd Ed.). London: John Wiley & Sons, Ltd.

Watson, R.T. (2005). *Data Management: Databases & Organizations,* (5th, Ed.). San Francisco: Wiley, USA.

Section 1
Data Mining Studied in Management and Government

Chapter 1

Before the Mining Begins:
An Enquiry into the Data for Performance Measurement in the Public Sector

Dries Verlet
Ghent University, Belgium

Carl Devos
Ghent University, Belgium

ABSTRACT

Although policy evaluation has always been important, today there is a rising attention for policy evaluation in the public sector. In order to provide a solid base for the so-called evidence-based policy, valid en reliable data are needed to depict the performance of organisations within the public sector. Without a solid empirical base, one needs to be very careful with data mining in the public sector. When measuring performance, several unintended and negative effects can occur. In this chapter, the authors focus on a few common pitfalls that occur when measuring performance in the public sector. They also discuss possible strategies to prevent them by setting up and adjusting the right measurement systems for performance in the public sector. Data mining is about knowledge discovery. The question is: what do we want to know? What are the consequences of asking that question?

INTRODUCTION

Policy aims at desired and foreseen effects. That is the very nature of policy. Policy needs to be evaluated, so that policy makers know if the specific policy measures indeed reach – and if so, how, how efficient or effective, with what unintended or unforeseen effects, etc. – these intended results and objectives. However, measuring policy effects

is not without disadvantages. The policy evaluation process can cause side effects.

Evaluating policy implies making fundamental choices. It is not an easy exercise. Moreover, policy actors are aware of the methods with which their activities – their (implementation of) policy – will or could be evaluated. They can anticipate the evaluation, e.g. by changing the official policy goals – a crucial standard in the evaluation process – or by choosing only these goals that can be met and avoiding more ambitious goals that are more difficult to reach. In this context, policy actors

DOI: 10.4018/978-1-60566-906-9.ch001

behave strategically (Swanborn, 1999). In this chapter, we focus on these and other side effects of policy evaluation. However, we also want to bring them in a broader framework.

Within the public sector, as elsewhere, there is the need to have tools in order to dig through huge collections of data looking for previously unrecognized trends or patterns. Within the public sector, one often refer to "official data" (Brito & Malerba, 2003, 497). There too, knowledge and information are cornerstones of a (post-) modern society (Vandijck & Despontin, 1998). In this context data, mining is essential for the public sector. Data mining can be seen as part of the wider process of so called Knowledge Discovery in Databases (KDD). KDD is the process of distillation of information from raw data, while data mining is more specific and refers to the discovery of patterns in terms of classification, problem solving and knowledge engineering (Vandijck & Despontin, 1998).

However, before the actual data mining can be started, we need a solid empirical base. Only then the public sector has a valid and reliable governance tool (Bouckaert & Halligan, 2008). In general, the public sector is quite well documented. In recent decades, huge amounts of data and reports are being published on the output and management of the public sector in general. However, a stubborn problem is the gathering of data about the specific functioning of specific institutions within the broad public sector.

The use of data and data mining in the public sector is crucial in order to evaluate public programs and investments, for instance in crime, traffic, economic growth, social security, public health, law enforcement, integration programs of immigrants, cultural participation, etc. Thanks to the implementation of ICT, recording and storing transactional and substantive information is much easier. The possible applications of data mining in the public sector are quite divers: it can be used in policy implementation and evaluation, targeting of

specific groups, customer-cantric public services, etc. (Gramatikov, 2003).

A major topic in data mining in the public sector is the handling of personal information. The use of such information balances between respect for the privacy, data integrity and data security on the one hand and maximising the available information for general policy purposes on the other (cf. Crossman, G., 2008). Intelligent data mining can provide a reduction of the societal uncertainty without endangering the privacy of citizens.

During the past decades, the functioning and the ideas about the public sector changed profoundly. Several evolutions explain these changes. Cornforth (2003, o.c. in Spanhove & Verhoest, 2007,) states that two related reforms are crucial. First, government create an increasing number of (quasi-)autonomous government agencies in order to deliver public services. Secondly, there is the introduction of market mechanisms into the provision of public services. Doing so, there is also a raising attention for criteria such as competition, efficiency and effectiveness (Verhoest & Spanhove, 2007). Spurred by "Reinventing Government" from Osborne & Gaebler (1993), in the public sector too, performance measurement was placed more on the forefront. The idea is tempting and simple: a government organisation defines its "products" (e.g. services) and develops indicators to make the production of it measurable. This enables an organisation – thanks to the planning and control cycle – to work on a good performing organisation (De Bruijn, 2002). In this way, a government can function optimally.

The evaluation of performance within the public sector boosted after the hegemony of the New Public Management (NPM) paradigm. An essential component of NPM is "explicit standards and measures or performance" (Hood, 1996, 271). Given the fact that direct market incentives are absent in government performance – as a result of which bad or too expensive performances are sanctioned by means of decreasing sale or income and corrective action is inevitable – the performance of the public sector needs elaborate and constant evaluation. So, bad or too expensive performances can be steered. It is often recommended that the public sector needs to use, as much as possible, the methods of the private sector, although the specific characteristics of the public sector must be taken into account. However, the application within the public sector not always goes smoothly (Modell, 2004).

There are a lot of reasons why one can plead to better evaluate the performance of the public, apart from NPM. One of those arguments is that better government policy will also reinforce the trust in public service. Although the empirical material is scarce, there are important indications that the objective of an increas of public trust in policy making and government is not reached, even sometimes on the contrary, if it the publication of performance measurements is not handled carefully (Hayes & Pidd, 2005).

Other reasons for more performance measurement speak for themselves. The scarce tax money must be applied as useful as possible; citizens are entitled to the best service. The attention for efficiency and effectiveness of the public service has been on top of the political and media agenda. For this reason, citizens and their political representatives ask for a maximal "return on investment". Therefore, there is political pressure to pay more attention to measuring government policy. The citizen/consumer is entitled to qualitative public service.

Measuring government performances, a booming business, is not an obvious task. What is, for example, effectiveness? Roughly and simple stated, effectiveness is the degree in which the policy output realizes the objectives – desired effects (outcome) – independent from the way that this effect is reached. That means that many concepts must be filled in and be interpreted. As a result, effectiveness could become a kind of super value, which includes several other values and indicators (Jorgenson, 2006). The striving towards "good governance" also encompasses a lot of interpretations, which refers to normative questions (Verlet, 2008). These interpretations and others of for example efficiency, transparency, equity, etc. are stipulated by the dominating political climate and economic insights, and by the broader cultural setting.[1] "Good governance" is a social construction (Edwards & Clough, 2005) without a strong basis in empirical research. Indicators for governance seem – according to Van Roosbroek – mainly policy tools, rather than academic exercises. (Van Roosbroek, 2007).

There are many studies about government performance, from which policy makers want to draw conclusions. For this reason all kinds of indicators and rankings see the light, which compare the performances of the one public authority to another. Benchmarking then is the logical consequence. How such international and internal rankings are constructed is often unclear. Van de Walle and others analysed comparative studies. Their verdict is clearly and merciless: the indicators used in those rankings generally measure only a rather limited part of the government functioning, perceptions of the functioning had to pass for objective measurements of performance. The fragmentation of the responsibility for collecting data is an important reason for the insufficient quality of the used indicators. As a result, comparisons are problematic. Hence, they stress the need for good databases that respect common procedures and for clear, widely accepted rules about the use and interpretation of such data. These rules shoud enable us to to compare policy performances in different countries and so to learn from good examples. The general rankings contain often too much subjective indicators, there are few guarantees about the quality of the samples and that there are all to often inappropriate aggregations (Van de Walle, Sterck, Van Dooren & Bouckaert, 2004; Van de Walle, 2006; Luts, Van Dooren & Bouckaert, 2008).

An important finding based on those meta-analysis is that when it comes down to the public sector, there is a lack on international comparable data enabling us to judge the performance in terms of, among others, efficiency and effectivity, besides other elements of "good" governance. Although such comparisons can be significant, they say little about the actual performance of the public sector in a specific country. Their objectives and contexts are often quite different. They sometimes stress to much some specific parameters, such as the number of civil servants, and they fail to measure the (quality of the) output/outcome of public authorities sufficiently. The discussion about the performance of the public sector is however an inevitable international one, which among other things, was reinforced by the Lisbon-Agenda. In 2010 the EU must be one of the most competitive economic areas (Kuhry, 2004). One important instrument to reach this is a "performance able government".

This attention for the consequences of measuring the impact of government policy is not new. Already in 1956, Ridgway wrote about the perverse and unwanted effects measuring government performances can have. There are some more recent studies about it. Smith (1995) showed that there is consensus about the fact that performance measurement can also have undesirable effects. Moreover, those undesirable effects also have a cost, which is frequently overlooked when establishing measurement systems (Pidd, 2005a). But the attention to the unforeseen impact of policy evaluations remains limited. It is expected that this will change in the coming years, because of increased attention for evaluation. The evaluation process itself will more and more be evaluated.

The current contribution consists of three parts. In the second paragraph, we discuss the general idea of the measurement of performance of governments. In the third paragraph we go into some challenges concerning the measurement of government policy and performance. In the fourth and final part, we focus on the head subject: which negative effect arise when measuring the performance of the public sector? We also discuss

several strategies to prevent negative effect when measuring performance in the public sector.

This contribution deals with questions that rise and must be solved before we begin the data mining. The central focus is on the question what kind of information is needed and accurate to evaluate government performance and on how me must treat that information. Before the mining can begin, we need to be sure that the data could deliver us where we are looking for. Data mining is about knowledge discovery. The question is: what do we want to know? What are the consequences of asking that question? Does asking that question has an influence on the data that we need in order to give the answer?

MEASURING PERFORMANCE IN THE PUBLIC SECTOR

The objective is clear: to depict the performance of actors within the public sector. But what is "performance"? It surely is a multifaceted concept that includes several elements. That makes it cumbersome to summarise performance in one single indicator. Also the relation between process and outcome is important (Van de Walle & Bouckaert, 2007). Van de Walle (2008) states we cannot measure performance and effectiveness of the government only by balancing outputs and outcomes with regard to certain objectives. This is because objectives of governments are generally vague and sometimes contradictory. The government is a house with a lot of chambers. Given the fact that most policy objectives are prone to several interpretations, plural indicators are required. The relation between the measured reality and the indicators used is frequently vague. Effects are difficult to determine. And even if it is possible to measure them, it still simple is quit difficult to identify the role of the government in the bringing about the effects in a context with a lot of actors and factors (De Smedt el al., 2004). At all this, we also must distinguish between deployed resources

Figure 1. The production process and public sector

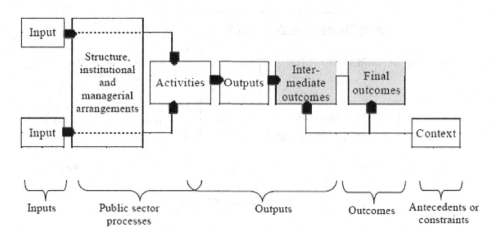

(input), processes (throughput), products (output) and effects (outcome). It is self-explanatory that we had to bear in mind the specific objective(s) and the context in which the evaluation takes place.

The evaluation of performance can only be done well if there is sufficient attention for the complexity of the complete policy process. We can represent the production process in the public sector as in Figure 1 (OECD, 2007, 16).

At the centre of the production process are efficiency and effectiveness. What are those concepts about? Efficiency indicates the relation between the deployed resources (input) and the delivered products or service (output) (I/O). Productivity is the inverse of efficiency. Efficiency indicates the quantity of input necessary per unit of output, whereas productivity is a criterion to quantify the output that one can realise per unit input (O/I). Effectiveness refers to the cause and consequence relation between output and outcome. Does policy had the aimed effect (within the postulated period)? To what extent are there desired or undesirable side effects? In short: efficiency is about doing things right, while effectivity is about doing the right things.

Along the input side for policy evaluation, it is essential to get a clear picture of the several types of resources. Along the output side, the problem for the public sector is that its services generally are not available on the free market, so it is generally quit difficult to calculate their (market) value. For this reason, physical product indicators frequently are used which are an (in) direct measure for production. This opens a lot of choices, and a lot of data to work with. In these tasks, data-mining could be of great assistance.

Contrary to output, it is often not easy to attribute outcomes to actions performed by the government (Hatry et al., 1994). Several other (f)actors, outside the control of a government, can play a role. What is the part of government actions in the coming about of desired outcome, what is the part of other actions and actors?[2] Do we need to measure output or outcomes? Policy evaluation research involves therefore a thorough study of all possible cause/consequence relations.

Information alone is not sufficient. It is assumed in traditional evaluation research that the efficiency shows itself by balance input and output against each other. However, that gives little information about the causal link between both. Using the words of Pawson and Tilley (1997) a "realistic evaluation" is not obvious. Besides, efficiency and effectiveness are only two criteria. Other criteria are also important when evaluating the public sector: legal security, legitimacy,

Figure 2. The performance measurement and its possible consequences

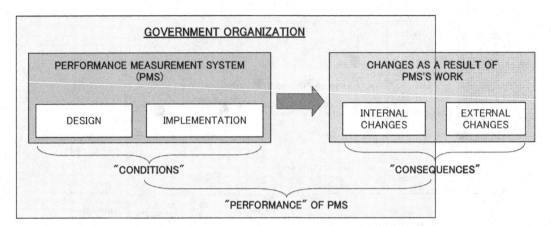

equity, transparency, accountability, etc. (Smith, 1995). Efficiency and effectiveness are specific aspects of "good governance". Although today much emphasis is particularly laid on efficiency and effectiveness, good governance is far more than that (Verlet, 2008). The over-emphasis of efficiency and effectiveness takes away the visibility on other values and criteria.

When speaking of policy or performance measurement systems, we must distinguish two dimensions: the conditions and the consequences. The conditions are related to the design and the implementation of the measurement system, whereas the consequences are related to the results of the functioning of such a system. The consequences can be internal and external. Internal consequences are for example changes in attitudes of employees, increase of the efficiency and changes in the assignment of resources. External changes situate themselves outside the organisational borders and refer to e.g. changes in the perception of citizens and changes in the societal setting. These concepts are brought together in the overview mentioned in Figure 2 (Hiraki, 2007, 5).

Before discussing the central question on the undesirable effects of evaluating government policy, we first deal with some particular issues of the process of public policy evaluation.

On Which Level Do We Measure the Performances of the Government?

We can distinguish between the analyses of government performance at three levels: the macro, meso or micro level (Callens, 2007). This is related to the objective of the analysis: do we want to analyse the production process of the government entirely (macro), in a specific government sector (sectoral) or a specific service to end users (micro)?

On first sight, the idea of an overall index is very interesting. Such an index could allow us, for example, to compare the position of Flanders with a number of regions or countries in order to make a ranking. Callens (2007) reports four examples of such an overall index, more specific the rankings produced by the European Central Bank, the Institute for Management Development, the World Economic Forum and the World Bank.

The main problem with making such general performance indicators is one of aggregation. The complexity of a government can not be reduced in a single indicator. Such a general indicator insufficiently takes into account for example the administrative culture, the differences in the state structures, et cetera.

In a so-called sectorial study, one compares for example the efficiency and the effectiveness of a specific sector in a country or region with these of that sector in other countries or regions. A classic example is the research from the Netherlands Institute for Social Research about the performance of the public sector (Kuhry, 2004). The aim of this study was to analyse the differences in productivity, quality and effectiveness of the services organised by the government between the Netherlands and other developed countries. They studied four policy fields: education, health care, law and order and public administration. Besides, the OECD is also very active in the field of sector studies. (For an overview: OECD, 2007, 38).

When using a micro-approach, one compares specific public services. For example there are comparative studies of fire services, hospitals, schools, prisons, courts, nursery and services concerning registry of births, deaths and marriages (e.g. Bouckaert 1992; Bouckaert 1993; Van Dongen, 2004).

Do We Measure Perception or Reality?

The problem with indicators is that they frequently do wrong to the complexity of social choices which underpin the policy. It's crucial to keep actual performance and the perception of performance separated. Unfortunately, we currently lack good general measurement systems of actual performance of the public sector which allow for useful comparisons between governments (Van de Walle & Bouckaert, 2007). Therefore, in many studies government policy users – citizens – are asked what they think or feel of the public services. Perception becomes important. We must be very careful with subjective indicators.

One of the reasons therefore is that a negative attitude of the population towards government can lead to a negative perception of the performance of that government. This attitude has possibly more to do with the general cultural context, than with the government in question (Van de Walle, Sterck, Van Dooren & Bouckaert, 2004). So we must take

into account that expectations can influence the perception to an important degree.

Which Value Indicators Can be Used for the Measurement of Public Service?

In the market sector, the production volume can be inferred easily from the market value of the goods or services in question. Time series can be constructed, taking into account the price index. This way, one can develop value indicators. Services produced by the public sector, are generally not negotiated on the free market. Therefore, their market value is not known. The value of this type of production cannot be expressed in money. For this reason, in most cases physical product indicators are used (Kuhry, 2004).

This is a generic term, which is related to several types of indicators, which can be considered as direct or indirect measures for production. We can be distinguished between:

- *Performance indicators.* These indicators are related to the provided end products, e.g. the number diplomas delivered by an education institution.
- *User indicators.* These indicators are related to the consumers of the services, e.g. the number of students.
- *Process indicators.* These indicators concern the performed activities or intermediary products, e.g. the number of teaching hours.

The problem remains that it is very difficult to measure purely collective goods/services. An alternative is to proportion the deployed resources to the GDP (Kuhry, 2004). Not only the volume, but especially the measurement of the quality of the government policy is quite difficulty. What is the quality of defence? There is a large dispute about the definition of quality (Eggink & Blank, 2002). Those authors depict a possible trade-off between quality and efficiency. If quality is not sufficiently reflected in the standards of production, then low quality norms can qualify themselves as very efficient. However, this trade-off is not a regularity, efficiency and quality can go together (Van Thiel & Leeuw, 2003; cf. infra).

Which Quality Guidelines Can be Used?

Which, well-defined quality guidelines had to be used to analyse the data to incorporate in the evaluation research? Examples of such criteria can be found in the research done by the Netherlands Institute for Social Research (cf. supra), Eurostat or OECD. In any case, it is crucial to use qualitatively good data if we want to build a reliable and valid measurement instrument. Besides, the quality of data is a crucial factor when talking about the (possible) negative effects of performance measurement systems (cf. infra).

EFFECTS OF PERFORMANCE MEASUREMENT

Introduction and the Good Side of Performance Measurement

In this section we deal with the core of this chapter and focus on the unintended and 'perverse' or negative impact of policy evaluation. More specific we deal with the impact of measuring performance. When analysing performance measurement, we see a predominating output orientation, although from a policy point of view it might be more interesting to focus on the eventual impact of the government action (outcome). As noted, measuring outcome is difficult, especially the attribution of the role of the different actors. Hence, the attention goes out to output, which is more easy measurable and to which corrective action is easier (De Bruijn, 2002). Hereafter, like

in most literature, we focus on the measurement of output.

Within the vast literature on performance measurement and performance measurement systems, the number of contributions on negative or perverse impact of performance measurement is rather limited. However, the attention for these effects is not new or unknown see for example the analysis of Ridgway (1956). We share the impression of Pidd (2005a) that just like performance measurement itself, the existence of such perverse effects appears to be unconventional. It seems to be inherent to and accepted in the performance measurement, as if they are unavoidable. However, perverse effect has direct and indirect costs that often are not taken into account. In some sectors they are more taken into consideration than in others. Within a number of specific policy sectors, such as the health care, we find relatively much attention to the unintentional impact of measurement systems (Brans e.a., 2008). For a more general analysis of the problem, we can refer to the work of De Bruin (2002 and 2006) and Smith (1995).

Not only sector specific characteristics are relevant, it's obvious that the communication of performance measurement results is also important to explain the relevance and effects that performance measurement can have. It is thus essential to bear in mind both internal (e.g. regarding employees) as external (e.g. regarding the general public) communication (Garnet, et al., 2008). The communication itself can generate impact which is linked to performance measurement.

Although our attention goes out to the negative impact of performance measurement as to strategies to reduce this, it is obvious that performance measurement has also positive effects. As noted, this chapter is not against evaluation or performance measurement. Evaluation research can contribute to the steering of the behaviour of policy agencies (Swanborn, 1999). De Bruijn (2002) reports four functions of performance measurement. In the first place performance measurement contributes to transparency. It allows organisations to offer clarity concerning the products or services which they offer and the resources which they use to realise them. Secondly, an organisation can learn on the basis of performance measurement what is good and what should be improved. Thirdly, such a measurement allows for a judgment of the (administrative) functioning of an organisation, what contributes to better management because there is more objective and explicit accountability.

In analysis about performance measurement impacts Smith (1995) notes that the impact shows itself on the internal management of organisations within the public sector, also when evaluations are clearly aimed at external stakeholders (e.g. citizens). Therefore, we focus on the impact of performance measurement on the organisation itself, and not for example on modifying attitudes of citizens towards those organisations.

Negative Effects of Performance Measurement

In this era where measurement, consulting and evaluation is popular and big business, the negative impact of performance measurement gets little attention. In his analysis Smith (1995) detected eight unwanted (negative) effects or dysfunctions of performance measurement.[3] According to Smith, they are mainly the result of a lack of congruence between the objectives of the agents and the objectives of principals. A same reasoning can be found in the work of De Bruijn (2006), who draws attention to the tensions between the professional (those who are active in the primary process) and the manager (who eventually wants to steer based on the performance measurement). A more general analysis of the (negative) impact of performance measurement can be found in the work of Bouckaert & Auwers (1999) and Van Dooren (2006).

The degree, in which specific (positive and negative) effects manifest themselves, is strongly depending on the structure and culture of a specific organisation. Also the quality of the indicators underpinning the performance data is essential (Brans et al., 2008). We discuss the effects in case of measurement. Sometimes, there is no measurement at all, because of the negative attitude towards such measurement or because of the expected negative effects. In this respect, the lack of such a measurement system can be seen as a negative effect as such. What are the most noted negative effects of performance measurement?

A Too Strong Emphasis on the Easily Quantifiable

In performance measurement systems, the emphasis often is on quantifiable phenomena. As a consequence, management also will have especially attention for quantifiable processes, at the expense of aspects of government policy that are not or less easy quantifiable. This is caused by the difficulty and disputes concerning the definition of quality and/or changes of the interpretation of it (Eggink and Blank, 2002).

Smith (1995) wrote in this context off a "tunnel vision". He gave the example of the health care in the UK. In that case, the strong emphasis on prenatal mortality rates led to changes in the nature of the service on maternity services, at the expense of not-quantifiable objectives. De Bruijn (2002) also refers to this problem by indicating that performance measurement potentially dissipates the professional attitude, by focussing on quantity in measuring the performance of especially measurable and easily definable aspects. The example which he quotes is that of museums, where a too strong focus on easily measurable data – such as the number of visitors – dominates other indicators and considerations, such as the artistic value of a collection.

This problem can be explained by the divergence between the objectives of an organisation and the measurement system. It is specific for the public sector. Characteristic for the public sector is that a whole range of objectives must be realised and that a lot of important objectives are reasonably difficult to quantify. In addition, objectives of organisations within the public sector reach frequently much further then the direct aim of the provision of services. For example, education must transfer not only more easy measurable knowledge and skills, but also attitudes, norms and values, et cetera.

Mostly, it is very difficult to inventory all activities and objectives. As a consequence, the importance attached to performance measurement of objective data can be reduced, while values can be more stressed. This requires a fitting policy culture. Policy measurement is not only about numbers and figures, it is also has to do with a specific normative view on what the public sector needs to be and do.

Too Little Attention to the Objectives of the Organisation as a Whole

This second problem is what Smith (1995) called sub-optimization. Actors responsible for a specific part of the broader organisation tend to concentrate on their particular objectives, at the expense of the objectives of the organisation as a whole. Especially for the public sector this is a severe problem, since a lot of policy entities are involved in the realisation of objectives. De Bruijn (2002) refers to this problem if he states that performance measurement can hamper the internal interchange of available expertise and knowledge. For example, the introduction of performance measurement in schools had a bad influence on the cooperation and mutual understanding between the schools in question.

Much depends on the type of activities of an organisation within the public sector. In addition the central government can avoid this problem, to a certain extent, by a good harmonisation between the different sections, e.g. by means of general service charters that are translated into more operational charters (Verlet, 2008).

Too Much Attention for Short-Term Objectives

This problem also descends from the possible differences between the objectives of an organisation and what can covered by the performance measurement system. Smith called this problem myopia. It concerns a short-sighted view, in the sense that one pursues short-term objectives at disadvantage of legitimate objectives on the long run. Performance measurement is mostly only a snapshot in time. Activities can produce large advantage in the long term, but that is not always noticeable in the measurement system. Many performance measurement systems don't give us a picture of the performance over a longer period, nor of future (anticipated) consequences of current management action.

This effect is reinforced when executive staff and employees hold functions for a shorter period. Of course, also in this case the degree in which this problem arises depends strongly on the types of public services, the culture and the structure of an organisation. A way to handle this specific problem in performance measurement is having attention for processes concerning topics on a longer period, rather than solely measuring output.

A Too Strong Emphasis on Criteria for Success

This impact is what Smith (1995) called measure fixation. Spurred by performance measurement, an organisation feels inclined to overemphasis the criteria on which they will be judged. In this context Brans et al. (2008) pointed that performance measurement can lead to ritualism. This means that one tries to score well on the key indicators in order to satisfy interested parties. In this context, several authors refer to the concept of Power (1999) which deals with disengagement, a false impression of things: the representation doesn't correspond with the reality.

A too strong emphasis on criteria for success originates from the incapacity of a lot of measurement systems to map complex phenomena. Smith gave an example of reducing the waiting times in the health care, more specifically the objective that patients should wait no longer then two years for a surgical intervention. This had as unforeseen effect that the number of patients that had to wait for one year increased and that the initial intake of patients happened at a later moment. Patients arrived later on the waiting list.

A possible solution for this problem is to increase the number of criteria in order to assess the functioning of an organisation. However, we need to take into account that this can blur the focus and can lead to demoralizing. An alternative solution which Smith (1995) suggests, is the recognition that most measurements are proxies for output and that the ultimate arbitrators of the quality of the output are the customers of the organisation. In order to make this happen, we need a clear picture of who those customers are and what their expectations and needs are. Moreover, we must keep in mind that the perception of the functioning of an organisation is not necessarily a good indicator for its actual functioning (Verlet, Reynaert & Devos, 2005).

Misrepresentation of Performance

This effect refers to intentional manipulation of data. As a result, reported behaviour does not correspond with actual behaviour. It is self-evident that the incentive to use these reprehensible practices is the largest when there is a strong emphasis on performance indicators. The possibilities for a wrong reproduction of the performance are often high in the public sector (Smith 1995). This because the organisations in question frequently supply the data and indicators needed for the evaluation of their own performance (or lack of it). Here too we can refer to the difficulty to map complex phenomena precise and reliable, so datamining could be a solution. Possible problems

can occur during aggregating or disaggregating data on performance (Van Dooren, 2006). Smith (1995) made a distinction between two types of misrepresentation: creative reporting and fraud. The difference between both is sometimes difficult. This shortcoming of a wrong reproduction of the performances can be reduced by (internal and external) audit and with introduction of the possibility for sanctions when misrepresentation comes on the track.

Poor Validity and Reliability

Under this denominator we include the effects which Bouckaert and Auwers (1999, 77) considered as pathologies referring to the false perceptions of volume and numbers. More specific, they discuss convex and concave measurement instruments, when respectively higher and lower values are noted compared to reality. It is clear that these problems do not originate particularly from the tension between managers/professional within an organisation, but are due to the very measurement as such.

Wrong Interpretations

The production process of public services is mostly quite complex. Moreover, actors themselves have to operate in a complex environment. Therefore even if it is possible to map performances perfectly, it is still not obvious to translate the signals in the data. It speaks for itself that these wrong interpretations are a real problem when using performance indicators.

The performances of several organisations are frequently compared with each other. However, this is not self-evident, because they might have very different objectives, resources, institutional and cultural contexts, et cetera. Correctly handling performance data is a skill. By restricting the number of indicators, one can counteract slightly the problem of the wrong interpretation of data, although this can in itself generate other perverse effects.

Gaming

This negative effect of performance measurement concerns intentional manipulating behaviour to secure strategic advantage. Whereas misrepresentation is about the reported behaviour, gaming is about the manipulation of actual behaviour. In the work of De Bruijn (2006) we find an example of how performance measurement can lead to strategic behaviour. It has to do with performance measurement of a service within the Australian army, which must provide housing to soldiers who have been stationed far from home. The performance indicator used is the number of soldiers that agreed with housing after maximum three offers. After introducing this indicator, quite soon the full 100% of the soldiers agreed after maximum three offers. The explanation was simple. The service first informally offered housing to the soldiers. Only when the employees of the service were rather certain that the soldier would agree with the offer, they did the formal offer. It is a matter of strategic behaviour: the performances are only on paper, the societal meaning of it is limited.

How to reduce gaming? In the first place one can, according to Smith (1995), counteract gaming by taking into account a broad pallet of performance indicators. Other possibilities are benchmarking or offering executive managers career perspectives on a shorter term. This can lead however to myopia (cf. supra).

Petrifaction

Petrifaction or fossilization refers to the discouragement of innovation because of a too rigid measurement. A lot of performance measurement systems have the inclination to reward constantly reproducing the existing. The need to select on advance performance indicators and objectives, can contribute to the blindness for new threats

and possibilities. In the same context gaming can germinate. The danger of petrifaction originates from inevitable time lag between setting up performance measurement and the possibility/difficulty to adjust the measurement system. By consequence, a kind of meta control mechanism is necessary in order to safeguard the adequacy of performance indicators.

This petrifaction of organisations can be thwarted by providing incentives for anticipating new challenges and innovative behaviour, even if these activities do not contribute directly to the current performance indicators.

Reinforces Internal Bureaucracy

Performance measurement needs time and resources. As it happens, a sound performance measurement demands a precise recording of inputs, processes, outputs, outcomes and additionally takes into account the ever changing surrounding factors (cf. supra). It speaks for itself that such a measurement demands extra resources and people of the public administration. Gathering, providing, analysing, constructing, interpreting ... the needed data are sometimes quite complex and demanding. They generate the need for a specific department, making the administrative process more complex.

Hamper Ambitions/Cherry Picking

That performance measurement possibly hampers the ambitions of an organisation, originates from the fact that organisations can force up their performance, for example in terms of output, by optimising the input. More specific, one can choose to select the input in such a way so that these require minimal throughput. In this context one can talk about "cherry picking". For an example we can refer to education, where a school can better its output (e.g. in terms of percentage succeeded students), by using strict selection criteria for allowing students (De Bruijn, 2006).

This negative side effect also can be called "cream-skimming", skimming the target group by especially addressing to subgroups which are easy to reach. According to Swanborn (1999) this effect can also manifest itself by self-selection from the target group. Under this denominator we can also mention the negative impact polarisation (Van Dooren, 2006). The situation that this author outlines is one in which certain forms of service or files are ricocheted because they are considered as hopeless in view of putting up standards. Rather then investing in these problem cases, one can opt for to ricochet these.

Can Punish Good Performance

Although performance measurement systems should stimulate good performance, it can also punish good performance. Describing this negative effect, De Bruijn (2002) refers to the work of Bordewijk and Klaassen (2000) who indicated that investing in transparency and efficiency is not without risks. Organisations which invest in transparency can possibly be sanctioned by means of a budget reduction. Control and transparency could learn that equal performance can be realised with less resources. A similar organisation which does not invest in transparency and efficiency is rewarded with the same budget for equal performance.

A GENERAL EXPLANATION OF NEGATIVE EFFECTS AND GLOBAL STRATEGIES TO PREVENT THOSE

According to Smith and De Bruijn, negative impact finds its origin in a mismatch between the objectives of principals/management on the one hand and those of the agents/professionals on the other. De Bruijn (2002, 2006) sees two general reasons behind the negative effects of performance measurement.

In the first place, he states that professionals could pervert the performance measurement systems and that they consider themselves legitimised to do so. This has several reasons. First of all, they consider performance measurement as poor measurements because - certainly in the public sector – there is a trade-off between several (competitive) values. Public performances are plural and this is not always reflected in the measurement systems. Moreover, a lot of professionals consider performance measurement as unfair, because they don't give sufficient account to the fact that performances are in many cases the result of co production. A third and last legitimating ground is the opinion that performance measurement is in it mostly static, whereas performances are dynamically of nature.

A second general reason is that the more managers want to steer by performance measurement, the less effectively performance measurement will be. De Bruijn (2006) talks about "the paradox of increasing perverse effects": the more the management wants to influence the primary process using performance measurement, the more negative effect will occur. The rationalization of this paradox is twofold. In the first place, professionals will try to "protect" themselves from the performance measurement. Secondly, he states that the more the functioning of performance measurement is tangible, the less justice is done to the plural, co-productive and dynamic character of the performances. Moreover, De Bruijn (2002) says that this paradox is particularly difficult. If professionals does not conform to the measurement system and screen off themselves, then this can be an incentive for strategic behaviour, which results in a performance measurement that is not effective. If one is willing to conform on the other hand, negative effect can still occur, for example a too strong emphasis on criteria for success, as a result of which measuring is also not effective.

Both Smith (1995) and De Bruijn (2002, 2006) reflect about strategies to counteract and reduce as much as possible the negative impact of performance measurement. An element in both studies is the use of subjective indicators in the form of satisfaction measurements. De Bruin sees this as an alternative appraisal system, besides performance measurement. We do not agree at this point, in the sense that those appraisals also can be an inherent part of the performance measurement systems. The perception of the functioning of a service can exert a substantial influence on the functioning of this service (Stipak, 1979). There is little doubt about the idea that such subjective indicators – e.g. 'are you happy with the opening hours …' – alone are not the only truths.

Nevertheless, to our opinion such indicators are crucial in the measurement of performance, although prudence in using them is in order. Yet, the use of subjective indicators has been frequently used in policy evaluation based on the simple assumption that such indicators also are good measures for the quality of the service. Besides other reasons, the lack of knowledge or visibility of a service can systematically bias the subjective evaluation of that service (Trent et al., 1984). Those considerations need attention, before the information produced by subjective indicators can be used in the policy evaluation (Anderson, et al., 1984). Subjective indicators can give several types of policy-relevant information to the policy makers. If these subjective indicators are by themselves sufficient to assess the quality of the service is, however, another question (Stipak, 1979).

There are a number of other strategies which can make performance measurement better. According to De Bruin (2006), one can accept a diversity of (even competitive) definitions of products. Moreover, the fact that target variables are mutually competitive is in itself not a problem (Swanborn, 1999). Using a variety of product definitions offers a number of advantages: it can reduce conflicts, it offers a richer picture of the achieved performance, it moderates perverting behaviour and can also be interesting for management. The diversity of product definitions can be favourable for the authority of the results. If an organisation scores for example on the basis of all product definitions bad/good, the conclusion is based on a firm argument.

Another advice of De Bruijn (2006) is the prohibition on a monopoly of "semantics". Performance measurement can have a concealing meaning and different meanings to different people. This problem increases if the distance between the producer and the recipient of the data and figures produced by performance measurement grows. The larger this distance, the more difficult it is to interpret and the higher also the alleged hardness of the data will be. This prohibition on a monopoly of semantics can be realised by making clear agreements between for example the managers and the professionals.

Limiting the functions and the forums, to which performance measurement is used, frequently helps performance measurement. The more functions and forums the measurement has, the higher also the chance on the paradox of increasing perverse effects. Therefore, clear appointments are essential for the success of performance measurement and especially for avoiding negative effects. A similar recommendation can be found in the work of Smith (1995), according to whom negative effects can be thwarted by involving employees at all levels in the development and the implementation of performance measurement systems. He pleads for a flexible use of performance indicators and not to use them only as a control mechanism.

De Bruin (2006) is in favour of a strategic selection of the products that will be visualised by the measurement system. As such, one can opt for a heavy or a light measurement.[4] The selection of the products is a strategic choice, mostly motivated by the striving towards completeness - although this frequently leads to an overload of information and such a measuring is not cost effective - whereas with an intelligent selection of a more limited number of products, one can exert influence on the organisation as a whole. Furthermore, there is a difference between the operationalization of plural products (for example giving education) versus simple products (for example the number of repeaters). It is chosen simple products and only a limited number of plural products.[5] In a sense, contrary to this, in the work of Smith (1995) it is argued to quantify each objective. For Smith, a critical attitude is needed towards the design of performance measurement systems: we should ask ourselves what can and can not be measured.

Another strategy is the management of the competitive approaches product and process. He means that it is essential for performance measurement not only to focus on the output, but also to look at the processes or throughput. It is important to give sufficient attention the so-called black box in which input is translated to output (Pawson & Tilley, 1997). Moreover, the risk on negative affects is higher if product indicators are used (Brans, et al., 2008). That is an extra reason to incorporate process indicators in the evaluation.

The essence of the strategies suggested by De Bruijn (2002) are a distant/reserved use, space and trust on the one hand and agreeing on rules of the game on the other side. Moreover, Smith (1995) gives a number of suggestions which are especially relevant when objectives are rather vague and the measurement of the output is problematic. In that case, he emphasises the use of subjective indicators, by measuring the satisfaction of customers. In the same context it is better to leave the interpretation of performance indicators to experts and to do a conscientiously audit.

CONCLUSION

Nobody disputes that in public policy, evaluation – using objective indicators – has become increasingly important. Within the framework of the growing complexity of the policy environment and in view of the need for obvious accountability, policy makers strive to an evidence-based policy that must guarantee (the impression of) a high return on public investment.

How these criteria and goals of policy evaluation in general and measuring performances in particular can be met, which functions one can or must impute on these evaluations and which forums they can be discussed at, … is object of discussion. These discussions are related to the criteria of good governance and of moral and democratic legitimacy.

Given that policy evaluation questions whether and how objectives are obtained, taking into account the means deployed, it seems logical that the choices of objectives and resources prevail, or are extern or prior to, the evaluation. Policy evaluation can lead to policy-learning and to the strengthening of accountability processes and is therefore by nature beneficial. However, the need for objective, quantified evaluation entails dangers and risks. Calculating policy outcomes can have influence on the choice of policy objective and therefore on the formulation of the problem. Evaluation can influence the policy process on an unforeseen, improper manner. Objectives (problem solutions) can be chosen in such a way to maximise the chances of a good evaluation.

The negative effect of performance measurement originates to an important degree from the tension between managers and the professionals, between those who deliver policy and those who measure and evaluate this deliverance these professionals could fear a loss of autonomy because of policy evaluation (Swanborn, 1999) and therefore try to influence the evaluation process. Not only are these relations important for the success of good measurement and policy learning. As we have shown, the measurement in itself can have negative effects.

These negative effects are important in the debate about performance measurement and the way we deal with data: what data should be gathered? What can we do with it? How should we analyse it? How can we publish or comment the analysis? Reminding the words of Ridgway - "the cure is sometimes worse than the disease" (1956, p.240) – we should bear in mind that evaluation is not good by definition. Ridgway dealt with the question if it was appropriate at all to use quantitative measurement instruments in order to analyse and evaluate performance in the public sector. Half a century later, the usefulness of quantifying the performance within the public sector seems not to be the main subject of discussion. But more then 50 years after his conclusion, we can agree that the perverse impact of performance measurement is insufficiently recognised. Fortunately, there are possible strategies to reduce specific perverse impact. Taking care of perverse effects is therefore an important task, and a difficult one.

Policy evaluation serves a noble objective in which "good" governance is of the first and most importance. In that respect, it is a means to an end. However, since it has become big business with many people making money out of it, since governments can no longer do without evaluating their performances, since the political pressure to evaluate is increasing, it sometimes has become an end in itself. Who will evaluate the evaluation? If we want to make public policy better and more accountable, we should look – more than we have done in the past – at the mechanisms that are used to bring about these effects. There is probably no such thing as a true "objective" evaluation.

In this chapter, we have demonstrated that asking the question 'what data do we need?' in order to start the analysis of that data, including data mining, has a severe impact on the precise nature of that data, and therefore, on the knowledge that data mining can produce. Performance measurement is inevitable, so we need data to analyse. But looking for data, trying to translate policy in quantitative standards that can be measured, could change the reality that is captured inside the data, because it influences policy makers and their actions. Therefore, attention needs to pay to the precise way in which we measure, in this case policy performance, and gather data. If we do not take these influences into account, if we are not aware of them, data mining will be applied on data

that is less representative of the reality of which we like to know more about.

Once we have solid empirical data, and the above posed difficulties are dealt with, the actual data mining can begin. However, also data mining must be a mean to an end. As with the use of all data, human (critical) judgment remains a critical factor (Mead, 2003). As noted by Siegel (cited in Mead, 2003), making data gathering integral to an organization's daily operational fabric tends to be far more difficult than designing and building the system. Gathering qualitative data by and about the public sector is an important en necessary step towards data mining in the public sector. However, we had to be taking into account the specific characteristics of the public context (cf. Kostoff & Geisler, 1999).

REFERENCES

Anderson, B., Ryan, V., & Goudy, W. (1984). Consistency in subjective evaluations of community attributes. Social Indicators Research, 14(2), 165–175. doi:10.1007/BF00293408doi:10.1007/BF00293408

Bouckaert, G. (1992). Productivity analysis in the public sector: the case of fire service. *International review of Administrative Sciences, 58*(2), 175-200.

Bouckaert, G. (1993). Efficiency measurement from a management perspective: a case of the civil registry office in Flanders. *International review of Administrative Sciences, 59*(1), 11-27.

Bouckaert, G., & Auwers, T. (1999). Prestaties meten in de overhead. Brugge, Belgium: Die Keure.

Brans, M., Giesbers, S., & Meijer, A. (2008). Alle ogen op de ziekenhuizen gericht? De effecten van openbaarheid van prestatiegegevens. Bestuurswetenschappen, 62(2), 32–52.

Brito, P., & Malerba, D. (2003). Mining official data. Intelligent Data Analysis, 7, 497–500.

Callens, M. (2007). *Efficiëntie en effectiviteit in de publieke sector.* Unpublished paper. Brussels: Studiedienst van de Vlaamse Regering.

Crossman, G. (2008). Nothing to hide, nothing to fear? International Review of Law Computers & Technology, 22(1/2), 115–118. doi:10.1080/13600 860801925003doi:10.1080/13600860801925003

De Bruijn, H. (2002). Prestatiemeting in de publieke sector. Strategieën om perverse effecten te neutraliseren. Bestuurswetenschappen, 56(2), 39–159.

De Bruijn, H. (2006). Prestatiemeting in de publieke sector. Tussen professie en verantwoording (2e druk). Den Haag, The Netherlands: Lemma.

De Peuter, B., De Smedt, J., & Van Dooren, W. (2007). Handleiding beleidsevaluatie. Deel 2: monitoring van beleid. Brussels: Steunpunt Beleidsrelevant Onderzoek – Bestuurlijke Organisatie Vlaanderen.

De Smedt, J., Conings, V., & Verhoest, K. (2004). De integratie van de beleids-, contract- en financiële cyclus. Het agentschapsperspectief: De managementsrapportage in de beheersovereenkomst in het kader van de koppeling van de cycli. Onderzoeksrapport, Beter Bestuurlijk Beleid. Brussels: Steunpunt Beleidsrelevant Onderzoek – Bestuurlijke Organisatie Vlaanderen.

Edwards, M., & Clough, R. (2005). *Corporate Governance and Performance: An Exploration of the Connection in a Public Sector Context.* Issues paper 1. Retrieved October 1, 2008, from http://www.canberra.edu.au/corpgov-aps/pub/Issues-PaperNo.1_GovernancePerformance Issues.pdf

Eggink, E., & Blank, J. L. (2002). Efficiëntie in de publieke sector. Beleidswetenschap, 16(2), 144–161.

Garnet, J., Marlowe, J., & Pandey, S. (2008). Penetrating the Performance Predicament: Communication as a Mediator or Moderator of Organizational Culture's Impact on Public Organizational Performance. Public Administration Review, 68(2), 266–281. doi:10.1111 /j.1540-6210.2007.00861.xdoi:10.1111/j.1540-6210.2007.00861.x

Gramatikov, M. (2003). *Data Mining Techniques and the Decision Making Process in the Bulgarian Public Administration.* Paper presented at the NISPACee Conference, 10-12 April 2003, Bucharest, Romania.

Hatry, H., Gerhart, C., & Marshall, M. (1994). Eleven Ways to Make Performance Management More Useful to Public Managers. International City/County Management Association [Washington, DC]. Public Management, (September): 15–18.

Hayes, M., & Pidd, M. (2005). *Public Announcement of Performance Ratings: implications for Trust Relationships.* Retrieved August, 15, 2008, from http://www.lancs.ac.uk/staff/smamp/ working%20paper%20on%20trust.pdf

Hiraki, T. (2007). *Factors affecting the "performance" of performance measurement systems: an analysis of the Japanese Practice.* Paper presented at the EGPA conference, EGPA Study Group on productivity and quality in the public sector, Madrid, Spain.

Hood, C. (1996). Exploring variations in public management reform of the 1980's. In H. Bekke, J. Perry, & T. Toonen (Eds.), Civil service systems in comparative perspective (pp. 268–287). Bloomington, IN: Indiana University Press.

Jorgenson, T. (2006). Value consciousness and public management. *International journal of organiszation theory and behavior, 9*(4), 510-536.

Kostoff, R., & Geisler, E. (1999). Strategic Management and Implementation of Textueal Data Mining in Government Organizations. Technology Analysis and Strategic Management, 11(4), 493–525. doi:10.1080/095373299107302 doi:10.1080/095373299107302

Kuhry, B. (Ed.). (2004). Prestaties van de publieke sector. Den Haag, The Netherlands: SCP Nederland.

Luts, M., Van Dooren, W., & Bouckaert, G. (2008). Internationale rangschikkingen gerangschikt. Een meta-analyse van rangschikkingen van publieke sectoren. Leuven, Belgium: Steunpunt beleidrelevant onderzoek-bestuurlijke organisatie Vlaanderen.

Modell, S. (2004). Performance measurement myths in the public sector: a research note. Financial Accountability & Management, 20(1), 39–55. doi:10.1111/j.1468-0408.2004.00185.x doi:10.1111/j.1468-0408.2004.00185.x

OECD. (2007). *OECD project on Management in Government: Comparative Country Data. Issues in Output Measurement for "Government at a Glance"*. OECD GOV Technical Paper 2 (Second Draft).

Osbourne, D., & Gaebler, T. (1993). Reinventing Government. How the Entrepreneurial Spirit is Transforming the Public Sector. Harmondsworth, UK: Penguin Books.

Pawson, R., & Tilley, N. (1997). Realistic Evaluation. London: Sage.

Pidd, M. (2005). Perversity in Public Service Performance Measurement. International Journal of Productivity and Performance Management, 54(5/6), 482–493. doi:10.1108/17410400510604601 doi:10.1108/17410400510604601

Ridgway, V. (1956). Dysfunctional Consequences of Performance Measurements. Administrative Science Quarterly, 1(2), 240–247. doi:10.2307/2390989 doi:10.2307/2390989

Smith, P. (1995). On the unintended consequences of publishing performance data in the public sector. International Journal of Public Administration, 18(2&3), 277–310. doi:10.1080/01900699508525011 doi:10.1080/01900699508525011

Spanhove, J., & Verhoest, K. (2007). Corporate governance vs. Government governance: translation or adoption? Paper, EIASM, 4th workshop on corporate governance, Brussels, 15-16 November 2007.

Stipak, B. (1979). Are there sensible ways to analyse and use subjective indicators of urban service quality. Social Indicators Research, 6(4), 421–438. doi:10.1007/BF00289436 doi:10.1007/BF00289436

Swanborn, P. G. (1999). Evalueren: het ontwerpen, begeleiden en evalueren van interventies: een methodische basis voor evaluatie-onderzoek. Amsterdam: Boom.

Trent, R., Stout-Wiegand, N., & Furbee, P. (1984). The nature of the connection between life course and satisfaction with community services. Social Indicators Research, 15(4), 417–429. doi:10.1007/BF00351447 doi:10.1007/BF00351447

Van de Walle, S. (2006). The State of the World's Bureaucracies. Journal of Comparative Policy Analysis, 8(4), 439–450. doi:10.1080/13876980600971409 doi:10.1080/13876980600971409

Van de Walle, S. (2008). Comparing the performance of national public sectors: Conceptual problems. International Journal of Productivity and Performance Management, 57(4), 329–338. doi:10.1108/17410400810867535 doi:10.1108/17410400810867535

Van de Walle, S., & Bouckaert, G. (2007). Perceptions of Productivity and Performance in Europe and The United. International Journal of Public Administration, 30(11), 1123–1140. doi:10.108 0/01900690701225309doi:10.1080/019006907 01225309

Van Dongen, W. (2004). *Kinderopvang als basisvoorziening in een democratische samenleving. Scenario's voor de toekomstige ontwikkeling van de dagopvang voor kinderen jonger dan drie jaar.* Brussel: Centrum voor Bevolkings - en Gezinsstudie.

Van Dooren, W. (2006). *Performance measurement in the Flemish public sector: A supply and demand approach.* Leuven: published doctoral dissertation, K.U. Leuven, Belgium.

Van Roosbroek, S. (2007). Rethinking governance indicators: What can quality management tell us about the debate on governance indicators? Paper EGPA annual conference. Study Group: Performance and Quality, Madrid, September 19-22, 2007.

van Thiel, S., & Leeuw, F. (2003). De prestatieparadox in de publieke sector. Beleidswetenschap, 17(2), 123–144.

Vandewalle, S., Sterck, M., & Van Dooren, W. (2004). What you see is not necessarily what you get, een verkenning van de mogelijkheden en moeilijkheden van internationale vergelijkingen van publieke sectoren op basis van indicatoren. Leuven, Belgium: Instituut voor de Overheid.

Vandijck, E. & Despontin, M. (1998). Hoe komen we te weten wat we weten? Data mining. *VTOM, Vlaams tijdschrift voor overheidsmanagement, 3*(3), 21-25.

Verhoest, K., & Spanhove, J. (2007). Inleiding tot het themanummer: Deugdelijk bestuur en government governance. [VTOM]. Vlaams Tijdschrift voor Overheidsmanagement, 4(1), 2–6.

Verlet, D. (2008) *Good governance, corporate governance, government governance: what's in a name? Een theoretische situering van Beter Bestuurlijk Beleid in Vlaanderen.* Brussel, Studiedienst van de Vlaamse Regering, SVR-nota 2008/4.

Verlet, D., Reynaert, H., & Devos, C. (2005). Burgers in Vlaamse grootsteden. Tevredenheid, vertrouwen, veiligheidsgevoel en participatie in Gent, Brugge en Antwerpen. Brugge, Belgium: Vanden Broele.

Zondergeld-Hamer, A. (2007). Een kwestie van goed bestuur. Openbaar Bestuur, 17(10), 5–10.

KEY TERMS AND DEFINITIONS

Efficiency: Indicates the relation between the deployed resources (input) and the delivered products or service (output) (I/O). It is about the quantity input necessary per unit of output (I/O).

Effectiveness: Concerns the cause and consequence relation between output and outcome. Does policy had the aimed effect (within the postulated period)? To what extent are there desired or undesirable side effects?

Evaluation: Evaluation is the systematic and objective determination of the worth or merit of an object".

Input: The financial, human, and material resources required to implement an operation.

Output: The products, capital goods and services which result from a development intervention; may also include changes resulting from the intervention which are relevant to the achievement of outcomes.

Outcome: The likely or achieved short-term and medium-term effects of an intervention's outputs.

Performance: The degree to which an operation or organisation (…) operates according to specific criteria/standards/guidelines or achieves results in accordance with stated goals or plans.

Performance Measurement: A system for assessing performance of development interventions against stated goals.

Productivity: The inverse of efficiency, it is to quantity the output one can realise per unit input (O/I).

Throughput: The processes involved when converting inputs into outputs within the organisation.

ENDNOTES

1   For example Zondergeld-Hamer (2007) discuss the role of religious expectations.

2   For example the increase of the life expectancy in good health (effect) can be related to the number of vaccinations, the number of persons reached with prevention campaigns (output) or with the quantity of government funds (input). It is not because the indicators increase in the same direction and with the same speed that the life expectancy can be explained only by the preventive policy. Also the progress in medicine (to which governments contribute by means of education and R&D), the rise in living standard (to which governments contribute by means of economic stimuli) resulting in healthier feeding habits, better housing and faster medical treatment have their influence.

3   More specific: tunnel vision, suboptimization, myopia, measure fixation, misrepresentation, misinterpretation, gaming and ossification. Of course, further in the text we discuss the interpretation of these concepts.

4   The distinction between them can be made by whether or not there is a link to a kind of sanctioning to the appraisal on the basis of the performance measurement systems.

5   It is attractive for the professionals, it gives them space and it is for managers also easier to settle scores on simple products. Moreover, a focus on simple products can have a positive impact on plural products. Finally, the good behaviour of professionals can be rewarded by a restricted selection of products. For a more detailed argumentation we can refer to De Bruin (2002, pp.152-154).

Chapter 2
Measuring the Financial Crisis in Local Governments through Data Mining

José Luis Zafra-Gómez
Granada University, Spain

Antonio Manuel Cortés-Romero
Granada University, Spain

ABSTRACT

In local government, the financial analysis is focused on evaluating the financial condition of municipalities, and this is normally accomplished via an analytic process examining four dimensions: sustainability (or budgetary stability), solvency, flexibility and financial independence. Accordingly, the first goal the authors set out to achieve in this chapter is to determine the principal explanatory factors for each of the above dimensions. This is done by examining a wide range of ratios and indicators normally available in published public accounts, with the aim of extracting the most significant explanatory variables for sustainability, solvency, flexibility and financial independence. They use a rule induction algorithm called CHAID, which provides a highly efficient data mining technique for segmentation, or tree growing. The research sample includes 877 Spanish local authorities with a population of 1000 inhabitants or more. The developed model presents a high degree of explanatory and predictive capacity. For the levels of budgetary sustainability the most significant variables are those related to the current margin, together with the importance of capital expenditure in the budgetary structure. On the other hand, the short-term solvency depends on the liquid funds possessed by the entity. The flexibility, however, depends mainly on the financial load per inhabitant of the municipality, on the total sum of fixed charges. Finally, financial independence depends fundamentally on the transfers that the entity receives and on the fiscal pressure, among other elements.

DOI: 10.4018/978-1-60566-906-9.ch002

INTRODUCTION

In the context of private enterprise, profitability is the main variable analyzed and monitored by researchers and company managers. At the theoretical level, the DuPont Model establishes the relationships between profitability and a group of variables and accounting ratios such as asset turnover, sales margin and financial leverage. However, in the public sector and even more specifically in the area of local government this concept is overshadowed by other magnitudes that reflect the success or otherwise of management performed in the public interest. Interest is thus focused on evaluating the financial condition of municipalities, and this is normally accomplished via an analytic process examining four dimensions: sustainability (or budgetary stability), solvency, flexibility and financial independence (Groves et al., 2003).

Accordingly, the first goal we set out to achieve in this chapter is to determine the principal explanatory factors for each of the above dimensions. This is done by examining a wide range of ratios and indicators normally available in published public accounts, with the aim of extracting the most significant explanatory variables for sustainability, solvency, flexibility and financial independence. We seek to quantify these relationships and their explanatory variables and thus obtain the relevant profiles, i.e., the combinations of economic-accounting features of the best municipalities with respect to their levels of sustainability, solvency, flexibility and financial independence (Zafra-Gómez et al., 2009a; 2009b; 2009c).

In this context, drawing up a body of rules making it possible to determine the probability of an organization presenting a better or worse financial condition is a crucial issue. The importance for the public manager is determined by the fact that the latter officer must be aware of the variables to be controlled when seeking a stable financial situation with regard to the four elements being considered. Moreover, the utility

of this methodology is that it provides a control instrument for municipal supervisory agencies (central or regional government) as those local authorities that face an Emergency Financial Condition would be obliged to draw up a viability plan to improve it, and their autonomy would be reduced by the supervision by such agencies. Taxes would have to be increased, within legal limits, and/or the services provided would have to be cut back, with the ensuing loss of popularity. Another real consequence that would affect the financial condition of such local authorities would be the denial to them of access to indebtedness facilities for investment projects. At the other extreme, those authorities presenting an excellent financial condition would be subjected to fewer controls and supervision, and thus their autonomy would increase; they would have greater access to certain forms of financial assistance and to indebtedness facilities.

This analysis makes use of a rule induction algorithm called CHAID (Chi-squared Automatic Interaction Detector, Kass, 1980), which provides a highly efficient data mining technique for segmentation, or tree growing, so that a tree of rules may be derived to describe different segments within the data in relation to the output (dependent) variable, allowing us to classify local governments according to the different values of their accounting ratios (explanatory variables or predictors).

The chapter begins with a review of the main empirical studies carried out to measure financial crises affecting local authorities. We go on to outline our methodological proposal to achieve the above aims, explaining the analytic technique to be applied, and then describe the sample and the variables. Subsequently, the main results of the analysis are discussed, firstly by means of an exploratory analysis, and then from an explanatory viewpoint. Finally, we highlight the most important issues raised in this chapter and suggest future areas for investigation.

HOW SHOULD FINANCIAL CRISES IN LOCAL GOVERNMENT BE MEASURED?

The study of municipal financial crises is a research objective that, while not a novel one, remains topical and continues to attract researchers around the world. Today, projects to evaluate fiscal distress continue to be developed in various US States (Khola et al., 2005). In Australia, as observed by Dollery et al. (2006), various local authorities are experiencing severe or chronic fiscal stress, while in the UK, the Audit Commission published a paper in February 2007 in which it was commented that "the assessment focuses on the importance of having sound and strategic financial management to ensure that resources are available to support the council's priorities and improve services".

Traditionally, the studies undertaken concerning the areas of budgetary, financial and economic information have tended to be based on the analysis of the financial situation of the organization in question. However, in recent years, such studies have been addressed in the framework of a broader concept, known as the financial condition. A growing volume of research in this respect is being carried out, with the aim of acquiring greater information about aspects that characterize the development of public activities.

The principal objective of our study of financial condition is to determine a means of measuring the financial crises that affect municipalities. Traditionally, financial condition is taken to be the ability of a government to provide services and to meet its future obligations (GASB, 1987); it can be measured by considering the situation of its net assets, its budget balance or the net cash position (GASB, 1999). Thus, if the institution is capable of meeting its debts and, at the same time, providing acceptable levels of services, we may say that it is in good financial health. For Groves et al. (2003), financial health results from various elements, which can be measured by means of four magnitudes that are related to cash solvency, budget solvency, long-run solvency and service-level solvency. Cash solvency is understood to be the entity's ability to generate sufficient liquidity to pay its short-term debts. Budget solvency is its ability to obtain sufficient budgetary income without entering into deficit. Long-run solvency concerns a government's ability to respond adequately to all its long-term obligations, while service-level solvency is defined as expressing the entity's capacity to provide the level and quality of services necessary for the wellbeing of the community in question. These four concepts of solvency embrace what the above authors have termed the financial factor.

The financial factor reflects the condition of the government's internal finances. For other authors, this concept is focused on the study of its assets and of liabilities (which may be of immediate effect or could have to be met at some future time), together with an analysis of income and expenditure trends and of the particular factors that characterise institutions when they acquire financial liabilities, within a particular time span and a specific, clearly-bounded economic dimension or space (Copeland & Ingram, 1983; Berne, 1992; Clark, 1990, 1994; Groves et al., 2003).

For Greenberg and Hiller (1995) and CICA (1997), the financial condition of an organization can be measured by means of a series of indicators related to its sustainability, flexibility, vulnerability and short-term solvency.

Sustainability refers to an organization's ability to maintain, promote and protect the social welfare of the population, employing the resources at its disposal. Flexibility is understood as a body's capability to respond to changes in the economy or in its financial circumstances, within the limits of its fiscal abilities, a capability that depends on the degree to which it is able to react to such changes, via modifications to tax rates, public debt or transfers. Finally, vulnerability is understood to be an organization's level of dependence on external funding received via transfers and grants.

Figure 1. Elements of financial condition

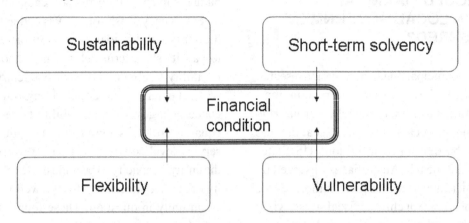

This is the context in which we put forward the following proposal for a financial performance model based on the concept of financial condition. To measure the financial factor, let us consider some of the definitions proposed by the above-mentioned authors. On the one hand, it is necessary to measure the concepts of short-run solvency (the capability to generate short-run liquidity) and of budget solvency (the capability to respond to budgetary obligations) (Groves et al., 2003). This concept is divided into the more specific aspects of flexibility, sustainability and vulnerability (Greenberg and Hillier, 1995; CICA, 1997). Finally, we measure long-run solvency by studying whether, in the course of the financial years that are under study, the local authority officers have been capable of improving the authority's financial condition.

However, the problem of measuring the above lies in the fact that four different elements must be addressed, in each of which each local authority may present different levels. Thus in predicting financial condition we must obtain a valuation of each of the elements of which it is constituted.

In view of these considerations, a study of the financial condition of local authorities requires an individualized analysis of each of its constituent elements, as these components are very heterogeneous. Therefore, we considered the application

of the CHAID methodology to each of the four elements that constitute the financial condition: one to examine an entity's budgetary sustainability, another for its short-term solvency, another for its flexibility (or indebtedness) and, finally, one for its levels of financial independence from other entities.

METHODOLOGICAL PROPOSAL: CHAID

The phenomenon to be studied requires us to establish certain rules for the behaviour of the different elements that constitute the financial condition of a local authority, using a specific data set. Such a study can be carried out, among other means, using decision trees, which provide a set of rules that are hierarchies in such a way that the final decision can be taken through the implementation of logical decisions, from the tree trunk towards the leaves.

In fact, a great many algorithms are capable of generating rules based on decision trees, including CLS (Hunt et al., 1966), ID3 (Quinlan, 1979), CART (Breiman et al., 1984) and C4.5 (Quinlan, 1993). In the present chapter, we implemented the algorithm known as CHAID (Chi-squared Automatic Interaction Detector), which is simple to apply and widely used. This classification mechanism, originally proposed by Kass (1980), has been used extensively by many authors in different studies to derive a tree of rules which help understanding of many phenomena (Santín, 2006; Galguera, 2006; Grobler, 2002; Strambi, 1998). It was also extended to ordinal dependent variables by Magidson (1993), who illustrated how this extension could be used to take advantage of fixed scores such as profitability, for each category of the dependent variable when such scores are known, as well as how to estimate meaningful scores when category scores are unknown.

As a segmentation tool, CHAID presents important benefits: firstly, the technique is not based on any specific probabilistic distribution, but solely on chi squared goodness-of-fit tests, from contingency tables. These, given an acceptable sample size, almost always function well. Secondly, it makes it possible to determine a variable to be maximized. This is very desirable, and not always possible with other segmentation techniques. Thirdly, classification by segments is always straightforward to interpret, as its results provide intuitive rules that are readily understood by non experts – which is not the case, for example, with Cluster Analysis. Fourthly, this technique ensures that the segments always have statistical meaning; they are all different, and are the best possible, given the data provided. Accordingly, the classifications made using the rules found are mutually exclusive, and so the decision tree identifies a single response based on a calculation of the probabilities of belonging to a certain class.

Finally, the CHAID unlike other algorithms such as CART (Breiman et al., 1984) is capable of constructing non-binary algorithms, i.e. it can present more than two branches, or data divisions, according to the categories to be explained, for each node. The algorithm performs non-symmetrical partitions that are optimal for each explicative variable, and which are derived from contingency tables based on the chi-squared statistic. After a series of iterations, the algorithm establishes the point at which the structure created is optimum, by demanding a level of significance for each branch created.

CHAID provides a set of rules[1] that can be applied to a new (unclassified) dataset to predict which records will have a given outcome. Using the significance of a chi-squared test, CHAID evaluates all of the values of each potential explanatory variable, by merging those values that are judged to be statistically homogeneous (similar) with respect to the dependent variable (target) and maintaining all the others, which are heterogeneous (dissimilar). It then selects the best predictor to form the first branch in the decision tree, such that each leaf node is made up of a group of homogeneous values of the selected field. This process continues recursively until the tree is fully grown.

Let us now examine in detail the methodological process to be followed to apply the technique. A complete description of this algorithm with a tutorial reference is showed by Kass (1980), Biggs (1991) and Goodman, L. A. (1979). Also, Santin (2006) uses a simplification of this application.

Binning of Continuous Explanatory Variables

In the first step, continuous explanatory variables are automatically discretized or binned into a set of ordinal categories. This process is performed once for each continuous explanatory variable in the model. Discretization can be done through various machine learning algorithms for building decision trees or decision rules, in particular by the CHAID algorithm, which we apply. We are aware that there are several methods for binning into a set of categories, for example, the one proposed by Berka (1998), which will be studied in future research, to compare results with those described in this chapter.

Merging Categories for Explanatory Variables

All the explanatory variables are merged to combine categories that are not statistically different with respect to the dependent variable, and each final category of an explanatory variable X represents a leaf node if that variable is used to split the node. For each explanatory variable X, the algorithm finds the pair of categories of X that is least significantly different (indicated by the largest p-value) with respect to the dependent variable Y. The method used to calculate the p-value is the chi-squared test:

$$\aleph^2 = \sum_{j=1}^{J} \sum_{i=1}^{I} \frac{\left(n_{ij} - \hat{m}_{ij} \right)^2}{\hat{m}_{ij}}$$

where $n_{ij} = \sum_{n} f_n I\left(x_n = i \wedge y_n = j \right)$ is the ob-

served cell frequency and $\hat{m}_{ij}$ is the expected estimated cell frequency for cell $\left(x_n = i, y_n = j \right)$ under the null hypothesis of Independence. The corresponding *p value* is given by $p = \Pr\left(\aleph_d^2 > X^2 \right)$, where $\aleph_d^2$ follows a chi-squared distribution with degrees of freedom $d = (J-1)(I-1)$. The frequency associated with case n is noted by f_n.

Then, it merges into a compound category the pair that gives the largest *p-value*, and calculates the *p-value* based on the new set of categories of X. This represents one set of categories for X. The process is repeated until only two categories remain. Then, the sets of categories of X generated during each step of the merge sequence are compared, to find the one for which the *p-value* in the previous step is the smallest. That set is the set of merged categories for X to be used in determining the split at the current node.

Splitting Nodes

Once the categories have been merged for all the dependent variables, the algorithm selects the explanatory variable with the largest association with the dependent variable, the one for which the chi-squared test has the smallest p-value, and if this value is less than or equal to the α split (the split threshold), then that variable is used as the split variable for the current node. Each of the merged categories of the split variable defines a leaf node of the split. After the split is applied to the current node, the leaf nodes are examined to see if they warrant splitting by applying the merge/split process to each in turn. This process continues recursively until the tree is fully grown.

RESULTS OF THE MODEL

Support

The support for a scored record is the weighted number of records in the data in the scored record's assigned terminal node (t), i.e., the number of records of each rule. $N_{w,j}(t)$ is the weighted number of records in node t with category j (or the number of records if no frequency or case weights are defined):

$$N_{w,j}\left(t \right) = \sum_{i \in t} w_i f_i j(i)$$

and $N_{w,j}$ is the weighted number of records in category j (any node):

$$N_{w,j} = \sum_{i \in T} w_i f_i j(i)$$

Response (Confidence)

The confidence for a scored record is the proportion of weighted records in the data in the scored record's assigned terminal node (t) that belong to a selected category j, modified by the Laplace correction (Margineantu, 2001), with k being the number of categories:

$$Response\left(\%\right) = \frac{N_{f,j}\left(t\right)+1}{N_f\left(t\right)+k}$$

The level of confidence (%) of each rule (terminal node) shows the proportion of records of each rule that belong to a selected category j. The level of confidence of a set of rules can also be defined as the proportion of records of this rule set belonging to a given category j.

Index

The index of each of the rules obtained for a given category j is obtained as the ratio between the level of confidence for each rule (terminal node) and the level of confidence of the category j in the total sample (i.e., 25%, as the sample is divided into quartiles).

Therefore, it is obtained by dividing the proportion of records that present category j in each terminal node (rule) into the proportion of records presenting category j in the total sample (25%). Thus, it represents the increased probability of belonging to the selected category j that contains the records presenting the characteristics defined for each rule. By accumulation, thus, the index of a set of rules can be obtained as the ratio between the proportion of records presenting category j in this rule set and the corresponding proportion to be found within the total sample (25%).

Gain

The gain for each terminal node (rule) can be defined, in absolute terms, as the number of records in a selected category j. For a set of rules or terminal nodes, and in percentage terms, the gain summary provides descriptive statistics for the terminal nodes of a tree, and shows the weighted percentage of records in a selected category j:

$$Gain\left(\%\right) = g\left(t,j\right) = \frac{\sum_{i \in t} f_i x_i\left(j\right)}{\sum_{i \in t} f_i}$$

where $x_i(j) = 1$ if record x_i is in category j, and 0 otherwise.

Risk Estimates

Risk estimates describe the risk of error in predicted values for specific nodes of the tree and for the tree as a whole. The risk estimate $r(t)$ of a node t is computed as:

$$r\left(t\right) = \frac{1}{N_f} \sum_j N_{f,j}\left(t\right)$$

where $N_{f,j}(t)$ is the sum of the frequency weights for records in node t in category j (or the number of records if no frequency weights are defined), and N_f is the sum of frequency weights for all records in the sample.

The risk estimate $R(T)$ for the tree (T) is calculated by taking the sum of the risk estimates for the terminal nodes $r(t)$:

$$R\left(T\right) = \sum_{t \in T} r\left(t\right)$$

where T' is the set of terminal nodes in the tree.

ANALYZING THE FINANCIAL CONDITION OF LOCAL AUTHORITIES IN SPAIN USING CHAID

Sample

The database contains economic, financial and budgetary data from 877 local authorities with a population of 1000 inhabitants or more, for the period 1992-1999 (Source: Directorate General for Financial Coordination with Local Authorities – Spanish Ministry of Economy and Finance). The data were provided by the latter Directorate and are available from them on request.

The final sample was constituted of 6200 cases, once the appropriate filtering had been performed for cases in which we did not possess all the values for the variables defined. In addition, taking into account the considerable standard deviation of many of the variables and their nature of ratio variables, as well as the assumption that the sample collection may include mistakes due to the lack of precision which can be assumed to be inherent in the accounting of small corporations, it was decided to remove the extreme cases, these being defined as those in which the standard deviation for each variable was exceeded by five times or more. We must be aware that the extreme cases were actually disposed of in some cases because they lacked economic sense, were municipalities with fewer than 1.500 people who practically do not follow any strict accounting or budgetary. Not help us to predict variables that warn us of the financial crisis.

Variables

The aim of this research was to identify the most significant explanatory variables of sustainability, solvency, flexibility and financial independence. Accordingly, four models were created, with each of these parameters, in turn, being taken as the dependent variable. As possible explanatory variables, we used a set of ratios and indicators commonly applied by local authority managers and analysts. The definitions of the variables used are shown in the Appendix 1, emphasizing those whose behaviour we set out to explain in the models created.

Dependent Variables Categorized

Each of the dependent variables to be studied is categorized into quartiles, in order to obtain an indication of the presence of the local authorities in each of these quartiles, which define four budgetary situations (numbered 1 to 4, in rising order according to the values of the dependent variable). This categorization into quartiles is applied by many authors in studies which use the CHAID technique such as Santín (2006), Dills (2005) and Gonzalez et al. (2002). In our chapter, what is especially interesting is the focus on the first and fourth quartiles, which represent the best and the worst budgetary situations (success and failure profiles).

Descriptive Analysis

Table 1 shows the descriptive analysis performed for the whole set of variables employed in this analysis.

ANALYSIS AND RESULTS

Exploratory Analysis

Firstly, we perform an exploratory analysis of the variables considered to be dependent, and their relation with the other variables, for each of the elements constituting the financial condition.

The first aspect to be analyzed is that of budgetary sustainability. For this purpose, we use the variable *Index of non financial budget result* (BR), as defined above and which describes the entity's capacity or need for self-funding of its

Table 1. Descriptive analysis of the variables employed in the chapter

VARIABLE	MEAN	STANDARD DEVIATION	MEDIAN
I. Implementation of expenditure	0.83	0.13	0.85
I. Implementation of current expenditure	0.92	0.06	0.93
I. Implementation of capital expenditure	0.69	0.29	0.7
I. Implementation of receipts	0.86	0.14	0.87
I. Implementation of current receipts	0.99	0.12	0.99
I. Implementation of capital receipts	182.49	9500.67	0.83
Index of Current budget payments	0.92	0.06	0.93
Index of Current budget receipts	0.84	0.12	0.86
I. Public expenditure per capita	82145.83	71982.30	70813.31
I. Current expenditure per capita	53508.89	51083.62	46848.49
I. Significance of current costs	0.66	0.14	0.67
Index of Expenditure rigidity	0.92	0.07	0.93
I. Significance of current receipts	0.77	0.14	0.79
Index of Taxation receipts	0.43	0.15	0.42
Index of Fiscal pressure	548769392.99	1318568835.10	111396668.00
I. Receipts from current transfers	0.41	0.14	0.4
Index of Gross savings	0.17	0.13	0.16
I. Capital expenditure per capita	23919.09	24111.47	17525.88
I. Significance of capital expenditure	0.29	0.14	0.27
Index of Capital funding	0.62	0.56	0.54
Index of Net savings	0.1	0.17	0.11
I. Significance of financial load	0.08	0.07	0.06
I. Financial load per capita	7367.07	13112.46	4198.30
I. Weight of financial load	0.11	0.11	0.08
I. Significance of cash surplus	0.13	0.33	0.09
Index of Immediate liquidity	0.86	3.66	0.39
Index of Income results	0.43	0.35	0.39
Index of Expenditure results	0.19	0.2	0.14
Mean receipts lapse	214.97	955.45	112.14
Mean payment lapse	170.69	442.61	112.21
Current self-funding margin	0.9	0.17	0.89
Outstanding debt of governing political party	34173767.26	200323652.57	-600000.00
Index of available cash	0.01	0.1	0.01
Index of staff costs	0.44	0.1	0.44
Index of current transfers effected	0.08	0.07	0.07
I. Public expenditure per capita	23862.70	24476.24	20839.90
I. Goods and services expenses per capita	21949.84	19416.06	18501.73
I. Financial expenses per capita	2842.44	5076.91	1628.92
I. Current receipts per capita	64955.36	58964.43	55594.33

continued on following page

Table 1. continued

VARIABLE	MEAN	STANDARD DEVIATION	MEDIAN
I. Investment per capita	23919.09	24111.47	17525.88
I. Short-term solvency	2.27	5.04	1.44
I. Coverage of the financial load	11.97	336.52	1.08
Index of self funding	2.09	0.98	1.81
Index of fixed charges	0.48	0.17	0.46
Index of coverage of expenditure	0.97	0.12	0.98
Sum of current receipts	874227925.02	2076623202.40	211944650.00
Index of current self funding	1.53	0.57	1.41
Index of non financial budget result	1.03	0.15	1.02

budget (non-financial surplus or deficit), without needing to resort to indebtedness. The second element is that of solvency, which is measured using the variable *short-term solvency* (STS), as defined above. This variable expresses the entity's capacity to meet its short-term obligations from the liquid funds at its disposal and from receipts pending. The third aspect to be taken into account is that of flexibility, which measures the levels of local authorities' indebtedness. For this purpose, we use the variable *index of the weight of financial load* (FL), which reflects the local authority's capacity to meet the obligations of its debts, i.e. capital repayment plus interests, from its current receipts. Finally, we measure the level of financial independence of local authorities, which determines whether the entity employs more or less of its own resources (via taxation). This aspect is studied by means of the variable *index of taxation receipts* (TR). In all of the above cases, the variables are categorized by quartiles, such that the variable takes values from 1 to 4.

Exploratory Analysis of Correlations; the Most Important Explanatory Variables

The exploratory analysis of correlations between each of the explanatory variables and the depen-

dent variable is shown in Table 2, Table 3, Table 4, and Table 5, including the mean values for each of the categories of the target variable and the F-test statistic of independence[2]. The tables include only the main variables, i.e. those presenting the greatest explicative power (F-test) in relation to the dependent variable being studied.

Table 2 shows that the variables with the greatest explanatory capacity of the Index of non financial budget result are the index of available cash, the index of gross and net savings, the index of capital funding and the current self-funding margin. On the contrary, other variables, such as the index of implementation of capital expenditure, the index of current budget receipts and the index of coverage of the financial load do not contribute explanatory capacity.

Be that as it may, there are many variables that enable us to identify differences regarding the output variable, and a model is needed to help summarize the body of information available and organize it so that it may be useful for explanatory and predictive purposes.

For Short-term solvency, the most influential variables are the index of gross savings, the net savings index and the margin of current self-funding, while on the contrary, little information is provided by the index of current transfers and

Table 2. Analysis of means and correlations of the variables with BR

INDEPENDENT VARIABLES	Mean (BR 1)	Mean (BR 2)	Mean (BR 3)	Mean (BR 4)	F value	p-level
Index of available cash	-0.037	-0.004	0.018	0.07	374.443	0.000
Index of Gross savings	0.107	0.139	0.175	0.247	374.155	0.000
Index of Capital funding	0.404	0.552	0.634	0.877	217.955	0.000
Index of Net savings	0.04	0.074	0.114	0.177	198.025	0.000
Current self-funding margin	0.96	0.926	0.886	0.823	198.025	0.000
I. Significance of capital expenditure	0.349	0.3	0.278	0.234	186.141	0.000
I. Implementation of current receipts	0.952	0.974	0.995	1.039	173.282	0.000
I. Implementation of capital receipts	0.756	0.728	0.696	0.56	149.25	0.000
I. Significance of current costs	0.607	0.654	0.673	0.704	147.346	0.000
I. Implementation of receipts	0.81	0.857	0.873	0.913	145.067	0.000
I. Implementation of expenditure	0.851	0.85	0.832	0.773	135.803	0.000

Table 3. Analysis of means and correlations of the variables with STS

INDEPENDENT VARIABLES	Mean (STS 1)	Mean (STS 2)	Mean (STS 3)	Mean (STS 4)	F test	p-level
I. Gross savings	0.111	0.155	0.179	0.223	210.875	0.000
I. Net savings	0.027	0.087	0.121	0.171	209.644	0.000
Margin of current self-funding	0.973	0.913	0.879	0.829	209.644	0.000
I. Implementation of expenditure	0.872	0.849	0.812	0.773	194.261	0.000
Index of fixed charges	0.548	0.49	0.456	0.417	187.619	0.000
Budget result	0.983	1.001	1.038	1.095	186.036	0.000
I. Implementation of current receipts	0.945	0.979	1.002	1.033	172.355	0.000
I. Immediate liquidity	0.009	0.351	0.624	2.46	149.14	0.000
Index of coverage of expenditure	1.01	0.988	0.962	0.93	136.598	0.000
I. Weight of financial load	0.141	0.108	0.093	0.079	87.954	0.000
I. Implementation of capital expenditure	0.753	0.727	0.655	0.605	87.21	0.000
I. Expenditure results	0.246	0.21	0.179	0.14	84.184	0.000
I. Significance of financial load	0.1	0.081	0.074	0.065	64.291	0.000

the index of implementation, among others (see Table 3).

The exploratory analysis reveals that levels of indebtedness (see Table 4), measured by the variable weight of financial load, are related to the variables index of fixed charges, index of net savings and the margin of current self-funding, among others. Most of the variables that do not present any significant relation with levels of indebtedness are those concerning the entity's cash balances.

From the prior analysis of the correlations between the variables to be studied and the other financial variables, we conclude that the variables that are most strongly related to the index of taxation receipts are the index of current transfer

Table 4. Analysis of means and correlations of the variables with FL

INDEPENDENT VARIABLES	Mean (FL 1)	Mean (FL 2)	Mean (FL 3)	Mean (FL 4)	F test	p-level
Index of fixed charges	0.39	0.427	0.463	0.631	909.483	0.000
Index of net savings	0.178	0.148	0.12	-0.041	654.583	0.000
Margin of current self-funding	0.822	0.852	0.88	1.041	654.583	0.000
I. Financial expenses per capita	459.435	1556.618	3254.434	6099.29	440.142	0.000
I. Significance of capital expenditure	0.344	0.312	0.278	0.228	204.321	0.000
Index of self funding	2.473	2.202	1.918	1.751	176.59	0.000
I. Fiscal pressure	150117608.6	346863643.9	687511143.1	1010585176	136.887	0.000
Sum of current receipts	259526767.1	573008187.9	1094860540	1569516206	127.217	0.000
I. Receipts from current transfers	0.456	0.426	0.389	0.376	103.949	0.000
I. Gross savings	0.19	0.18	0.173	0.125	76.659	0.000
I. Taxation receipts	0.388	0.424	0.461	0.441	67.208	0.000
I. Significance of cash surplus	0.208	0.152	0.122	0.045	66.217	0.000
I. Income results	0.345	0.428	0.481	0.466	48.897	0.000

Table 5. Analysis of the means and correlations of the variables with TR

INDEPENDENT VARIABLES	Mean (TR 1)	Mean (TR 2)	Mean (TR 3)	Mean (TR 4)	F test	p-level
I. Receipts from current transfers	0.551	0.451	0.376	0.268	2258.757	0.000
I. Self funding	3.138	2.096	1.722	1.388	1674.978	0.000
I. Current self funding	2.101	1.576	1.35	1.106	1449.906	0.000
I. Significance of current receipts	0.645	0.745	0.81	0.883	1245.019	0.000
I. Significance of current expenditure	0.567	0.643	0.692	0.737	546.56	0.000
I. Significance of capital expenditure	0.389	0.302	0.254	0.216	514.909	0.000
I. Fiscal pressure	81067990.31	298395143.2	753019452.8	1062594986	190.489	0.000
I. Income results	0.307	0.378	0.463	0.571	181.776	0.000
I. Capital funding	0.803	0.684	0.578	0.401	157.176	0.000
I. Goods and services expenses per capita	16853.073	19130.939	21636.683	30178.654	149.447	0.000
I. Current receipts per capita	49095.334	56725.752	65284.625	88715.71	140.204	0.000
Sum of current receipts	195821007	560565257.2	1238412657	1502112779	138.721	0.000
I. Implementation of capital expenditure	0.781	0.71	0.663	0.585	132.056	0.000

receipts, the index of self funding (both current and total), and the index of the significance of current receipts. Again, we find there is least relation, in this respect, with the variables related to the entity's level of short-term solvency.

In short, it can be seen that the variables most closely related to the indicators used to measure each of the indicators of financial condition are the index of gross savings, the index of net saving and the index of implementation of expenditure.

PREDICTIVE ANALYSIS WITH CHAID: SUCCESS AND FAILURE PROFILES FROM EACH ELEMENT OF FINANCIAL CONDITION

Results Obtained with the Rules for Each Element of Financial Condition

With CHAID modelling, the sample is segmented using a classification tree to create a set of terminal nodes, with routes from the origin node (the whole sample) that constitute the profiles or rules for each of the categories defined in the variable to be explained[3]. Moreover, it should be taken into account that the main aim of the chapter is not to classify all cases that may arise in the environment, but to offer recommendations to local authorities regarding the main variables that influence the financial condition, as well as to ascertain the most suitable values for them.

In the case of the study of budgetary sustainability, we are particularly interested in the profiles of the local authorities located in the extreme quartiles, i.e. in BR=4 (high level of sustainability) and in BR=1 (low sustainability), and in turn, within each of these categories, we focus on the most important profiles, which are those presenting the highest classificatory and predictive capacities in terms of the level of confidence

Accordingly, on the basis of the general rule tree, we filter out the rules obtained for the categories BR=1 and BR=4, and after ordering them by level of confidence and gain, the most important rules in each category are selected. The end result, thus, is that we have the rules for the highest sampling decile in each category, representing 620 local authorities. The principal rules selected, in both cases, are illustrated in the Figure 2, which show the corresponding support and confidence levels.

Thus, the main explanatory variables coincide with those identified previously in the exploratory analysis of correlations and, therefore, these

are the variables that must be controlled by the local authorities if sustainability is to be improved.

The different rules for BR=4 indicate the levels within which these variables should be situated in order to ensure budgetary sustainability, with a high level of probability. Thus, for example, Rule 13 indicates that when the index of gross savings is higher than 0.334 and the index of the significance of capital expenditure is lower than 0.272, 100% (confidence) of the 118 (support) local authorities in the sample present very good levels of sustainability (upper quartile, BR=4).

At the other extreme, we have the profiles of the authorities with the lowest levels of sustainability. For example, Rule 2, for a sampling support of 155 authorities, indicates that there is a 99.4% probability that the authorities with a gross savings index of less than 0.018, an index of capital funding of less than 0.747 and an index of the significance of capital expenditure of over 0.162 will present very low levels of budgetary sustainability (lower quartile, BR=1).

It would be possible to analyze all the selected rules in the tables in the same way, and thus obtain a series of profiles and/or recommendations providing local authorities with quantitative control measures for obtaining high levels of budgetary sustainability[4].

For the case of the second element of financial condition considered, that of short-term solvency, the main rules obtained were those shown in Figure 3. These tables show that the worst situations with respect to short-term solvency occur when liquid funds are scarce, when payments are made promptly and when more expenditure is implemented. On the other hand, for local authorities to have good levels of short-term solvency, they need a high index of liquidity, to receive payments promptly (in approximately three months), to make their payments in about six months, to achieve substantial budgetary receipts and, in most cases, to have a moderate level of fixed expenses.

The rules that most precisely determine when a local authority may have greater or lesser flex-

Figure 2. Principal rules obtained for BR=4 and BR=1

RULES FOR BR=4

Rule 1 (108; 0.963)
If I. gross savings > 0.070 and <= 0.135 and I. capital funding > 1.046

Rule 2 (66; 0.955)
If I. gross savings > 0.135 and <= 0.190 and I. significance of capital expenditure <= 0.117 and I. capital expenditure per capita <= 5763.515

Rule 4 (95; 0.905)
If I. gross savings > 0.190 and <= 0.225 and I. significance of capital expenditure <= 0.162

Rule 5 (158; 1.0)
If I. gross savings > 0.225 and <= 0.334 and I. significance of capital expenditure <= 0.162

Rule 7 (80; 1.0)
If I. gross savings > 0.225 and <= 0.334 and I. significance of capital expenditure > 0.162 and <= 0.235 and I. capital funding > 0.446

Rule 13 (118; 1.0)
If I. gross savings > 0.334 and I. significance of capital expenditure <= 0.272

RULES FOR BR=1

Rule 2 (155; 0.994)
If I. gross savings <= 0.018 and I. capital funding <= 0.747 and I. significance of capital expenditure > 0.162

Rule 4 (113; 0.85)
If I. gross savings > 0.018 and <= 0.070 and I. capital funding <= 0.351

Rule 5 (133; 0.857)
If I. gross savings > 0.018 and <= 0.070 and I. capital funding > 0.351 and <= 0.747 and I. significance of capital expenditure > 0.200

Rule 7 (130; 0.992)
If I. gross savings > 0.070 and <= 0.135 and <= 0.642 and I. significance of capital expenditure > 0.235 and I. capital funding <= 0.45

Rule 11 (97; 0.979)
If I. gross savings > 0.135 and <= 0.190 and I. significance of capital expenditure > 0.359 and I. capital funding <= 0.544

Figure 3. Principal rules obtained for STS=1 and STS=4

RULES FOR STS=1

Rule 3 (89; 0.764)
If I. immediate liquidity <= 0.049 and I income results> 0 and Mean payment lapse > 57.403 and <= 160.353 and I. Implementation of expenditure > 0.878

Rule 4 (72; 0.917)
If I. immediate liquidity <= 0.049 and I income results> 0 and Mean payment lapse > 160.353 and <= 262.65 and Mean receipts lapse <= 186.209

Rule 6 (130; 0.869)
If I. immediate liquidity <= 0.049 and I. income results > 0 and Mean payment lapse > 262.650

Rule 7 (69; 0.913)
If I. immediate liquidity > 0.049 and <= 0.128 and Mean payment lapse > 93.692 and <= 196.967 and Mean receipts lapse <= 112.1

Rule 9 (79; 0.975)
If I. immediate liquidity > 0.049 and <= 0.128 and Mean payment lapse > 196.967 and Mean receipts lapse <= 247.690 and I. significance of current receipts <= 0.790

Rule 10 (71; 0.803)
If I. immediate liquidity > 0.049 and <= 0.128 and Mean payment lapse > 196.967 and Mean receipts lapse <= 247.690 and I. significance of current receipts > 0.790

Rule 14 (120; 0.808)
If I. immediate liquidity > 0.128 and <= 0.203 and Mean payment lapse > 196.967 and Mean receipts lapse <= 247.690

Rule 15 (74; 0.811)
If I. immediate liquidity > 0.203 and <= 0.285 and Index of coverage of expenditure > 0.976 and Mean payment lapse > 112.202 and Mean receipts lapse <= 130.786

RULES FOR STS=4

Rule 6 (134; 1.0)
If I. immediate liquidity > 1.125 and <= 1.909 and Mean receipts lapse > 93.862 and Mean payment lapse <= 112.202

Rule 9 (345; 1.0)
If Index of immediate liquidity > 1.909 and Index of income results> 0 and Index of fixed charges <= 0.427

Rule 10 (85;0.965)
If Index of. immediate liquidity > 1.909 and Index of income results> 0 and Index of fixed charges > 0.427 and <= 0.492

Rule 11 (71; 1.0)
If Index of immediate liquidity > 1.909 and Index of income results> 0 and Index of fixed charges > 0.492

Figure 4. Principal rules obtained for FL=1 and FL=4

RULES FOR FL=1

Rule 3 (367; 0.951)
If I. weight of GF <= 121.894 and I. income results> 0

Rule 6 (231; 0.944)
If I. weight of GF > 121.894 and <= 419.274 and I. Current receipts per capita > 28593.622 and Outstanding debt of governing political party > -1.742.320 and <= 533.754

Rule 7 (103; 0.806)
If I. weight of GF > 121.894 and <= 419.274 and I. Current receipts per capita > 28593.622 and Outstanding debt of governing political party > 533.754

RULES FOR FL=4

Rule 4 (128; 0.781)
If I. Financial expenses per capita > 3087.972 and <= 4197.914 and I. Current receipts per capita <= 49704.129

Rule 7 (91; 0.956)
If I. Financial expenses per capita > 4197.914 and <= 6113.369 and I. Current receipts per capita <= 62098.372 and I. fixed charges > 0.669

Rule 8 (68; 0.853)
If I. Financial expenses per capita > 4197.914 and <= 6113.369 and I. Current receipts per capita > 62098.372 and <= 100892.467 and I. net savings<= 0.004

Rule 10 (66; 0.924)
If I. Financial expenses per capita > 6113.369 and <= 26328.526 and I. fixed charges > 0.427 and <= 0.530

Rule 13 (215; 0.991)
If I. Financial expenses per capita > 6113.369 and I. fixed charges > 0.530 and I. income results> 0 and I. I. Implementation of current receipts <= 1.012

Rule 14 (74; 0.905)
If I. Financial expenses per capita > 6113.369 and I. fixed charges > 0.530 and I. income results> 0 and I. Implementation of current receipts 1.012

ibility are shown in Figure 4. We find that the determinant variable, with respect to the rules determining the highest and lowest levels of indebtedness, is that of financial expenditure on the total population. It can also be seen that in order to obtain the best results (FL=1), rules with fewer variables are needed, and so they present a lower degree of complexity than does the analysis of local authorities with lower levels of flexibility (FL=4). In addition to this variable, the authorities presenting worse levels of flexibility are also characterized by higher values of the variables fixed charges, low net savings and low current receipts per capita. In consequence, such local authorities must seek resources via indebtedness. Those presenting the highest values for flexibility are notable for presenting high levels of current receipts per capita and moderate levels of accumulated debt.

Finally, we show the rules for the element independence. From the analysis of the worst results, we conclude that in most cases, the local authorities need to have high levels of receipts from current transfers, together with relatively low values for the variable significance of current receipts and, in some cases, low levels of fiscal pressure (See Figure 5).

The local authorities presenting the best results, with respect to financial independence, are characterized by low levels of receipts from current transfers, significant current receipts and relatively high indices of fiscal pressure. In addition to these variables, in some rules there is a low index of capital funding and moderate financial expenditure per capita.

It can be said that the fact that the greater or lesser independence of local authorities largely depends on the transfers received from other entities and on the importance attained by the sum of current receipts. In conclusion, the variables that seem to predict a better or worse financial condition are the index of gross savings, the index of significance of capital expenditure and the index of fixed charges. These are the main variables that public sector managers should monitor in order to ensure good financial condition.

Figure 5. Principal rules obtained for TR=1 and TR=4

RULES FOR TR=1

Rule 2 (73; 1.0)
If I. receipts from current transfers > 0.440 and <= 0.481 and I. significance of current receipts <= 0.573

Rule 5 (222; 0.995)
If I. receipts from current transfers > 0.533 and <= 0.603 and I. significance of current receipts <= 0.706

Rule 7 (408; 1.0)
If I. receipts from current transfers > 0.603 and I. significance of current receipts <= 0.861 and I. fiscal pressure <= 77,070,262

RULES FOR TR=4

Rule 3 (181; 0.95)
If I. receipts from current transfers <= 0.230 and I. significance of current receipts > 0.750 and I. fiscal pressure > 111,391,233 and <= 576,599,338

Rule 4 (222; 1.0)
If I. receipts from current transfers <= 0.230 and I. significance of current receipts > 0.750 and I. fiscal pressure > 576,599,338

Rule 6 (99; 0.949)
If I. receipts from current transfers > 0.230 and <= 0.289 y 15) I. significance of current receipts > 0.750 and I weight of GF > 780.623 and <= 2206.967

Rule 10 (133; 0.992)
If I. receipts from current transfers > 0.289 and <= 0.329 and I. fiscal pressure > 77,070,262 and I. capital funding <= 0.544 and I. significance of current receipts > 0.861

Table 6. Estimation of risks with the total for BR

Real/Predicted	BR=1	BR =2	BR =3	BR =4
BR =1	1290	217	8	35
BR =2	380	859	208	103
BR =3	113	325	796	316
BR =4	37	44	327	1142
RISKS	Correct 4087 (65.02%)		Incorrect 2113 (34.08%)	

Goodness of the Element of Financial Condition

To illustrate the goodness of the rule of the evaluated element, the following matrix of incorrect classification shows the cases correctly and incorrectly classified by the general model (See Table 6).

The total risk, that is, the sum of all the risks from all the terminal nodes (rules) is 34.08%, and this is representative of the percentage of cases classified incorrectly when all the model rules are used for classification or prediction, and this also enables us to determine the overall level of confidence provided by the model (65.02%). The error rate is much lower than the initial 75% which is found without sample segmentation (the 75% represents the proportion of cases that do not belong to a specific selected category). Therefore,

the rule model does contribute explanatory and predictive capacity.

However, as our interest mainly lies in the rules for BR=4 and BR=1, and in particular for the ones described above, within each of these categories, if we make our prediction using these rules exclusively, the error rate is reduced considerably. Thus, Table 7 shows that for the six rules selected for BR=4, with a sampling support of 620 local authorities, the probability of an accurate prediction increases to 97.5% (confidence or response), which is equivalent to an index of 389.98%, i.e. almost four times higher than with the 25% of the total sample (the percentage of local authorities with BR=4 in the not segmented sample). In other words, 620 local authorities presented the above-stated levels of variables for the six rules of BR=4, and of these authorities, 97.5% achieved high

Table 7. Gain, index and response with the rules selected for BR=4 and BR=1

Nodes	Percentile	Percentile: n	Gain: n	Gain (%)	Response (%)	Index (%)
6 Rules Decile BR=4	10	620	604	39	97.5	389.98
6 Rules Decile BR=1	10	620	590	38.06	95.15	380.61

Table 8. Estimation of risks with the total model for STS

Real/Predicted	STS=1	STS=2	STS=3	STS=4
STS=1	974	459	77	40
STS=3	332	745	461	12
STS=3	110	271	1051	118
STS=4	25	47	337	1141
RISKS	Correct 3911 (63.08%)		Incorrect 2289 (36.92%)	

levels of sustainability (BR=4). This also means that the model presented accounts for 39% (gain) of all the local authorities in the total sample with a sustainability of BR=4. The level of confidence in the six rules defined for BR=4 is thus 97.5%, while the individual level of confidence for each of these rules is as shown in Figure 2.

This table also shows the level of confidence for each of the six rules obtained for BR=1, with the corresponding gain and index indicators, for each of which similar goodness analyses could be made. The charts in Appendix (i.e. *Appendix 2*) illustrate the gains, responses and indices for the set of rules obtained for the classification of the category BR=4. Note that for the tenth percentile, the values coincide with those given in Figure 2.

The Responses Chart indicates the level of confidence in the rules; thus, for example, for the rules addressed in 10% of the sample (the highest decile), the level of confidence in them is 97.5%. The higher the level of the chart with respect to the 25% benchmark (the confidence in the prediction for the category BR=1, using the not segmented sample), the higher the model's predictive and classificatory capacity.

With respect to the second of the elements that constitute financial condition, the estimation of risks correctly classifies 63.08% of the cases, in contrast to the level of risk assumed in the unsegmented model (75%). Hence, it improves the prediction and classification results by reducing this risk to 36.92% (See Table 8).

With respect to the risks for the two categories of greatest interest (STS=1 and STS=4), the rate of accurate prediction rises considerably, with the response (confidence) rate reaching 99.6%, with a gain of 39.84%, while the index value approaches 400% for the case of local authorities with the highest level of short-term solvency. For the case of the authorities with the poorest short-term solvency, the index of response is lower than for those situated in the higher quartile, but in general the model produces very satisfactory classifications (See Table 9).

For the element of flexibility, concerning the goodness of fit, note that the risk continues to decrease and that accurate predictions are made for 64.19% of cases, this value being similar to that obtained with the two previous models (See Table 10).

On examination of the rules that represent the best and the worst results related to the entity's

Table 9. Gain, index and response with the rules selected for STS=4 and STS=1

Nodes	Percentile	Percentile: n	Gain: n	Gain (%)	Response (%)	Index (%)
4 Rules Decile STS=4	10	620	618	*39.84*	*99.6*	*398.41*
8 Rules Decile STS=1	10	620	537	*34.63*	*86.58*	*346.34*

Table 10. Estimation of risks with the total model for FL

Real/Predicted	FL=1	FL=2	FL=3	FL=4
FL=1	1271	254	15	10
FL=2	317	851	324	58
FL=3	93	366	783	308
FL=4	55	109	311	1075
RISKS	Correct 3980 (64.19%)		Incorrect 2220 (35.81%)	

flexibility, we see that, once again, the success rate exceeds 91%. Both the gain and the index present results similar to those achieved with the models measuring sustainability and short-term solvency (See Table 11).

With respect to the goodness of the element vulnerability, the following table shows that this model produces the greatest reduction in risk, with success rates exceeding 81% (See Table 12).

Finally, the goodness of this element in the principal profiles within quartiles of 1 (upper decile of rules for TR=1) and 4 (upper decile of rules for TR=4), we see that the model achieves a similar level of response to the others, with the local authorities in the highest decile being located at 97.7%, while those in the lowest decile even higher (99.9%) (See Table 13).

We now show the charts illustrating the goodness of the modelling of the different elements that make up the financial condition (see Appendix 2). The Gain Index Chart is interpreted in a similar way, with the model presenting better goodness as the curve is higher. For example, the same 97.5% confidence in the rules for the highest decile represents a probability of accurate prediction 3.89 times higher than the initial 25% corresponding to the not segmented sample. The

charts below illustrate the gain, the response and the index values for the whole set of rules obtained by the model for the success category (STS=4). In all three figures, the gain of the curve above the initial slope reflects the substantial improvement in predictive capacity achieved from applying the rules obtained. The following charts show the behaviour with respect to the different percentiles. The three figures show the elevation of the curve above the initial slope, reflecting the substantial improvement in predictive and explanatory capacity achieved with the use of the rules obtained. It is only shown for rules obtained for FL=1, the most relevant category. Chart 4 illustrates the Gain, Index and Response values for the set of rules for TR=4. Again, it can be seen that the rules model obtained makes an important contribution to prediction for the financial independence of local authorities.

In summary, we can conclude that the variables that most influence the Index of non financial budget result are the current margin between budget receipts and expenses, and the levels of capital expenditure. The variables which have most influence on a local authority's capacity to manage its level of debt are related to the financial costs per capita that must be borne, the

Table 11. Gain, index and response with the rules selected for FL=4 and FL=1

Nodes	Percentile	Percentile: n	Gain: n	Gain (%)	Response (%)	Index (%)
6 Rules Decile FL=4	10	620	569	36.7	91.74	366.98
3 Rules Decile FL =1	10	620	586	37.79	94.48	377.91

Table 12. Estimation of risks with the total model for TR

Real/Predicted	TR=1	TR =2	TR =3	TR =4
TR =1	1151	321	46	32
TR =2	73	1248	179	50
TR =3	4	178	1204	164
TR =4	1	0	117	1432
RISKS	Correct 5035 (81.21%)		Incorrect 1165 (18.79%)	

Table 13. Gain, index and response with the rules selected for TR=4 and TR=1

Nodes	Percentile	Percentile: n	Gain: n	Gain (%)	Response (%)	Index (%)
4 Rules Decile TR=4	10	620	606	39.08	97.7	390.81
3 Rules Decile TR =1	10	620	619	39.96	99.9	399.60

impact of fixed charges on the entity's funding structure and its current receipts. Thus, the level of financial independence of an entity depends, in most cases, on the levels of transfers received from higher levels of the public sector, and on the weight attained by current receipts in the sum of the entity's total receipts.

CONCLUSION AND DISCUSSION

The detection and rectification of financial crises in local authorities is of fundamental interest for public-sector managers. Nevertheless, in deciding whether a local authority has managed well or badly, it is necessary to take into account a series of external factors that are influential in this respect. In general, for all countries, the proposed model represents an advance in the maximization of benchmarking, which is an essential process in

public-sector management. In general, a control system of these characteristics makes it possible to advise different types of users of the existence of financial tensions; such users might include public-sector managers in authorities responsible for supervising the financial situation of town and city councils, or senior officers in such councils who need to know how resources are being managed, and how this is done in comparable councils.

In order to determine whether a local authority is experiencing a financial crisis, we consider the concept of financial condition, which is measured by means of different elements, including short-term solvency (the capacity to generate liquidity in the immediate future) and budgetary solvency (the capacity to meet budgetary obligations). This concept can be divided into other, more specific, aspects, such as those of flexibility, sustainability and vulnerability (Greenberg and Hillier 1995; CICA 1997). Finally, long-term solvency is measured through the incorporation of a considerable period of time into the indicators considered.

However, there is a problem concerning the measurement of the elements that constitute financial condition, namely the non-existence of an instrument that can be used to measure the different aspects that make it up, bearing in mind the large body of variables that can be applied for this purpose, as well as the need to take a long-term view. We propose a means of overcoming this problem, by applying data mining using the CHAID algorithm. This methodology enables us to create non-binary decision trees, with multiple branches for each node, providing occurrence probabilities via exclusionary rules, and is especially suitable for large sample sizes, for which, in principle, no model has yet been established for the phenomenon in question. The financial condition, in the terms defined in the present chapter, provides the characteristics necessary for such an application.

The results obtained from applying the above methodology to evaluating financial independence, short-term solvency, flexibility and budgetary sustainability are highly satisfactory. The models derived, for all the Spanish local authorities analyzed, produced a success rate of over 63%, while in the case of financial independence, over 80% accuracy was achieved. Clearly, the model developed presents a high degree of explanatory and predictive capacity.

For the specific cases of the worst and best values, i.e. the first and fourth quartiles for each of the elements of financial condition analyzed, an even higher rate of accuracy was recorded, ranging from 86% (for the case of the local authorities with the worst situation regarding short-term solvency) to 99.9% (for those authorities with the highest levels of financial independence). The results also suggest that the characterization of the financial condition by means of four models is a good method, as the main rules created by means of the different decision trees are made up of variables that differ depending on the element

to be analyzed. Thus, for the levels of budgetary sustainability, the most significant variables are those related to the current margin (gross savings), together with the importance of capital expenditure in the budgetary structure, while on the other hand, the short-term solvency depends on the liquid funds possessed by the entity, on the time elapsing before payments are made and received, and on the fixed charges to be met. The flexibility, however, depends on the financial load per inhabitant of the municipality, on the total sum of fixed charges, and on certain variables related to the implementation of current receipts. Finally, financial independence depends fundamentally on the transfers that the entity receives (an aspect that is predictable) and on the fiscal pressure, among other elements.

On the basis of the results reported here, it would be useful in the future to include other lines of research based on the introduction of variables concerning the social and economic context, as well as variables related to the way in which public services are managed, as these factors influence the characterization of local authorities' financial behaviour. Furthermore, we recommend the consideration of other algorithms, within the data mining method, that could make it possible to achieve higher success rates and thus reduce the risks involved, by considering all the local authorities in question in order to classify and predict financial behaviour in local government.

From the methodological point of view, it would be appropriate to apply other algorithms to compare the stability and prediction power of the model created, in particular, the advanced version C5.0 (Chesney, 2009), which improves how missing values are dealt with. In addition, we are aware that the automatic discretization of the continuous explanatory variables could represent a strongly impacting pre-processing statement, one that might not be necessary in certain other tree algorithms. However, since our goal is to measure the four elements of the financial condition, such an extension of the study would lead to the word limits of a book chapter being exceeded. Therefore we have focused on the implementation of the CHAID method to each of the above four elements, to obtain preliminary results as a starting point for future research on which we are currently working, such as the use of Neural Networks or the Support Vector Machine (SVM).

REFERENCES

Berka, P., & Bruha, I. (1998). *Principles of Data Mining and Knowledge Discover, Nantes, France*. Berlin: Springer.

Berne, R. (1992). *The relationship between financial reporting and the measurement of financial condition.* Government Accounting Standard Board, Research Report, (18), Nolwalk, CT.

Biggs, D., Ville, B., & Suen, E. (1991). A method of choosing multiway partitions for classification and decision trees. *Journal of Applied Statistics, 18*(1), 49–62. doi:10.1080/02664769100000005

Breiman, L., Friedman, J. H., Olshen, R. A., & Stone, C. J. (1984). Classification and regression tree., Monterey, CA: Wadsworth and Brooks-Cole.

Chesney, T., & Penny, K. (2009). Data mining trauma injury data using C5.0 and logistic regression to determine factors associated with death. *International Journal of Healthcare Technology and Management, 10*(1/2), 16–26. doi:10.1504/IJHTM.2009.023725

(1997). *CICA - Canadian Institute of Chartered Accountants*. Toronto, Canada: Indicators of Government Financial Condition.

Clark, T. (1990). *Monitoring Local Governments*. Dubuque, IA: Kendal Hunt Publishing.

Clark, T. (1994). Municipal Fiscal Strain: Indicator and Causes. *Government Finance Review, 10*(3), 27–29.

Copeland, R. E., & Ingram, R. (1983). *Municipal Financial Reporting and Disclosure Quality*. Reading, MA: Addison-Wesley.

Dills, A. K. (2005). Does cream-skimming curdle the milk? A study of peer effects. *Economics of Education Review, 24*, 19–28. doi:10.1016/j.econedurev.2004.01.002

Directorate General for Financial Coordination with Local Authorities, Spanish Ministry of Economy and Finance, *(1992-1999)*.

Dollery, B., Crase, L., & Byrnes, J. (2006, September). Local Government Failure: Why Does Australian Local Government Experience Permanent Financial Austerity? *Australian Journal of Political Science, 41*(3), 339–353. doi:10.1080/10361140600848952

Galguera, L., Luna, D., & Mendez, M. P. (2006). Predictive segmentation in action: using Chaid to segment loyalty card holders. *International Journal of Market Research, 48*(4), 459–479.

GASB. (1987). Concepts Statement N° 1 of Governmental Accounting Standards Board: Objectives of Financial Reporting, Norwalk, CT.

(1994). *GASB*. Norwalk, CT: Service Efforts and Accomplishments Reporting.

Gonzalez, A., Correa, A., & Acosta, M. (2002). Factores determinantes de la rentabilidad financiera de las pymes. *Revista Española de Financiación y Contabilidad, 31*(112), 395–429.

Goodman, L. A. (1979). Simple models for the analysis of association in cross-classifications having ordered categories. *Journal of the American Statistical Association, 74*, 537–552. doi:10.2307/2286971

Greenberg, J., & Hillier, D. (1995). *Indicators of Financial Condition for Governments*. Paper presented at the 5th Conference of Comparative International Governmental Accounting Research, Paris-Amy, France.

Grobler, B. R., Bisschoff, T. C., & Moloi, K. C. (2002). The CHAID-technique and the relationship between school effectiveness and various independent variables. *International Studies in Educational Administration, 30*(3), 44–56.

Groves, M., Godsey, W., & Shulman, M. (2003). *Evaluating Financial Condition: A handbook of Local Government* (3rd ed.). Washington, DC: The International City/County Management Association.

Hunt, E. B., Marin, J., & Stone, P. J. (1966). *Experiments in Induction*. New York: Academic Press.

Kass, G. V. (1980). An exploratory technique for investigating large quantities of categorical data. *Applied Statistics, 29,* 119–127. doi:10.2307/2986296

Kloha, P., Weissert, C. S., & Kleine, R. (2005). Developing and testing a composite model to predict local fiscal distress. *Public Administration Review, 65*(3), 313–323. doi:10.1111/j.1540-6210.2005.00456.x

Magidson, J. (1993). The use of the new ordinal algorithm in CHAID to target profitable segments. *The Journal of Database Marketing, 1,* 29–48.

Margineantu, D., & Dietterich, T. (2001). Improved class probability estimates from decision tree models. In Nonlinear Estimation and Classification, (pp. 169–184).

Quinlan, J. R. (1979). Discovering rules by induction from large collection of examples. In Michie, D. (Ed.), *Expert Systems in the Microelectronic Age* (pp. 168–201). Edinburgh, UK: Edinburgh University Press.

Quinlan, J. R. (1993). *C4.5: Programs for machine learning*. San Mateo, CA: Morgan Kaufmann.

Santín, D. (2006). La medición de la eficiencia de las escuelas: una revisión crítica. *Hacienda Pública Española / Revista de Economía Pública, 177*(2), 57-82.

SPSS. (2006). *AnswerTree algorithm summary*. Retrieved from http://www.spss.com/download, (login required)

Strambi, O. & Karin-Anne, T. (1998). Trip generation modeling using CHAID, a criterion-based segmentation modeling tool. *Journal of the Transportation Research Board,* (1645), 24-31.

Zafra-Gómez, J. L. López-Hernandez, A.L. & Hernández-Bastida, A. (2009) Developing a Model to Measure Financial Condition in Local Government: Evaluating Service Quality and Minimizing the Effects of the Socioeconomic Environment: An Application to Spanish Municipalities. *The American Review of Public Administration*. Retrieved from http://arp.sagepub.com/cgi/rapidpdf/

Zafra-Gómez, J. L., López-Hernández, A. M., & Hernández-Bastida, A. (2009). Evaluating financial performance in local government. Maximising the benchmarking value. *International Review of Administrative Science, 75*(1), 151–167. doi:10.1177/0020852308099510

Zafra-Gómez, J. L., López-Hernandez, A. M., & Hernández-Bastida, A. (2009, May). Developing an alert system for local governments in financial crisis. *Public Money & Management, 29*(3), 175–181.

KEY TERNS AND DEFINITIONS

Data Mining: (also called data or knowledge discovery): The process of analyzing data from different perspectives and summarizing it into useful information by finding correlations or patterns among multiple fields in large relational databases.

CHAID: A decision tree technique used for classification of a dataset. It provides a set of rules for application to a new (unclassified) dataset to predict which records will have a given outcome.

Rule Induction: The extraction of useful if-then rules from data based on statistical significance.

Local Government: An administrative body that may span one or several geographic areas. It may also refer to a city or village.

Financial Condition: The ability of a government body to provide services and to meet its future obligations. This concept can be measured by considering the situation of its net assets, its budget balance or the net cash position.

Flexibility: An entity's capacity to respond to changes in the economy or in its financial circumstances, within the limits of its fiscal abilities. This capacity is reflected in the degree to which it is able to react to such changes, via public debt.

Sustainability: An organization's ability to maintain, promote and protect the social welfare of the population, employing the resources at its disposal.

Independence: An organization's level of dependence on the external funding received via transfers and grants.

Short-Run Solvency: An entity's ability to generate sufficient liquidity to pay its short-term debts.

Long-Run Solvency: A government's ability to respond adequately to meet its long-term obligations.

ENDNOTES

1   Each rule is derived from a particular route defined by the tree, until each terminal node (t) is reached. Therefore, there are as many rules as there are terminal nodes in the tree.

2   F-Test. This test is based on the ratio of the variance between the groups and the variance within each group. If the means are the same for all groups, you would expect the F ratio to be close to 1 since both are estimates of the same population variance. The larger this ratio, the greater the variation between groups and the greater than chance that a significant difference exists (See Ipiña, S. *Inferencia estadística y análisis de datos.* Madrid. Pearson. 2008).

3   The population segmentation, carried out taking into account the different levels of the explanatory variables, produces a global model that is structured as a tree, with a large number of rules or local authority profiles, although for the purposes of the present study only the most important have been selected.

4   It is not necessary to describe the main rules obtained for BR=2 and BR=3, as it is the extreme quartiles, indicative of success and failure profiles, that are the most interesting and useful. For the same reason, these quartiles are also omitted for the other three models examined in this study.

APPENDIX 1 (FIGURE 6, FIGURE 7)

Figure 6. Indicators for analysis of the financial factor in the financial condition (1)

VARIABLE	FORMULATION
Index of implementation of expenditure	Net recognized obligations / Definitive credits
Index of implementation of current expenditure	Current budget net recognized obligations / Current budget definitive credits
Index of implementation of capital expenditure	Capital budget net recognized obligations / Capital budget definitive credits
Index of implementation of receipts	Net extinguished receivables / Final previsions
Index of implementation of current receipts	Current budget net extinguished receivables / Current budget final previsions
Index of implementation of capital receipts	Capital budget net extinguished receivables / Capital budget final previsions
Index of current budget payments	Current budget liquid payments made / Net recognized obligations
Index of current budget receipts	Current budget payments received / Net extinguished receivables
Index of public expenditure per capita	Net recognized obligations / No. of inhabitants
Index of current expenditure per capita	Net recognized obligations Chaps. 1-IV / No. of inhabitants
Index of significance of current expenditure	Net recognized obligations Chaps. 1-IV / Net recognized obligations
Index of significance of current receipts	Current net extinguished receivables / Net extinguished receivables
Index of taxation receipts	Extinguished receivables Chaps. I-III / Current net extinguished receivables
Index of gross savings	Gross savings / Current net extinguished receivables
Index of capital expenditure per capita	Net extinguished receivables Chaps. VI-VII / No. of inhabitants
Index of significance of capital expenditure	Net extinguished receivables Chaps. VI-VII / Net recognized obligations
Index of capital funding	Net extinguished receivables Chaps. VI-VII / Recognized obligations Chaps. VI-VII
Index of net savings	Net savings / Current net extinguished receivables
Index of significance of financial load	Net recognized obligations Chaps. III and IX / Net recognized obligations
Index of financial load per capita	Net recognized obligations Chaps. III and IX / No. of inhabitants
Index of accumulated debt per capita	Debt balance of the corporation per capita
Index of indebtedness over current receipts	Outstanding debts owed at year end / Current receipts
Index of the weight of financial load	Net recognized obligations Chaps. III and IX / Current net recognized obligations
Index of immediate liquidity	Liquid funds / Obligations pending payment
Index of short-term solvency	Liquid funds and obligations pending receipt / Obligations pending payment
Mean receipts lapse	(Obligations pending receipt / Net extinguished obligations) x 365
Mean payment lapse	(Obligations pending payment / Net recognized obligations) x 365
Index of significance of cash surplus	General expenses cash surplus / Obligations pending payment
Index of year-end liquidity	Difference between current budget payments received and paid
Index of current financial independence	Current recognized obligations / Recognized receivables Chaps. I-III and V
Index of total financial independence	Net recognized obligations / Recognized receivables Chaps. I-III, and V, VI, VIII and XI
Index of non financial budget result	Net recognized obligations Chaps. I-VII / Net recognized receivables Chaps. I-VII
Index of fiscal pressure	Net recognized receivables Chaps. I-III per capita
Index of current transfer receipts	Recognized obligations Chaps. I-III / Recognized obligations Chaps. I-IV

Figure 7. Indicators for analysis of the financial factor in the financial condition (2)

VARIABLE	FORMULATION
Index of gross savings	(Net recognized receivables Chaps. I-IV – Net recognized obligations Chaps. I, II and IV) / Net recognized receivables Chaps. I-IV
Index of income results	Current budget receivables pending payment / Total receivables pending payment
Index of expenditure results	Current budget obligations pending payment / Total obligations pending payment
Margin of current self funding	Recognized receivables Chaps. I-IV and IX / Recognized receivables Chaps. I-V
Index of available cash	(Current budget receipts – Current budget payments made) / Net recognized obligations
Index of staff costs	Recognized obligations Chap. I / Current recognized obligations
Index of current transfers effected	Recognized obligations Chap. IV / Current recognized obligations
Index of staff costs per capita	Recognized obligations Chap. I per capita
Index of expenditure on goods and services, per capita	Recognized obligations Chap. II per capita
Index of financial expenditure per capita	Recognized obligations Chap. III per capita
Index of investment per capita	Recognized obligations Chap. VI per capita
Index of coverage of financial load	Margin of current receipts (Income Chaps. I-V – Expenses Chaps. I-IV) / Financial payments (Expenses Chaps. III and IX)
Index of fixed charges	Recognized obligations Chaps. I-III and IX / Recognized receivables Chaps. I-V
Index of coverage of expenditure	Total recognized receivables / Net recognized receivables
Sum of current receipts	Sum of recognized receivables Chaps. I-V
Index of current receipts per capita	Recognized receivables Chaps. I-V / No. of inhabitants

Budget chapters of expenses and receipts

EXPENSE BUDGET	INCOME BUDGET
Chapter I: Staff costs	Chapter I: Direct taxes
Chapter II: Goods and services	Chapter II: Indirect taxes
Chapter III: Financial costs	Chapter III: Fees and public charges
Chapter IV: Current transfers	Chapter IV: Current transfer receipts
Chapter VI: Investment costs	Chapter V: Patrimonial receipts
Chapter VII: Capital transfer costs	Chapter VI: Sales of real investments
Chapter VIII: Financial asset costs	Chapter VII: Current transfer receipts
Chapter IX: Financial liability costs	Chapter VIII: Receipts from financial assets
	Chapter IX: Receipts from financial liabilities

APPENDIX 2 (FIGURE 8)

Figure 8. Gain, Index and Response with the Rules Obtained for BR=4 (number 1); for STS=4 (number 2); for FL=1 (number 3); for TR=4 (number 4)

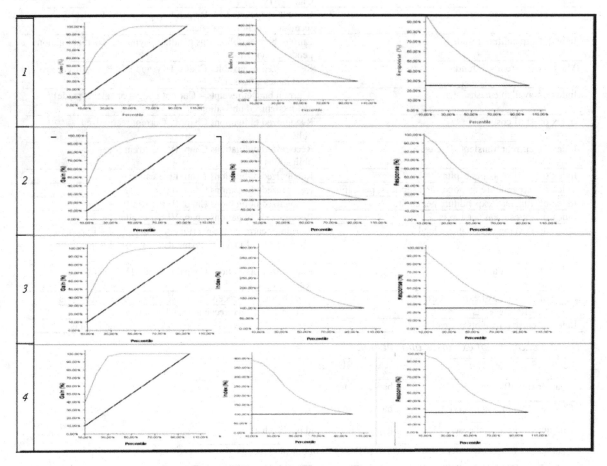

Chapter 3
Data Mining Using Fuzzy Decision Trees:
An Exposition from a Study of Public Services Strategy in the USA

Malcolm J. Beynon
Cardiff University, UK

Martin Kitchener
Cardiff Business School, UK

ABSTRACT

The chapter exposits the strategies employed by the public long-term care systems operated by each U.S. state government. The central technique employed in this investigation is fuzzy decision trees (FDTs), producing a rule-based classification system using the well known soft computing methodology of fuzzy set theory. It is a timely exposition, with the employment of set-theoretic approaches to organizational configurations, including the fuzzy set representation, starting to be discussed. The survey details considered, asked respondents to assign each state system to one of the three 'orientations to innovation' contained within Miles and Snows' (1978) classic typology of organizational strategies. The instigated aggregation of the experts' opinions adheres to the fact that each long-term care system, like all organizations, is "likely to be part prospector, part defender, and part reactor, reflecting the complexity of organizational strategy". The use of FDTs in the considered organization research problem is pertinent since the linguistic based fuzzy decision rules constructed, open up the ability to understand the relationship between a state's attributes and their predicted position in a general strategy domain - the essence of data mining.

INTRODUCTION

With data storage increasing at a phenomenal rate, traditional *ad hoc* mixtures of data mining tools are no longer adequate. In one response, some attention has been given to the potential for soft computing frameworks to provide flexible information processing capability that can exploit the tolerance of imprecision, uncertainty, approximate reasoning, and partial truth in knowledge discovery (Mitra *et al.*, 2002). This chapter extends that line of enquiry

DOI: 10.4018/978-1-60566-906-9.ch003

by providing an early and detailed exposition of the data mining potential of a soft computing methodology that is based on fuzzy set theory, henceforth FST (Zadeh, 1965).

Since its introduction in 1965, FST is closely associated with uncertain reasoning and is the earliest and most widely reported constituent of soft computing (Mitra *et al.*, 2002). Of particular interest in this exposition of data concerning public policy and strategy, FST incorporates opportunities to develop techniques that incorporate vagueness and ambiguity in their operation, and it allows outputs to be presented in a highly readable and easily interpretable manner (Zhou and Gan, 2008). While data mining encompasses the typical tasks of; classification, clustering, association and outlier detection, here its role in rule-based classification is considered.

Previous FST-based research in organizational and policy contexts is limited but includes: explaining constitutional control of the executive of parliamentary democracies in US states (Pennings, 2003), and the evaluation of knowledge management capability of organizations (Fan *et al.*, 2009). Ragin and Pennings (2005) give a discussion of FST in social research, in their introduction to a special issue of the journal *Sociological Methods & Research*. This acknowledges the need to continually validate this new methodology (FST), through its continued application. A pertinent study by Fiss (2007), considered the whole issue of the employment of a set-theoretic approach to organizational configurations, including the progression from a crisp to fuzzy set representation, and the latter's potential for undertaking appropriate analysis.

The context of the exposition presented in this chapter is a study of the strategies employed by the public long-term care systems operated by each U.S. state government. The main dataset was collected from a survey of experts in this area (including academics, government officials, and service providers). The survey asked respondents to assign each state system to one of the three 'orientations to innovation' contained within

Miles and Snows' (1978) classic typology of organizational strategies: prospectors, defenders, and reactors. Briefly, these strategic groups describe different orientations to strategy from the more consistently innovative prospectors, to reactors that typically innovate only after coercion. The instigated aggregation of the experts' opinions adheres to the fact that each long-term care system, like all organizations, is "likely to be part prospector, part defender, and part reactor, reflecting the complexity of organizational strategy" (Andrews *et al.*, 2006).

In this chapter, the aggregated expert assignments are assessed using a fuzzy decision tree (FDT) analysis of state long-term care system characteristics. The pertinence of this analysis is that, with the federal system existing in each U.S. state, the decision rules constructed are in respect of the state's governing organization's management attitudes to healthcare. FDT is a data mining technique which benefits from the general methodology FST (Yuan and Shaw, 1995; Mitra *et al.*, 2002). The overriding remit of, decision trees, within crisp and fuzzy environments, is with the classification of objects described by a data set in the form of a number of condition and decision attributes.

A decision tree, in general, starts with an identified root node, and paths are constructed down to leaf nodes, where the attributes associated with the intermediate nodes are identified through a measure to preferentially gauge the classification certainty of certain objects down that path. Each path down to a leaf node forms an '*if.. then..*' decision rule, used to classify those objects whose condition attribute values satisfy the condition part of that rule. Beyond FDT, other rule based classification methods include, amongst others, RIPPER (Cohen, 1995; Thabtah *et al.*, 2006) and rough set theory (Beynon *et al.*, 2000).

The development of decision trees in a fuzzy environment furthered the readability of the now constructed '*if.. then..*' fuzzy decision rules (Zhou and Gan, 2008). The potential appropriateness of

FDTs in organization research can be gauged from the recent statement by Li *et al.* (2006, p. 655);

"Decision trees based on fuzzy set theory combines the advantages of good comprehensibility of decision trees and the ability of fuzzy representation to deal with inexact and uncertain information."

Their findings also highlight that FDTs may not need extensive data to operate or intensive computing powers, pertinent to the analysis undertaken in this chapter.

The specific FDT technique employed here was presented in Yuan and Shaw (1995) and Wang *et al.* (2000). It attempts to include the cognitive uncertainties evident in the data values (condition and decision attribute values), in the creation of concomitant sets of fuzzy '*if.. then..*' decision rules, whose condition and decision parts, using concomitant attributes, can be described in linguistics terms (such as low, medium or high). This FDT technique has been used in Beynon *et al.* (2004a) to investigate the audit fee levels of companies, and Beynon *et al.* (2004b) to investigate the songflight of the Sedge Warbler.

The use of FDTs in the considered organization research problem is pertinent since the linguistic based fuzzy decision rules constructed open up the ability to understand the relationship between a state's attributes and their predicted position in a general strategy domain - the essence of data mining. In general, linguistic variables are often used to denote words or sentences of a natural language (Zadeh, 1975a, 1975b, 1975c). Its utilisation is appropriate for data mining where information may be qualitative, or quantitative information may not be stated precisely (Wang and Chuu, 2004; Fan *et al.*, 2009), often the case in organizational and policy research.

The contribution of this book chapter is the clear understanding of the advantages of the utilization of FDTs in data mining in organizational and policy research, including; the formulation of attribute membership functions (MFs), fuzzy

decision tree construction, and inference of produced fuzzy decision rules. A small hypothetical example will also be included to enable the reader to comprehend the included analytical rudiments of the technique employed, and the larger previously described application demonstrates the potential interpretability allowed through the use of this data mining approach.

BACKGROUND

The background of this chapter covers; the rudiments of fuzzy set theory, the fuzzy decision tree (FDT) approach considered, and a tutorial presentation on the application of FDTs on a small example data set.

Fuzzy Set Theory

In fuzzy set theory (Zadeh, 1965), a grade of membership exists to characterise the association of a value x to a set S. The concomitant membership function (MF), defined $\mu_S(x)$, has range [0, 1]. The domain of a numerical attribute can be described by a finite series of MFs that each offers a grade of membership to describe a value x, which form its concomitant fuzzy number (Kecman, 2001).

Further, the finite set of MFs defining a numerical attribute's domain can be denoted a linguistic variable (Herrera *et al.*, 2000). Zadeh (1975a-c) offer an early insight on the concept of a linguistic variable, where each MF, within a set of MFs, denotes a linguistic term. Different types of MFs have been proposed to describe fuzzy numbers, including triangular and trapezoidal functions. Yu and Li (2001) highlight that MFs may be, advantageously, constructed from mixed shapes, supporting the use of piecewise linear MFs (see also Dombi and Gera, 2005). The functional form of a piecewise linear MF, (in the context of the jth linguistic term T_j^k of a linguistic variable A_k), is given through a visual representation in Figure 1, which elucidates their general structure.

The general form of a MF presented in Figure 1 shows how the value of a MF is constrained within 0 and 1. In Figure 1, a piecewise triangular MF is shown, based on five *defining values* $[\alpha_{j,1}, \alpha_{j,2}, \alpha_{j,3}, \alpha_{j,4}, \alpha_{j,5}]$. The implication of these specific defining values is also illustrated, including the idea of associated support, $[\alpha_{j,1}, \alpha_{j,5}]$ in Figure 1. Further, the notion of dominant support can also be considered, where a MF is most closely associated with an attribute value, the domain $[\alpha_{j,2}, \alpha_{j,4}]$ in Figure 1.

These definitions of support and dominant support, along with the defining values, are closely associated with the commonly used concept of the α-cut, in particular the defining values are when α equals 0, 0.5 and 1 (Kovalerchuk and Vityaev, 2000). Moreover, the issue becomes the assignment of values to the defining values, to enable the creation of the MFs required to describe a numerical attribute. As Fiss (2007) suggests, talking about FST in an organization research context, FST is a superior way (over crisp set theory) of offering substantive knowledge on a numerical attribute, with meaningful values required for the defining values.

Beyond this technical exposition of the rudiments of FST, and general positive elucidation of this methodology presented in the introduction, Ragin and Pennings (2005, p. 425) present four claims on the applicability of FST to social research:

1. FST permits a more nuanced representation of categorical concepts by permitting degrees of membership in sets rather than binary in-or-out membership.
2. FST can be used to address both diversity and ambiguity in a systematic manner, through set calibration and set-theoretic relations.
3. More verbal theory in the social sciences is formulated explicitly in set-theoretic

terms. The FST approach provides a faithful translation of such theory.
4. FST enables researchers to evaluate set-theoretic relationships such as intersection and inclusion and, thereby, necessity and sufficiency. Set theoretic relationships are very difficult to evaluate using conventional approaches such as the general linear model.

Aspects of these claims will become apparent in the technical description of the FDT technique employed (next given), and in its employment in a small example, and larger state strategy problem later given.

Fuzzy Decision Trees

Following the realization of the decision tree approach to data mining in the 1960s (Hunt *et al.*, 1966), the introduction of fuzzy decision trees (FDTs) was first loosely referenced in the late 1970s (Chang and Pavlidis, 1977), with early formulizations of FDTs including; derivatives of the well known ID3 approach (Quinlan, 1979) utilizing fuzzy entropy (Ichihashi *et al.*, 1996), and other versions of crisp FDT techniques (see Pal and Chakraborty, 2001; Olaru and Wehenkel, 2003).

This section outlines the technical details of the FDT approach introduced in Yuan and Shaw (1995). With an inductive fuzzy decision tree, the underlying knowledge related to a decision outcome can be represented as a set of fuzzy '*if.. then..*' decision rules, each of the form;

If $(A_1$ is $T_{i_1}^1)$ and $(A_2$ is $T_{i_2}^2)$ ... and $(A_k$ is $T_{i_k}^k)$

then D is D_j,

where $A_1, A_2, .., A_k$ and D are linguistic variables for the multiple antecedents (A_i's) and consequent (D) statements used to describe the considered objects, and $T(A_k) = \{T_1^k, T_2^k, ... T_{S_i}^k\}$ and $\{D_1, D_2,$

Figure 1. General definition of piecewise linear MF (including the required defining values [$\alpha_{j,1}$, $\alpha_{j,2}$, $\alpha_{j,3}$, $\alpha_{j,4}$, $\alpha_{j,5}$])

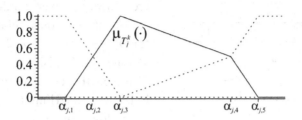

..., D_L} are their respective linguistic terms. Each linguistic term T_j^k is defined by the MF $\mu_{T_j^k}(x)$,

which transforms a value in its associated domain to a grade of membership value to between 0 and 1. The MFs, $\mu_{T_j^k}(x)$ and $\mu_{D_j}(y)$, represent the grade of membership of an object's antecedent A_j being T_j^k and consequent D being D_j, respectively.

A MF $\mu(x)$ from the set describing a fuzzy linguistic variable Y defined on X, can be viewed as a possibility distribution of Y on X, that is $\pi(x) = \mu(x)$, for all $x \in X$ the values taken by the objects in U (also normalized so $\max_{x \in X} \pi(x) = 1$). The possibility measure $E_\alpha(Y)$ of ambiguity is defined by $E_\alpha(Y) = g(\pi) = \sum_{i=1}^{n} (\pi_i^* - \pi_{i+1}^*) \ln[i]$, where $\pi^* = \{\pi_1^*, \pi_2^*, ..., \pi_n^*\}$ is the permutation of the normalized possibility distribution $\pi = \{\pi(x_1), \pi(x_2), ..., \pi(x_n)\}$, sorted so that $\pi_i^* \geq \pi_{i+1}^*$ for $i = 1, ..., n$, and $\pi_{n+1}^* = 0$. In the limit, if $\pi_2^* = 0$, then $E_\alpha(Y) = 0$, indicates no ambiguity, whereas if $\pi_n^* = 1$, then $E_\alpha(Y) = \ln[n]$, which indicates all values are fully possible for Y, representing the greatest ambiguity.

The ambiguity of attribute A (over the objects $u_1, ..., u_m$) is given as: $E_\alpha(A) = \frac{1}{m} \sum_{i=1}^{m} E_\alpha(A(u_i))$,

where $E_\alpha(A(u_i)) = g(\mu_{T_s}(u_i) / \max_{1 \leq j \leq s}(\mu_{T_j}(u_i)))$, with $T_1, ..., T_s$ the linguistic terms of an attribute (antecedent) with m objects. When there is overlapping between linguistic terms (MFs) of an attribute or between consequents, then ambiguity exists.

For all $u \in U$, the intersection $A \cap B$ of two fuzzy sets is given by $\mu_{A \cap B} = \min[\mu_A(u), \mu_B(u)]$. The fuzzy subsethood $S(A, B)$ measures the degree to which A is a subset of B, and is given by, $S(A, B) = \sum_{u \in U} \min(\mu_A(u), \mu_B(u)) / \sum_{u \in U} \mu_A(u)$. Given fuzzy evidence E, the possibility of classifying an object to the consequent D_i can be defined as, $\pi(D_i | E) = S(E, D_i) / \max_j S(E, D_j)$, where the fuzzy subsethood $S(E, D_i)$ represents the degree of truth for the classification rule ('if E then D_i'). With a single piece of evidence (a fuzzy number for an attribute), then the classification ambiguity based on this fuzzy evidence is defined as: $G(E) = g(\pi(D | E))$, which is measured using the possibility distribution $\pi(D | E) = (\pi(D_1 | E), ..., \pi(D_L | E))$.

The classification ambiguity with fuzzy partitioning $P = \{E_1, ..., E_k\}$ on the fuzzy evidence F, denoted as $G(P | F)$, is the weighted average of classification ambiguity with each subset of partition: $G(P | F) = \sum_{i=1}^{k} w(E_i | F) G(E_i \cap F)$, where $G(E_i \cap F)$ is the classification ambiguity with fuzzy evidence $E_i \cap F$, and where $w(E_i | F)$ is the

Table 1. Example small data set

Object	T1	T2	T3	D
u_1	31	38	15	12
u_2	32	15	26	14
u_3	40	52	20	16
u_4	24	22	30	20
u_5	29	35	12	38

weight which represents the relative size of subset $E_i \cap F$ in F: $w(E_i | F) =$

$$\sum_{u \in U} \min(\mu_{E_i}(u), \mu_F(u)) \Big/ \sum_{j=1}^{k} \left(\sum_{u \in U} \min(\mu_{E_j}(u), \mu_F(u)) \right)$$

In summary, attributes are assigned to nodes based on the lowest level of classification ambiguity. A node becomes a leaf node if the level of subsethood is higher than some truth value β assigned to the whole of the FDT. The classification from the leaf node is to the decision group with the largest subsethood value. The truth level threshold β controls the growth of the tree; lower β may lead to a smaller tree (with lower classification accuracy), higher β may lead to a larger tree (with higher classification accuracy).

Fuzzy Decision Tree Analyses of Example Data Set

In this section a FDT analysis is described on a small example data set, consisting of five objects described by three conditions (T1, T2 and T3) and one decision (D) attribute, see Table 1.

Using the data set presented in Table 1, the example FDT analysis next exposited, starts with the fuzzification of the individual attribute values. Throughout this analysis, and pertinent to the later applied FDT analysis, the level of fuzzification employed here is with three MFs (linguistic terms) designated to represent the linguistic variables for each of the attributes, condition (T1, T2 and T3) and decision (D), see Figure 2 for the case of the decision attribute D.

In Figure 2, three MFs, $\mu_L(D)$ (labelled D_L - Low), $\mu_M(D)$ (D_M - Medium) and $\mu_H(D)$ (D_H - High), are shown to cover the domain of the decision attribute D, the concomitant defining values are, for D_L: $[-\infty, -\infty, 14, 18, 22]$, D_M: $[14, 18, 22, 30, 40]$ and D_H: $[22, 30, 40, \infty, \infty]$. An interpretation of these MFs, as mentioned, could then simply be the associated linguistic terms of the three MFs being, low (L), medium (M) and high (H).

For the three condition attributes, T1, T2 and T3, their fuzzification is similarly based on the creation of linguistic variables, each described by three linguistic terms (three MFs), see Figure 3.

The sets of MFs described in Figure 3 are each found from a series of defining values, in this case for; T1 - $[[-\infty, -\infty, 18, 26, 28], [18, 26, 28, 38, 40], [28, 38, 40, \infty, \infty]]$, T2 - $[[-\infty, -\infty, 26, 34, 40], [26, 34, 40, 52, 54], [40, 52, 54, \infty, \infty]]$ and T3 - $[[-\infty, -\infty, 12, 14, 18], [12, 14, 18, 23, 24], [18, 23, 24, \infty, \infty]]$.

Applying these MFs, in Figures 2 and 3, on the example data set in Table 1, achieves a fuzzy data set version, see Table 2.

In Table 2, each condition attribute, T1, T2 and T3, is described by three values associated with the three linguistic terms (L, M and H). Also shown, in bold, is the largest of the fuzzy values from each triplet of MFs (associated with a single fuzzy variable), indicating the most dominant linguistic term each condition value is associated with (for the individual objects). The same is presented for the decision attribute D.

The fuzzy data set represented in Table 2 is suitable for its FDT-based analysis. For the construction of a FDT (using the FDT technique described earlier), the classification ambiguity of each condition attribute with respect to the decision attribute is first considered, namely the evaluation of the $G(E)$ values. Before this was undertaken, a threshold value of $\beta = 0.800$ was used throughout this construction process, associated with the required level of subsethood required for a node to designate a leaf node (see later).

Figure 2. Fuzzification of decision attribute D using three MFs (labeled D_L - Low, D_M - Medium and D_H - High)

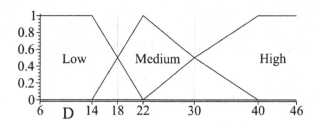

Figure 3. Fuzzification of condition attributes, T1, T2 and T3, using three MFs in each case

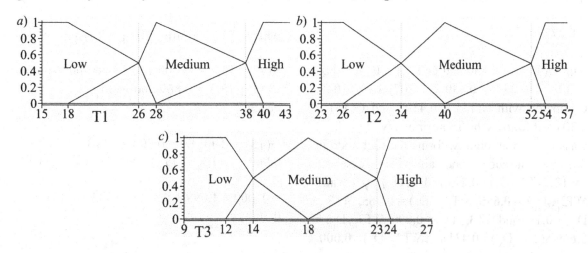

Table 2. Fuzzy data set using three MFs for each condition and decision attribute

Object	T1 = [$T1_L$, $T1_M$, $T1_H$]	T2 = [$T2_L$, $T2_M$, $T2_H$]	T3 = [$T3_L$, $T3_M$, $T3_H$]	D = [D_L, D_M, D_H]
u_1	[0.000, **0.850**, 0.150]	[0.167, **0.833**, 0.000]	[0.375, **0.625**, 0.000]	[**1.000**, 0.000, 0.000]
u_2	[0.000, **0.800**, 0.200]	[**1.000**, 0.000, 0.000]	[0.000, 0.000, **1.000**]	[**1.000**, 0.000, 0.000]
u_3	[0.000, 0.000, **1.000**]	[0.000, **0.500**, 0.500]	[0.000, **0.800**, 0.200]	[**0.750**, 0.250, 0.000]
u_4	[**0.625**, 0.375, 0.000]	[**1.000**, 0.000, 0.000]	[0.000, 0.000, **1.000**]	[0.250, **0.750**, 0.000]
u_5	[0.000, **0.950**, 0.050]	[0.417, **0.583**, 0.000]	[**1.000**, 0.000, 0.000]	[0.000, 0.100, **0.900**]

The evaluation of a $G(E)$ value is shown for the attribute T1 ($= g(\pi(D| T1))$), where it is broken down to the fuzzy labels L, M and H, so for L; $\pi(D| T1_L) = S(T1_L, D_i) / \max_j S(T1_L, D_j)$, considering D_L, D_M and D_H with the information in Table 1:

$$S(T1_L, D_L) =$$

$$\sum_{u \in U} \min(\mu_{T1_L}(u), \mu_{D_L}(u)) \Big/ \sum_{u \in U} \mu_{T1_L}(u)$$

$= (\min(0.000, 1.000) + \min(0.000, 1.000) + \min(0.000, 0.750)$
$+ \min(0.625, 0.250) + \min(0.000, 0.250)) / (0.000 + 0.000 + 0.000 + 0.625 + 0.000)$

$=$

$$(0.000 + 0.000 + 0.000 + 0.250 + 0.00)\Big/0.625$$

$= 0.250 \big/ 0.625 = 0.400,$

whereas $S(T1_L, D_M) = 1.000$ and $S(T1_L, D_H) = 0.000$. Hence $\pi = \{1.000, 0.400, 0.000\}$, giving $\pi^* = \{1.000, 0.400, 0.000\}$, with $\pi_4^* = 0$, then:

$$G(T1_L) = g(\pi(D \mid T1_L)) = \sum_{i=1}^{2} (\pi_i^* - \pi_{i+1}^*) \ln[i]$$

$$=$$

$$(1.000 - 0.400)\ln[1] + (0.400 - 0.000)\ln[2] + (0.000 - 0.000)\ln[3]$$

$$= 0.277,$$

with $G(T1_M) = 0.430$ and $G(T1_H) = 0.207$, then $G(T1) = (0.277 + 0.430 + 0.207)/3 = 0.3048$. Compared with $G(T2) = 0.4305$ and $G(T3) = 0.3047$, it follows the T3 attribute, with the least classification ambiguity, forms the root node in this case. The subsethood values in this case are; for T3: $S(T3_L, D_L) = 0.273$, $S(T3_L, D_M) = 0.073$ and $S(T3_L, D_H) = \mathbf{0.655}$; $S(T3_M, D_L) = \mathbf{0.965}$, $S(T3_M, D_M) = 0.175$ and $S(T3_M, D_H) = 0.000$; $S(T3_H, D_L) = \mathbf{0.659}$, $S(T3_H, D_M) = 0.431$ and $S(T3_H, D_H) = 0.000$.

In each case the linguistic term with largest subsethood value (shown in bold), indicates the possible augmentation of the path. For $T3_L$, its largest subsethood value is 0.655 ($S(T3_L, D_H)$), below the desired truth value of 0.800 hence requires further consideration of its augmentation. For $T3_M$, its largest subsethood value is 0.965 ($S(T3_M, D_L)$), above the desired truth value of 0.800, and so is a leaf node, with classification to D_L. For $T3_H$, its largest subsethood value is 0.659 ($S(T3_H, D_L)$), hence is also not able to be a leaf node and further possible augmentation needs to be considered.

With only three condition attributes considered, the possible augmentations of $T3_L$ and $T3_H$ are with either T1 or T2. In the case of $T3_L$, where with $G(T3_L) = 0.334$, the ambiguity with partition evaluated for T1 ($G(T3_L$ and $T1 \mid D)$) or T3 ($G(T3_L$ and $T2 \mid D)$) has to be less than this value. In the case of T1:

$$G(T3_L \text{ and } T1 \mid D) = \sum_{i=1}^{k} w(T1_i \mid T3_L) G(T3_L \cap T1_i)$$

Starting with the weight values, in the case of $T3_L$ and $T1_L$, it follows:

$$w(T1_L \mid T3_L) =$$
$$\sum_{u \in U} \min(\mu_{T1_L}(u), \mu_{T3_L}(u)) \Big/ \sum_{j=1}^{k} \left(\sum_{u \in U} \min(\mu_{T1_j}(u), \mu_{T3_L}(u)) \right)$$

$$= (\min(0.000, 0.375) + \min(0.000, 0.000) + \min(0.000, 0.000)$$
$$+ \min(0.625, 0.000) + \min(0.000, 1.000)) \Big/ \sum_{j=1}^{k} \left(\sum_{u \in U} \min(\mu_{T1_j}(u), \mu_{T3_H}(u)) \right)$$

where $\sum_{j=1}^{k} \left(\sum_{u \in U} \min(\mu_{T1_j}(u), \mu_{T3_L}(u)) \right) = 1.525$, so $w(T1_L \mid T3_L) = 0.000/1.525 = 0.000$. Similarly $w(T1_M \mid T3_L) = 0.869$ and $w(T1_H \mid T3_L) = 0.131$, hence:

$$G(T3_L \text{ and } T1 \mid D) = 0.000 \times G(T3_H \cap T1_L) +$$
$$0.869 \times G(T3_H \cap T1_M) + 0.131 \times G(T3_H \cap T1_H)$$

$$= 0.000 \times 1.099 + 0.869 \times 0.334 + 0.131 \times 0.366$$

$$= 0.338,$$

similarly, $G(T3_L$ and $T2 \mid D) = 0.462$. With $G(T3_L$ and $T1 \mid D) = 0.338$, the lowest of these two values, but not lower than the concomitant $G(T3_L) = 0.334$ value, there is no lessening of ambiguity with the augmentation of either T1 and T2 to the path $T3_L$.

In the case $T3_H$, there is $G(T3_H) = 0.454$, and $G(T3_H$ and $T1 \mid D) = 0.274$ and $G(T3_H$ and $T2 \mid D) = 0.462$, with the lowest of these the $G(T3_H$ and $T1 \mid D) = 0.274$ less than $G(T3_H) = 0.454$, so less ambiguity would be found if the T1 attribute was augmented to the T3 = H path. The subsequent subsethood values in this case for each new path are; $T1_L$; $S(T3_H \cap T1_L, D_L) = 0.400$, $S(T3_H \cap T1_L, D_M) = \mathbf{1.000}$ and $S(T3_H \cap T1_L, D_H) = 0.000$; $T1_M$; $S(T3_H \cap T1_M, D_L) = \mathbf{0.894}$, $S(T3_H \cap T1_M, D_M) = 0.319$ and $S(T3_H \cap T1_M, D_H) = 0.000$; $T1_H$: $S(T3_H \cap T1_H, D_L) = \mathbf{1.000}$, $T1_M$: $S(T3_H \cap T1_H, DF_M) = 0.500$ and $S(T3_H \cap T1_H, D_H) = 0.000$.

Figure 4. FDT for example data set with three MFs describing each condition attribute

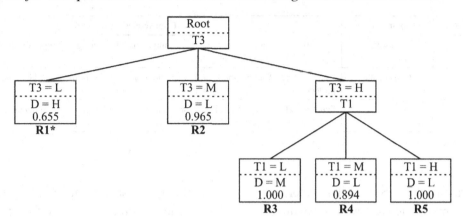

These subsethood results show all three paths end in leaf nodes (largest subsethood value above 0.800 in each case - shown in bold), hence there is no further FDT construction required. The resultant FDT in this case is presented in Figure 4.

The tree structure in Figure 4 clearly demonstrates the visual form of the results described previously. Only shown in each node box is the truth level associated with the highest subsethood value to a decision attribute linguistic term. There are two levels of the tree showing the use of only two of the three considered condition attributes, T1 and T3. There are five leaf nodes which each have a defined fuzzy decision rule associated with them.

One of the rules, **R1***, is indicated with a *, since the largest truth value associated with this rule is less than the 0.8 truth threshold value imposed. In the case of this path of the FDT, there was no further ability to augment it with other nodes (condition attributes), to improve the subsequent classification ambiguity. By their very nature, the fuzzy decision rules are readable (interpretable), for example, the rule **R4** can be written as:

R4: "If T3 = H and T1 = M then D = L (0.894)".

In a more readable (interpretable) form this rule can be further written as:

R4: "If T3 is high and T1 is medium then D is low with truth level 0.894".

Inspection of the objects in Table 2, in terms of their fuzzy values, shows the object u_2 satisfies the condition part of the rule **R4**, and with its known dominant association to D = L, this rule correctly classifies this object.

FUZZY DECISION TREE ANALYSIS OF PUBLIC SERVICES IN THE USA

The starting point for the analysis presented in this chapter is that while it is known that variation exists among the strategies adopted by US states' long term care (LTC) systems, little analysis has been conducted to extend knowledge of this phenomenon. The conception of strategy employed here follows Miles and Snow's (1978) formulation of strategic stance as resting on organizational orientation towards innovation that is considered unlikely to change substantially in the short term (Zajac and Shortell, 1989). The first task of this study is to conceptualize what strategy 'means' in the context of state LTC systems. We begin by introducing the distinctive context of this study and then argue the relevance of Miles and Snow's classic conception of strategic groups.

Table 3. State Medicaid LTC Systems' Strategic Stances

Strategic Stance	Response Type	Characteristics
Prospector	Innovate	Proactive research & experimentation, innovative budgeting, attempts to colonize 'policy space' & budgets of other agencies
Defender	Consolidate	Little research & experimentation, later adoption of innovations, defend existing budget and protect existing service/policy portfolio.
Reactor	Wait	Seldom makes adjustment of any sort until forced to do so by environmental pressures e.g., consumer advocacy, regulation or litigation

Source: Developed from Boyne and Walker (2004, p. 244)

In contrast to the U.S. hospital sector, state LTC administrations deliver few services directly but are the primary strategic bodies with responsibility for spending Medicaid budgets devolved from the federal government (Crisp *et al.*, 2003). State LTC administrations are, therefore, among the most public organizations in the U.S. because they are owned by state governments, funded by government, and subject to high degrees of political influence (Bozeman, 1987). This set of contextual features might suggest limited strategic 'space' for state LTC administrations. However, considerable strategic choice is demonstrated by studies of inter-state variations in state LTC systems which highlight significant differences in policies such as provider regulation and cost control.

From the early 1980s, after decades of consumer advocacy for more Medicaid resources to be spent on home and community-based services (HCBS e.g., home healthcare) as an alternative to institutional care provided in nursing homes, some states began to introduce innovative 'rebalancing' policies such as moratoria on the building of new nursing homes and the development of new HCBS programs such as personal care. Considerable inter-state variation persists in rebalancing efforts such that in 2004, Oregon spent 70 percent of its Medicaid LTC budget on home care services while Mississippi spent only 5 percent (Kitchener *et al.*, 2004).

This brief outline of the field of Medicaid LTC systems demonstrates that analysts recognize

variation among states strategies. This 'ground-up' conception of strategy resonates well with Miles and Snow's (1978) formulation of strategic stance as resting on organizational orientation towards innovation which is considered unlikely to change substantially in the short term (Zajac and Shortell, 1989; Mouritzen, 1992). This contention is supported by early public service applications of Miles and Snow's work (Nutt and Backoff, 1995; Walker and Ruekert, 1987), and much general management research.

To operate their innovation-based conception of strategy, Miles and Snow (1978) introduce a typology of strategic stances that include: (1) prospectors that innovate early and consistently, (2) defenders that tend more towards stability, and (3) reactors that innovate little and typically only when coerced to do so (see Table 3). Here, we omit Miles and Snow's original 'analyzer' group on the basis of previous assessments that it represents an intermediate category (Zahra and Pearce, 1990; Boyne and Walker, 2004). While we argue that the resulting (reduced) framing of the extent to which a state LTC system is an innovative prospector, consolidating defender, or passive reactor maintains the taxonomic criterion of conceptual exhaustiveness, this is essentially a matter for empirical testing.

Previous applications of Miles and Snow's strategy framework in public service settings have typically used one of three approaches to assign organizations to strategic stances based on assessments of issues such as 'whether strategy anticipates events or reacts to them' and 'orientation towards change/status quo' (Wechlser and Backoff, 1986). The first involves experts assigning all organizations in the field to strategic stances based on perception and experience. The second approach involves the assigning of units to stances based on a variety of statistical techniques that compare units' characteristics taken from archival sources (Shortell and Zajac, 1990). A third approach involves asking organizational participants (typically senior managers) to assess the strategic stance of their own organization. While more simple approaches result in the assignment of organizations to a single strategic stance this misses the fact that, in reality, "they are likely to be part prospector, part defender, and part reactor, reflecting the complexity of organizational strategy" (Andrews *et al*., 2006).

Each of the three approaches to strategy measurement outlined above rests on the basic assumption that when compared with other organizations of its type, prospectors would be more proactive in terms including: innovations in budget use and service mix (Bourgeois, 1980); being 'first movers' to new circumstances (perhaps indicated by innovation awards); and attempting to invade the policy and/or budget 'space' of other agencies (Downs, 1967). Defenders, whether in the absence of strategy or by conscious, would tend to maintain existing budget distributions and services, wait until innovations had been evaluated, and protect their own boundaries rather than seeking to colonize other agencies. Reactors would typically: alter existing distribution and services patterns only under duress, adopt innovations last, and be inward looking.

Our perceptual measure of state LTC strategic stance was derived from an email survey of a purposive sample of experts with nation-wide knowledge of the field of state LTC systems. In June 2007, participants were asked to assign each state to one of the strategy groups using a basic instrument that provided a brief description of the three stances, listed the states, and asked respon-

dents to assign each state to a stance category. We began by assuming that the perceptual ratings were ordinal and that disagreement among raters by one category was less serious than across two categories (e.g., that disagreement is greater if two respondents rated a state Prospector and Reactor, rather than if they if rated a state as Prospector and Defender). A final group of 13 raters was established using two criteria: (1) respondents who rated all states, and (2) those with an average agreement rate of 0.5.

Using the judgements made by the 13 experts, sets of association values can be evaluated for each state towards the three strategic stances. These association values are evaluated by the number of experts that categorised a state to each of the stances, Prospector, Defender or Reactor, divided by the number of experts who made a judgement on that state. For example, when considering the 13 experts, for the state KY (Kentucky), the respective breakdown of their judgements is, 0 to Prospector, 2 to Defender and 11 to Reactor, giving the respective association values of 0.000, 0.154 and 0.846. Using these sets of association value for each state, a visual elucidation of the strategic stances of all the 51 states is given in Figure 5, for when the opinions of 13 experts were expressed.

In Figure 5, the levels of association to the strategic stances, Prospector, Defender and Reactor, of a state are represented as a simplex coordinate (circle) in a simplex plot (equilateral triangle). The vertices (corners) of the presented simplex plot denote where there is total association to a single strategic stance. The dashed lines presented inside the simplex plot partition its domain to where there is largest association to one of the strategies (indicated by the nearest vertex label), as well as the ordered association. Also present in Figure 5 are shaded regions which show the area where there will be at least 50% association to one stance (majority association to one stance over the other stances).

The results in Figure 5 show the majority of the states have strategic stances which are part

Figure 5. Association details of strategic stances of US states, using 13 experts' opinions

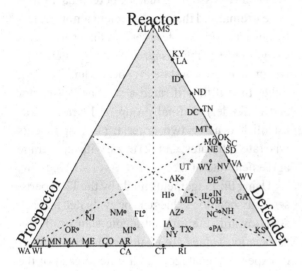

beds), state politics (senate voting records), and state government munificence (state finances).

To enable an FDT analysis of this data, the fuzzification of the eight characteristics is necessary. Within an applied problem, it is important to undertake an understandable mechanism for their fuzzification (Fiss, 2007).

The impact of the level of fuzzification of the characteristics directly impacts on the potential size of the developed FDT, where low level of fuzzification (low numbers of linguistic terms (MFs) associated with each state characteristics) may induce larger FDT, than if a higher level of fuzzification is given (high numbers of linguistic terms (MFs) associated with each characteristic). Mitra *et al.* (2002) directly considers this point, highlighting that a smaller/compact tree is; more efficient both in terms of storage and time requirements, tends to generalize better to unknown test cases, and leads to the generation of more comprehensible linguistic rules.

Here, the fuzzification of the characteristics is next described, with the defining values $[\alpha_{j,1}, \alpha_{j,2}, \alpha_{j,3}, \alpha_{j,4}, \alpha_{j,5}]$ necessary to be found for each characteristic. For a characteristic, the list of attribute values was first discretized into three groups, using equal frequency discretization (whereby each groups is made up of the same number of states (objects)). The result of this discretization is the evaluation of the defining values, $\alpha_{j,2}$ and $\alpha_{j,4}$ (cut points found from the discretization). The other three defining values, $\alpha_{j,1}, \alpha_{j,3}$ and $\alpha_{j,5}$, they are the mean values from the attributes values in each of the groups previously identified.

Based on this fuzzification process, the MFs associated with the linguistic terms for a linguistic variable form of the numerical characteristics can be constructed, see Figure 6.

In Figure 6, the sets of defining values are shown which describe the MFs defining the concomitant linguistic terms, here termed, Low, Medium and High (forming linguistic variable) for each of the eight characteristics. The explicit interpretation of these terms needs to be taken in

Prospector, Defender and Reactor. Interestingly, there is a dearth of states' with mostly Prospector and Reactor stance associations; instead there is a predominance of associations including the Defender stance. Indeed, this predominance of the Defender stance is shown by the breakdown of the states to their most dominant (largest) stance association; with 13 expert opinions; 14 Prospector, 28 Defector and 9 Reactor. In the case of '50% plus majority' association (states in shaded regions), the breakdown is; 13 Prospector, 25 Defector and 9 Reactor (four states not in shaded regions).

In this study, eight state LTC characteristics were considered (see Table 4). The first two measures (innovative programmes and innovate policies) were created specifically for this analysis. Both measures assign a score to each state based on the number of innovative HCBS initiatives (programs and policies respectively) operated by the state LTC system. The other six characteristics are those most commonly used in previous studies of variation in the performance of LTC systems and including measures of need (aged population and disability rate), service supply (nursing home

Table 4. State characteristics, measures, and sources

Label	Characteristics	Measure
C1	Innovative LTC Programs	Combined score from 1 point each for: Money Follows the Person, Cash & Counselling, Better jobs Better Care, National Governors Association Research grants, Demonstration projects, Medicaid state Plan personal care optional program, Medicaid Alzhiemers programs, state-only funded programs, Medicaid waivers
C2	Innovative LTC Policies	Combined score from 1 point each for: generous eligibility on Medicaid HCBS waiver programs; lower than average waiting list on waiver program; existence of formal Olmstead Plan; CON/moratorium on nursing home expansion; nursing home complaints; % long-term care; operating Medically needy eligibility policy; value of real choice systems change grants). Score 0-9
C3	Liberal state politics	Americans for Democratic Action, index of state senators' liberal voting records
C4	State Government Wealth	State government (revenue – expenditure) + Debt
C5	State's Need for Elderly LTC	% aged population (65+)
C6	State's Need for Disability LTC	Disability rate
C7	State Wealth	Income per capita
C8	Institutional Bed Supply	Nursing home beds per 1,000 population

Figure 6. Membership functions of the linguistic terms, describing the linguistic variable forms of the eight characteristics describing the states

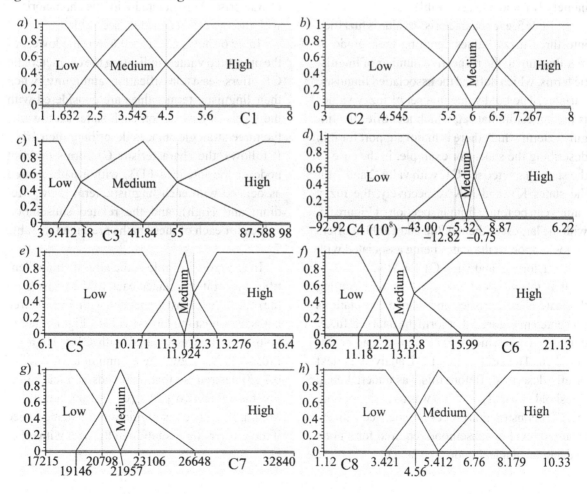

Table 5. Characteristic values and their fuzzification with majority linguistic term presented for KY and MN

State	KY			MN		
Char	Value	Fuzzy Values	Term	Value	Fuzzy Values	Term
C1	2	[**0.788**, 0.212, 0.000]	Low	7	[0.000, 0.000, **1.000**]	High
C2	6	[0.000, **1.000**, 0.000]	Medium	5	[**0.762**, 0.238, 0.000]	Low
C3	10	[**0.966**, 0.034, 0.000]	Low	45	[0.000, **0.880**, 0.120]	Medium
C4	−7.5	[0.143, **0.857**, 0.000]	Medium	−33.1	[**0.847**, 0.153, 0.000]	Low
C5	11.7	[0.179, **0.821**, 0.000]	Medium	11.1	[**0.589**, 0.411, 0.000]	Low
C6	17.76	[0.000, 0.000, **1.000**]	High	10.52	[**1.000**, 0.000, 0.000]	Low
C7	18587	[**1.000**, 0.000, 0.000]	Low	25579	[0.000, 0.151, **0.849**]	High
C8	5.89	[0.000, **0.823**, 0.177]	Medium	6.76	[0.000, **0.500**, **0.500**]	Medium/High
Stance		[0.000, 0.154, **0.846**]	Reactor		[**0.923**, 0.077, 0.000]	Prospector

the context of the ordinal and continuous state characteristics. An example of the impact of this fuzzification process is made for two states, namely KY and MN, see Table 5.

In Table 5, each characteristic value is fuzzified into three fuzzy values denoting their grade of membership to the respective number of linguistic terms, which defined the associatied linguistic variable. The bold value in a set of fuzzy values is the largest in that set, which identifies the linguistic term which there is major support for it in describing the state. For example, in the case of the state characteristic C1, with value 2 and 7 for the states KY and MN respectively, the fuzzy values can be found from inspection of Figure 6a, with the largest of them 0.788 and 1.000, it offers major support to the states being associated with Low C1 for KY and High C1 for MN.

It is the series of fuzzy values representing the state characteristics and stance associations presented in Figure 5 that form the data set (fuzzy data set), from which a FDT analysis can be undertaken. The start of this FDT analysis is next briefly described. Before this was undertaken, a threshold value of $\beta = 0.700$ was used throughout this FDT construction process, associated with the required level of subsethood required for a node to designated a leaf node (see later).

Following the FDT analysis given on the small example data set earlier, the start of the FDT analysis is with the evaluation of the root node (with characteristic), associated with the characteristic with the lowest $G(E)$ value, see Table 6.

Table 6 shows $G(C1) = 0.636$ is the lowest of the presented values, indicating the characteristic C1 offers least classification ambiguity, when their linguistic term values are considered with the levels of association each state has towards the three strategic stances describing their LTC. It follows, the characteristic C1 forms the root node of the intended FDT, with a path created associated with each linguistic term (Low, Medium and High), and the related subsethood values for each of these paths presented in Table 7.

In each row in Table 7, the largest value identifies the strategic stance each of the paths from the root node is most associated with. For all three paths, amongst the largest values, highlighted in bold, only that associated with C1 = High (to Prospector) is above the minimum truth level of 0.7 (β) desired, so that path ends at a leaf node. For the other two paths (C1 = Low and C1 = Medium), a check is required to be made to see if the further augmentation of the path with other

Table 6. Classification ambiguity values (G(·)) associated with fuzzy forms (linguistic variables) of the state characteristics, C1, ..., C8

	C1	C2	C3	C4	C5	C6	C7	C8
G(·)	0.636	0.796	0.708	0.755	0.724	0.759	0.722	0.732

Table 7. Subsethood values of C1 paths to strategy stances, Prospector, Defender and Reactor

C1	Prospector	Defender	Reactor
Low	0.156	0.612	**0.477**
Medium	0.422	**0.645**	0.387
High	**0.731**	0.449	0.258

state characteristics will continue the reduction in classification ambiguity.

This construction process is continued, until each path results in a leaf node, either because a required level of subsethood has been achieved or it is not appropriate for any further augmentation of characteristics. The resultant FDT is presented in Figure 7.

There are nine leaf nodes in the FDT, which each have a defined fuzzy decision rule associated with them. One of the rules, **R6***, is indicated with a *, since the largest truth value associated with this rule is less than the 0.7 truth threshold value imposed. In the case of this path of the FDT, there was no further ability to augment it with other nodes to improve the subsequent classification ambiguity. By their very nature, the fuzzy decision rules are readable (interpretable), for example, the three rules **R1**, **R4** and **R9** can be written as:

R1: "If C1, C7 and C3 are Low then LTC Strategic Stance of a state is Prospector (0.059), Defender (0.428) and **Reactor (0.810)**"

R4: "If C1 is Low and C7 is Medium then LTC Strategic Stance of a state is Prospector (0.248), **Defender (0.907)** and Reactor (0.571)"

R9: "If C1 is High then LTC Strategic Stance of a state is **Prospector (0.731)**, Defender (0.449) and Reactor (0.258)"

In Figure 5, the relative association of the states to the three strategic stances was exposited. In Figure 8 the relative associations of the fuzzy decision rules are considered. To achieve these relative associations, for each fuzzy decision rule, the three subsethood values associating a state to the three strategic stances are normalised so they sum to one, allowing their representations as a simplex coordinates in a simplex plot.

In each simplex plot shown in Figure 8, a fuzzy decision rule is shown (represented as a star), along with the states that satisfy the conditions of that rule (using the simplex coordinates presented in Figure 5).

The fuzzy decision rule **R1** is considered to exposit these results. This reports truth levels to Prospector, Defender and Reactor, of 0.059, 0.428 and 0.810 (normalized to 0.045, 0.330 and 0.625) with its largest association to the Reactor strategic stance. Further inspection of the simplex plot covering the rule **R1** shows three out of the five states, whose majority linguistic terms for each state characteristic satisfy the conditions of this rule, are also most associated with the Reactor stance. While this is not a stipulation, all five states are roughly clustered in the top right hand region of the simplex plot. One of these states is KY whose fuzzified state characteristics were reported in Table 5, where the levels of strategic stance associations are given. Similar clusters of states are shown associated with each fuzzy decision rule.

Figure 7. FDT for US states' health service strategy positions

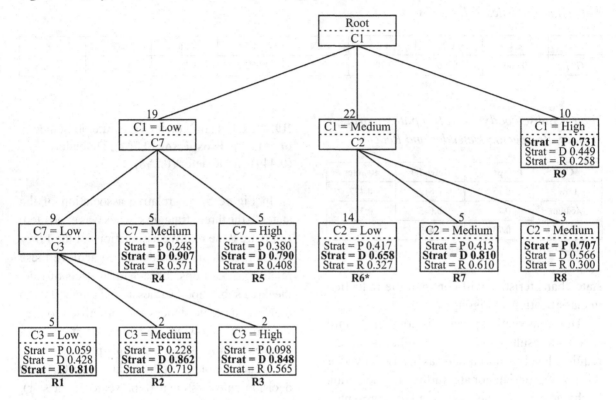

FUTURE TRENDS

While fuzzy set theory (FST), is well known in many fields of study, it has had limited impact in the area of organizational and policy research. It is not surprising then that the fuzzy decision tree (FDT) approach has not properly formally been applied in this area. With the resultant fuzzy '*If.. then..*' decision rules constructed, being readable and interpretable, it offers a novel way forward to gain inference in this area.

It will be interesting to note how FDT and other alternative fuzzy approaches can be employed within the fields of organization and policy research in the future. In the case of FDT and other FST based techniques, how pertinent their application is will depend greatly on how acceptable the readability and interpretability associated with FST techniques is.

CONCLUSION

The recent discussion of set-theoretic approaches in organization research, with the inclusion of the understanding of fuzzy set theory (FST), is a demonstration of the potential for FST based approaches to be further employed in organizational and policy research. The detailed discussion and analysis presented in this chapter presents a concrete example of one way in which FST can usefully be employed in both organizational and policy research.

The fuzzy decision tree (FDT) approach described is, of course, only one of a number of approaches that operate within a fuzzy environment. As this chapter demonstrates, however, FDTs is an approach to data mining that offers considerable potential to organizational and policy researchers as it brings together a relatively well known

Figure 8. Simplex plots exhibiting decision rules' position with the three strategic stances

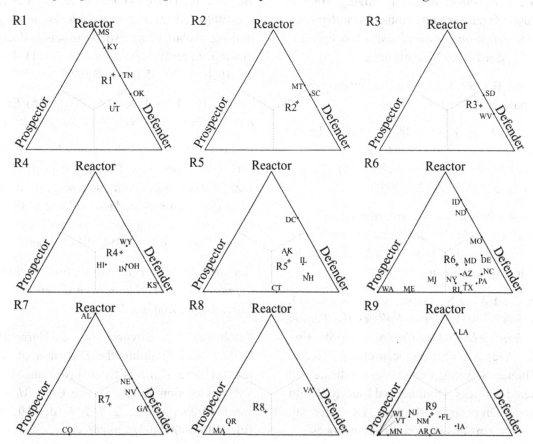

technique, the crisp 'original' form of decision trees, and its development in a fuzzy environment.

REFERENCES

Andrews, R., Boyne, G. A., & Walker, R. M. (2006). Strategy Content and Organizational Performance: An Empirical Analysis. *Public Administration Review*, 66(1): 52–63. doi:10.1111/j.1540-6210.2006.00555.x

Beynon, M., Curry, B., & Morgan, P. (2000). Classification and Rule Induction Using Rough Set Theory. *Expert Systems: International Journal of Knowledge Engineering and Neural Networks*, 17(3), 136–148. doi:10.1111/1468-0394.00136

Beynon, M. J., Buchanan, K., & Tang, Y.-C. (2004b). The Application of a Fuzzy Rule Based System in an Exposition of the Antecedents of Sedge Warbler Song Flight. *Expert Systems: International Journal of Knowledge Engineering and Neural Networks*, 21(1), 1–10. doi:10.1111/j.1468-0394.2004.00258.x

Beynon, M.J., Peel, M.J., & Tang, Y.-C. (2004a). The Application of Fuzzy Decision Tree Analysis in an Exposition of the Antecedents of Audit Fees. *OMEGA - International Journal of Management Science, 32*(2), 231-244.

Bourgeois, L. (1980). Performance and Consensus. *Strategic Management Journal, 1*, 227–248. doi:10.1002/smj.4250010304

Boyne, G., & Walker, R. (2004). Strategy content and public service organizations. *Journal of Public Administration: Research and Theory, 14*(2), 231–252. doi:10.1093/jopart/muh015

Bozeman, B. (1987). *All organizations are public.* San Francisco, CA: Jossey-Bass.

Chang, R. L. P., & Pavlidis, T. (1977). Fuzzy decision tree algorithms. *IEEE Transactions on Systems, Man, and Cybernetics, 7*(1), 28–35. doi:10.1109/TSMC.1977.4309586

Cohen, W. (1995). Fast effective rule induction. In *Proceedings of the 12th international conference on machine learning,* (pp. 115–123). Los Altos, CA: Morgan Kaufmann.

Crisp, S., Eiken, S., Gerst, K., & Justice, D. (September 2003). *Money Follows the Person and Balancing Long-Term Care Systems: State examples.* A report for the US Department of Health and Human Services, Centers for Medicare and Medicaid Services, Disabled and Elderly Health Programs Division. Washington, DC: Medstat. http://www.cms.hhs.gov/promisingpractices/mfp92903.pdf

Dombi, J., & Gera, Z. (2005). The approximation of piecewise linear membership functions and Łukasiewicz operators. *Fuzzy Sets and Systems, 154,* 275–286. doi:10.1016/j.fss.2005.02.016

Downs, A. (1967). *Inside bureaucracy.* Boston: Little Brown.

Fan, Z.-P., Feng, B., Sun, Y.-H., & Ou, W. (2009). Evaluating knowledge management capability of organizations: a fuzzy linguistic method. *Expert Systems with Applications, 36,* 3346–3354. doi:10.1016/j.eswa.2008.01.052

Fiss, P. C. (2007). A Set-Theoretic Approach to Organizational Configurations. *Academy of Management Review, 32*(4), 1160–1198. doi:10.2307/20159362

Herrera, F., Herrera-Viedma, E., & Martinez, L. (2000). A fusion approach for managing multi-granularity linguistic term sets in decision making. *Fuzzy Sets and Systems, 114*(1), 43–58. doi:10.1016/S0165-0114(98)00093-1

Hunt, E. B., Marin, J., & Stone, P. T. (1966). *Experiments in Induction.* New York: Academic Press.

Ichihashi, H., Shirai, T., Nagasaka, K., & Miyoshi, T. (1996). Neuro-fuzzy ID3: a method of inducing fuzzy decision trees with linear programming for maximising entropy and an algebraic method for incremental learning. *Fuzzy Sets and Systems, 81,* 157–167. doi:10.1016/0165-0114(95)00247-2

Kecman, V. (2001). *Learning and Soft Computing: Support Vector Machines, Neural Networks, and Fuzzy Logic.* London: MIT Press.

Kitchener, M., Beynon, M., & Harrington, C. (2004). Explaining the Diffusion of Medicaid Home Care Waiver Programs Using VPRS Decision Rules. *Health Care Management Science, 7*(3), 237–244. doi:10.1023/B:HCMS.0000039386.59886.dd

Kovalerchuk, B., & Vityaev, E. (2000). *Data Mining in Finance: Advances in Relational and Hybrid Methods.* Amsterdam: Kluwer Academic Publishers.

Li, M.-T., Zhao, F., & Chow, L.-F. (2006). Assignment of Seasonal Factor Categories to Urban Coverage Count Stations Using a Fuzzy Decision Tree. *Journal of Transportation Engineering, 132*(8), 654–662. doi:10.1061/(ASCE)0733-947X(2006)132:8(654)

Miles, R. E., & Snow, C. (1978). *Organizational strategy, structure and process.* New York: McGraw-Hill.

Mitra, S., Konwar, K. M., & Pal, S. K. (2002). Fuzzy Decision Tree, Linguistic Rules and Fuzzy Knowledge-Based Network: Generation and Evaluation. *IEEE Transactions on Systems, Man and Cybernetics. Part C, Applications and Reviews, 32*(4), 328–339. doi:10.1109/TSMCC.2002.806060

Mouritzen, P. (1992). *Managing cities in austerity*. London: Sage.

Nutt, P., & Backoff, R. (1995). Strategy for Public and Third Sector Organizations. *Journal of Public Administration: Research and Theory, 5*, 189–211.

Olaru, C., & Wehenkel, L. (2003). A complete fuzzy decision tree technique. *Fuzzy Sets and Systems, 138*, 221–254. doi:10.1016/S0165-0114(03)00089-7

Pal, N. R., & Chakraborty, S. (2001). Fuzzy Rule Extraction From ID3-Type Decision Trees for Real Data. *IEEE Transactions on Systems, Man, and Cybernetics Part B, 31*(5), 745–754. doi:10.1109/3477.956036

Pennings, P. (2003). Beyond dichotomous explanations: Explaining constitutional control of the executive with fuzzy-sets. *European Journal of Political Research, 42*, 541–567. doi:10.1111/1475-6765.00095

Quinlan, J. R. (1979). Discovery rules from large examples: A Case Study. In Michie, D. (Ed.), *Expert Systems in the Micro Electronic Age*. Edinburgh, UK: Edinburgh University Press.

Ragin, C. C., & Pennings, P. (2005). Fuzzy Sets and Social Research. *Sociological Methods & Research, 33*(4), 423–430. doi:10.1177/0049124105274499

Shortell, S., & Zajac, E. (1990). Perceptual and archival measures of Miles and Snow's strategic types: A comprehensive assessment of reliability and validity. *Academy of Management Journal, 33*, 817–832. doi:10.2307/256292

Thabtah, F., Cowling, P., & Hammoud, S. (2006). Improving rule sorting, predictive accuracy and training time in associative classification. *Expert Systems with Applications, 31*, 414–426. doi:10.1016/j.eswa.2005.09.039

Walker, O., & Ruekert, R. (1987). Marketing's role in the implementation of business strategies: A critical review and conceptual framework. *Journal of Marketing, 51*, 15–33. doi:10.2307/1251645

Wang, R. C., & Chuu, S. J. (2004). Group decision-making using a fuzzy linguistic approach for evaluating the flexibility in a manufacturing system. *European Journal of Operational Research, 154*(3), 563–572. doi:10.1016/S0377-2217(02)00729-4

Wang, X., Chen, B., Qian, G., & Ye, F. (2000). On the optimization of fuzzy decision trees. *Fuzzy Sets and Systems, 112*(1), 117–125. doi:10.1016/S0165-0114(97)00386-2

Wechsler, B., & Backoff, R. W. (1986). Policy making and administration in state agencies: Strategic management approaches. *Public Administration Review, 46*, 321–327. doi:10.2307/976305

Yu, C.-S., & Li, H.-L. (2001). Method for solving quasi-concave and non-cave fuzzy multi-objective programming problems. *Fuzzy Sets and Systems, 122*(2), 205–227. doi:10.1016/S0165-0114(99)00163-3

Yuan, Y., & Shaw, M. J. (1995). Induction of fuzzy decision trees. *Fuzzy Sets and Systems, 69*(2), 125–139. doi:10.1016/0165-0114(94)00229-Z

Zadeh, L. A. (1965). Fuzzy Sets. *Information and Control, 8*(3), 338–353. doi:10.1016/S0019-9958(65)90241-X

Zadeh, L. A. (1975a). The concept of a linguistic variable and its application to approximate reasoning (Part I). *Information Sciences, 8*, 199–249. doi:10.1016/0020-0255(75)90036-5

Zadeh, L. A. (1975b). The concept of a linguistic variable and its application to approximate reasoning (Part II). *Information Sciences*, *8*, 301–357. doi:10.1016/0020-0255(75)90046-8

Zadeh, L. A. (1975c). The concept of a linguistic variable and its application to approximate reasoning (Part III). *Information Sciences*, *9*, 43–80. doi:10.1016/0020-0255(75)90017-1

Zahra, S. A., & Pearce, J. A. (1990). Research evidence on the Miles-Snow typology. *Journal of Management*, *16*, 751–768. doi:10.1177/014920639001600407

Zajac, E. J., & Shortell, S. M. (1989). Changing generic strategies: Likelihood, direction and performance implications. *Strategic Management Journal*, *10*, 413–430. doi:10.1002/smj.4250100503

Zhou, S.-M., & Gan, J. Q. (2008). Low-level interpretability and high-level interpretability: a unified view data-driven interpretable fuzzy system modelling. *Fuzzy Sets and Systems*, *159*, 3091–3131. doi:10.1016/j.fss.2008.05.016

KEY TERMS AND DEFINITIONS

Condition Attribute: An attribute that describes an object. Within a decision tree it is part of a non-leaf node, so performs as an antecedent in the decision rules used for the final classification of an object.

Decision Attribute: An attribute that characterises an object. Within a decision tree is part of a leaf node, so performs as a consequent, in the decision rules, from the paths down the tree to the leaf node.

Decision Tree: A tree-like structure for representing a collection of hierarchical decision rules that lead to a class or value, starting from a root node ending in a series of leaf nodes.

Induction: A technique that infers generalizations from the information in the data.

Leaf Node: A node not further split, the terminal grouping, in a classification or decision tree.

Linguistic Term: One of a set of linguistic terms, which are subjective categories for a linguistic variable, each described by a membership function.

Linguistic Variable: A variable made up of a number of words (linguistic terms) with associated degrees of membership.

Path: A path down the tree from root node to leaf node, also termed a branch.

Membership Function: A function that quantifies the grade of membership of a variable to a linguistic term.

Node: A junction point down a path in a decision tree that describes a condition in an if-then decision rule. From a node, the current path may separate into two or more paths.

Root Node: The node at the top of a decision tree, from which all paths originate and lead to a leaf node.

Chapter 4
The Use of Data Mining for Assessing Performance of Administrative Services

Zdravko Pečar
University of Ljubljana, Slovenia

Ivan Bratko
University of Ljubljana, Slovenia

ABSTRACT

The aim of this research was to study the performance of 58 Slovenian administrative districts (state government offices at local level), to identify the factors that affect the performance, and how these effects interact. The main idea was to analyze the available statistical data relevant to the performance of the administrative districts with machine learning tools for data mining, and to extract from available data clear relations between various parameters of administrative districts and their performance. The authors introduced the concept of basic unit of administrative service, which enables the measurement of an administrative district's performance. The main data mining tool used in this study was the method of regression tree induction. This method can handle numeric and discrete data, and has the benefit of providing clear insight into the relations between the parameters in the system, thereby facilitating the interpretation of the results of data mining. The authors investigated various relations between the parameters in their domain, for example, how the performance of an administrative district depends on the trends in the number of applications, employees' level of professional qualification, etc. In the chapter, they report on a variety of (occasionally surprising) findings extracted from the data, and discuss how these findings can be used to improve decisions in managing administrative districts.

INTRODUCTION

The aim of this research was to assess the performance of 58 Slovenian administrative districts (state government offices at local level), which provide

DOI: 10.4018/978-1-60566-906-9.ch004

administrative services for eight state ministries. These administrative tasks are commonly organised in four departments of each administrative district. The research covered only one of them – the departments for environment and spatial planning, whose task is to issue various permits (planning permits, building permits and others) upon applications, under the laws and supervision of Ministry for environment and spatial planning. The following three hypotheses were set at the beginning of the research:

- The administrative districts have very different productivity.
- The level of employee education has the major influence on productivity.
- The increased number of applications results in longer times for processing.

The analysis showed several findings of interest. Among them it was found that the organizational productivity among administrative districts varied enormously, up to the ratio of 10: 1. Also, the number of new applications plays a major role in predicting the future trends in productivity. Level of education of employees, and to a lesser degree their age and gender, also influence the productivity.

In our experience, machine learning methods proved to be a very efficient tool for quick, automatic and holistic analysis of large sets of different data. It was especially effective at exposing most characteristic patterns of behavior. According to our experience in this study, the analyses with classical statistical methods is much more rigid and more costly in that it requires more time for recognizing various hidden patterns of behavior such as ones generated by machine learning methods. In this sense, machine learning is particularly good at data exploration stage when hypotheses are formulated. Of course, when we get to the question of proving statistical significance of hypotheses, then we face essentially the same problems as in classical statistics.

BACKGROUND

Among practitioners, there is unfavourable and prevailing general opinion (shared also by professionals and politicians) that the work performance

at administrative services cannot be measured. The authors of this paper and an emerging group of innovative public managers which participated with data gathering and discussions during the present research have organized "committee for quality". Members of this committee do not share this opinion and believe that the performance of these services can gradually be more systematically measured and managed, very much like all those in the private sector (Asbjorn, 1995). This committee was a facilitator of new ideas in this respect.

The main idea was to analyse the available statistical data (Annual reports of Administrative statistics 1996–1999) relevant to the performance of the administrative districts with tools of machine learning, to obtain clear relations between various parameters of administrative districts and the performance. These machine learning tools include those that are usually employed in data mining. Additional objective was to set the requirements for better performance measurement system and suggest the need for new ways of decision making by public managers in the fields of strategic planning and performance management (including performance based budgeting and performance based pay).

The main data analysis tool used in this study was the method of regression trees, one of rather common machine learning techniques (Witten and Frank 2005). We will describe this technique in more detail in Section 3.

Developing and Organizing Data for Analysis

All 58 administrative districts, which employ more than 3000 administrative workers, provide administration services at local level for eight state ministries. The performance of these districts is not properly measured, monitored and thus not well managed.

Data sets that were used for the analysis were gathered for the period of four years: 1996–99, from various sources (Administrative statistics, and quarterly reports by Ministry of Interior; these are specially designed questionnaires, interviews, etc.).

Structuring the Domain of Investigation

The first step in the development of a data base for the analysis was to classify and standardize various different administrative services as much as possible. The existing official quarterly reports and administrative statistics regarded and presented various administrative services from all departments as equally demanding, which is far from reality. If we want to exercise any serious performance assessment, we must first establish the common denominator for these various services. In this study, one of the authors (Z.P.) carried out this task by conducting several meetings with representative experts from the departments for environment and spatial planning (which was the focus of the research). It was agreed to classify the administrative services into five groups.

Also, the time needed to process different types of applications were defined by taking the average time estimates by these experts. On this basis, the relative ratios were calculated, taking as the base the group of services which demanded the least time – basic service). By multiplying each administrative service with its ratio, all the services provided can be expressed in *units of basic services*, which made it possible to compare the productivity between all five groups of administrative services. These ratios per one service were:

A. Planning permit 1.99 (32.4 hrs)
B. Building permit 1.77 (28.8 hrs)
C. Permit for use 2.26 (36.8 hrs)
D. Registration of construction work 1.00 (16.3 hrs) – basic unit of service
E. Other permits 1.34 (21.8 hrs)

Data Collection and Cleaning

The next step was to gather as much data as possible about all the possible attributes (parameters) that may effect, or are in any way related to the performance of administrative districts.

For the benefit of expressing the average and each single organization's productivity in costs per unit of various administrative services (which is best understood by the customers – taxpayers; and should be even more by budget authorities), the approximate costs were estimated - 20.000 EUR per year per worker (approximately one half of this amount represents the salary and another half material costs).

The next task was to "clean" the data from official administrative statistics, by eliminating errors (noise) from the existing data. The most common errors were found when data was extracted from quarterly reports, where the numbers of unsolved cases at the end of each quarter were simply added together and presented in annual reports (instead the end of the fourth quarter only).

The final data sets that were used for the analysis were organized in electronic spreadsheets and included the following groups of attributes:

1. Annual structure and number of different classified administrative services (solved cases per year = "production" per year in % for four year period)
2. Annual "production" expressed in units of basic services
3. "Production" cost per basic service for four year period
4. Number of new applications and unsolved cases per year for four year period
5. Number of employees, age, gender, level of education for four year period
6. Presence of performance measurement and stimulation measures for four year period
7. Population served by administrative unit
8. Various other derived indexes (trends) and some other performance indicators (such as

Table 1. Average time spent for administrative services (productivity) in years 1996–99

	1996	1997	1998	1999
Number of employees in dept. 58 AD	555	574	568	544
Available working hours: 6,5 hrs x 20 days x 10 months (approx.) x number of workers	721.500	746.200	738.400	707.200
Number of services performed (expressed in basic units)	117.489	118.236	105.647	101.162
Hours per basic unit of service	6.14	6.31	6.99	6,99
Hours per planning permit	12.19	12.56	13.91	13.91
Hours per building permit	10.87	11.17	12.37	12.37
Hours per permit for use	13.88	14.26	15.80	15.80
Hours per other permits	8.23	8.46	9.37	9.37

denied applications or overturned decision on higher level)

Then a table of classified administrative services was constructed. The rows in the table correspond to the 58 administrative districts. For each row in the table, there were four groups of columns corresponding to the four years 1996–1999. Each column contained 5 different classified services (A–E). By learning the share of different services of each administrative district (from the questionnaires) in the four years and the number of employees, we were able to calculate the average production time and cost for all services in the given year.

Nearly all the data sets needed some quality improvement which is quite usual experience (see Table 1).

The experts from the administrative districts gave their estimated average (standard) time of 16.30 hours per basic unit of services, while these calculations showed this to have been a gross underestimate by the factor of 2,466 (the actual average time for basic unit was found to be only 6,61 hours). This additionally adds to the conclusion that the understanding of the work processes in administrative districts is very weak.

DATA MINING METHOD USED IN THE ANALYSIS

For this study we have chosen to use Machine Learning (ML) methods (Witten & Frank 2005; Mitchell 1997; Weiss & Kulikowski 1991) for data analysis. We could have chosen for our analysis more traditional, classical statistical methods. However, we found ML tools more appropriate for this study. The reason is that our primary interest was exploratory data analysis, where we try to extract relations, possibly tentative and largely speculative, from the data. These relations that result from ML-based analysis should be understood as hypotheses, not necessarily as definite, statistically significant findings.

Generating hypotheses is harder to do in the classical statistical framework than with ML techniques because the latter are more flexible in enabling automatic generation (not only testing) of hypotheses. For example, classical numerical regression methods are usually limited to linear regression functions, whereas regression tree techniques in ML typically result in non-linear models. Here we may also consider the so-called model trees with linear regression in the leaves. Therefore, regression trees are a much more expressive hypothesis language than the one used by classical numerical regression. The class of models generated by regression tree techniques is much larger than that of linear regression. Classical statistical methods, on the other hand, may have advantage in that they are easier for rigorous statistical testing of the significance of hypotheses. Simply, the much larger multiplicity of possible hypotheses in regression trees makes it harder to avoid over fitting of hypotheses to data, and to evaluate the hypotheses' statistical significance.

An approach to the handling of multiplicity of hypotheses considered by the search for a model, called EVC (extreme value correction) was developed by Mozina et al. (2006), but applying this technique in ML techniques is quite complicated. It requires an approximation of the distribution of accuracy over the (usually large) set of trees considered by a tree induction algorithm. By way of a summary, ML is more flexible and effective for generating material for further interpretation and research. The price for this greater flexibility is, of course, that there is danger of misinterpreting the results of ML. The results should usually be interpreted very cautiously.

As it will become clear later, learning to make accurate numerical predictions is very hard in our domain (many attributes and small number of examples), therefore the ability of ML techniques to generate more versatile models is more valuable than numerical prediction accuracy. ML models offer more ways of meaningful interpretation of the relations in the domain. They enable the expert to explore the domain, consider patterns that appear in induced hypotheses, and gain unexpected insights about the domain.

The particular ML technique used in our study is the learning of regression trees from data (Breiman et al. 1986; Witten & Frank, 2005). In most of our analyses we used an early implementation of regression tree learning RETIS by A. Karalić (Karalić 1991). A more recent implementation of regression tree learning is part of the Orange system for ML (Demsar, Zupan & Leban, 2004). A particularly powerful practical feature of Orange is the intelligent data visualization module that

can be used for initial "visual" analysis of the data at the stage where the "data miner" develops the "feel" for the data (Leban et al., 2006).

The choice of regression trees among many other ML techniques was in our case justified by the following properties of our data mining problem:

1. the class (or "target variable", i.e. the variable that we want to predict) was given: the productivity of an administrative district measured as the cost of basic unit of service; this fact makes some other data mining approaches, such as unsupervised learning (e.g. inducing association rules) less appropriate;

2. the target variable was numerical; therefore classification learning methods (such as decision trees, or rules) would be less appropriate because they would require at least the discretization of the numerical class variable;

3. we were interested in detecting complex, non-linear patterns, which is handled by regression trees, but not with, say, multivariate linear regression.

Of course there are a number of ML techniques that we considered as alternatives to regression trees. These alternatives include decision trees (which would require the discretization of the target variable), or if-then rules with either numerical predictions or, again, discretized target variable, or neural networks, or variants of Support Vector Machines, etc. As explained above, the choice of regression trees fits the properties of our data mining problem the most directly and naturally. Discretization of the target variable, required by decision trees, would either lead to loss of information on the order of discrete values, or to the difficulty of non-standard decision tree learning with ordinal class. Our major requirement regarding the data mining technique also was that the results of learning be easy to understand and interpret by a human expert. This makes methods like neural networks less appropriate. We could here continue to analyze in depth various aspects of the choice of the data mining method, and find that some alternatives would be quite viable and would lead to similar general findings as regression trees. But the main contribution of this paper is the analysis of public administrative services data; therefore we will instead concentrate in this paper more on this application.

In the following we describe more precisely how our data mining problem was formulated as a regression tree learning task. Induction of regression trees can be viewed as a method for automatic knowledge acquisition from data. Regularities that are present in the analyzed data are automatically extracted from the data. In the context of machine learning, the data is interpreted as examples drawn from the domain of investigation, and the true regularities in the domain are hopefully extracted from the examples. In the case of learning regression trees, the data has the form of a table, and the extracted regularities are represented in the form of a *regression tree*. Each row of the data table is viewed as an example for learning.

In our case study, each administrative district represents an example for learning. The columns of the data table correspond to the *attributes* that are used to describe the examples. In our case study, the number of employees is one of the attributes. There is a selected distinguished attribute, called the target variable, or *class*. A learned regression tree extracted from the data specifies the mapping from the attributes to the class. More formally, let the class be y, and the attributes be $x_1, x_2,...,$ x_m. Then the learned regression tree defines a function $y = f(x_1, x_2,..., x_m)$. The attributes can be discrete (nominal) or continuous (numerical). In the case of regression trees, the class is continuous. In our analysis, the class is typically the average time in an administrative district needed to accomplish the basic administrative task (cost of basic service). This is a continuous variable. This choice of class attribute is the most natural because in our analysis we are most interested

in the district's performance depending on the attributes of an administrative district.

In a regression tree, there are selected attributes assigned to the internal nodes of the tree. The branches stemming from an internal node correspond to possible values of the attribute at the node. Class values, i.e. numbers, are assigned to the leaf nodes of the tree. A regression tree learning algorithm constructs such a tree from the given data table in such a way that the tree minimizes the expected prediction error when predicting the class value given the attribute values. The algorithm attempts to select the most "informative" attributes and inserts them at the highest levels in the tree. The most "informative" attributes are those that have the highest influence on the class value, so they are the most important in predicting the class.

A regression tree is used for prediction of the class value for a given new case as follows. We start at the root node and consider the attribute at the root. We then proceed down the tree along the branch that corresponds to the new case's value of this attribute, which leads to the next internal node. At the next node, we repeat the same action. We thus progress down-words along a path of the tree until a leaf node is encountered. The class value assigned to that leaf is our predicted class value for the given case. We will show a number of examples of regression trees, along with their interpretation, in the section on the results of the analysis.

In our experiments, we sometimes used the variation of regression trees with linear regression at the leaves that is model trees. In such a tree, a linear regression formula is assigned to a leaf node, instead of a single numerical value. This regression formula is then used to *compute* the class value (instead of just reading the class value at the leaf). This variety of regression tree learning can be viewed as *structured* linear regression. That is, the tree assigns separate regression formulas to different subspaces of the problem domain. The subspace covered by a regression formula is defined by the conditions along the path from the root to the leaf at which the formula appears. Although model trees are an attractive possibility, in our study they generally turned out to be less useful than the usual, "point-value" trees, and model trees' prediction accuracy was somewhat inferior. The reason for this is probably the fact that linear regression in the leaves was unreliable because of shortage of learning data.

Regression tree learning programs typically also have the built in simplification mechanism called "pruning". This mechanism prunes those leaves of the tree and corresponding branches that have low degree of significance. This simplifies the induced trees which makes trees less complex and thus easier to comprehend and to interpret key patterns in the trees. The pruning also tends to improve the predictive accuracy of regression trees because it largely reduces the effect of "noise" (errors) in the learning data.

PERFORMANCE ANALYSIS WITH REGRESSION TREES

Studying regression trees that resulted from the mining of administrative districts data, we can draw valuable conclusions about various patterns of behavior among 58 administrative districts (departments).

It should be noted that, as usual in data mining, the mining was not done in "one shot", but it was a complex, iterative process that involved many experiments where our data mining tool was applied with various parameter settings (e.g. degree of tree pruning) to different versions of data. In this process, several learning problems were formulated and re-formulated, and induced trees were interpreted by the domain expert where new ideas about problem formulations appeared. The data for various formulations of the leaning problem were refined or re-interpreted. For example, subsets of attributes were pre-selected according to the domain expert's (Z. P.) opinion,

and new (derived) attributes were added, such as "trend attributes" that indicate the changes of attribute values between different years.

One interesting question is whether further experimentation with other parameter settings and reformulations of the learning task might lead to predictors with higher accuracy than that attained in this paper. On this note, a rather firm conclusion of our experience in this study is that it is unlikely that further experiments could lead to substantial improvements in predictive accuracy.

Examples of induced regression trees and their interpretation, together with findings of interest, are shown on the following pages. In these experiments, we varied the class attribute and the set of other attributes selected in individual cases from the whole data table.

Impact of Unsolved '96 and New Applications '97 on Productivity '97

Here RETIS induced a relation between the number of unsolved applications from the previous year and the current year, and the productivity expressed as cost of basic administrative service (see Figure 1).

The generated regression tree offers the following findings:

a. The single most influential attribute is the number of new applications in '97, the next is the number of employees, then the combined number of unsolved from the previous plus new applications from the current year, and the number of unsolved from the previous year.

b. The cluster of 21 administrative districts on the left lower part of the regression tree offers an interesting picture. This is the group of larger administrative districts with more than 8 employees in the department. The subgroup of 13 with more than 1346 applications per year has higher productivity than the other 8 by about 25%. The further distinction in

Figure 1. Cost of basic service depending on the four attributes mentioned in the right top corner

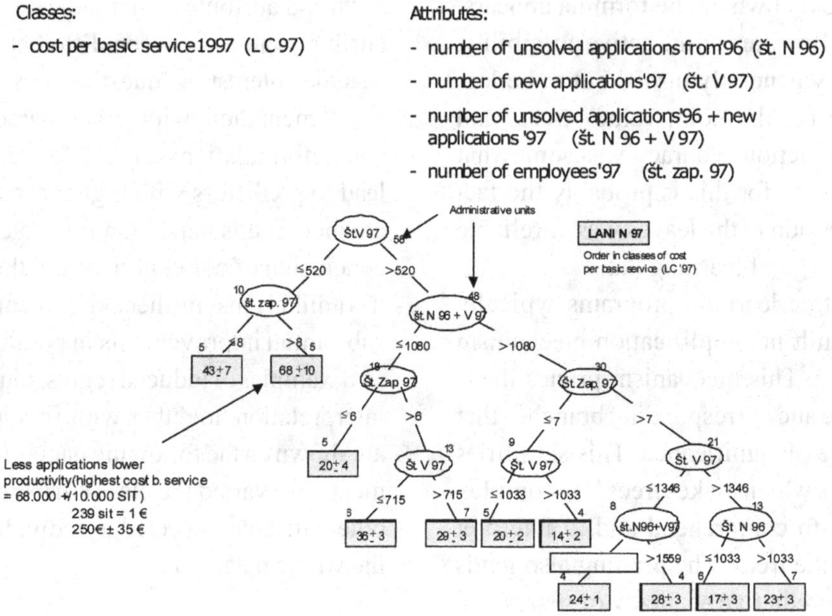

productivity between the two subgroups is the amount of unsolved cases from the previous year. Those ones from the subgroup with the highest number of unsolved cases show about 20% lower productivity. These findings show the hidden rule; too many unsolved cases produce kind of "panic" effect which occurs when the number of "orders" (new and old applications) exceeds an optimal number which appears to be around 250 - 300.

c. The lowest productivity (cost of basic service = 242.68 – 326.35 EUR) is shown by 5 administrative districts which employ 8 or more workers and received up to 520 new applications in 1997 (1 EUR = 239 SIT).

Relations between Productivity Trends and Trends of New Applications '98–'99

Here the selected attributes and class were relevant for studying the trends between productivity and

trends in new applications (Figure 2). The findings are: For the majority of the administrative districts (43) it seems to hold: if the index of new applications is from 86 to 114 than the index of basic service cost is between 73 and 139. The tree hints inverse correlation with slightly greater dispersion on the cost side. In other words, this pattern shows direct dependency between new applications and productivity. This phenomenon is further clarified in the graph of Figure 3 where inverse correlation is clearly indicated.

Productivity, Throughput and Education Level of Employees in 1996

The tree in Figure 4 shows how the cost per basic service is affected by the percentages of cases solved in 1 month, more than one month, and the average education level of the employees. The findings are:

Figure 2. Relations between productivity trends and trends in new applications 98-99

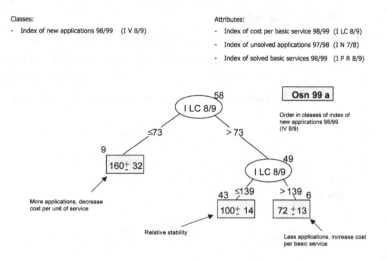

Figure 3. Indexes of new applications and cost per basic service

Graph: Relation between 98/99 indexes of new applications (series 1) and costs per basic unit (series 2)

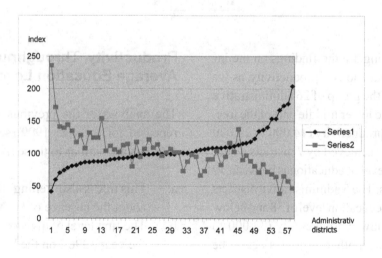

a. The first division is made on the throughput performance (percentage of cases solved within one month). We would expect from the group of 21 administrative districts with faster throughput on the right side of the tree to have also higher productivity than the group of the remaining 37 on the left side. The machine learning analysis proves this expectation wrong. The share of the most productive ones (cost per unit around 20.000 SIT = 83.68 EUR) is equal in both groups (1/3), while the least productive ones (cost around 40.000 SIT = 167.36 EUR) have a higher share in the group of 21 with the fastest throughput.

Figure 4. Cost per basic service dependence on throughput and education of employees in 1996

Classes:

- Cost per basic service '96 (LC 96)

Attributes:

- % of solved cases within 1 month '96 (% R 1mes.96)
- % of solved cases within 1 month - 2 month '96 (% R 1-2mes.96)
- % of solved cases within 2 month + month '96 (% R 2+mes.96)
- Average education level of employees '96 (st. izobr.)

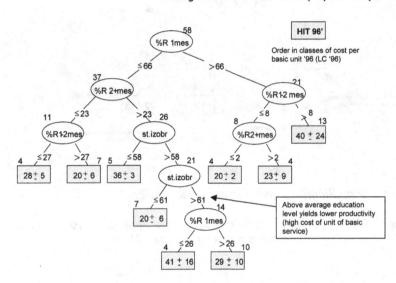

b. Very interesting are the findings on the influence of education on productivity, as we can see from the group of 26 administrative districts in the lower middle part of the tree. The highest productivity (14.000 to 26.000 sit – 20 ± 6) is achieved by 7 districts where the average level of education is between 59 and 61 points. The 5 administrative districts with average education level of 58 and below attain much lower productivity (33.000 to 39.000 sit), with other attributes being the same. The 14 districts (in the low center of the tree) with highest level of education – 62 points or more, show the lowest productivity (especially 4 districts that solve only 26% or less cases in one month, with cost per unit 25.000 to 57.000 sit = 104.60 – 238.50 EUR). This finding presents an urgent challenge for the HRM specialists.

Productivity, Throughput and Average Education Level in 1999

The analysis of the previous section was here repeated for the year 1999 (see Figure 5). The findings are similar to those of year 1996:

a. This tree is also "telling" the same sad story about the absence of HRM.

b. The first level of division is the same as for the year 1996 - on the basis of 66% solved cases in 1 month. Only 14 districts meet this criterion (in 1996, 21 districts). This reflects a decline in performance.

c. On the left lower side of the regression tree, the previously found paradox appears again. The 17 districts with education level of 63 and less has the productivity in terms of cost from 18.000 to 32.000 sit = 75,31 – 133,89 EUR per basic service, while the other 7 administrative districts with education level of

64 and more show much lower productivity with costs of basic service from 29.000 to 55.000 sit = 121,34 – 230,13 EUR. Similar but not as significant relation is seen for the group of 12 administrative districts next to the right.

d. By observing the group of 14 administrative districts on the very right side of the tree, we can see 6 administrative districts that solve between 67% and 78% of cases within 1 month, to have the lowest productivity with costs 41.000 to 87.000 sit = 171.55 – 364.02 EUR, while the other 8 administrative districts with even better throughput cycle show much better productivity with costs for basic service of 16.000 to 38.000 SIT = 66.95 – 159.00 EUR. It looks that the throughput cycle is not in direct correlation with productivity. This relation was examined by tracing same data "by hand", and the results showed that the throughput cycle is a very stable attribute. For example some administrative districts experienced drop of applications by 50% which was followed by the lowering of productivity by almost the same percentage, while the rate of throughput cycle remained the same. Obviously the workers themselves regulate how many applications they process simultaneously at the one cycle time.

Accuracy of Induced Regression Tree Models

In the foregoing sections, we studied regression tree models induced from the data. We were mainly interested in qualitative relations between various parameters indicative of the productivity of administration districts. On the other hand, the generated tree models can also be used for numerical prediction. For example, by using such a tree we could answer questions like: What would be the cost of basic service in a given administrative district if the number of new applications increased from 600 to 700?

A regression tree answers such questions by a numerical prediction. An important question is how reliable the tree's predictions are? Of course, only predictions for new cases (not the cases already seen among the existing data) are of true interest. We estimated the accuracy of trees' numerical predictions on new cases by computing the following frequently used measures of accuracy of numerical prediction (Witten & Frank 2005):

a. Mean squared error:

$$MSE = \frac{1}{N} \sum_i (x_n(i) - x_d(i))^2$$

Here $x_n(i)$ is the predicted class value of test case i, and $x_d(i)$ is its true value.

b. Relative mean squared error:

$$RMSE = \frac{N \times MSE}{\sum_i (\bar{x} - x_d(i))^2}, \text{ where}$$

$$\bar{x} = \frac{1}{N} \sum_i x_d(i)$$

c. Relative error: $RE = \frac{\sqrt{MSE}}{\bar{x}}$

To compute these measures of accuracy as estimates of performance on new cases, we used the method of leave-one-out (Witten & Frank 2005). This is a standard accuracy estimation method used when the number of learning examples is relatively small (in our case N=58 which is considered as small). In this method, one of the N learning examples is excluded from the learning set, a regression tree is computed from the remaining (N-1) examples, and the tree is applied to predict the class value of the excluded case as if this was a new case. This is repeated over all the N learning cases, each time one of the cases being used as a new, not yes seen case.

Figure 5. Cost per basic service dependence on throughput and education of employees in 1999

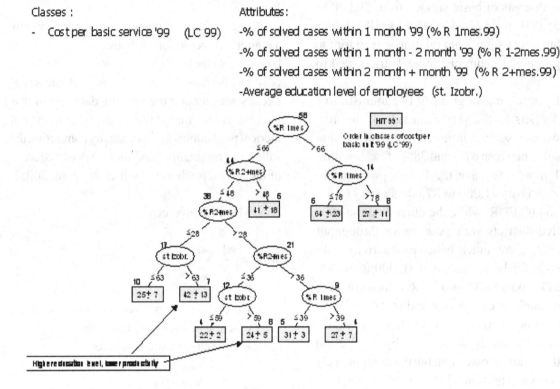

The following average values over all the generated trees were obtained: *MSE*=12.61, *RMSE*=30.86%, *RE*=23%. Although *RE* is not bad, these accuracy estimates indicate that the generated regression trees cannot be really recommended to be used for numerical prediction. Therefore the use of generated regression trees should be mainly limited to qualitative analysis that aims at formulating interesting hypotheses in the domain, as we did in the foregoing sections. These hypotheses can then be used as useful qualitative indicators combined with indicative quantitative thresholds, when managing administrative districts with the aim at improved productivity.

As already stated, predictive accuracy of the induced trees is hardly sufficient for making reliable numerical predictions. Therefore the main value of these trees is as "food for thought" for the domain expert, as an aid to help her or him to develop the intuitive understanding of the domain of exploration. It would be interesting to consider the question of statistical significance of the hypotheses (correlations) indicated by regression trees: is the distribution of class values in a leaf statistically significantly different from the distribution in the whole domain. In the case of tree learning, this is however not straightforward to answer, and we avoid it because such results are typically misleading. A statistical test is intended to essentially answer the question: what is the probability of obtaining the observed class distribution in a leaf by chance when randomly sampling from the data in the whole domain? Such an analysis is sometimes provided in applications of tree learning.

However, the results are usually not useful and are misinterpreted. The reason is that in the process of inducing a tree from the data, the induction algorithm considers *many* hypotheses in a subspace of all possible hypotheses that have the form of a decision or regression tree. The resulting leaf is a result of the tree learning algorithm's choice among the many hypotheses involved. This choice by the algorithm already aimed at optimizing the chances of the statistical test to succeed. This violates a basic assumption of the test – namely that what is tested is a single hypothesis defined prior to collecting observations, and not to test whether a significant hypothesis exists among the many hypotheses considered. A way to compensate for this multiplicity of hypotheses would be, to use the Bonferroni correction. This however requires at least the knowledge of the number of competing hypotheses among which the learner selected the final tree. This number is, however, not provided by decision tree learning algorithms and it is not easy to estimate.

HOW FINDINGS MAY HELP TO IMPROVE DECISION MAKING

Relative absence of scientific and analytical research of processes in Slovenian public administration, is the main reason why their performance is spontaneous and decision making is often mainly political and aimed to serve the employees, not the clients (Pečar, 2002).

Data mining and machine learning results from this research may benefit managerial decision making in several ways, both on the macro and micro levels. The processes of management on the macro level include mainly tasks of political decision making (law, policy, strategy, etc.). Major such process is legislature, for which are responsible: the Parliament, political parties, and the Government, mostly the Ministry of Public administration and Ministry of finance. These groups of decision makers need to know more about performance measurement as an important vehicle for New Public Management (Hood 1998, Hood & Peters 2004). On this basis, they should promote policies to develop performance measuring systems for better decision making

not only in administrative districts, but in public services in general.

Many findings in this paper can directly benefit the processes of decision making of administrative districts in:

- Human resource management
- Strategic planning
- Operational planning
- Performance management

Useful Findings Concerning Inputs of Administrative Processes

The optimal amount of applications. The number of applications (new and unsolved) has very significant correlation with productivity. To attain the highest productivity (cost of basic service between 50 and 120 EUR, there have to be more than 176 new applications per year per employee, or more than 243 new and unsolved applications together per year per employee.

Education of employees. Higher level of education is generally in correlation with higher productivity, except for the anomaly where the group with the highest education shows below average productivity. This pattern of behavior should be further analyzed. A new hypothesis has emerged: that those with higher education feel that their job is more secure and the absence of a measuring system additionally lowers their motivation.

Gender. Gender has a small influence on productivity. In our data, an optimal percentage of males in the structure of employees are between 6 and 24%.

Age. Influence of age on productivity is small, up to 10%. In our data, there is an indication of an optimal average age in the range from 39 to 42 years.

Useful Findings about the Performance of Processes

Productivity standards, performance measurement. The old administrative statistics in Slovenia neglected the huge differences between various administrative services. This research presents the first effort to classify time standards for various services, as a necessary precondition for measuring productivity. The time standards (productivity) for various services were previously unknown. Productivity is influenced significantly by the number of new applications and unsolved ones from the previous year "orders".

The size of administrative districts. The size of an administrative district also influences the productivity. Productivity increases with the size, with the exception of the largest districts, where productivity slightly falls. According to our data, an optimal size of administrative district is between 21.000 to 43.000 inhabitants.

Time of processing: from receiving an application to mailing the decision. Data on »through-put« was available only in 3 intervals – within 1 month, between 1 to 2 months, and more than 2 months. The average processing time in the four year period analyzed was more stable than productivity. Nearly half of administrative districts solved 67% or more cases within one month, but their productivity varied significantly. The time of processing (through-put) is not necessarily in correlation with productivity.

Motivation for employees. 25% of administrative districts reported to practice stimulative pay (the law allows only 3% share of wages as stimulative pay). Considering this information as a binary attribute, the machine learning analysis did not find this attribute to influence productivity. Only two administrative districts measure individuals' productivity with their own standards. Overall, stimulation is small and shows no influence on productivity.

Useful Findings about Outputs of Processes

Solved cases. The rate of solved cases is in strong correlation with the trend of "orders". Higher numbers of denied cases is in slight relation with higher productivity.

Decisions overturned. Our data indicates that higher productivity does not produce more decisions which can be overturned on a higher level of decision making. Thus there was no correlation detected between productivity and decisions overturned.

Testing Current Hypotheses

At the beginning of this research, three hypotheses were set. Concerning these hypotheses we can conclude the following:

Hypothesis 1: Administrative districts have very different efficiency (productivity) of work processes. This hypothesis was proven correct. Organizational efficiency (productivity) of administrative districts varies extremely, up to the ratio of 1: 10.

Hypothesis 2: The level of employees' education has major influence on efficiency. The research findings show general positive influence of higher level of education on increased productivity, but an interesting behavioral pattern was found, where the highest (above average) level of education often lowers the productivity. Here the additional hypothesis evolves (and should be explored further) – that higher educated employees feel their job is more secure than those of lower educated ones, and fully exploit this advantage.

Hypothesis 3: The increased number of applications results in longer time for processing. The analysis proved this hypothesis to be wrong. The administrative districts with highest numbers of applications per employee show the highest level of productivity and often highest share of cases solved within one month (throughput).

CONCLUDING REMARKS, FUTURE TRENDS AND SUGGESTED RESEARCH

The early expert opinion of production time for administrative services from the administrative districts proved to be way off – by almost a factor of 3 (exactly by 2,466). This adds the prevailing conclusion that the understanding of the work processes in administrative districts is very weak. The findings of this research attracted the attention of the ministries and support for further research was given. The next step was to define the standard time values for most of 350 various administration services provided by administrative districts. The government also passed a law, that every public organization must monitor the efficiency (productivity) and this should be important for promotions and stimulative pay.

Also the methodology of administrative statistics was changed. By first trial of computerized analyses of all production data for 9-month period in 2006, the results showed a similar situation as in this preliminary research. Different productivity was found in all departments. The computerized analyses made possible to track also the productivity of individuals. These differences naturally exceeded organizational ones by far. The government officials than decided not to reveal all the data, but to track the results of analyses in longer period and at the same time look for the solutions of workers mobility from one district to another. However the study had a positive effect on the awareness of public managers and policy makers.

The use of data mining has proven its benefits and should become an essential part of many future decision support systems not only in private, but also in public sector. Its main benefits are demonstrated in quick analysis and diagnosis of multivariable situations, and detection of more or less hidden behavior patterns.

A prerequisite for using such data mining tools is well organized data bases of comprehensive measurements. This way data mining and machine learning (as an increasingly important managerial tool) can significantly add new value to the generic task – decision making in areas of strategic planning and performance management.

REFERENCES

Asbjorn, R. (1995). *Performance Management*. Boca Raton, FL: Chapman & Hall.

Breiman, L., Friedman, J. H., Olshen, R. A., & Stone, C. J. (1984). *Classification and Regression Trees*. Belmont, CA: Wadsforth International Group.

Demšar, J., Zupan, B., & Leban, G. (2004). *Orange: From Experimental Machine Learning to Interactive Data Mining*. White Paper (www.ailab.si/orange), Faculty of Computer and Information Science, University of Ljubljana, Slovenia.

Hood, C. (1998). *The Art of State*. Oxford, UK: Oxford University Press.

Hood, C., & Peters, G. (2004). The Middle Aging of New Public Management: Into the Age of Paradox? *Journal of Public Administration: Research and Theory, 14*(3), 267–282. doi:10.1093/jopart/muh019

Karalić, A. (1991). *Regression tree inductive system – Retis*. Ljubljana, Slovenia: Faculty of Computer and Information Science.

Leban, G., Zupan, B., Vidmar, G., & Bratko, I. (2006). VizRank: data visualization guided by machine learning. *Data Mining and Knowledge Discovery, 13*(2), 119–136. doi:10.1007/s10618-005-0031-5

Ministry of International affairs of the Republic of Slovenia (1996-1999). *Annual reports of Administrative statistics*, Slovenia.

Mitchell, T. M. (1997). *Machine Learning*. Boston: McGraw-Hill.

Mozina, M., Demsar, J., Zabkar, J., & Bratko, I. (2006). Why is rule learning optimistic and how to correct it. *Lecture Notes in Compututer Sc. (ECML '06)*, pp. 330-340. Berlin: Springer.

Pečar, Z. (2002). *A model of Assessing the Efficiency of Work Processes in Public Administration Using Some Methods of Artificial Intelligence*. PhD thesis, Kranj, Faculty of Management Sc.

Weiss, S. M., & Kulikowski, C. A. (1991). *Computer Systems that Learn*. San Francisco: Morgan Kaufmann.

Witten, I., & Frank, E. (2005). *Data Mining: Practical Machine Learning Tools and Techniques* (2nd ed.). Amsterdam: Elsevier.

KEY TERMS AND DEFINITIONS

Public Administration: Public administrative bodies at different levels of government, in this study – administrative districts (orig. "Upravne enote")

Administrative Services: Services provided by public administration, in our case different permits upon application.

Basic Unit of Administrative Services: The least time consuming administrative service, used in the study as basic unit (for expressing time values by ratios for all other administrative services).

Performance Management: Managerial task of monitoring, understanding and improving performance of workers.

Productivity Analysis: Studying relations between outputs – amount of administrative services produced, and inputs – working hours used (and other resources); often expressed in costs of producing a unit of output.

Data Mining: Discovering regularities, or knowledge, from typically large sets of data using techniques such as machine learning

Machine Learning: An area of artificial intelligence concerned with methods that enable computers to improve their performance by learning from experience, or data; an important aspect of this, central to this paper, is the capability of machine learning methods to discover general laws from data

Induction of Regression Trees: A machine learning technique for extracting from data a (non-linear) dependence between a numerical "target" variable and other variables in the system

Chapter 5
Productivity Analysis of Public Services:
An Application of Data Mining

Aki Jääskeläinen
Tampere University of Technology, Finland

Paula Kujansivu
Tampere University of Technology, Finland

Jaani Väisänen
Tampere University of Technology, Finland

ABSTRACT

Productivity is a key success factor in any organization. In order to improve productivity, it is necessary to understand how various factors affect it. The previous research has mainly focused on productivity analysis at macro level (e.g. nations) or in private companies. Instead, there is a lack of knowledge about productivity drivers in public service organizations. This study aims to scrutinize the role of various operational (micro level) factors in improving public service productivity. In particular, this study focuses on child day care services. First, the drivers of productivity are identified in light of the existing literature and of the results of workshop discussions. Second, the drivers most conducive to high productivity and the specific driver combinations associated with high productivity are defined by applying methods of data mining. The empirical data includes information on 239 day care centers of the City of Helsinki, Finland. According to the data mining results, the factors most conducive to high productivity are the following: proper use of employee resources, efficient utilization of premises, high employee competence, large size of day care centers, and customers with little need for additional support.

INTRODUCTION

Productivity improvement is high on the agenda in many public organizations. It is necessary to improve the productivity of public services in order to satisfy increasing demand with limited resources. Productivity is commonly regarded as an organization's key success factor. On the level of national economy, productivity improvement has been linked to many economic and social phenomena, such as economic growth and high standard of living (Miller, 1984;

DOI: 10.4018/978-1-60566-906-9.ch005

Sink, 1983). Research in various disciplines typically applies different approaches in productivity studies, for instance, national economists are more interested in macro level perspectives, whereas researchers of industrial management and business economics typically examine productivity at micro level (Käpylä et al., 2008).

Productivity is a traditional research topic on which there is a rich body of literature. In a recent Finnish study examining the current status of productivity research, it was concluded that the effects of various factors on productivity are verified too rarely (Käpylä et al., 2008). Productivity effects are often studied at macro level, e.g. national level (e.g. Lambsdorff, 2003; Skans, 2008). In order to improve productivity by managerial means, the drivers of productivity must be identified. These drivers can be utilized for different purposes, such as identifying development targets. Many initiatives of productivity improvement have proven to be inefficient and have met with resistance among employees due to the implementation of harsh decisions (e.g. job cuts) as the only means to improve productivity. However, many different factors may in practice affect productivity. These factors should somehow be connected to micro level organizational operations in order to identify concrete development targets (e.g. improving the division of labor).

The understanding of the role and the significance of various productivity drivers is still in its infancy. This study seeks to establish what role various managerial (micro level) factors play in improving public service productivity. In this study, productivity improvement is examined from the point of view of service provides. The research questions are the following:

- What are the drivers of productivity?
- Which drivers are best related to high productivity?
- Which specific driver combinations are associated with high productivity?

In particular, this study focuses on child day care services. The first question is answered in light of the literature and the results of workshop discussions. The second and third questions are examined by applying data mining methods. Since the specific productivity driver combinations are beforehand unknown, data mining methods will provide a relatively easy way of gaining insight into the relationships between these various drivers. The empirical data includes information on 239 municipal day care centers of the City of Helsinki, Finland.

First, we summarize the relevant literature on the productivity of public services in general. Then follows a discussion of factors contributing to productivity specifically in child day care services. The data and measures used in this study are presented with a brief description of the data analysis methods used. Finally, the results of the empirical examination are reported. In addition, conclusions (including the contribution and limitations of the study and future research suggestions) are presented at the end of this chapter.

ASSUMED DRIVERS OF PRODUCTIVITY

Literature on Productivity of Public Services

Productivity is traditionally defined as the ratio between output (e.g. the quantity of services produced) and input (e.g. the number of employees needed for such production) (Sink, 1983). This definition is interpreted slightly differently in different research disciplines. According to Pritchard (1995), all commonly used productivity definitions can be classified into one of three categories:

- The economist/engineer approach, where productivity is seen as an efficiency measure (outputs/inputs)

- The approach where efficiency (outputs/inputs) and effectiveness (outputs/goals) are evaluated simultaneously
- The broad approach, which comprises everything enabling an organization to function better.

The wider approach, including both efficiency and effectiveness, is in its meaning quite close to the concept of performance (e.g. Kaydos, 1999). The service productivity literature has opted for a wider examination of productivity by underlining factors such as the quality of service (Sahay, 2005), utilization of service capacity (Grönroos & Ojasalo, 2004) and the role of customers in service provision (Martin et al., 2001). In the context of public services, productivity has been related to the cost-efficiency and quality of services (Faucett & Kleiner, 1994; Hodgkinson, 1999). Several theoretical models of service productivity can be found (Grönroos & Ojasalo, 2004; Johnston & Jones, 2004; Parasuraman, 2002).

A typical feature of services is that they cannot be stored (Grönroos, 1984). Services are often consumed simultaneously with their production. Therefore, the poor quality of services can hardly be concealed. Numerous studies have been conducted on the connections between quality, productivity and profitability. Conflicting thoughts have been voiced on the issue (He et al., 2007; Huff et al., 1996). According to Reichheld and Sasser (1990), reducing defects means greater loyalty, which is related to productivity in service companies. High customer satisfaction (which can be assumed to indicate high quality) reduces the need for resources since there will be less reworking, returns and complaints (Huff et al., 1996; Westlund & Löthgren, 2000). On the other hand, it can be argued that increasing customer satisfaction means more work and costs, thereby reducing productivity. This is a common view in economics, for instance. (Anderson et al., 1997) It seems that the role of quality in productivity is dependent on how the productivity concept is understood. If the wider approach related to efficiency and effectiveness is applied, poor quality will obviously mean a decline in productivity. According to Anderson et al. (1997), productivity and customer satisfaction are positively related to profitability in any industry. Based on their results they also concluded that simultaneous attempts to improve productivity and customer satisfaction while pursuing better profitability are more difficult in services than in manufacturing operations. In other words, increasing productivity may decrease customer satisfaction and vice versa. The results of the research by He et al. (2007) corroborated this. They concluded that service companies need to strike a balance between productivity and customer satisfaction improvements in order to achieve optimal profitability.

While the role of employees in the provision of services is often visible to the customers, factors such as employee satisfaction and employee turnover may affect service outputs. Appelbaum et al. (2005) identified a positive link between low employee satisfaction and low productivity. According to the study by Westlund and Löthgren (2000), employee satisfaction has a positive impact on customer satisfaction as well as on productivity. Many factors possibly causing decrease in productivity have been linked to employee turnover. It has been estimated that it takes at least a year before a new employee has adapted to a new task and realized his/her productivity potential (Kransdorff, 1995). When an employee is lost for some reason, it takes an average of four years to replace competence losses (Hall, 1992). Costs may be generated through numerous factors (e.g. interruption in work processes, recruitment and training) (Dess & Shaw, 2001; Sutherland, 2002).

The competence of employees may also be a factor affecting productivity. According to the resource-based view of a firm, the internal resources of an organization such as competencies determine the success of the organization (Penrose, 1995). A connection has been established between proper human resource management practices and improved productivity (Delaney & Huselid, 1996; Xu et al., 2006). However, the positive impact of competence improvement on productivity is not straight-forward. Even though it has been estimated that an investment in intellectual capital (includes also other intangible resources in addition to competence) can yield twice the benefit compared to a similar investment in a physical asset (Abernethy & Wyatt, 2003), the findings of a study by Väisänen et al. (2007) suggest that investments in intellectual capital have a positive impact on productivity only in the long-term.

Factors related to capacity utilization are fundamental to productivity examination since they are directly linked with the output/input ratio. The efficient utilization of service provision resources is demanding, since inputs may not adapt directly to the fluctuation in demand (Sahay, 2005). One essential factor behind resource utilization appears to be linked to employee absenteeism. If sickness absences could be reduced it would be possible to compensate for the labour shortage caused by the rapid aging of the workforce in many industrialized countries (Böckerman & Ilmakunnas, 2008). According to Miller et al. (2008), there is only limited literature on the impact of employee absenteeism on productivity. They studied the impact in schools and identified that teacher absences reduce productivity by having a negative effect on students' grades. The effect of absenteeism on productivity has also been studied by Allen (1983). He suggested that productivity effects depend on the job: if it is difficult to find replacement workers or to reassign workers from other positions, the productivity effects are more severe.

It is a characteristic of service production that customers are often active participants. Consequently, a customer may affect productivity (positively or negatively) (Ojasalo, 2003). Customer involvement also causes variation in service provision, and it may therefore be difficult to standardize service outputs (McLaughlin & Coffey, 1990). A service providing unit with customers urgently needing special services may

need more inputs for providing certain standard outputs (e.g. the number of provided care days).

In light of the literature the following factors may be summarized to have an effect on public service productivity: quality, customer satisfaction, employee satisfaction, employee turnover, employee competence, capacity utilization, absences of employees and customers. In addition to the studies examining the factors affecting productivity, there is a lot of research on those factors without the productivity link, but focusing on the relationships between different productivity drivers. Some key findings of these studies are now briefly presented.

Several factors may affect service quality. According to Xu et al. (2006), attention must be paid to employee competence to ensure the desired level of quality performance as perceived by customers. Employee turnover has also been studied in relation to quality. Low employee satisfaction has frequently been mentioned as a key factor causing resignations (see e.g. Hom & Kinicki, 2001; Lum et al., 1998). In the study by Hurley and Estelami (2007), it was found that employee turnover predicts customer satisfaction as effectively as employee satisfaction. High employee turnover may cause loss of experienced employees and established customer relationships which, in turn, may be detrimental to the customer.

Many factors have been linked to employee absenteeism. There is evidence that job dissatisfaction increases sickness absences (Brown & Sessions, 1996; Farrell & Stamm, 1988). Böckerman and Ilmakunnas (2008) found evidence that adverse working conditions are linked with job dissatisfaction which, in turn, is related to sickness absences. They also concluded that improvement of working conditions is an essential way to reduce sickness absences. According to a study by Lehtonen (2007), educational activities and competence development may help in improving employee satisfaction. In the study by Steel and Rentsch (1995), it was found that high educational level indicates lower level of absenteeism. They also stated that good employee commitment is linked to fewer sickness absences. Lehtonen (2007) also identified a link between high educational level and small number of sickness absences. This may be because assignments requiring high education are more challenging and compelling. People may well work even when they are sick.

Productivity Drivers of Child Day Care Services – Workshop Discussions

Child day care centers account for a large proportion of the costs of public services in Finland. For example, at the Social Services Department of the City of Helsinki they account for around one fifth of the total costs. Therefore, it can be argued that the understanding of factors affecting productivity in the context of child care is relevant from the perspective of national economy. From the perspective of the Social Services Department there was a clear managerial need to gain deeper understanding on productivity drivers and their role in improving productivity. This would provide better understanding on the performance measures used – what is the role and relevance of different measures in managing productivity. This would also guide in planning the way the services are provided – what kind of units are ideal for proving the services. Initially, there were understanding and presumptions on these issues but a lack of knowledge based on the in-depth analysis of various quantitative measures. From the point of view of research on data mining, child day care services were a suitable context. They have by far the highest unit volume in the service production of the Social Services Department. The large number of units providing similar services offers rich empirical data for the research setting of this paper.

The productivity drivers and their assumed relationships in child care services were identified by combining the results of the literature review (see above) with knowledge obtained through workshops. Three representatives of child day care services and two employees from the financial department were involved in three workshops held in spring 2007. In addition, one of the authors participated in the workshops as a facilitator. The purpose of these workshops was to identify factors affecting productivity in order to support the productivity improvement of child day care services. This research setting made it possible to utilize the knowledge and long experience of the personnel working in the organization studied.

In practice, different productivity drivers identified through the review of the literature were presented and evaluated in the context of child day care. All the discussions were documented for research purposes. As a result, a figure representing the drivers of productivity and their relationships was drawn. On the basis of this work the model for productivity drivers in child day care services was constructed (see Figure 1). It is used as a framework for the empirical part of this study.

Figure 1 includes both direct and indirect drivers of productivity. Employee resources, the utilization of premises and additional support need are examples of factors assumed to directly affect the level of productivity. Indirect productivity drivers may affect productivity but only through another productivity driver. Employee satisfaction and the absences of children are examples of the indirect productivity drivers in the model.

RESEARCH METHODS

Data and Measures

The empirical data was gathered from the City of Helsinki, Finland. More specifically, this study focuses on municipal child day care services. The child day care services are classical services with close interaction between a service provider and a customer. This means that the provision of services is very employee-intensive. Since employees are the key input resources, it is necessary to pay at-

Figure 1. Assumed drivers of productivity and their relationships

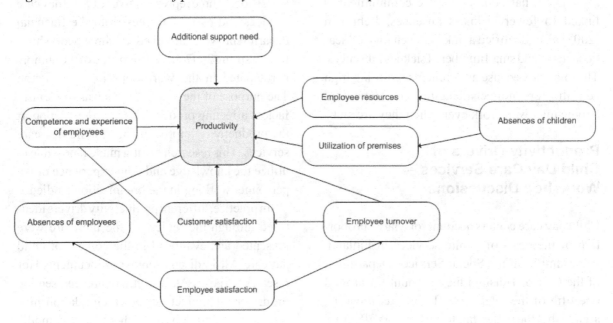

tention to human resources management. There are both educational and caring professionals working in day care centers. In general, the employees in the centers are very experienced – more than 2/3 of employees have worked more than 10 years. Another relevant characteristic of child day care relates to the actual service process. Even though customers (both children and their parents) have clearly an impact on the provision of services, the service process is rather standard – in general there is a low level of customization that depends on a child.

There are 17 day care district in the Helsinki region, with a total of 279 day care centers. The empirical data used in this study excludes Swedish language day care centers (31 centers). This was because they are typically smaller and constitute a separate entity. In addition, nine centers providing 24-hour services were excluded, because they are quite different in terms of costs and personnel structure compared to typical day care centers. Finally, information for the years 2006 and 2007 related to 239 day care centers was taken for examination.

The measures used in this study are summarized in Table 1. The main reason for choosing these measures for the factors identified previously (see Figure 1) is that they were already widely used in the day care services of the City of Helsinki. Thus, they were considered cost efficient. It was not considered reasonable to take new measurements for the purposes of this study, for example, due to the tight time schedule and limited human resources. However, due to the foregoing, some of the factors identified (i.e. employee satisfaction and employee turnover) could not be included in the empirical examination, because the authors were unable to obtain such data from the day care management. In addition, most of the information required needed some modification and manual work from both the representatives of day care management and the authors before it was suitable for analysis. Finally, the data included in the study contains eight possible drivers of productivity. The measures used in this study are discussed more thoroughly in the following.

Productivity is measured by the average cost of calculated care day. The measure is calculated

Table 1. Measures for productivity and proposed drivers of productivity

Measurement objective	Measure
Productivity	Cost of calculated care day (€)
Customer satisfaction	Customer satisfaction according to a survey (scale 1–5)
Absences of employees	Percentage of days lost through sickness (%)
Employee satisfaction	–
Employee turnover	–
Employees' working experience	Percentage of employees worked less than 10 year within the day care center (%)
Employee's competence	Employee competence according to welfare survey
Utilization of premises	Degree of utilization of premises (%)
Employee resources	Number of children per number of employees (ratio)
Absences of children	Percentage of days lost through sickness per child (%)
Additional support need	Percentage of S2 children (%)

as follows: total costs divided by the number of calculated days of care (the content of which is defined by regulation). The weighting of the output is dependent on the age of the children, likewise the need for special care services. The information needed was taken from two different data sources. Total costs were taken from the AdeEko data system, and the number of days from the Effica/DW data system. The information is calculated monthly at day care center level. Moving average values are used. It should be noted that a high measurement result indicates low productivity and vice versa. The *customer satisfaction* measure is based on a customer satisfaction survey. The survey includes 12 questions, answered on a Likert scale 1–5. The questionnaire is intended for the parents of all children in day care in Helsinki. Data is collected at a day care center level every second year. Thus, in this study, the average result describing customer satisfaction with the respective day care centers was used. Moreover, the information on customer satisfaction in 2006 was also used for 2007.

The *absences of employees* is measured as an average percentage of days lost through sickness in a year. The measure is calculated as follows: the number of sickness days divided by the total number of working days (during a year). Person-

nel having more than 60 days a year lost through sickness were excluded from this study. This is the maximum number of sickness days (in a year) during which an employee continues to receive full salary. The information used in this study describes sickness absences at day care center level in 2006 and 2007 and is available in the Hijat information system data base.

The data needed for *employees' working experience* is available in the Hijat information system data base. It was decided to use the percentage of employees who have worked less than 10 years in the day care center as a measure for working experience. The information is available at day care center level for both years. The measure for *employees' competence* is based on a working welfare questionnaire. One of the main components of the questionnaire focuses on the competence of employees (5 questions). Each employee estimates his or her own competence using a Likert scale 1–5. The average values of day care centers (calculated according to the individual responses) were used in this study for both 2006 and 2007. However, the day care centers with fewer than five responses were excluded.

The *utilization of premises* is simply measured by the degree of utilization of premises, more specifically by dividing the number of children by the places available. The exact result is calculated as an average degree per month. However, June and July are excluded from the examination as these months are typically holiday periods and do not represent the usual situation. The information is available in the Effica/DW data system. The number of children per number of employees was used as a measure for the utilization of *employee resources*. The information is provided by the Effica/DW data system and calculated every month at the level of day care centers.

The *absences of children* is measured by the percentage of days lost through sickness per child. This information is gathered at day care center level monthly and held in the Effica/DW data system. In this study, the average percentage of the year is used. *Additional support need* is measured using the percentage of S2 children. S2 children refer to the children who do not speak Finnish or Swedish (the official native languages) as their first language and receive teaching of Finnish language. This information is not embedded in the calculated day of care discussed above. An average percentage per year is calculated in each day care center. The information is available at the Effica/DW data system.

In addition to the variable described above, the data used in this study includes three other variables: first, a variable referring to the division of the day care center (a division may include one or more centers), second, a variable referring to the region of the day care center (a region may include one or more divisions) and, third, a variable describing the size of the day care center (measured by the number of calculated places at the end of the year).

Analysis Methods

The data were examined using various data mining methods to ensure that the proper productivity drivers are identified. For directed data mining methods (see e.g. Kudyba & Hoptroff, 2001) the obvious output variable is productivity itself.

Prior to the data mining process, an exploratory data analysis was performed to gain insight into the distribution shapes of the variables as well as possible outliers and relationships within the data.

The data mining tasks were carried out by SAS Enterprise Miner tool. The data mining tools used in this study included decision trees and cluster analysis (see e.g. Giudici, 2004). Decision trees gave the authors insight into which productivity drivers are best related to high productivity. Additionally, tree models form the structure of the model from the actual data itself, rather than having a researcher specifying it *a priori*. Tree models recursively divide a set of n statistical units according to a chosen division rule intended to maximize the homogeneity of the response variable. At each step of the tree model, the procedure splits the observations according to the variable that best explains the target variable (Giudici, 2004, p. 100, Han & Kamber, 2006; Hand et al., 2001), which in this case is productivity. Additionally, performing cluster analysis on the whole data served to reveal a set of clusters where productivity is high, along with the drivers that are associated to that specific cluster. Cluster analysis aims to find a set of groups where observations within groups are as homogenous as possible, i.e. finding which observations in a data set are similar (Aldenderfer & Blashfield, 1984; Romesburg, 2004). In this case, we wanted to find out whether day care centers with high productivity have some other factors in common.

The main motivation for such techniques in this study was the relatively easy interpretation of both techniques. The tree models are commonly depicted as tree-like diagrams with the contents of each data subset clearly defined. This makes the results more usable for the any interested audience – e.g. the day care center managers – that may not have a strong background in statistics or data mining.

In this study, only the direct linkages between various drivers and productivity were examined. Thus, indirect effects (e.g. absences of children

Table 2. Summary statistics

Measure	Year	Mean	Std Dev.	Min	Max	N
Cost of calculated care day (€)	2006	46.59	4.32	39.23	74.82	238
	2007	48.13	5.70	38.03	102.40	239
Customer satisfaction according to a survey	2006	4.21	0.10	3.81	4.44	239
Percentage of days lost through sickness (%)	2006	3.16	1.59	0.14	12.54	237
	2007	4.09	1.49	0.90	8.80	239
Percentage of employees having worked less than 10 years within the day care center (%)	2006	27.75	17.55	0.00	88.89	237
	2007	28.99	17.66	0.00	100.00	236
Employee competence according to welfare survey	2006	3.84	0.32	2.69	4.66	213
	2007	3.80	0.41	2.91	4.49	138
Degree of utilization of premises (%)	2006	91.05	14.08	43.50	170.50	231
	2007	95.70	15.35	44.00	200.00	239
Percentage of days lost through sickness per child (%)	2006	4.23	0.98	1.60	10.50	237
	2007	4.17	0.83	2.10	7.00	239
Number of children per number of employees (ratio)	2006	4.59	0.46	2.24	6.32	237
	2007	4.60	0.48	2.10	6.40	239
Percentage of S2 children (%)	2006	11.36	10.12	0.00	47.70	237
	2007	12.05	10.42	0.00	46.50	239

– utilization of premises – productivity) were not included.

RESULTS

Description of the Data

Table 2 contains descriptive information related to the productivity measure and the eight possible productivity drivers. The size of the day care center varies from 21 places to 147 places in the year 2006; the corresponding figures being 21 and 154 in the year 2007.

Before analyzing the relationship between productivity and various drivers, it is essential to understand how productivity differs in the day care centers included in the study. In Figure 2 and Figure 3 the distributions of the productivity measure for 2006 and 2007 are presented.

Visual examination reveals the existence of extreme positive outliers in the productivity data for both 2006 and 2007 samples. Since we used tree models and clustering it is recommended to remove such outliers from the data (Giudici, 2004). The MAD (Median Absolute Deviation) procedure was used to filter out any outliers from the data set (for more information on MAD, please refer to Pearson, 2005). Since the data set is rather small compared to many other data mining sets, a moderate factor of 9 deviations from the median was chosen. After the filter outliers procedure the Distributions for productivity look as presented in Figure 4 and Figure 5.

Even though there still seem to be some unusually high observations in the 2007 productivity variable, no more filtering was done to ensure a suitable amount of observations for analyses.

Data Mining Results

First, we applied a decision tree model to both 2006 and 2007 datasets with measured productivity as a target variable. Several tree structures were

Figure 2. Distribution of productivity in 2006

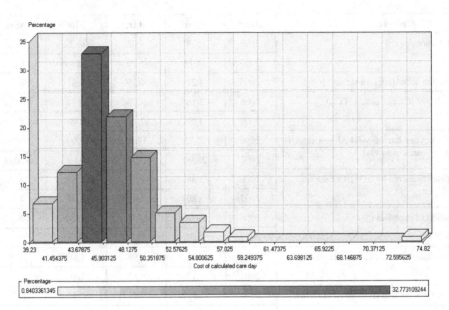

Figure 3. Distribution of productivity in 2007

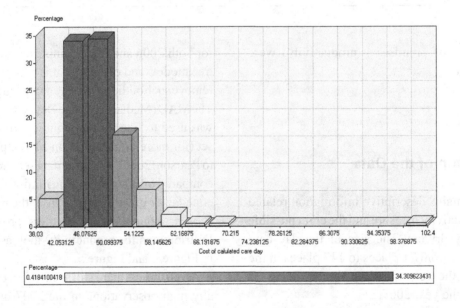

tested before the final result with the following criteria: (a) only binary splits were allowed to maintain the readability of the tree, as well as allowing a suitable amount of observations per leaf; (b) a minimum of 20 observations per leaf

was determined. Figure 6 presents the selected tree model for the 2006 sample.

In 2006, the most differentiating factor is the number of children per single employee with higher number yielding better productivity. Additionally, employee competence has an impact

Figure 4. Distribution of productivity in 2006 after the MAD procedure

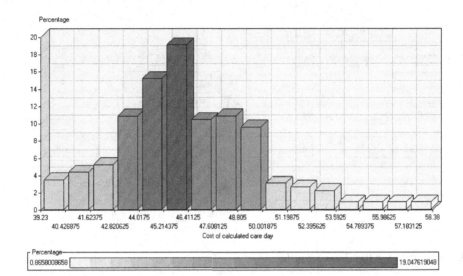

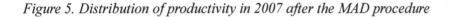

Figure 5. Distribution of productivity in 2007 after the MAD procedure

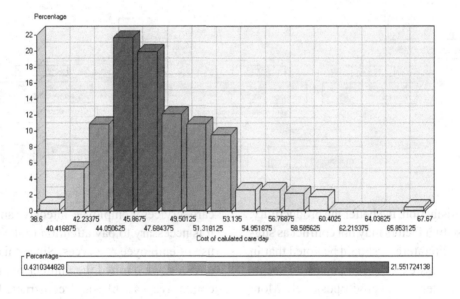

on productivity, but even if the employee competence is high, the benefits are not fully realized, if the utilization of premises is not high as well. With less competent personnel, smaller improvements in productivity are seen in centers with fewer S2 children. Correspondingly, Figure 7 presents the selected tree model for the 2007 data set.

As in 2006, in 2007 the single most decisive factor in differentiating the productivity of a random day care center is the number of children per employee; the higher the number, the better the productivity. Furthermore, large day care centers seem to be more productive than smaller ones, most probably due to economies of scale. Even in large day care centers the higher the

Figure 6. Decision tree for the 2006 sample

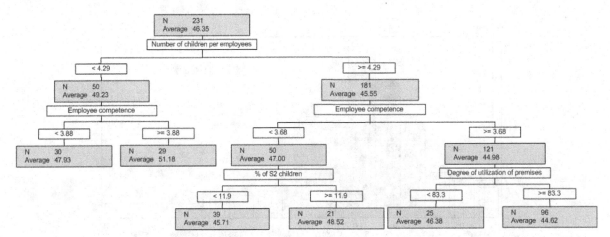

Figure 7. Decision tree for the 2007 sample

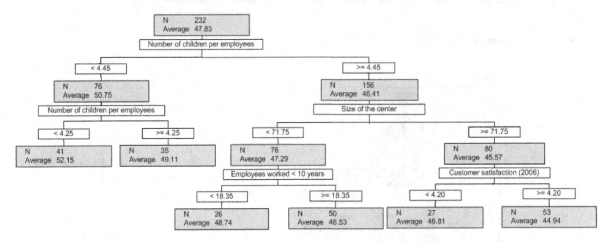

customer satisfaction, the better the productivity. Hence, these two factors may not conflict as suggested in the literature. It should be noted that in small centers less experienced personnel seems to affect the center's productivity positively. More experience may mean more costs since salaries tend to rise over the career. However, long experience does not necessarily increase the outputs.

To sum up, in both 2006 and 2007 samples the number of children per employees (i.e. the measure of employee resources) has the greatest impact on productivity. This makes sense, as the main amount of costs to the day care center accrues from employee salaries. The provision of day

care services is employee-intensive and therefore it is necessary to pay attention to the productive use of employee resources. Since this should be obvious, we omitted the number of children per employees variable, and constructed the same decision trees as before. Figure 8 presents the tree for the 2006 sample and Figure 9 presents the tree for the 2007 sample.

When the number of children per employees variable was removed from the tree, the utilization of premises rose out as the single most determining factor affecting productivity in 2006. Afterwards the number of S2 children becomes important with smaller number of S2 children yielding

Figure 8. Decision tree for the 2006 sample with the number of children per employees variable removed

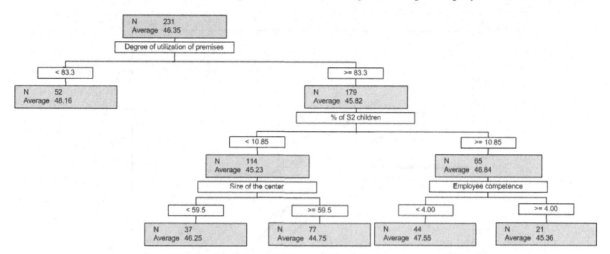

Figure 9. Decision tree for the 2007 sample with the number of children per employees variable removed

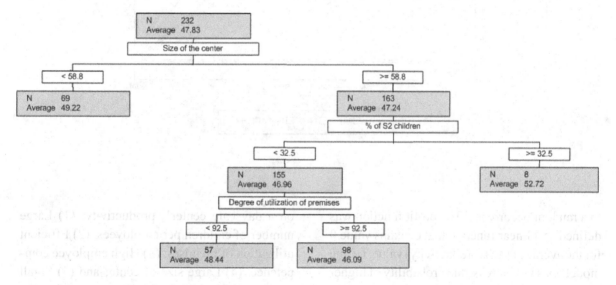

better productivity. Still, even with the smaller number of S2 children, smaller day care centers do not seem to be any more productive that the average day care center in the sample. On the other hand, if the number of S2 children is large, competent personnel may provide some additional productivity. This is an understandable result since competent personnel are needed to take care of children needing extra support.

In the 2007 sample the size of the day care center is the most discriminating factor in deter-

mining the centers' productivity. Similar to the 2006 sample, the number of S2 children has an effect on productivity here as well.

This study was set out to find the specific factors that affect productivity rather than concentrating on the actual fiscal amounts. To assess the accuracy of the models, SAS Enterprise Miner allows the user to assign a profit function to each of the obtained models (see e.g. Matignon, 2005). The main idea behind the assessment was not to compare the models between each other but rather

Figure 10. Cumulative profit functions for all four tree models with zero baselines

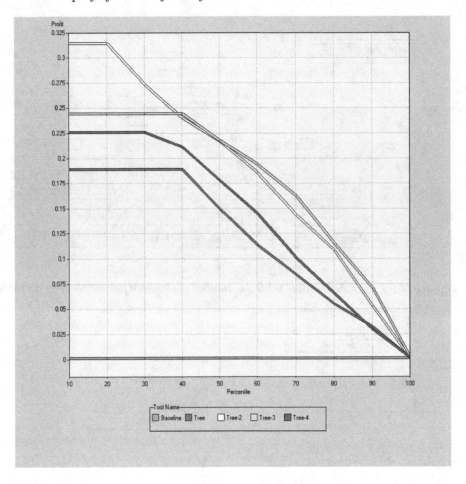

to a random occurrence. The profit function was defined as a linear function that contains value 0 for the average target (productivity) value, i.e. the model does not increase the probability of higher than average productivity. For the maximum productivity occurring in each of the samples, the profit function contains value 1. As can be seen from Figure 10, for the first three deciles, the cumulative profit values for all the models ranged between values 0.188 and 0.272 (random guess would give us the value 0). This implies that our models return better than average productivities, and can be used to extract factors affecting productivity.

In summary, the tree models clearly suggest that the following items have positive influence on a day care center's productivity: (1) Large number of children per employees; (2) Efficient utilization of premises; (3) High employee competence, (4) Large size of center and (5) Small number of S2 children. Measures related to the use of employee resources and the utilization of premises could have been used as alternative measures of productivity since they are clearly linked to output/input ratio. Therefore, it is natural that they are strongly linked to productivity. It seems to be more efficient to provide services in large centers. The need for high employee competence makes sense, likewise the small number of S2 children. More inputs are needed in providing services for S2 children. However,

Figure 11. Input means plot for the 2006 sample

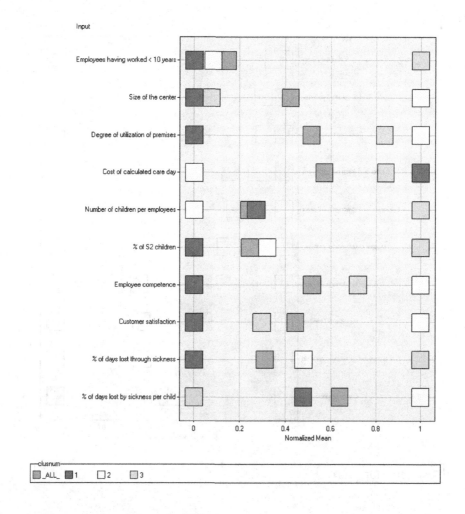

these inputs do not have an effect on the output of the measure used in this study.

To gain more insight into how the day care centers in the sample differ from each other, a cluster analysis was performed on both samples. Because of the small number of observations available, and for easier interpration of the results, three clusters were used. Cluster analysis does not predict the behavior of any variable, nor does it classify other variables according to the values of others, but rather describes the similarities of values within the data set. This is used to find similarities between those day care centers with high productivity.

The input means plots for both 2006 and 2007 samples are presented in Figure 11 and Figure 12, respectively. The input means plots rank the normalized input means for each variable in each cluster relative to the overall input means. This way we can easily spot any clusters that are associated with higher than average productivity.

In the 2006 data only one cluster (Cluster 2) has a smaller than average cost per day. By examining cluster 2 more closely, we can extract factors associated with that factor. The input means plot presents the clusters, and the normalized factor the means associated with each cluster.

The analysis shows, that day care centers in Cluster 2:

Figure 12. Input means plot for the 2007 sample

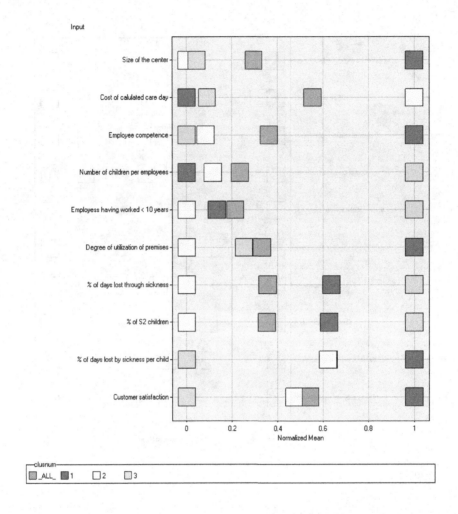

- have average personnel experience
- are larger than average
- utilize the premises well
- have lower than average number of children per employees
- have approximately average amount of S2 children
- have highly competent personnel
- rank very well in customer satisfaction survey
- have slightly more personnel sick days than average
- have more children sick days than average.

It is not surprising that large day care centers seem to be more productive than smaller ones due to economies of scale. The utilization of premises is in the core of productivity phenomenon and it was assumed to have a positive impact on productivity. A slight surprise is that it is not necessary to have many children per employee in order to achieve high productivity.

Cluster analysis in the 2007 sample revealed two clusters with above average productivity (Clusters 1 and 3). Interestingly, in Cluster 1, the size of the day care center is well above average and in Cluster 3 below average. Since the variables in the input means plot are listed in order of importance, and since the tree models suggested that large day care centers are more productive, we classified the clusters as "small productive day care centers" (Cluster 3) and "large productive day care centers" (Cluster 1).

According to the results presented in Figure 12, small productive day care centers (Cluster 3):

- *have less than average competent personnel*
- *have very high number of children per employees*
- *have less experienced personnel*
- *utilize the premises as average*
- *have high number of personnel sick days*
- *have high number of S2 children*
- *have very low number of children sick days*
- *score lower than average in customer satisfaction surveys.*

In small day care centers, there seem to be a need for high number of children per employee in order to achieve high productivity. Employees with high level of competence or long working experience are not necessities. In addition, small productive day care centers appear to require a small number of children's sicknesses. It is necessary to have all the children present in order to utilize the resources well in striving for the maximum number of outputs.

Instead, large productive day care centers (Cluster 1):

- have highly competent personnel
- have lower than average number of children per employees
- have approximately average experienced personnel
- have very intensively utilized premises
- have a large amount of personnel sick days (not as high as small productive day care centers)
- have a large number of S2 children (not as many as small productive day care centers)

- have greater than average number of children sick days
- score higher than average in customer satisfaction surveys.

Large productive day care centers seem to have highly competent personnel with average experience. These units are productive even if they do not have many children per employee. However, the utilization of premises needs to be high. A rather surprising result in light of the existing literature is that large productive day care centers (and small units too) do not need to have a small number of personnel sickness days.

CONCLUSION

This study provided answers to the three questions posed. First, a literature review and knowledge obtained through workshops were used to arrive at a theoretical framework presenting the assumed drivers of productivity. The framework was used as a basis for the empirical examination. Second, a large data sample was used in the examination of the linkages between assumed drivers and productivity. Both decision trees and cluster analysis were applied. According to the results, the drivers that are most closely related to high productivity are the following: proper use of employee resources, efficient utilization of premises, high employee competence and customers with little need for additional support. In addition, the large size of centers seems to have a positive impact on productivity. Third, this study failed to provide a clear answer to the question: which specific driver combinations are associated to higher productivity? Instead, the cluster analysis revealed that various driver combinations may contribute to high productivity in the day care center. According to the results, it is easier to achieve high productivity in large day care centers. Hence, productivity may be high even if there are not many children per employee. In light of this, it can be argued that productivity could be improved in a more human way by paying attention on the size of day care centers. Interestingly, customer satisfaction seems to be higher in large and productive day care centers. A surprising result of this study is that productivity can be high even if there are many sickness absences among employees.

Prior research has paid a lot of attention to productivity improvement and measurement. However, there is a lack of knowledge about productivity drivers. In addition, most of the productivity research has focused on the macro level examination or the context of traditional (e.g. manufacturing) companies. This study contributes to productivity research by providing new knowledge about the drivers of productivity in the context of public services. The results help to better understand the phenomenon and various factors related to it. The results of this study rely on a large amount of empirical data. To the best of the authors' knowledge, this type of data has not earlier been used in service productivity research. The information may also be useful in practice. The managers of child day care services can utilize the results when investing in productivity improvement. The development work can be targeted at the right factors, i.e. drivers best related to high productivity.

Also it should be noted that not all the productivity affecting factors (e.g. center size and customer structure) may be controlled by day care center managers but by higher level managers and the politicians. The impacts of the improvements may be substantial. Due to the large number of service providing units, small improvements in the right factors may yield substantial savings of public money. If the cost of care day could be reduced by one or two euros in every municipal day care center of the City of Helsinki, yearly savings of several million euros could be achieved. Furthermore, this study demonstrates that data mining could well be a practical and useful method for analyzing and managing productivity in various public organizations. However, this requires that

an organization already uses measures and surveys rather extensively. In addition, there have to be high number of organizational units that use the similar set of measures in order to have sample size large enough.

There are some issues that should be considered when interpreting the results of this study. First, some criticism can be made regarding the measures used. Measures were not available for all the potential drivers of productivity. In addition, the validity of the measures is not optimal. Validity refers to the extent to which a test measures what a researcher wishes to measure (e.g. Emory, 1985, p. 94). We chose to use measures that were available, not the most valid ones. For example, the measure for productivity does not include all output aspects. Especially factors related to the quality of service are not very well captured by the measure. On the other hand, the practicality (cost vs. benefits) of the measures is high. It is not untypical that indirect measures have poor validity but can provide some information regarding an important phenomenon that otherwise could not be described at all (Lönnqvist 2004, 96). Second, the empirical data does not provide the most typical data mining research setting, because the size of the sample was not very large. On the other hand, the sample actually includes the whole population (typical day care centers at Helsinki Region). Contextual issues depending on the region should not affect the results of this study. The main purpose was not to generalize the results, but to understand the phenomenon in this specific context. However, the results may also be useful for other public service organizations (e.g. elderly care). There are similarities between different public services since they all need many personnel with close contact to clients. In light of the findings of this study, it seems that in improving productivity of these kinds of services it is necessary to focus on utilizing service providing capacity, managing human resources and anticipating the needs of different customers. It is also necessary to pay attention to the size of service providing units. It should also be noted that high customer satisfaction (an indicator of service quality) is not necessarily in conflict with high productivity.

This study represents a small attempt to understand productivity and various productivity drivers in the context of public service organizations. More research is needed. Many issues were excluded from the scope of this study. First, the study explored the direct linkages between different productivity drivers and productivity. However, the indirect relationships were not taken into account. To be able to understand the phenomenon more profoundly, these complicated relationships need to be analyzed. Second, this study did not take into account the possible time lag between drivers and productivity. Thus, an important topic for further analysis is the examination of a longer period of time. For example, adding the results for 2008 would allow an examination of a three-year period. Third, this study was based quantitative data and statistical methods. More detailed information on the productive day care center is valuable. Hence, a fruitful avenue for further research is in-depth case studies (e.g. interviews) in high productivity organizations. Fourth, this study only used data on one region (a large municipal organization). It would be interesting to carry out the same analysis in the context of other similar organizations. The characteristics of different organizations and regions may have an effect on the role of different productivity drivers.

ACKNOWLEDGMENT

This study was carried out as a part of a larger research project, the aim of which is to design new productivity measures for the City of Helsinki, Finland. The authors are grateful to the representatives of the organization for their input and efforts in providing the data needed in this study. The authors also acknowledge the financial support by the Finnish Work Environment Fund and the City of Helsinki.

REFERENCES

Abernethy, M., & Wyatt, A. (2003). *Study on the measurement of intangible assets and associated reporting practices*. Prepared for the European Communities Enterprise Directorate General.

Aldendefrer, M., & Blasfield, R. (1984). *Cluster Analysis*. London: SAGE.

Allen, S. G. (1983). How much does absenteeism cost? *The Journal of Human Resources*, *18*(3), 379–393. doi:10.2307/145207

Anderson, E. W., Fornell, C., & Rust, R. T. (1997). Consumer satisfaction, productivity, and profitability: differences between goods and services. *Marketing Science*, *16*(2), 311–329. doi:10.1287/mksc.16.2.129

Appelbaum, S., Adam, J., Javeri, N., Lessard, M., Lion, J. P., Simard, M., & Sorbo, S. (2005). A case study analysis of the impact of satisfaction and organizational citizenship on productivity. *Management Research News*, *28*(5), 1–26. doi:10.1108/01409170510629023

Böckerman, P., & Ilmakunnas, P. (2008). Interaction of working conditions, job satisfaction, and sickness absences: evidence from a representative sample of employees. *Social Science & Medicine*, *67*(4), 520–528. doi:10.1016/j.socscimed.2008.04.008

Brown, S., & Sessions, J. G. (1996). The economics of absence: theory and evidence. *Journal of Economic Surveys*, *10*(1), 23–53. doi:10.1111/j.1467-6419.1996.tb00002.x

Delaney, J., & Huselid, M. (1996). The impact of human resource management practices on perceptions of organizational performance. *Academy of Management Journal*, *39*(4), 949–969. doi:10.2307/256718

Dess, G. G., & Shaw, J. D. (2001). Voluntary turnover, social capital and organizational performance. *Academy of Management Review, 26*(3), 446–456. doi:10.2307/259187

Emory, C. W. (1985). *Business research methods* (3rd ed.). Homewood, Illinois: Irvin.

Farrell, D., & Stamm, C. L. (1988). Meta-analysis of the correlates of employee absence. *Human Relations, 41*(3), 211–227. doi:10.1177/001872678804100302

Faucett, A., & Kleiner, B. H. (1994). New developments in performance measures of public programmes. *International Journal of Public Sector Management, 7*(3), 63–70. doi:10.1108/09513559410061768

Giudici, P. (2004). *Applied data mining: statistical methods for business and industry.* Chichester, UK: John Wiley & Sons.

Grönroos, C. (1984). A service quality model and its marketing implications. *European Journal of Marketing, 18*(4), 36–44. doi:10.1108/EUM0000000004784

Grönroos, C., & Ojasalo, K. (2004). Service productivity: towards a conceptualization of the transformation of inputs into economic results in services. *Journal of Business Research, 57*(4), 414–423. doi:10.1016/S0148-2963(02)00275-8

Hall, R. (1992). The strategic analysis of intangible resources. *Strategic Management Journal, 13*(2), 135–144. doi:10.1002/smj.4250130205

Han, J., & Kamber, M. (2006). *Data mining: concepts and Techniques.* San Francisco: Morgan Kaufmann.

Hand, D., Mannila, H., & Smyth, P. (2001). *Principles of Data Mining.* Cambridge, MA: MIT Press.

He, Y.-Q., Chan, L.-K., & Wu, M.-L. (2007). Balancing productivity and consumer satisfaction for profitability: statistical and fuzzy regression analysis. *European Journal of Operational Research, 176*(1), 252–263. doi:10.1016/j.ejor.2005.06.050

Hodgkinson, A. (1999). Productivity measurement and enterprise bargaining – the local government perspective. *International Journal of Public Sector Management, 12*(6), 470–481. doi:10.1108/09513559910301342

Hom, P. W., & Kinicki, A. J. (2001). Toward a greater understanding of how dissatisfaction drives employee turnover. *Academy of Management Journal, 44*(5), 975–987. doi:10.2307/3069441

Huff, L., Fornell, C., & Anderson, E. W. (1996). Quality and productivity: contradictory and complementary. *Quality Management Journal, 4*(1), 22–39.

Hurley, R. F., & Estelami, H. (2007). An exploratory study of employee turnover indicators as predictors of customer satisfaction. *Journal of Services Marketing, 21*(3), 186–199. doi:10.1108/08876040710746543

Johnston, R., & Jones, P. (2004). Service productivity. towards understanding the relationship between operational and customer productivity. *International Journal of Productivity and Performance Management, 53*(3), 201–213. doi:10.1108/17410400410523756

Käpylä, J., Jääskeläinen, A., Seppänen, S., Vuolle, M., & Lönnqvist, A. (2008). *Tuottavuuden kehittäminen Suomessa: haasteet ja tutkimustarpeet.* Helsinki, Finland: Finnish Work Environment Fund. (In Finnish)

Kaydos, W. (1999). *Operational performance measurement: increasing total productivity.* Delray Beach, FL: St. Lucie Press.

Kransdorff, A. (1995). Exit interviews as an induction tool. *Management Development Review*, *8*(2), 37–40. doi:10.1108/09622519510084260

Kudyba, S., & Hoptroff, R. (2001). *Data mining and business intelligence: a guide to productivity*. Hershey, PA: Idea Group Publishing.

Lambsdorff, J. G. (2003). How corruption affects productivity. *Kyklos*, *56*(4), 457–474. doi:10.1046/j.0023-5962.2003.00233.x

Lehtonen, V.-M. (2007). Henkilöstöjohtamisen tehostaminen valtionhallinnossa henkilöstötilinpäätösinformaation avulla – empiirinen tutkimus Suomen valtionhallinnossa tuotettavan henkilöstötilinpäätösinformaation arvosta johtamisessa. Helsinki, Finland: Svenska handelshögskolan. (In Finnish)

Lönnqvist, A. (2004). *Measurement of intangible success factors: case studies on the design, implementation and use of measures*. Tampere, Finland: Tampere University of Technology.

Lum, L., Kervin, J., Clark, K., Reid, F., & Sirola, W. (1998). Explaining nurse turnover intent: job satisfaction, pay satisfaction or organizational commitment? *Journal of Organizational Behavior*, *19*(3), 305–320. doi:10.1002/(SICI)1099-1379(199805)19:3<305::AID-JOB843>3.0.CO;2-N

Martin, C. R., Horne, D. A., & Chan, W. S. (2001). A perspective on client productivity in business-to-business consulting services. *International Journal of Service Industry Management*, *12*(2), 137–157.

Matignon, R. (2005). *Neural Network Modeling Using SAS Enterprise Miner*. Bloomington, IN: AuthorHouse.

McLaughlin, C. P., & Coffey, S. (1990). Measuring productivity in services. *International Journal of Service Industry Management*, *1*(1), 46–64. doi:10.1108/09564239010002847

Miller, D. M. (1984). Profitability = productivity + price recovery. *Harvard Business Review*, *62*(3), 145–153.

Miller, R. T., Murnane, R. J., & Willett, J. B. (2008). Do worker absences affect productivity? The case of teachers. *International Labour Review*, *147*(1), 71–89. doi:10.1111/j.1564-913X.2008.00024.x

Ojasalo, K. (2003). Customer influence on service productivity. *S.A.M. Advanced Management Journal*, *68*(3), 14–19.

Parasuraman, A. (2002). Service quality and productivity: a synergistic perspective. *Managing Service Quality*, *12*(1), 6–9. doi:10.1108/096045202104

Pearson, R. (2005). *Mining imperfect data: dealing with contamination and incomplete records*. SIAM.

Penrose, E. (1995). *The theory of the growth of the firm*. Oxford, UK: Oxford University Press. doi:10.1093/0198289774.001.0001

Pritchard, R. D. (1995). *Productivity measurement and improvement: organizational case studies*. Westport, CT: Praeger Publishers.

Reihheld, F. F., & Sasser, W. E. (1990). Zero defections: quality comes to services. *Harvard Business Review*, *68*(5), 105–111.

Romesburg, C. (2004). *Cluster analysis for researchers*. Raleigh, NC: Lulu.

Sahay, B. S. (2005). Multi-factor productivity measurement model for service organization. *International Journal of Productivity and Performance Measurement*, *54*(1), 7–22. doi:10.1108/17410400510571419

Sink, D. S. (1983). Much ado about productivity: where do we go from here. *Industrial Engineering (American Institute of Industrial Engineers)*, *15*(10), 36–48.

Skans, O. N. (2008). How does the age structure affect regional productivity? *Applied Economics Letters*, *15*(10), 787–790. doi:10.1080/13504850600749123

Steel, R. P., & Rentsch, J. R. (1995). Influence of cumulation strategies on the long-range prediction of absenteeism. *Academy of Management Journal*, *38*(6), 1616–1634. doi:10.2307/256846

Sutherland, J. (2002). Job-to-job turnover and job-to-non-employment movement – a case study investigation. *Personnel Review*, *31*(6), 710–721. doi:10.1108/00483480210445980

Väisänen, J., Kujansivu, P., & Lönnqvist, A. (2007). Effects of intellectual capital Investments on productivity and profitability. *International Journal of Learning and Intellectual Capital*, *4*(4), 377–391. doi:10.1504/IJLIC.2007.016334

Westlund, A., & Löthgren, M. (2001). The interactions between quality, productivity and economic performance: the case of Swedish pharmacies. *Total Quality Management*, *12*(3), 385–396. doi:10.1080/09544120120034528

Xu, K., Jayaram, J., & Xu, M. (2006). The effects of customer contact on conformance quality and productivity in Chinese service firms. *International Journal of Quality & Reliability Management*, *23*(4), 367–389. doi:10.1108/02656710610657585

KEY TERMS AND DEFINITIONS

Driver: Productivity drivers relate to different factors having an effect on the level of productivity.

Measure: Measures are used to provide relevant, quantitative information for managerial purposes.

Productivity: Productivity refers to the ratio between output and input used to produce the output.

Productivity Management: Productivity management refers to various managerial activities which aim to improve productivity.

Public Service: Public services include various functions like social care, health care and education that are organized by central and local government and funded with tax revenues.

Section 2
Data Mining as Privacy, Security and Retention of Data and Knowledge

Chapter 6

Perceptions of Students on Location-Based Privacy and Security with Mobile Computing Technology

John C. Molluzzo
Pace University, USA

James P. Lawler
Pace University, USA

Pascale Vandepeutte
University of Mons-Hainaut, Belgium

ABSTRACT

Mobile computing is a maturing technology with benefits for consumers. The purpose of this chapter is to furnish research on the perceptions of non-information systems students in both America and Europe on the impact of mobile computing devices on privacy and security. The chapter expands upon earlier research on only the perceptions of information systems students in America on mobile computing privacy and security. This research indicates a higher level of knowledge of the features of mobile computing, but lower levels of knowledge of inherent issues of mobile computing and consumer privacy and of precaution with mobile computing devices. Findings imply an inadequacy in general curriculum, and especially in data mining curriculum, but also an opportunity to improve the curricula. This research will benefit educators attempting to improve their pedagogy with syllabi summarized in the chapter that integrates contemporary issues of privacy and security with mobile computing technology.

INTRODUCTION

The authors of the chapter describe the benefits of mobile computing devices for both American and European consumers in the context of location-based services. They discuss the benefits of location-based services as constrained by the challenge of concerns of privacy and security with the devices. The data mining of information on consumers by business firms and by governments, as consumers interact

DOI: 10.4018/978-1-60566-906-9.ch006

and transact with location-based services on organizational and governmental applications on the devices, is a concern cited by the authors in this chapter, consistent with the theme of the Handbook.

The focus of the chapter is on the findings of the authors on perceptions of privacy and security of location-based services. The findings are from a survey of European and American students who were proxy for consumers of mobile computing. From the findings, the authors furnish a foundation for integrating location-based privacy and security into data mining and general curricula of schools for undergraduate and graduate students who are the current and future consumers of mobile computing, so that privacy and security might be perceived as critical facets of pervasive computing in society, a perception that might not be evident in the curricula pedagogy of schools.

The objectives of the chapter are to discuss the benefits and concerns of location-based services with mobile computing devices, the perceptions of privacy and security of the devices by proxy students, and the proposed solutions and trends with mobile computing devices and services that might be integrated into curricula of schools. The research in this chapter is important to the field, because curricula of schools might not be current with organizational and governmental practices of data mining that impact, if not intrude on, privacy and security of mobile computing technology. The research helps educators by informing them of the perceptions of non-information systems students who might not be as knowledgeable of privacy and security threats as information systems students.

The Appendix following the chapter will be especially helpful to instructors considering syllabi of privacy regulation and security of mobile computing technology.

BACKGROUND

Mobile computing applications on mobile computing devices (MCDs), such as cellular phones, laptops, personal digital assistants (PDAs), tablets, and other devices, are advancing in beneficial features for consumers. Browsing information and news, game playing, instant messaging, personal and professional e-mailing, and photo and text messaging are frequent features on the devices (M: Metrics Inc., 2006). These devices have advanced from basic cellular phones and PDAs to light computing devices interfaced to the Internet with information-rich and location-based or enabled services. Innovations in mobile computing have advanced from cellular payment systems to high speed networks in Europe, which is considered further along in the development of the devices than in America (Lundquist, March, 2007). Mobile computing with location-enabled services is considered by pundits as *the* killer application (Lundquist, April, 2007) and *the* technical trend of 2007 integral to consumers (Castells et al., 2007). Miniature mobile computing is contributing to a new period of pervasive computing (Denne, 2007).

Data mining involves searching and finding hidden patterns in large databases of mostly public data to generate profiles based on personal data and behavior patterns of citizens and consumers (Tavani, 2004). Data mining analysis methods evaluate the potential of current customer profiles in order to facilitate future customer prospecting and sales. Much of the data that is mined today is either public or semi-public – our supermarket purchases, surfing habits, salary, location, and other such information. The main ethical issues in data mining are that consumers are not generally aware their data is being gathered, do not know the uses to which the data will be made, or have not consented to the use of such data.

Presently, in the United States, there are limited legal restrictions on the use of personal data for data mining. Other than the protection of healthcare data under the 1996 Health Insurance Portability and Accountability Act (HIPPA), financial data under the 1999 Gram-Leach-Bliley Act, or the protection of children while on-line under the Children's Online Privacy Protection

Act (COPPA), there are no federal laws that protect data mined by firms and organizations. On the other hand, the European Union's European Directive 95/46/EC strictly controls the gathering and use of private data by firms and organizations operating within the European Union (European Directive 95/46/EC, 1995).

Location-based privacy is the freedom to limit control of one's whereabouts. This concept is derived from the notions of *accessibility* privacy (knowing one's location can be construed as a type of intrusion) and *informational* privacy (one's location can be construed as private information). Location data gathered from cell phone and other GPS enabled devices are not clearly protected by either United States federal law or European Union legislation (Molluzzo & Lawler, 2007). Where one is located and when are not the only things that can be inferred from geographic positioning system (GPS) data. Studies by Eagle and Pentland (2006) and others have indicated that diverse social patterns for individuals and groups, such as when one leaves home for work, when one leaves work for home, when one plans a circle of friends, and so on, can be inferred from cell-phone data. This process has become known as *reality mining*.

CONCERNS AND ISSUES

The benefits of location-based services are coupled, however, with concerns about control of personal and private information on the mobile devices and by perception of frequent incidents on the devices of likely identity theft and intrusion on the privacy of consumers (Grossman, 2007). Privacy activists, such as the Electronic Privacy Information Center and the European Commission, cite fundamental issues in the mismanagement, marketing and mining of information on consumers. They cite issues in the monitoring of consumers by business and carrier firms and by governments from information retained from

interactions or transactions (Eggen, 2006). The monitoring is increased in the field of collective intelligence that is integrating information from mobile computing devices and from the Internet. This level of monitoring might enable further decreased expectation of privacy, in an increased Big Brother environment more Orwellian than the level of data mining, if collective intelligence is misused by governments or by business firms.

Issues may include employee monitoring (Hamblen, 2007). RFID is not infrequently considered by pundits and researchers as synonymous with surveillance (Curtin et al. 2007). Further issues include networks and systems behind the services that might be hacked by intruders, phishers, spammers and stalkers (Brandt, 2006) but not disclosed by firms when they learn of the hacking. Firms might lose mobile devices having information on customers because of internal loss or theft (Pratt, 2007). Firms might lose customers because of this (Romano & Fjermestad, 2007). Clearly the benefits of location-enabled services can be considered paltry when contrasted with issues on privacy and security (Stross, 2006).

The impact of the concerns on location-based services may eventually hinder the deployment of mobile computing in the marketplace and in society. Concerns of access of information or of location beyond the carrier, firm or government and beyond known collaborators in the absence of the knowledge of consumers are considerations in the design of location-enabled services on governmental and organizational applications. Consumers continue to have concerns about information interacted on the Internet (Sraeel, April, 2007). Consumers may not have confidence in the privacy and security of location services on their mobile computing devices or in regulation already considered by legislators to not include MCDs (Hines, 2007). The lack of confidence may impede pervasive computing as a trend if improved control of information and of privacy is not implemented in the field by information systems practitioners.

RESEARCH AND SOLUTIONS

This chapter introduces a framework for practitioners and instructors in integrating issues of location-related privacy with mobile computing, so that pervasive computing continues in society to be a bona fide trend.

In 2007 research (Molluzzo & Lawler 2007), the authors analyzed the knowledge of undergraduate and graduate *information system students* of the impact of mobile computing on location-based privacy. In this chapter, the research is extended to *non-information systems undergraduate students*, in the United States and in Europe. Both non-information systems and information systems populations are Generation Y, Millennial or Net Generation students under the age of 28, but are effectively knowledgeable consumers of mobile computing devices to be proxy in exploratory research and in initial study of consumers in society. The extension of the research to non-information systems students is important to the field, inasmuch as information systems students may be more experienced on factors of privacy and security because of their potential further knowledge of the technology. Such experience may be different, if not less, with non-information systems students and inevitably limiting in the knowledge of these students in privacy and security and in technology, which might argue that pedagogy be improved in schools of universities educating non-information students on contemporary issues of technology.

The survey was administered on-line to students at Pace University in the United States in November, 2007. These students were mostly first and second year undergraduates taking an introductory computing course that is required of all students at the university. In the spring of 2007, the survey was administered to the European students, all of whom were undergraduate business majors at the University of Mons, Belgium, using hard-copy. There were 75 completed United States surveys and 19 completed European surveys. The survey instructions asked the respondents to limit their responses to their experience using mobile computing devices (MCDs), excluding dedicated audio devices, such as the iPod. The survey was administered anonymously – the respondents' names were not collected by the authors.

The survey was divided into several sections:

- Background Questions to gather demographic data;
- Objective Questions on the importance of using mobile devices for various purposes;
- Knowledge Questions on respondent awareness of the privacy issues of location-based data collection;
- Concern and Control Questions about the protection of consumer privacy by government and wireless providers; and
- Summary Question to gauge the respondents' overall concern for privacy.

These questions were based on and were equivalent essentially to those in the 2007 survey (Molluzzo & Lawler, 2007).

BACKGROUND QUESTIONS

Of the European students, 13 were female and 6 were male; of the United States students, 49 were female (65%) and 26 (35%) were male students, which is close to the general Pace University population of approximately 60% female and 40% male students. The academic majors of the United States students were varied: business (48%), liberal arts (13%), computing (8%), nursing (4%), and other (27%), which again reflects the general Pace University undergraduate population of students. The European students were all business majors. The average age of the United States students was 19, while the average age of European students was 22. European students reported using their mobile devices for an average of 6 hours per day. United States students reported using their mobile devices on average for 7 hours per day.

Table 1. Frequency of use (percents)

Use	Frequently or Very Frequently
Games	10
Emergency	35
Search	60
Media	63
Business/School	69
Social Contacts	83

Table 2. Use of MCD Features (percents)

Use	Frequently or Very Frequently
E-Banking	16
Driving Directions	19
Destination Guides	29
Photo/Video Sharing	33
Weather	34
Instant Messaging	61
E-Mail	65
Text Messaging	76

For the below analysis, European and United States groups of students were asked the following questions:

Objective Questions

The survey attempted to discern how students use their MCDs. Therefore, objective questions were asked regarding the respondents use of MCDs.

Frequency of Use: Respondents were asked to "rate how frequently you use your Mobile Computing Device" and for what reasons. The answers were based on a five-point Likert scale. Each entry in the table, see Table 1, is a percent of those answering the question either "Frequently" or "Very Frequently. The most frequently used service is for Social Contacts with Business/School not far behind it. The lowest used service was for Games.

Use of Location-Enabled features of MCD: Respondents were asked to "rate the frequency with which you use the location-enabled features of your mobile computing device." The answers were based on a five-point Likert scale. Table 2 indicates the percent of respondents answering "Frequently" or "Very Frequently". The least used features were driving directions and e-banking, possibly because of the low average age of the students. Also, possibly because of the low average age of the students, texting was the most frequently used feature, with e-mail and instant messaging following.

Private Information: Respondents were asked "What private information do you store on your mobile computing device(s)?" A list of possible data was presented. Although some personal information is inevitably stored on a MCD, it is interesting to note that some respondents save highly confidential data on their MCD. For example, three people (out of the 75 United States students) store their social security numbers, five people store unencrypted account passwords, three people store credit card numbers, and five store bank account numbers.

Knowledge Questions

Privacy: The respondents were asked several questions that rate their knowledge about various privacy concerns using MCDs. The answers were based on a five-point Likert scale. The only statement with which a majority of respondents "Agree" or "Strongly Agree" (55%) is that a "location-based mobile computing device can monitor your exact location." Even this number is very low considering that GPS technology is constantly in the news. Table 3 indicates the results. It is very interesting that such large percentages of students do not consider wireless Internet access (53%) and GPS systems (64%) as possible threats to their privacy.

Table 3. Privacy (percents)

Question	Agree or Strongly Agree
GPS Can Intrude on Privacy	36
MCD Location Data Can Be Marketed to Other Firms	46
Wireless Internet Access Can Intrude on Privacy	47
Email Can Intrude on Privacy	48
Provider Can Monitor Exact Location	55

Table 4. Wireless provider policies (percents)

Question	No
Was your MCD ever misplaced or stolen?	68
Do you know what your provider will do if your information in compromised?	74
Have you expressly Opted-out on your mobile contract?	78
Do you know the procedure your provider uses to safeguard your personal information?	80
Do you read the privacy policies before signing the contract?	100

Wireless Provider Policies: The respondents were asked several questions on their relationship with their wireless provider. These were Yes - No questions. The respondents' answers here are in line with the Privacy questions in Table 3, which indicate a low degree of awareness of important privacy issues when using MCDs. This set of questions indicates a high degree of complacency and lack of knowledge among the respondents regarding the actual privacy policies of their mobile carriers. For example, 100% do not read their carrier's privacy policy; and 74% do not know what their provider will do if their information is compromised. The results are indicated in Table 4, where numbers represent percents who answered No to the questions.

Table 5. Trust and advertising (percents)

Question	Agree or Strongly Agree
I like the idea of mobile advertising messages.	7
I like the idea of mobile advertising if the advertising is meaningfully personalized to me.	15
I am concerned about location-based privacy when using my MCD.	25
I am comfortable that my provider will protect my privacy.	30
I am confident that government regulations will protect my privacy.	34
I am concerned about identity theft.	56

Concern and Control Questions

Trust and Advertising: The respondents were asked to "rate their level of agreement with the given statement." The answers were based on a five-point Likert scale. See Table 5. Respondents show mistrust that their provider (30% Agree or Completely Agree) or the government (34% Agree or Completely Agree) will protect their privacy. A fairly low percentage, 56%, either Agree or Completely Agree that they are concerned about identity theft. Interestingly, however, only 25% Agree or Completely Agree that they are concerned about location-based privacy. It seems the respondents do not yet consider location-based data to be personal information.

Mobile advertising did not get a strong vote of confidence from the respondents. Only 7% of the respondents either Agree or Strongly Agree that they would like mobile advertising messages. Even if the advertising were targeted and personalized, only 15% of the respondents Agree or Strongly Agree. Both results speak to a lack of trust among students of Internet and mobile-based advertising.

Protecting Your Mobile Device: The respondents were asked how they protect their mobile device? They were provided with a list and were asked to check all that apply. Not many respondents encrypt data on their MCD. Only 12% encrypt all data, 10% encrypt all business-related data, and 11% encrypt all sensitive data. Also, only 17% use encryption when connected to a wireless network. However, 44% lock access to their MCD using a strong password, and 32% set the MCD to auto-lock when not in use for a specified time. Many respondents, 62%, keep their MCD hidden when traveling, but only 29% do not access private or business data in public places. Finally, only 30% of respondents remove all data on their MCD before discarding or turning it in.

Summary Question: Respondents were asked "which of the following statements best describes your feelings about privacy?": I feel strongly about privacy (41%); I feel strongly about privacy but may benefit from surrendering my privacy at times if my privacy is not abused by a firm or service (54%); and I do not feel strongly about privacy (5%).

These questions are based on categorization of subjects into *privacy fundamentalists* (first question), *privacy pragmatists* (second question), and *privacy unconcerned* (third question) from extant field research (Westin, 1996). In a Harris poll conducted in 2003 (Taylor, 2003), the percentage of respondents in the three categories were 26%, 64% and 10%. The distribution from our results was 41%, 54% and 5%. This indicates that our population of students might be more informed about privacy issues than the general population, or in the intervening four years the general population has been made more aware of privacy issues.

It is to be noted that the only students who do not feel strongly about privacy were from Europe. Only two European students out of 19 students (10.5%) consider themselves privacy fundamentalists as compared to 41% of students in the United States. This could be a result of the fairly strict privacy laws of the European Union, as defined in Directive 95/46/EC (European Directive 95/46/EC, 1995).

This research also attempted to determine whether there are significant differences between

the 77 information systems students from the research in 2007 (Molluzzo & Lawler, 2007) and the non-information systems students from the present research. To determine if there were such differences, a chi-squared test for independence was determined to be suitable. Many of the questions in the survey utilized a 5-point Likert scale. However, the small sample sizes made the chi-squared test for significant differences using the five Likert categories unusable. Therefore, the 5-point scale was compressed in the study. The three lowest Likert scores (Strongly Disagree, Disagree, and Neutral) were converted to 0 and the two highest (Agree and Strongly Agree) were converted to 1. This enabled use of the chi-squared test for independence on 2x2 tables, which did yield valid results. It is to be noted that all significance measures are for two-sided p-values.

Information Systems vs. Non-Information Systems Students

MCD Use: There were statistically significant differences between information systems and non-information systems students at the $p < .001$ level of significance in three of the uses of their MCD devices. These uses were for emergency, storing digital media, and e-banking, as indicated in Table 6.

Non-information systems students tend to use the social functions of their MCDs more than computing students. For instant messaging, text messaging, contacting family and friends there were significant differences in use at the $p < .001$ level. For social contact uses there was a significant difference at the $p < .01$ level.

There were also some significant differences in what students store on their MCDs. There is a difference at the $p < .001$ level of significance in storing their age and storing their school name. There is a difference at the $p < .01$ level in storing their place of employment.

In all the above cases, except for use in emergencies, non-information systems students tend

Table 6. Significant differences in uses between computing and non-computing students

Use	p <.001	p <.01	p <.05
Emergency	***		
Storing Digital Media	***		
E-banking	***		
Instant messaging	***		
Texting	***		
Contacting Family and Friends	***		
Social Contacts		**	
Storing User's Age	***		
Storing User's School Name	***		
Storing User's Place of Employment		**	

Table 7. Significant differences in privacy awareness between computing and non-computing students

Question	p <.001	p <.01	p <.05
Wireless Access can intrude on Privacy	***		
GPS Can Intrude on Privacy	***		
I am Concerned About Identity Theft	***		
MCD's Can Monitor My Exact Location			*
I Like the Idea of Mobile Advertising			*

Table 8. Significant differences in control questions between computing and non-computing students

Question	p <.001	p <.01	p <.05
Encrypt All Data Stored on MCD			*
Encrypt All Sensitive Data Stored on MCD	***		
Encrypt All Business Data Stored on MCD		**	
Use Encryption When Connecting to a Wireless Network	***		
Remove All Data Stored on MCD Before Discarding or Handing In			*

to use their MCDs for the reasons indicated more than information systems students. These uses, such as storing digital media, using MCDs for social contacts and storing personally identifiable information, such as age and place of employment, indicate that non-information systems students are more apt to use their MCDs for social reasons.

Privacy Awareness: There was a significant difference between information systems and non-information systems students in the awareness of how MCDs can affect privacy, as indicated in Table 7. Information systems students were significantly more aware (at the p <.001 level) that wireless access and GPS services can intrude on privacy. Non-information systems students were also significantly more concerned about identity theft (at the p <.001 level.) There was also a difference at the p <.05 level in the knowledge that an MCD can monitor your exact location.

Mobile Advertising: The only question related to wireless provider in which there was a significant difference between information systems and non-information systems students at the p <.05 level was whether they like the idea of mobile advertising, as indicated in Table 7. Non-

information systems students seem to like the idea more.

Control Questions: There were also significant differences in the ways the two groups protect their MCDs, as indicated in Table 8. In the use of encryption, either in storing sensitive data or connecting to a wireless network, there were differences at the p <.001 level of significance. Similarly, there was a difference at the p <.01 level in the encryption by the groups of business data on their MCDs. Also there was a difference at the p <.05 level of significance in encrypting all the data on their MCDs. In all the above cases, information systems students were more likely to use encryption. Finally, there was a difference at the p <.05 level of significance in whether the students remove all data on their MCD before discarding the device or returning it to the provider. Once again, information systems students were more likely to remove information from their MCDs.

The differences in results among information systems and non-information systems students show that information systems students are more aware of location-based privacy issues than is the general student population. Clearly the general population needs to be made aware of the privacy and security issues surrounding the use of MCDs. The importance of the present research is that the results indicate that pedagogy needs to be improved in schools of universities educating non-information systems students on issues of privacy and security of technology.

United States vs. European Students

This research further investigated the differences between United States and European students in their use of MCDs. Because of the small sample size of European students (n = 19), only results that were significant at the p <.01 or p <.001 levels, with one exception noted below, are indicated in Table 9. Even in these cases, it is not advisable to make generalizations from the results without caution.

On the use of MCDs for accessing weather, business/school, and family and friends; only one European student in all three categories answered yes (p <.001). The interpretation of this is not clear from the result. Further investigation is necessary in a larger sample of students. Several other MCD use differences were observed at the p <.01 level of significance, such as for emergencies, storing and sharing digital media, and searching. European student use is far less than that of United States students.

Only one other difference at the p <.05 level of significance was observed in the results. That is, European students are not as concerned about

Table 9. Significant differences between U.S. and European students

Uses		p <.001	p <.01	p <.05
	Weather	***		
	Contacting Business or School	***		
	Contacting Family and Friends	***		
	Emergency		**	
	Storing and Sharing Digital Media		**	
	Searching		**	
Concern Question	I Am Concerned About Identity Theft			*

identity theft as are their United States counterparts. This difference could be due to the European Union's stronger privacy laws (European Directive 95/46/EC, 1995).

FUTURE TRENDS

A trend emerging from the research in this chapter is the clear knowledge of information systems students of the fundamental functionality of mobile computing devices compared to a lesser knowledge of these issues by non-information systems majors. The non-information systems students were not as knowledgeable in both the processes and practices of mobile computing firms. These trends imply a likely lower sensitivity of non-information systems students to the larger impact of mobile computing technology on society as compared to information systems students.

Another trend from the research is an inconsistency in the higher knowledge of both groups of students in the processes of location-based mobile computing technology in contrast to lower personal *precaution* with the technology. The students were not as diligent as expected in the confidentiality and protection of information on mobile computing devices, which is not distinct from the inconsistency of non-student subjects in follow-up of intrusions of privacy (Sraeel, May, 2007). Though they felt the generic importance of privacy, the students were not fully protective of their devices through recognized security techniques. This lower diligence in precaution was not an encouraging example for the management of the privacy and security of mobile computing technology. The trends imply a lower sensitivity to the non-technological impact of mobile computing as a societal tool, a theme that continues in the research.

Further trends from the research include the potential opportunity to improve the mobile computing syllabi of information systems and business or non-information systems instructors, in order to mitigate deficiencies in knowledge. The students may learn more of the impact of marketing, mining and business practices that mobile computing firms and retailers might apply from innovations in mobile computing technologies, if schools improved their information systems syllabi. Information systems students may also learn more of privacy and security issues and techniques with mobile technology (Taylor, 2007). Moreover, they may be encouraged as future practitioners and professionals by their instructors to be more sensitive to regulatory and societal themes. These trends imply minimally that an improvement is needed in mobile computing and information systems and business or non-information systems syllabi, which is furnished in the Appendix of this chapter.

Other trends to be elaborated from the research in the chapter include the clear knowledge of the fundamental functionality of mobile computing devices. The information systems students were knowledgeable in the *processes* of mobile computing firms. This knowledge was, however, indicated to be not as clear and to be lower in the probable privacy and security *practices* of the firms. The general student population seems to be much less aware of both the processes and practices of mobile computing firms. These trends imply a likely lower sensitivity to the larger impact of mobile computing technology on society.

A final trend of the research is an inconsistency in the higher knowledge of the information systems students in the processes of location-based mobile computing technology in contrast to lower personal *precaution* with the technology. These students were not as diligent as expected in the confidentiality and protection of information on mobile computing devices, which is not distinct from the inconsistency of non-student subjects in follow-up of intrusions of privacy (Sraeel, May, 2007). Though they felt the generic importance of privacy, the students were not fully protective of their devices through recognized security techniques. This lower diligence in precaution was not an encouraging example for the management of the privacy and security of mobile computing technology. The trends imply a lower sensitivity to the non-technological impact of mobile computing as a societal tool, a theme that continues in this research.

Limitations and Opportunities

The main limitations to the study described in this chapter are the scope and size of the study sample. To make more general conclusions the sample would need to be widened in scope to include the general population, not only college students, and would need to reflect the composition of the general population of MCD users in the United States and Europe. Also, to go beyond the preliminary study of this chapter, the number of subjects involved in the study would have to be increased to the point where reliable statistical analysis can be applied.

Each of the limitations described provides an opportunity for further research. A broad survey of the general population of the United States and Europe having a large enough sample would produce interesting results in that population's knowledge, uses and concerns about privacy and security in the use of their mobile computing devices. Moreover, similar studies done in other areas of the world would be of great interest.

Finally, there are other opportunities for further research. Inasmuch as it was noted, in Concern and Control Questions of the Research and Solutions section of the chapter, that the survey seems to be indicating students do not consider location-based data to be personal information, this attitude might soon change with the advent of new services, such as Google Latitude and Loopt, which allow monitoring of physical locations of others. In the same section, it was even noted that there is a lack of trust in mobile advertising. Future study might investigate the basis for the mistrust. Lastly, in the results of the research, in Protecting Your Mobile Device, it was noted that most of the students do not adequately protect their MCDs or remove sensitive information from those devices when they are discarded by them or returned by them to the providers. Why is the general population of students careless about the protection and the security of the information stored on MCDs? In what manner might the public be informed of the issues of non-protection and non-security? The field is ripe for new research.

CONCLUSION

The research in this chapter analyzed the learning and non-learning of non-information systems students on location-based privacy with mobile computing and compared these findings to an earlier study of information systems students. Also indicated in the research is a lower level of knowledge of non-information systems students of inherent data mining methods and practices that might intrude on privacy and security. Essentially non-information systems students are indicated to be less knowledgeable of organizational practices of privacy and security on mobile computing technology.

Overall, the importance of the results and the trends are in the necessity of improving non-information systems curricula, especially data mining curriculum, in universities integrating organizational and governmental practices of privacy regulation and security into societal-sensitive syllabi. The results of this chapter also indicate a number of challenges for personal privacy, security, how commercial Web sites and organizations handle the privacy of personal data, and how software is developed that incorporates privacy into the design phase of its development.

Data Security and Privacy Challenges: There are now location-aware applications that can let a person's circle of friends know her location. The social networking application Loopt (www.loopt.com) uses the GPS chip in a person's MCD to place her location on a map. She can then allow friends to see where she is and they can allow her to see where they are located. While this application and others like it, for example Google Lattitude (www.google.com/lattitude), allow a person to meet up with friends, there are a number of privacy concerns with its use. For example, after turning on the application, the user might forget to turn it off thus giving away her location when she does not want it known. Also, it is possible for someone else to turn on the application and monitor her location without her knowing it. Even if she does not allow anyone to use her phone, while surfing, it might be possible for an application to load onto her device, detect the presence of Loopt and turn it on without her knowledge. Although this last scenario is hypothetical, it is not outside the realm of possibility. For example, if a Web site uses Adobe Flash to place animations on a Web page, Flash can actually detect the computer's microphone and Webcam and make adjustments to them! (Adobe, 2009).

In addition to its real-time availability, one's location is stored in the application vendor's database. Both Loopt and Google Lattitude say that they do not store historical locations – only a user's last location. While this would prevent historical location data from being used by the application vendor and from it being subpoenaed by the government or a civil or criminal investigation, it is only company policy. Company policy can change, especially if user location data can be seen as a source of advertising revenue. In this situation, a vendor might decide to anonymize the location data and then use it or sell it to marketing companies so it can be mined for commercial purposes. However, even when anonymized, recent research has shown that the mined data can be linked to individuals (Bonneau, 2009). This shows that anonymity is not equivalent to privacy. Also, we cannot count on federal laws to help protect our location data. Paul Stephens, director of policy and advocacy at the Privacy Clearinghouse, recently remarked that "These location-tracking services have been available since about 2005 and the laws haven't caught up with the technology." (Farrell, 2009).

Research conducted at the MIT Media Lab has developed techniques that combine conversation, location, and temporal data to do social network analysis. The original experiment (Eagle and Pentland, 2006) involved collecting a huge amount of data from 100 mobile phones over nine months. The phones acted as wearable sensors giving the location and other data of their users. The analytic technique employed, called *reality mining* (http://reality.media.mit.edu/), can be used to predict the behavior of organizations, groups of individuals, and even to predict what a single user will do next. Many organizations, including telecommunications companies, have the computing power, data storage, data mining capacity, and expertise to duplicate the MIT experiment using their customer data. Therefore, in the not-too-distant future, it might be possible for such organizations to reality mine their customer data to make accurate predictions of individual behavior. This is certainly a point of concern that the public and government should be made aware of prior to its possible implementation.

Another area of concern is the spread of "spear phishing" attacks. A recent incident will illustrate the problem. In the fall of 2008, about 10,000 members of LinkedIn, a social networking site for professionals, were targeted by customized emails sent to specific individuals. The emails, which were made to look like they came from support@linkedin.com, asked the recipients to open a malicious attachment that supposedly contained the names of business contacts (Krebs, 2008). Such attacks are made possible by scammers mining the data contained in social networking sites. Once such data is linked with location data, spear phishing attacks will certainly arrive on cell phones and other mobile devices.

The research of this chapter also shows that the general public needs to be made more aware of privacy threats in general and in particular threats associated with mobile computing. As noted previously, most of the survey respondents in the chapter study were not aware of the possibility of the intrusiveness on privacy that their mobile devices can be. Apparently, most people are also either unaware or are complacent about data breaches. The Identity Theft Resource Center recently announced (ITRC, 2009) an increase of reported data breaches from 446 in 2007 to 656 in 2008, an increase of 47%. Possibly one of the largest and potentially most sensitive data breaches came in November of 2008 when Express Scripts, a company that manages drug benefits for health care providers, announced that extortionists were threatening to make public millions of health records, complete with names and social security numbers. Express Scripts posted a $1 million reward for the capture of the extortionists, but as of the writing of this chapter, the FBI has yet to capture them. (Express Scripts, 2009) Why is there no public outcry about such situations? It could be that efforts to inform the public about privacy breaches have actually backfired. The more than 300 federal and state privacy-related laws have resulted in a deluge of privacy notices (for example 224 notices were sent to Maryland residents from mid 2008 to mid-2009.) This information overload has perhaps caused consumers to care less about privacy protection (Gomes, 2009). The research in this chapter indicates that a possible solution is proper education of the public and computer professional though a curriculum that emphasizes privacy awareness.

Organizational Challenges: As described in a Motorola White Paper (Motorola, 2007), mobile devices are a productivity boon and an enterprise risk. MCDs enable a mobile work force. Those who use MCDs most are managers and sales and service personnel, who are the people most likely to access sensitive and proprietary data. This data is frequently stored on the user's MCD, which is a fact not very comforting because nearly 30% of organization-owned MCDs are lost every year. The data stored on those devices include passwords, employee records, sensitive emails, business plans and so on. Often the data is not encrypted. The solution to this security problem is to adopt stringent security standards and practices for all MCDs. At the very least an MCD should be accessible to only authorized users. All MCDs should be protected by requiring a strong password, which should be different from other passwords employed by the user of the MCD, and which should expire after a period of time. All data stored on the MCD should be encrypted automatically. The organization's information systems staff should also have the capability of remotely locking the device and erasing its contents should the employee quit the organization or should the device be lost or stolen.

The research described in this chapter has also revealed a number of challenges for organizations that use data obtained by people using MCDs. Organizations must earn the confidence of consumers on how their data is obtained and used. A recent Harris Poll (HarrisInteractive, 2008) showed that 59% of adults polled were not comfortable with Web sites using a person's online activity to tailor advertisements based on the person's interests. Clearly, online companies need to earn the confidence of consumers when using consumer data. Organizations must make more clear what data will be collected, how it will be used, how long it will be stored, and with whom the data will be shared. This needs to be done by making their privacy policies easily available and writing them in easy to understand language. The language used must avoid imprecise words that obfuscate the meaning of the privacy policies (Pollach, 2007).

It is also almost impossible for Web surfers to avoid having their data tracked and collected by Web sites. Almost all Web sites have only an opt-out option for data that they collect on the site's visitors. However, Jon Leibowitz, the chairman of the Federal Trade Commission, which oversees matters of online privacy and data collection, has warned online ad companies that he would like to see them obtain explicit permission from Web surfers to track them online (Davis, 2009). This is one of the few times that a high-ranking federal officer has expressly lobbied for an opt-in policy. It would, therefore, behoove the online ad industry to try to develop workable, understandable, and effective privacy policies before the federal government decides on regulations that might limit the effectiveness of these organizations.

Finally, the use of MCDs can have long-term and unintended effects on our society. The use of MCDs as an educational tool has been written about extensively. Students can access the many text, image, audio and video resources of the Web to enrich their classroom learning and textbooks. Nearly every school in the United States has many computers with Internet access. Some are "laptop schools", requiring all students to bring a laptop to every class. (This is a trend that will expand greatly with the advent of sub-$400 "netbooks".) Some are now experimenting using handheld devices for student Internet access. However, there is a downside to the use of MCDs among elementary and high school children. As reported in the New York Times (Kafner, 2009), many experts are concerned about the use of texting by teenagers. The average teenager in the fourth quarter of 2008 sent or received an average of 80 text messages a day. Assuming a normal teen is awake for 16 hours each day, this means the average teenager sends or receives 5 text messages each hour or one every 12 minutes – even during class time!

Psychologists are concerned that excessive use of texting means possible loss of sleep, and a possible shift in the way adolescents develop. Because keeping in touch with parents is made easy by texting, adolescents may not be separating from their parents sufficiently for their development into mature, autonomous adults. Excessive texting also makes it difficult for teens to enjoy moments of solitude and to have time to reflect because they are constantly hearing their phone announce the arrival of still another text message. Will excessive texting have a long-term effect on teens? This situation also has implications for the workforce of the future. Will organizations be able to recruit enough mature, independent individuals who can think creatively and independently?

In 2003 the Computing Research Association declared that to "enable trusted systems for important societal applications" is one of the four grand challenges of trustworthy computing (CRA, 2003). To achieve this goal, the authors of this chapter believe that privacy must be included as an integral component in the design stage of software. This is not, however, an easy task. The notion of privacy is very complex and involves a combination of personally, culturally, and socially constructed properties of relationships and groups (O'Sullivan, 2000). Thus, software developers need to move away from the notion that privacy can be accomplished by a small, discrete set of software settings and move towards a privacy calculus that controls the development of boundaries and the disclosure of confidences (Petronio, 2002). A first step in such a paradigm shift is the proper privacy education of software professionals.

REFERENCES

Adobe. (2009). *Adobe Flash Microphone Settings*. Retrieved May 25, 2009 from http://www.macromedia.com/support/documentation/en/flashplayer/help/settings_manager02.html

Bonneau, J., Anderson, J., Anderson, R., & Stajano, F. (2009) Eight Friends Are Enough: Social Graph Approximation via Public Listings. In *Second ACM Workshop on Social Network Systems*, Nuremburg, Germany.

Brandt, A. (2006). Privacy watch: Phishers put their lures on cell phones. *PC World*, (November 20), 1-2.

Castells, M., Fernandez-Ardevol, M., Qiu, J. L., & Sey, A. (2007). *Mobile Communication and Society: A Global Perspective* (p. 77). Cambridge, MA: The MIT Press.

CRA. (2003). *Four Grand Challenges in Trustworthy Computing*. Available at http://www.cra.org/reports/trustworthy.computing.pdf, last accessed on May 26, 2009.

Curtin, J., Kauffman, R. J., & Riggins, F. J. (2007). Making the 'MOST' out of RFID technology: A research agenda for the study of the adoption, usage and impact of RFID. *Information Technology and Management*, 8(92), 100.

Davis, W. (2009). *FTC's Leibowitz Opts For BT Opt-In*. Available at http://www.mediapost.com/publications/?fa=Articles.showArticle&art_aid=105954, last accessed on May 26, 2009.

Denne, S. (2007). After being over-hyped, RFID starts to deliver. *The Wall Street Journal*, (November 7), B5F.

Eagle, N., & Pentland, A. (2006). Reality mining: Sensing complex social systems. *Personal and Ubiquitous Computing*, 10(4), 255–268. doi:10.1007/s00779-005-0046-3

Eggen, D. (2006). Justice department database stirs privacy fears. *Washington Post*, (December 26), 2-3.

European Directive 95/46/EC. (1995). Available at http://www.cdt.org/privacy/eudirective/EU Directive. html, last accessed on May 1, 2009.

Express Scripts. (2009). Available at http://www.esisupports.com/, last accessed on May 29, 2009.

Farrell, M. B. (2009). *Cellphone tracking services: Friend finder or Big Brother?* Available at http://features.csmonitor.com/innovation/2009/05/01/cellphone-tracking-services-friend-finder-or-big-brother/, last accessed on May 26, 2009.

Gilbert, N. (2007). Dilemmas of privacy and surveillance: Challenges of technological change. *The Royal Academy of Engineering*, March.

Gomes, L. (2009). *The Hidden Cost of Privacy*. Available at http://www.forbes.com/forbes/2009/0608/034-privacy-research-hidden-cost-of-privacy.html, last accessed on May 26, 2009.

Grossman, L. (2007). Tag, you are it: They are cheap, they are tiny, and they are everywhere. But are RFID chips good for humanity? *Time*, (October 29), 57.

Hamblen, M. (2007). Privacy concerns dog information technology (IT) efforts to implement RFID: Employees often rebel against plans to include chips in corporate identification (ID) badges. *Computerworld*, October 15, 26.

HarrisInteractive. (2008). *Majority Uncomfortable with Websites Customizing Content Based Visitors Personal Profiles*. Available at http://www.harrisinteractive.com/harris_poll/index.asp?PID=894, last accessed on May 26, 2009.

Hines, M. (2007). Black hat exposes RFID security risk. *InfoWorld*, (March): 5, 9–10.

ITRC. (2009). *Data Breach Total Soars*. Available at http://www.idtheftcenter.org/artman2/publish/m_press/2008_Data_Breach_Totals_Soar.shtml, last accessed May 26, 2009.

Kafner, K. (2009). *Texting May Be Taking a Toll*. Available at http://www.nytimes.com/2009/05/26/health/26teen.html?scp=1&sq=texting&st=cse, last accessed on May 26, 2009.

Krebs, B. (2008). *Spear Phishing Scam Targets LinkedIn Users*. Available at http://voices.washingtonpost.com/securityfix/2008/10/spear_phishing_attacks_against.html?nav=rss_blog, last accessed on May 26, 2009

Lawler, J., & Molluzzo, J. C. (2006). A study of data mining and information ethics in information systems curricula. *Information Systems Journal*, *4*(34).

Lundquist, E. (2007). The next killer application?: It will be in the mobile segment, if CTIA Is Any Indication. *eWeek*, April 2/9, 6.

Lundquist, E. (2007). The view from Europe: United States lags in some areas, but hiring woes are similar. *eWeek*, (March 19), 9.

M: Metrics Inc. (2006). *United States Mobile Subscriber: Monthly Consumption of Content and Applications. M:Metrics Inc., Benchmark Survey*, April, 16.

Molluzzo, J., & Lawler, J. (2007). Integrating issues of location-based privacy with mobile Computing into international information systems curricula. *Information Systems Education Journal*, *6*(32).

Motorola. (2007). *Mobile Device Security: Securing the Handheld, Securing the Enterprise*, Motorola Technology Group.

O'Sullivan, P. (2000). What you don't know won't hurt me: Impression management functions of communication channels in relationships. *Human Communication Research*, *26*, 403–431. doi:10.1093/hcr/26.3.403

Petronio, S. (2002). *Boundaries of Privacy: Dialectics of Disclosure*. Albany, NY: State University of New York Press.

Pollach, I. (2007, September). What's Wrong with Online Privacy Policies? *Communications of the ACM, 50*(9), 103–108. doi:10.1145/1284621.1284627

Pratt, M. K. (2007). Your gadgets are springing leaks: Handheld electronics travel everywhere in your company, spilling data along the way. *Computerworld*, (March): 19, 34–36.

Romano, N. C. Jr, & Fjermestad, J. (2007). Privacy and security in the age of electronic customer relationship management. *International Journal of Information Security and Privacy, 1*(1), 103.

Sraeel, H. (2007). Protecting data on-line is a top priority for consumer. *Bank Technology News*, April, 8.

Sraeel, H. (2007). In the United States, privacy is not always convenient or wanted. *Bank Technology News*, May, 8.

Stross, R. (2006). Cellphone as tracker: X marks your doubts. *The New York Times*, Business Section, Sunday, November 19, 3.

Talukder, A. K., & Yavagal, R. P. (2007). *Mobile Computing: Technology, Applications and Service Creation*. New York: McGraw Hill.

Tavani, H. T. (2004). *Ethics and Technology: Ethical Issues in an Age of Information and Communication Technology*. Hoboken, NJ: John Wiley and Sons.

Taylor, C. (2007). As RFID tracking booms, privacy issues loom. *Business 2*, May 11, 1-3.

Taylor, H. (2003). *Most People Are "Privacy Pragmatists" Who, While Concerned about Privacy, Will Sometimes Trade It Off for Other Benefits*. Available at http://www.harrisinteractive.com/harris_poll/index.asp?PID=365, last accessed June 24, 2007.

Westin, A. F. (1996). *Harris-Equifax Consumer Privacy Survey*. Atlanta, GA: Equifax, Inc.

KEY TERMS AND DEFINITIONS

Curriculum Design: Methodology of analyzing current data mining and general curricula for expansion and integration of evolving governmental and organizational practices of mining on mobile computing devices that might impact if not intrude on privacy and security;

Data Mining: Method of evaluating data patterns of interactions and transactions on mobile computing devices for future marketing of more customized and personalized products and services and for further monitoring of movements of citizens, consumers and employees;

Location-Based Privacy: Method of defining personal and professional and otherwise private protected interactions and transactions on mobile computing devices that might be integrated into a broader definition of privacy covered in curricula;

Location-Based Security: Methodology of defining and enabling protective measures and routines on mobile computing devices that might be integrated into a broader definition of regulation and security covered in curricula;

Location-Based Services: Method of facilitating feature functionality of products, services and tools on mobile computing devices consistent with the evolution of pervasive technology;

Mobile Computing: Method of furnishing products, services and tools through increasingly pervasive and portable technology; and

Radio Frequency Identification Devices (RFID): Method of enabling immediate location-based services.

APPENDIX

Framework of Syllabi

Location-Based Privacy with Mobile Computing

Module 1: Architecture and Applications of Mobile Computing

Bluetooth
Global Positioning Systems (GPS)
Radio Frequency Identification Tags (RFID)
Short Messaging Services (SMS)
Wireless Application Protocols (WAP), Broadband (WiMax) and Local Area Networks

Module 2: Design and Development of Mobile Computing Applications

Graphical User Interface (GUI)
Java 2 Micro Edition (J2ME)
Multimedia
Palm Operating System (OS)
Symbian Operating System (OS)
Windows CE
Voice over Internet Protocol (VoIP)

Module 3: Privacy of Mobile Computing Applications – Enhancement to Syllabi

Citizen and Consumer Constructs

Definitions of Privacy
Functions of Privacy

Ethical Constructs

Ethics Management
Ethics of Profiling
Ethical Use and Mining of Consumer Data
Integrity Management
Levels of an Ethical Organization

Governmental Constructs – United States

United States Constitution
Court Decisions
Federal Legislation
State Legislation

Governmental Constructs – European Union

European Commission Directives
Member Nation Legislation

Methodological Constructs

Chief Privacy Officers (CPO)
Digital Identity, Identity Layers, Liability and Rights Management
Human Factor Failures
Platform for Privacy Preferences
Pretty Good Privacy (PGP)
Privacy Organization Standards
Privacy Policies

Technological Constructs

Privacy Aware Technologies (PAT)
Privacy Invasive Technologies
Privacy Software Technologies

Module 4: Security of Mobile Computing Architecture and Applications – Enhancement to Syllabi

Chief Security Officers (CSO)

Information Protection and Security

Authorization
Availability
Confidentiality
Integrity
Non-Repudiation
Public Key Infrastructure (PKI)

Security Protocols

Secured Socket Layers (SSL)
Transport Layer Security (TLS)
Wireless Transport Layer Security (WTLS)
Multifactor Security
Digital Watermark
Key Recovery
Smartcard Security

Mutual and Spatial Authentication
RFID Security
Mobile Agent Security

Security Techniques

Ciphering
Cryptography
Hashing Algorithms
Security Policies
Solutions and Threats to Security and Trust

Module 5: Mobile Computing Societal and Technological Trends

"Big Brother"
Biometrics
e-Passports
Loyalty and Travel Cards
National Identity Cards
Reality Mining
Privacy and Surveillance in Era of Terrorism

Reference Research Sites for Syllabi

www.bentley.edu/research
www.bsr.org – Business for Social Responsibility
www.cdt.org – Center for Democracy and Technology
www.corpwatch.org – Watchdog on the Web
www.depaul.edu/ethics - Institute for Business and Professional Ethics
www.ebnsc.org – Corporate Social Responsibility in Europe
www.epic.org – Electronic Privacy Information Center
www.esrc.ac.uk – Economic and Social Research Council in United Kingdom
www.ethics.org – Ethics Resource Center
www.ietf.org – The Internet Engineering Task Force
www.oecd.org – Organization for Economic Cooperation and Development
www.ponemon.org – Ponemon Institute LLC
www.privacyconference.co.uk – International Data Protection and Privacy Commissioners – United
    Kingdom
www.privacyinternational.com – Privacy International
www.privacyjournal.com – Privacy Journal
www.rfid-world.com – RFID World
www.w3.org/p3p/ - The Platform for Privacy Preferences
www.worldcsr.com – World Social Responsibility

Chapter 7
Privacy Preserving Data Mining:
How Far Can We Go?

Aris Gkoulalas-Divanis
Vanderbilt University, USA

Vassilios S. Verykios
University of Thessaly, Greece

ABSTRACT

Since its inception in 2000, privacy preserving data mining has gained increasing popularity in the data mining research community. This line of research can be primarily attributed to the growing concern of individuals, organizations and the government regarding the violation of privacy in the mining of their data by the existing data mining technology. As a result, a whole new body of research was introduced to allow for the mining of data, while at the same time prohibiting the leakage of any private and sensitive information. In this chapter, the authors introduce the readers to the field of privacy preserving data mining; they discuss the reasons that led to its inception, the most prominent research directions, as well as some important methodologies per direction. Following that, the authors focus their attention on very recently investigated methodologies for the offering of privacy during the mining of user mobility data. In the end of the chapter, they provide a roadmap along with potential future research directions both with respect to the field of privacy-aware mobility data mining and to privacy preserving data mining at large.

INTRODUCTION

The significant advances in data collection and data storage technologies have provided the means for the inexpensive storage of enormous amounts of data in data warehouses that reside in companies and public organizations. Despite the benefit of using this data per se (e.g. for maintaining up to date

profiles of the customers and record of their recent or historical purchases, maintaining an inventory of the available products, as well as their quantities and price, etc), the mining of these datasets with the existing data mining tools can reveal invaluable knowledge that was unknown to the data holder beforehand.

The extracted knowledge patterns can provide insight to the data holders and at the same time can be invaluable in tasks such as decision making and

DOI: 10.4018/978-1-60566-906-9.ch007

strategic planning. Moreover, private companies are often willing to collaborate with other entities who conduct similar business, towards the mutual benefit of their businesses. Significant knowledge patterns can be derived and shared among the collaborative partners with respect to the collective mining of their datasets. Furthermore, public sector organizations and civilian federal agencies usually have to share a portion of their collected data or knowledge with other organizations having a similar purpose, or even make this data and knowledge public. For example, the National Institute of Health (NIH) endorses research that leads to significant findings which improve human health and provides a set of guidelines which sanction the sharing of NIH-supported research findings with research institutions.

As it becomes evident, there exists an extended set of application scenarios in which information or knowledge derived from the data has to be shared with other (possibly untrusted) entities. Public agencies for example collect data for different purposes like population surveys, epidemiological and clinical studies, as well as various other social and economic experiments to answer a variety of problems that disturb the society as a whole. The sharing of data and/or knowledge may come at a cost to privacy, primarily due to two reasons: (a) if the data refers to individuals (e.g. as in customers' market basket data, medical data, preferences data and the like) then the disclosure of this data or any knowledge extracted from the data can potentially violate the privacy of the individuals if their identity is revealed to untrusted third parties, and (b) if the data regards business (or organizational) information, then the disclosure of this data or any knowledge extracted from the data may potentially reveal sensitive trade secrets, whose knowledge can provide a significant advantage to business competitors and thus can cause the data holder to lose business over his/her peers. The aforementioned privacy issues in the course of data mining are amplified due to the fact that untrusted entities (adversaries and data terrorists) may utilize other external and publicly available sources of information (e.g. the yellow pages, public reports) in conjunction with the released data or knowledge, in order to reveal even more protected sensitive information.

BACKGROUND

Since the pioneering work of Agrawal & Srikant (2000) and Lindell & Pinkas (2000), several approaches have been proposed for the offering of privacy in data mining. Most existing approaches can be classified along two broad categories: (a) methodologies that protect the sensitive data itself in the mining process, and (b) methodologies that protect the sensitive data mining results (i.e. the extracted knowledge patterns) that were produced by the application of data mining. The first category refers to methodologies that apply perturbation, sampling, generalization/suppression, transformation, etc. techniques to the original datasets in order to generate their sanitized counterparts that can be safely disclosed to untrusted third parties. The goal of this category of approaches is to enable the data miner to get accurate data mining results when is not provided with the real data.

As part of former category we highlight methodologies that have been proposed to enable a number of data holders to collectively mine their data without having to reveal their datasets to each other. On the other hand, the second category deals with distortion and blocking techniques that prohibit the disclosure of sensitive knowledge patterns derived through the application of data mining algorithms, as well as techniques for downgrading the effectiveness of the classifiers in classification tasks, such that they do not reveal any sensitive knowledge.

Vaidya, Clifton & Zhu (2006), and Aggarwal & Yu (2008) provide the different research directions that were investigated over the past eight years along with some of the methodologies that have been proposed along each direction. Giannotti & Pedreschi (2008) elaborate on methodologies that have been recently proposed for the offering of privacy in mobility data mining. In this chapter, we endeavor to present some of the most prevalent methodologies that have been proposed in privacy preserving data mining, along the aforementioned directions. In addition we pay particular attention to methodologies that have been recently proposed for the offering of privacy in the mining of user mobility data. In the end of the chapter, we provide a roadmap along with potential future research directions with respect to the field of privacy-aware mobility data mining and privacy preserving data mining at large.

MAIN THRUST OF THE CHAPTER

As we previously explained, privacy preserving data mining is a new research area inspired by the need of scientists to analyze, interrogate and utilize row collected data without harming the privacy of the subjects contained in the data itself. We may also consider privacy preserving data mining as a descendant of the so-called disclosure control and statistical databases research areas whose main focus was the protection of information stored in databases about human and artificial subjects from positive or negative compromise as well as the controlled publication of vast data collections mostly by government agencies to third party entities like private organizations.

In the sequel we give an overview of privacy preserving data mining approaches proposed for the protection of sensitive traditional forms of data like textual data. We have selected for presentation in this section techniques classified as perturbative, non-perturbative and secure multiparty computation. The second part in the main thrust is devoted to techniques related to protecting sensitive patterns from mining. In this part we focus our attention

on two paradigms, the so-called association rule hiding and classification rule hiding. The third and last part is cornerstone to the significance of our book chapter since it is related to addressing state-of-the-art issues in privacy preserving data mining like privacy aware mobility data mining. The approaches presented in this part include approaches like data perturbation and obfuscation, secure multipart computation approaches and sequential pattern hiding approaches.

PROTECTING TRADITIONAL SENSITIVE DATA DURING MINING

A wide range of methodologies have been proposed in the research literature to effectively shield the sensitive information contained in a dataset by producing its privacy-aware counterpart that can be safely released. The goal of all these privacy preserving methodologies is to ensure that the distorted (also known as *sanitized*) dataset (a) properly shields all the sensitive information that was contained in the original dataset, (b) has similar properties (e.g. first/second order statistics, etc) to the original dataset – possibly resembling it to a high extent – and (c) maintains reasonably accurate data mining results (when compared to those attained when mining the original dataset) when mined.

The protection of sensitive data from disclosure has been extensively studied in the context of *microdata* release, where methodologies have been proposed for the protection of sensitive information regarding individuals, which are recorded in a dataset. In microdata, we consider each record of the dataset to represent an individual for whom the values of a number of attributes are being recorded (e.g. name, date of birth, residence, occupation, salary, etc). Among the complete set of attributes, there exist some attributes that explicitly identify the individual (e.g. name, social security number, etc), as well as attributes which, once combined together or with publicly available external resources, may lead to the identification of the individual (e.g. address, gender, age, etc). The first type of attributes, also known as *identifiers*, must be removed from the data prior to its publishing. On the other hand, the second type of attributes, also known as *quasi-identifiers*, have to be handled by the privacy preservation algorithm in such a way that in the sanitized dataset, the knowledge of their values regarding an individual does no longer pose a threat to the identification of his or her identity.

The existing methodologies for the protection of sensitive microdata can be partitioned in the two following categories: (a) data modification approaches, and (b) synthetic data generation approaches. Willenborg & DeWaal (2001) further partition the data modification approaches in perturbative and non-perturbative, depending on whether they introduce false information in the attribute-values of the data (e.g. by the addition of noise based on a data distribution) or they operate by altering the precision of the attribute-values (e.g. by changing a value to an interval that contains it). In what follows, we provide some more information on each of these categories of approaches.

Perturbative Approaches

In data perturbation approaches the attribute-values of the original dataset are modified in a way that the released values are inaccurate. Several data perturbation approaches have been proposed in the research literature; the most prevalent ones can be partitioned under the following directions: (a) the addition of noise based on an underlying distribution (see Brand, 2002 for a detailed presentation of the methodologies in this direction), (b) the use of microaggregation, in which the data records are partitioned into groups of either fixed (see Domingo-Ferrer & Torra, 2005, and Defays & Nanopoulos, 1993) or variable (see Domingo-Ferrer & Mateo-Sanz, 2002, Laszlo & Mukherjee,

2005, and Sande, 2002) size, based on record similarity criteria; the average value for each attribute in each group is calculated and is then used to replace the exact attribute-value of each record that belongs to the group, and (c) the use of data swapping, in which the attribute-values of a set of records are exchanged (see Reiss, 1984).

Non-Perturbative Approaches

In non-perturbative approaches the attribute-values of the original data are altered in a way that affects the precision in which they are released in the sanitized dataset. The most prevalent non-perturbative methodologies are sampling and global recoding. In sampling (see Willenborg & DeWaal, 2001), only a portion of the original dataset is released. On the other hand, in global recoding, the exact attribute-values of the quasi-identifiers are replaced with less specific (more general) values that enable previously distinct data records to be combined after the *sanitization* process.

For example, in a categorical dataset attribute marital status can take the value "married" for one record and "divorced" for another record of the original dataset, while it can be substituted with "been married" in both records in the sanitized counterpart. Probably the most important approach that ecompases global recoding is K-anonymity (see Samarati, 2001 and Samarati & Sweeney, 1998). The *K*-anonymity principle requires that every record in the sanitized dataset is indistinguishable from at least K-1 other records with respect to a set of identifying variables that formulate the quasi-identifier. Several algorithms have been proposed to enforce K-anonymity, while several of its variations have been explored. Furthermore, although K-anonymity was originally proposed for disclosure control in the context of microdata, it has been successfully applied in different contexts and application areas, such as in mobility data mining (as we present later on).

Secure Multiparty Computation Approaches

The two previous categories of approaches aim at generating a sanitized dataset from the original one, which can be safely shared with untrusted third parties as it contains only non-sensitive data. Secure Multiparty Computation (SMC) provides an alternative family of approaches that can effectively protect the sensitive data. SMC considers a set of collaborators who wish to collectively mine their data but are unwilling to disclose their own datasets to each other. As it turns out, this distributed privacy preserving data mining problem can be reduced to the secure computation of a function based on distributed inputs and it thus solved by using cryptographic approaches.

Pinkas (2002) elaborates on former close relation that exists between privacy-aware data mining and cryptography. In SMC, each party contributes to the computation of the secure function by providing its private input. A secure cryptographic protocol that is executed among the collaborating parties ensures that the private input that is contributed by each party is not disclosed to the others. Most of the applied cryptographic protocols for multi-party computation result to some primitive operations that have to be securely performed: secure sum, secure set union, and secure scalar product. Clifton, et al. (2002) discusses these operations.

The operation of the secure protocols in the course of distributed privacy preserving data mining depends highly on the existing distribution of the data in the sites of the collaborators. Two types of data distribution have been investigated: In a horizontal data distribution, each collaborator holds a number of records and for each records he or she has knowledge of the same set of attributes as his/her peers. On the other hand, in a vertical partitioning of the data, each collaborator is aware of different attributes referring to the same set of records. Some representative SMC approaches that operate on horizontally partitioned datasets

can be found in the work of Inan et al. (2006), Jagannathan & Wright (2005), Jagannathan et al. (2006), Kantarcioglou & Clifton (2004), and Kantarcioglu & Vaidya (2003). On the other hand, some SMC approaches that assume a vertical data distribution have been proposed by Vaidya & Clifton (2002), Vaidya & Clifton (2003), Vaidya & Clifton (2004), Vaidya & Clifton (2005), Vaidya & Clifton (2006), and Yu et al. (2006). SMC has also been studied in the context of distributed K-anonymity. A secure K-anonymous protocol that assumes a vertical data partitioning was proposed by Jiang & Clifton (2005), while a secure protocol that ensures K-anonymity in a horizontal data partitioning can be found in the work of Zhong, et al. (2005).

PROTECTING SENSITIVE PATTERNS FROM MINING

In this section, we focus our attention on privacy preserving methodologies that protect the sensitive knowledge patterns that would otherwise be revealed after the course of mining the data. Similarly to the methodologies that we have presented so far for protecting the sensitive data prior to its mining, the methodologies of this category also modify the original dataset but in such a way that certain sensitive knowledge patterns are suppressed, when mining the data. In what follows, we discuss methodologies that have been proposed for the hiding of sensitive knowledge in the context of association and classification rule mining.

Association Rule Hiding

The association rule mining framework along with some computationally efficient heuristic methodologies for the production of association rules can be found in the work of Agrawal, et al. (1993) and Agrawal & Srikant (1994). Knowledge hiding, in the context of association rule mining, aims at sanitizing the original dataset such that (a) all the sensitive rules (as indicated by the data holder) that appear when mining the original dataset for association rules, do not appear when mining the sanitized dataset for association rules at the same (or higher) levels of support and confidence, (b) all the non-sensitive rules can be successfully mined in the sanitized dataset at the same (or higher) levels of support and confidence, and (c) no rule that was not initially found in the mining of the original dataset can be found in its sanitized counterpart, when mining the sanitized dataset at the same (or higher) levels of support and confidence.

The first goal simply states that all the sensitive association rules are properly hidden in the sanitized dataset. The hiding of the sensitive knowledge comes at a cost to the utility of the sanitized outcome. The second and the third goals aim at minimizing this cost. Specifically, the second goal requires that only the sensitive knowledge is hidden in the sanitized dataset and thus no other, non-sensitive rules are lost due to side-effects of the sanitization process. On the other hand, the third rule requires that no artifacts (i.e. false association rules) are generated by the sanitization process. To recapitulate, in association rule hiding the sanitization process has to be accomplished in a way that minimally affects the original dataset, preserves the general patterns and trends of the dataset, and achieves to conceal all the sensitive knowledge, as indicated by the data holder.

The problem of association rule hiding has been studied along three directions, namely (a) heuristic approaches, (b) border-based approaches, and (c) exact approaches. The first class of approaches collects time and memory efficient algorithms that heuristically select a portion of the transactions of the original dataset to sanitize, in order to facilitate sensitive knowledge hiding. Due to their efficiency and scalability, these approaches have been investigated by the majority of the researchers in the knowledge hiding field

of privacy preserving data mining. However, as in all heuristic methodologies, the approaches of this category take locally best decisions when performing knowledge hiding, which may not always be (and usually are not) globally best.

As a result, there are several circumstances in which these methodologies suffer from undesirable side-effects and may not identify optimal hiding solutions, even if they exist. Heuristic approaches can rely on a distortion (i.e. inclusion/exclusion of items from selected transactions) or on a blocking (i.e. replacing some of the original values in a transaction with question marks) scheme. Some distortion-based algorithms for association rule hiding can be found in the work of Atallah, et al. (1999), Dasseni, et al. (2001), Oliveira & Zaiane (2003), Verykios, et al. (2004), and Wu, et al. (2007). Some blocking-based algorithms can be found in the work of Saygin, et al. (2001), Saygin, et al. (2002), Pontikakis, et al. (2004), and Wang & Jafar (2005).

The second class of approaches collects methodologies that hide the sensitive knowledge by modifying the original borders in the lattice of the frequent (i.e. statistically significant) and the infrequent (i.e. statistically insignificant) patterns of the original dataset. In particular, the sensitive knowledge is hidden by enforcing the revised borders (which accommodate the hiding of the sensitive itemsets) in the sanitized database. The algorithms in this class differ in the borders they track, as well as in the methodology that they apply to enforce the revised borders in the sanitized dataset. An analysis regarding the use of borders in association rule mining can be found in the work of Mannila and Toivonen (1997). Two border-based approaches to association rule hiding can be found in the work of Sun & Yu (2005) and Moustakides & Verykios (2006).

Finally, the third class of approaches involves non-heuristic algorithms which conceive the knowledge hiding process as a *constraints satisfaction problem* (an optimization problem) that is solved through the application of integer or linear programming. This class of approaches differs from the previous two, primarily due to the fact that it collects methodologies that they can guarantee optimality in the hiding solution (provided that an optimal hiding solution exists). On the negative side, these approaches are usually several orders of magnitude slower than the heuristic ones, especially due to the runtime that is required for the solution of the constraints satisfaction problem by the integer/linear programming solver. Menon, et al. (2005) proposes an approach that combines a constraints satisfaction problem with a heuristic algorithm for data sanitization to improve the quality of the hiding solution. The proposed approach, although interesting, it may lead to suboptimal solutions even if optimal ones exist. A family of more advanced methodologies that guarantee optimality of the hiding solution can be found in the work of Gkoulalas-Divanis & Verykios (2006), Gkoulalas-Divanis & Verykios (2008), and Gkoulalas-Divanis & Verykios (2009).

Classification Rule Hiding

Privacy-aware classification has been studied to a substantially lower extent than privacy preserving association rule mining. Similarly to association rule hiding, classification rule hiding algorithms consider a set of classification rules as sensitive and proceed to protect them from disclosure by using either suppression-based or reconstruction-based techniques. In suppression-based techniques the confidence of a classification rule (measured in terms of the owner's belief regarding the holding of the rule when given the data) is reduced by distorting a set of attributes in the dataset that belong to transactions related to its existence. Some approaches that fall under this category are proposed by Chang & Moskowitz (1998), Clifton (2000), Johnsten & Raghavan (2000), Chen & Liu (2005), and Wang, et al. (2005).

A system that is based on former category of approaches was proposed by Moskowitz & Chang (2000). On the other hand, reconstruction-

based approaches target at reconstructing the dataset by using only those transactions of the original dataset that support the non-sensitive classification rules. The works of Natwichai, et al. (2005) and Natwichai, et al. (2006) fit in this category of approaches. Katsarou, et al. (2009) proposes an intermediate approach that performs reconstruction-based classification rule hiding through controlled data modification.

PRIVACY AWARE MOBILITY DATA MINING

The remarkable advances in telecommunications and in location tracking technologies, such as GPS, GSM and UMTS, have made possible the tracking of mobile devices (and thus their human companions) at an accuracy of a few meters, at an affordable cost. From this perspective, we have nowadays the means of collecting, storing and processing mobility data of unprecedented quantity, quality and timeliness. The movement traces, left by the mobile devices of the users, are an excellent source of information that can aid towards decision making in mobility-related issues, such as urban planning, traffic analysis, forecasting of traffic-related phenomena, and timely detection of problems that emerge from users' movement behavior. On the other hand, it becomes evident that on the wrong hands this type of emergent knowledge may lead to an abuse scenario, as the mobility data may reveal highly sensitive personal information. Some examples of misuse include, but are not limited to, user tailing, surveillance or even unsolicited advertising.

As a result, in the last few years, a set of privacy preserving methodologies have been proposed for the protection of sensitive data and/or knowledge related to user mobility. The existing so far methodologies can be partitioned in two broad categories: (a) methodologies that protect the sensitive data related to user mobility prior to the course of data mining, and (b) methodologies that hide sensitive knowledge patterns that summarize user mobility, which are identified as a result of the application of data mining. The first category of approaches collects data perturbation and obfuscation methodologies that distort the original dataset to facilitate privacy-aware data publication, as well as distributed privacy-aware methodologies for secure multiparty computation. On the other hand, the second category of approaches treats the mobility data as sequential data and applies a sequential pattern hiding strategy to prevent the disclosure of the sensitive sequential patterns in the course of sequential pattern mining. After the application of these approaches, only the non-sensitive patterns, summarizing user' movement behavior, survive the mining process, while the sensitive ones are suppressed in the data mining result. In what follows, we present in detail some of the approaches that have been proposed along each of these three categories.

Data Perturbation and Obfuscation

Data perturbation and obfuscation approaches aim at sanitizing a dataset containing user mobility data, in such a way that an adversary can no longer match the recorded movement of each user to a particular individual (thus reveal the identity of the user based on his or her recorded movement in the sanitized dataset). In what follows, we consider that user mobility is captured as a set of trajectories (one per user) that depict the locations and times in the course of his or her history of movement. We assume that these location/time recordings occur at a reasonably high rate that allows the tracking of user movement in the original dataset. For example, an adversary could use these recordings to track the user down to his/her house or place of work, even if the user trajectory was not accompanied by an explicit user identifier, such as the user id, the social security number or even the name of the user.

Hoh & Gruteser (2005) present a data perturbation algorithm that is based on the idea of path crossing. The proposed approach identifies when two nonintersecting trajectories that belong to different users are reasonably close to each other and generates a fake crossing of these two trajectories in the sanitized dataset. The goal of this approach is to prevent an adversary from successfully tracking a complete user trajectory in the sanitized dataset, and thus identifying the corresponding user. Provided that many crossings of trajectories exist in the sanitized dataset, the probability that an adversary succeeds in following the same individual prior and after a crossing of this user's trajectory with one or more other trajectories in the dataset, sufficiently deteriorates. As the authors demonstrate, path confusion can be formalized as a constrained nonlinear optimization problem which, when given the trajectories of two users within a bounded area where a crossing has to occur, it estimates the perturbed locations for each user such that their trajectories meet within a pre-specified time period.

To continue, at each generated fake user location towards the meeting of the two trajectories, the algorithm takes special care to keep the enforced perturbation of the exact user location within reasonable bounds. In order to achieve this, each perturbed (fake) location has to reside within a given perturbation radius (indicating the maximum allowable perturbation) from the original user location. As is expected, a larger radius increases the degree of privacy that is offered to the users but also deteriorates the utility of the sanitized dataset. Equivalently, a smaller radius offers less privacy to the users but achieves a better utility of the publicized data. Through experiments the authors prove that the proposed algorithm limits the duration in which an adversary can successfully track the same individual in the sanitized dataset.

Hoh, et al. (2007) introduces a new empirical measure for the quantification of privacy in a set of publicized location/time recordings. The proposed measure calculates the time that a user can be successfully tracked (by an adversary) based on the knowledge of his/her user trajectory. The proposed measure calculates the time that elapsed between two consecutive occasions where the adversary could not determine (at least with sufficient certainty) the next location/time recording in the trajectory of the user. By using this measure, the authors propose a path perturbation strategy that relies on data coarsening to exclude a limited amount of location/time recordings from a user trajectory. The applied coarsening strategy ensures that the corresponding user cannot be tracked (at least with sufficient certainty) by the adversary, for a time that exceeds a pre-specified time threshold (i.e. the maximum time to confusion). To achieve this goal, the perturbation algorithm discloses a location/time recording of a user trajectory (as it appears in the original dataset) to the sanitized dataset, only if the time that has passed since the last point of confusion is below the pre-specified time threshold.

Terrovitis & Mamoulis (2008) consider datasets that depict user mobility in the form of sequences of places that each user has visited in the course of his/her movement. For each user, the authors assume the existence of a transaction in the dataset that contains the list of places that this particular user has visited (e.g. based on his/her card transactions), set out in the order of visit. No other information of spatial or temporal nature (e.g. the exact time of each visit) is assumed to be provided. Based on this type of data, the authors propose a suppression technique that removes some of the places that were visited by specific users, in order to protect their identity from adversaries who hold partial information on the user trajectories. Specifically, an adversary is considered to be any individual who has knowledge of certain places that were visited by particular users, for whom he/she knows their identity. To exemplify, consider a bank which has many branches in a city. Each branch of the bank has some ATM machines that people can use to perform regular money transactions. Whenever a person uses the ATM of the bank this transaction is recorded.

Now assume that the bank manager has possession of the original dataset of user mobility, where he/she identifies that some of the users that appear in the dataset have visited certain branches of the bank. By using this information it is possible that the manager can figure out the identity of some of the users who are recorded in the dataset and then learn the other places that they have visited during their movement. To protect the privacy of the users when publicizing their movement data, the proposed methodology assumes that the data holder has knowledge of the sets of places (i.e. the projection of the dataset) that are known to each individual adversary. In our example, the data holder knows the branches of the bank that the bank manager controls. By using this information, the data holder can compute the probability by which the corresponding adversary can infer the identity of a user in the publicized dataset, based on the projection of the data that the adversary holds. The proposed suppression strategy operates in an iterative fashion to minimize the probability of a given adversary to associate (based on his/her data projection) a place that appears in the publicized data to the identity of a particular person. (Some other interesting approaches in this direction are proposed in the work of Pensa, et al. 2008, Nergiz, et al. 2008 & Abul, et al. 2008).

Secure Multiparty Computation

Secure multiparty computation has also been studied in the context of user mobility (and more generally on spatiotemporal) data. Inan & Saygin (2006) were the first authors to propose a privacy-aware methodology that clusters a set of spatiotemporal datasets, owned by different parties. To perform clustering, a similarity measure is necessary in order to quantify the proximity between two objects (e.g. the user trajectories), such that in the computed clustering solution, the co-clustered objects are more similar to one another than to objects belonging in different clusters. As part of this work, the authors propose a secure protocol that can be employed to enable the pairwise secure computation of trajectory similarity among all the trajectories of the different parties, thus building a global matrix of trajectory similarity. By using this matrix, a trusted third party can perform the clustering on behalf of the users and communicate the computed clustering results back to the collaborating parties. The proposed privacy preserving protocol supports all the necessary basic operations for the computation of trajectory similarity based on widely adopted trajectory comparison functions: (a) Euclidean distance, (b) longest common subsequence, (c) dynamic time warping, and (d) edit distance.

The protocol makes the following assumptions: (a) it assumes a semi-honest model in which all the parties follow the protocol but may also store any information that they receive from other parties in order to infer private data, (b) the parties do not mutually share any other kind of information, and (c) the mobility data that is to be clustered follows a horizontal partitioning. The proposed methodology operates as follows: (a) every involved party, including the trusted party, generates pairwise keys which are used to disguise the exchanged messages, (b) each party locally computes the trajectory similarity matrix (based on the commonly accepted trajectory comparison function) for its own trajectories and securely transmits it to the trusted party, (c) for every pair of trajectories that belong to the datasets of different parties, the two parties execute the protocol to compute the similarity of their trajectories, build a similarity matrix based on their trajectories, and subsequently transmit it to the trusted party, and (d) the trusted party uses the computed matrix of trajectory similarity based on the trajectories of all the collaborating parties, in order to perform trajectory clustering. An interesting observation is that by using this technique, the trusted party is free to choose any clustering algorithm, depending on the requirements of the data holders, in order to perform the clustering of the trajectories.

Sequential Pattern Hiding

The extraction of frequent patterns from mobility data has primarily concentrated on the sequential nature of such datasets by extracting frequent subsequences of user mobility (e.g. Cao, et al. 2005, Giannotti, et al. 2006). Giannotti, et al. (2007) proposed the integration of spatial and temporal information in the extracted mobility patterns by temporally annotating the extracted sequences, depicting frequent movement, with the transition times from one element (place of interest) to another. In a similar manner, the approaches that have been proposed for the hiding of frequent mobility patterns consider knowledge hiding in the form of sequential pattern hiding. In what follows, we present an approach that belongs in this category.

Abul, et al. (2007a) models the problem of trajectory hiding to that of sequential pattern hiding. The authors consider that pertinent to every sensitive sequence is a disclosure threshold that defines the maximum number of sequences in the sanitized database that are allowed to support the sensitive sequence. The sequence sanitization operation is based on the use of unknowns to mask selected elements in the sequences of the original dataset. As the authors prove, the problem of sanitizing a sequence from the original dataset, while introducing the least amount of unknowns, is NP-hard and thus one needs to resort to heuristics to identify an efficient solution. The proposed heuristic operates as follows: For each sensitive sequence, the algorithm searches all the sequences of the original database to identify those in which the sensitive sequence is a subsequence (a sequence S_1 is a subsequence of another sequence S_2 if it can be obtained by deleting some elements from S_2). For every such sequence of the original dataset, the algorithm examines in how many different ways this sequence becomes a subsequence of the sensitive one. Each "different way" (also called a matching) is counted based on the position of each element in the sequence that participates to the generation of the sensitive sequence.

Thus as an effect, for each element of the sequence coming from the original dataset, the algorithm maintains a counter depicting the number of matchings in which it is involved. To sanitize the sequence, the algorithm iteratively identifies the element of the sequence which has the highest counter (i.e. it is involved in most matchings) and replaces it by an unknown, until the sensitive sequence is no longer a subsequence of the sanitized one. As a result of this operation, the sensitive sequence becomes unsupported by the sanitized sequence. In order to enforce the requested disclosure threshold the algorithm applies this sanitization operation in the following manner: For each sensitive sequence, all the sequences of the original dataset are sorted in ascending order based on the number of different matchings that they have with the sensitive sequence. Then, the algorithm sanitizes the sequences in this order, until the required disclosure threshold is met in the privacy-aware version of the original dataset.

A similar approach to that of Abul, et al. (2007a), which operates by removing (instead of masking) elements from sequential mobility patterns and assumes an underlying network of user movement from which those patterns were extracted, is presented in the work of Abul, et al. (2007b).

FUTURE TRENDS

Data mining is a rapidly evolving field counting numerous conferences, journals and books that are dedicated to this area of research. As new forms of data come into existence, as well as new application areas and challenges arise, it becomes evident that innovative privacy preserving data mining methodologies will also have to be proposed to keep pace with this progress. The current applications of privacy preserving data mining are numerous, spanning from the offering of privacy

in the release of medical and genomic databases to the extraction of knowledge patterns that provide information related to homeland security. Mobility data mining, as well as privacy-aware stream data mining are among the most recent and prominent directions of privacy preserving data mining.

As spatiotemporal and geo-referenced datasets grow, a novel class of applications is expected to appear that will be based on the extraction of behavioral patterns of user mobility. Clearly, in these applications privacy is a major concern and thus novel privacy preserving methodologies will have to be proposed to protect those patterns that are sensitive with respect to the privacy of individuals. In what follows, we briefly present some future research directions both with respect to the field of privacy-aware mobility data mining and to privacy preserving data mining at large.

Privacy-Aware Mobility Data Mining

Spatiotemporal datasets present a new challenge to the privacy preserving data mining community due to their spatial and temporal characteristics. Few approaches have been proposed so far that achieve to address some of the special requirements of this type of data. A basic drawback of the existing methodologies is that they fail to treat space and time equally well. Instead, most of the approaches that have been proposed put their effort on the adequate treatment of either the spatial or the temporal dimension of the data, but not both. As a result, user mobility data is often transformed into sequential data, where the spatial component is reduced to a set of places of interests (events) and the time component (apart from providing the total ordering of these events in the sequence) is disregarded. Thus, we feel that there is plenty of room for research in this interesting and challenging area.

As presented earlier, privacy preserving data mining in the context of mobility data has been investigated towards three broad research directions: (a) data perturbation approaches, (b) distributed

(SMC) approaches, and (c) knowledge hiding approaches. Based on the number of published works per direction, it becomes evident that most of the research effort has been placed towards the development of data perturbation methodologies, while few approaches have been devised to support the other two directions. We believe that in the upcoming years, data mining researchers will put more effort in devising novel algorithms for the hiding of user mobility patterns, especially due to the urging need of these methodologies in various application contexts. The hiding of sensitive mobility patterns imposes far greater challenges than traditional knowledge hiding, since specially crafted algorithms are necessary to identify all the important correlations that exist within the datasets.

Furthermore, the mining of sensitive knowledge, depicted in the form of associations in mobility datasets, may allow for the use of different measures of pattern interestingness than the commonly employed support and confidence metrics. As an effect, new knowledge hiding techniques may have to be investigated that will successfully conceal this novel type of sensitive knowledge.

Privacy Preserving Data Mining

As mentioned earlier, privacy preserving data mining is a highly evolving area with a tremendous amount of applications and with many opportunities for research. A recent trend in this area is the exploring of new data types and novel domains of potential knowledge. The privacy-aware mining of mobility data is only one among the hot research directions. Another example of a research domain that is expected to receive a lot of attention in the upcoming years is the offering of privacy in the context of applications where data is released incrementally and in an unconditional rate.

In this challenging area of research, privacy preserving data mining methodologies have to be designed to handle streams of data rather than datasets containing historical recordings. Finally,

apart from domain-driven research, as the one presented in the above-mentioned examples, there is currently an urging need for the development of frameworks that will unify more advanced measures for the evaluation and the comparison of different privacy preserving data mining methodologies.

CONCLUSION

In this chapter, we presented an overview of privacy preserving data mining, one of the most popular directions in the data mining research community. In the first part of the chapter, we presented approaches that have been proposed for the protection of either the sensitive data itself in the course of data mining or the sensitive data mining results, in the context of traditional (relational) datasets. Following that, in the second part of the chapter, we focused our attention on one of the most recent as well as prominent directions in privacy preserving data mining: the mining of user mobility data. Although still in its infancy, privacy preserving data mining of mobility data has attracted a lot of research attention and already counts a number of methodologies both with respect to sensitive data protection and to sensitive knowledge hiding. Finally, in the end of the chapter, we provided some roadmap along the field of privacy preserving mobility data mining as well as the area of privacy preserving data mining at large.

REFERENCES

Abul, O., Atzori, M., Bonchi, F., & Giannotti, F. (2007a). Hiding Sequences. In *IEEE International Conference on Data Engineering Workshop* (pp. 147-156), Istanbul, Turkey.

Abul, O., Atzori, M., Bonchi, F., & Giannotti, F. (2007b). Hiding Sensitive Trajectory Patterns. In *IEEE International Conference on Data Mining Workshops* (pp. 693-698), Omaha, NE.

Abul, O., Bonchi, F., & Nanni, M. (2008). Never Walk Alone: Uncertainty for Anonymity in Moving Objects Databases. In *International Conference on Data Engineering* (pp. 376-385), Cancun, Mexico.

Aggarwal, C. C., & Yu, P. S. (Eds.). (2008). *Privacy Preserving Data Mining: Models and Algorithms.* New York: Springer-Verlag.

Agrawal, R., Imielinski, T., & Swami, A. (1993). Mining Association Rules between Sets of Items in Large Databases. In *ACM SIGMOD International Conference on Management of Data* (pp. 207-216), Washington, DC.

Agrawal, R., & Srikant, R. (1994). Fast Algorithms for Mining Association Rules in Large Databases. In *International Conference on Very Large Data Bases* (pp.487-499), San Francisco, CA.

Agrawal, R., & Srikant, R. (2000). Privacy Preserving Data Mining. In *ACM SIGMOD Conference on Management of Data,* (pp. 439-450), Dallas, TX.

Atallah, M., Bertino, E., Elmagarmid, A. K., Ibrahim, M., & Verykios, V. S. (1999). Disclosure Limitation of Sensitive Rules. In *IEEE Workshop on Knowledge and Data Engineering Exchange* (pp. 45-52), Chicago, IL.

Brand, R. (2002). Microdata Protection Through Noise Addition. In *Inference Control in Statistical Databases* []. New York: Springer-Verlag.]. *Theory into Practice, 2316,* 97–116.

Cao, H., Mamoulis, N., & Cheung, D. W. (2006). Discovery of Collocation Episodes in Spatiotemporal Data. In *International Conference on Data Mining* (pp. 823-827), Hong Kong, China.

Chang, L., & Moskowitz, I. S. (1998). Parsimonious Downgrading and Decision Trees Applied to the Inference Problem. In *Workshop on New Security Paradigms* (pp. 82-89), Charlottesville, VA.

Chen, K., & Liu, L. (2005). Privacy Preserving Data Classification with Rotation Perturbation. In *IEEE International Conference on Data Mining* (pp. 589-592), Houston, TX.

Clifton, C. (2000). Using Sample Size to Limit Exposure to Data Mining. *International Journal of Computer Security, 8*(4), 281–307.

Clifton, C., Kantarcioglou, M., Lin, X., & Zhu, M. (2002). Tools for Privacy Preserving Distributed Data Mining. *ACM SIGKDD Explorations, 4*(2), 28–34. doi:10.1145/772862.772867

Dasseni, E., Verykios, V. S., Elmagarmid, A. K., & Bertino, E. (2001). Hiding Association Rules by Using Confidence and Support. In *International Workshop on Information Hiding* (pp. 369-383), Pittsburgh, PA.

Defays, D., & Nanopoulos, P. (1993). Panels of Enterprises and Confidentiality: The Small Aggregates Method. In *Symposium on Design and Analysis of Longitudinal Surveys* (pp. 195-204). Ottawa, Canada: Statistics Canada.

Domingo-Ferrer, J., & Mateo-Sanz, J. M. (2002). Practical Data-Oriented Microaggregation for Statistical Disclosure Control. *IEEE Transactions on Knowledge and Data Engineering, 14*(1), 189–201. doi:10.1109/69.979982

Domingo-Ferrer, J., & Torra, V. (2005). Ordinal, Continuous and Heterogeneous K-anonymity Through Microaggregation. *Data Mining and Knowledge Discovery, 11*(2), 195–212. doi:10.1007/s10618-005-0007-5

Giannotti, F., Nanni, M., & Pedreschi, D. (2006). Efficient Mining of Temporally Annotated Sequences. In *SIAM International Conference on Data Mining*, Bethesda, MD, (pp. 346-357).

Giannotti, F., Nanni, M., Pinelli, F., & Pedreschi, D. (2007). Trajectory Pattern Mining. In *ACM SIGKDD International Conference on Knowledge Discovery and Data Mining* (pp. 330-339), San Jose, CA.

Giannotti, F., & Pedreschi, D. (Eds.). (2008). *Mobility, Data Mining and Privacy: Geographic Knowledge Discovery*. New York: Springer-Verlag. doi:10.1007/978-3-540-75177-9

Gkoulalas-Divanis, A., & Verykios, V. S. (2006). An Integer Programming Approach for Frequent Itemset Hiding. In *ACM Conference on Information and Knowledge Management* (pp. 748-756), Arlington, VA.

Gkoulalas-Divanis, A., & Verykios, V. S. (2008). Exact Knowledge Hiding Through Database Extension. In IEEE Transactions on Knowledge and Data Engineering.

Gkoulalas-Divanis, A., & Verykios, V. S. (2009). Hiding Sensitive Knowledge without Side Effects. In Knowledge and Information Systems.

Hoh, B., & Gruteser, M. (2005). Protecting Location Privacy through Path Confusion. In *International Conference on Security and Privacy for Emerging Areas in Communications Networks* (pp. 194-205), Athens, Greece.

Hoh, B., Gruteser, M., Xiong, H., & Alrabady, A. (2007). Preserving Privacy in GPS Traces via Uncertainty-Aware Path Cloaking. In *ACM Conference on Computer and Communications Security* (pp. 161-171), Alexandria, VA.

Inan, A., Kaya, S. V., Saygin, Y., Savas, E., Hintoglu, A., & Levi, A. (2006). Privacy Preserving Clustering on Horizontally Partitioned Data. *Data & Knowledge Engineering, 63*(3), 646–666. doi:10.1016/j.datak.2007.03.015

Inan, A., & Saygin, Y. (2006). Privacy-Preserving Spatiotemporal Clustering on Horizontally Partitioned Data. In *International Conference on Data Warehousing and Knowledge Discovery* (pp. 459-468), Krakow, Poland.

Jagannathan, G., Pillaipakkamnatt, K., & Wright, R. (2006). A New Privacy Preserving Distributed K-Clustering Algorithm. In *SIAM International Conference on Data Mining*, Bethesda, MD.

Jagannathan, G., & Wright, R. (2005). Privacy Preserving Distributed K-Means Clustering over Arbitrarily Partitioned Data. In *ACM SIGKDD Conference on Knowledge Discovery in Data Mining* (pp. 593-599), Chicago, IL.

Jiang, W., & Clifton, C. (2005). Privacy Preserving Distributed K-anonymity. In *IFIP 11.3 Working Conference on Data and Applications Security,* (pp. 166-177), Storrs, CT.

Johnsten, T., & Raghavan, V. V. (2000). Impact of Decision-Region Based Classification Mining Algorithms on Database Security. In *IFIP TC13 WG11.3 International Conference on Database Security* (pp. 177-191), Deventer, Netherlands.

Kantarcioglu, M., & Clifton, C. (2004). Privacy Preserving Distributed Mining of Association Rules on Horizontally Partitioned Data. *IEEE Transactions on Knowledge and Data Engineering, 16*(9), 1026–1037. doi:10.1109/TKDE.2004.45

Kantarcioglu, M., & Vaidya, J. (2003). Privacy Preserving Naïve Bayes Classification for Horizontally Partitioned Data. In *IEEE International Conference on Data Mining Workshop on Privacy Preserving Data Mining* (pp. 3-9), Melbourne, FL.

Katsarou, A., Gkoulalas-Divanis, A., & Verykios, V. S. (2009). Reconstruction-Based Classification Rule Hiding through Controlled Data Modification. In *IFIP Conference on Artificial Intelligence Applications & Innovations*, Thessaloniki, Greece.

Laszlo, M., & Mukherjee, S. (2005). Minimum Spanning Tree Partitioning Algorithm for Microaggregation. *IEEE Transactions on Knowledge and Data Engineering, 17*(7), 902–911. doi:10.1109/TKDE.2005.112

Lindell, Y., & Pinkas, B. (2000). Privacy Preserving Data Mining. *Journal of Cryptology, 15*(3), 36–54.

Mannila, H., & Toivonen, H. (1997). Levelwise Search and Borders of Theories in Knowledge Discovery. *Data Mining and Knowledge Discovery, 1*(3), 241–258. doi:10.1023/A:1009796218281

Menon, S., Sarkar, S., & Mukherjee, S. (2005). Maximizing Accuracy of Shared Databases when Concealing Sensitive Patterns. *Information Systems Research, 16*(3), 256–270. doi:10.1287/isre.1050.0056

Moskowitz, I., & Chang, L. (2000). A Decision Theoretic System for Information Downgrading. In *Joint Conference on Information Sciences*.

Moustakides, G. V., & Verykios, V. S. (2006). A Max-Min Approach for Hiding Frequent Itemsets. In *IEEE International Conference on Data Mining Workshops* (pp. 502-506), Hong Kong.

Natwichai, J., Li, X., & Orlowska, M. (2005). Hiding Classification Rules for Data Sharing with Privacy Preservation. In *International Conference on Data Warehousing and Knowledge Discovery* (pp. 468-477), Copenhagen, Denmark.

Natwichai, J., Li, X., & Orlowska, M. (2006). A Reconstruction-Based Algorithm for Classification Rules Hiding. In *Australasian Database Conference* (pp. 49-58), Hobart, Australia.

Nergiz, M. E., Atzori, M., & Yucel, S. (2008). Towards Trajectory Anonymization: a Generalization-Based Approach. In *ACM GIS Workshop on Security and Privacy in GIS and LBS*, Irvine, CA.

Oliveira, S. R. M., & Zaiane, O. R. (2003). Protecting Sensitive Knowledge by Data Sanitization. In *IEEE International Conference on Data Mining* (pp. 211-218), Melbourne, FL.

Pensa, R. G., Monreale, A., Pinelli, F., & Pedreschi, D. (2008). Pattern-Preserving K-Anonymization of Sequences and its Application to Mobility Data Mining. In *International Workshop on Privacy in Location Based Applications*, Malaga, Spain.

Pinkas, B. (2002). Cryptographic Techniques for Privacy Preserving Data Mining. *ACM SIGKDD Explorations, 4*(2), 12–19. doi:10.1145/772862.772865

Pontikakis, E., Theodoridis, Y., Tsitsonis, A., Chang, L., & Verykios, V. S. (2004). A Quantitative and Qualitative Analysis of Blocking in Association Rule Hiding. In *ACM Workshop on Privacy in the Electronic Society* (pp. 29-30), Washington, DC.

Reiss, S. P. (1984). Practical Data Swapping: The First Steps. *ACM Transactions on Database Systems, 9*, 20–37. doi:10.1145/348.349

Samarati, P. (2001). Protecting Respondents' Identities in Microdata Release. *IEEE Transactions on Knowledge and Data Engineering, 13*(6), 1010–1027. doi:10.1109/69.971193

Samarati, P., & Sweeney, L. (1998). *Protecting Privacy when Disclosing Information: K-Anonimity and its Enforcement Through Generalization and Suppresion (Technical Report)*. Menlo Park, CA: SRI International.

Sande, G. (2002). Exact and Approximate Methods for Data Directed Microaggregation in One or More Dimensions. *International Journal of Uncertainty. Fuzziness and Knowledge-Based Systems, 10*(5), 459–476. doi:10.1142/S0218488502001582

Saygin, Y., Verykios, V. S., & Clifton, C. (2001). Using Unknowns to Prevent Discovery of Association Rules. *SIGMOD Record, 30*(4), 45–51. doi:10.1145/604264.604271

Saygin, Y., Verykios, V. S., & Elmagarmid, A. K. (2002). Privacy Preserving Association Rule Mining. In *International Workshop on Research Issues in Data Engineering: Engineering E-Commerce/E-Business Systems* (pp. 151-163), San Jose, CA.

Sun, X., & Yu, P. S. (2005). A Border Based Approach for Hiding Sensitive Frequent Itemsets. In *IEEE International Conference on Data Mining* (pp. 426-433), Houston, TX.

Terrovitis, M., & Mamoulis, N. (2008). Privacy Preservation in the Publication of Trajectories. In *Intl. Conference on Mobile Data Management* (pp. 65-72), Beijing, China.

Vaidya, J., & Clifton, C. (2002). Privacy Preserving Association Rule Mining in Vertically Partitioned Databases. In *ACM SIGKDD International Conference on Knowledge Discovery and Data Mining* (pp. 639-644), Edmonton, AB.

Vaidya, J., & Clifton, C. (2003). Privacy Preserving K-Means Clustering over Vertically Partitioned Data. In *ACM SIGKDD International Conference on Knowledge Discovery and Data Mining,* (pp. 206-215), Washington, DC, USA.

Vaidya, J., & Clifton, C. (2004). Privacy Preserving Naïve Bayes Classifier for Vertically Partitioned Data. In *SIAM International Conference on Data Mining* (pp. 522-526), Lake Buena Vista, FL.

Vaidya, J., Clifton, C., Kantarcioglu, M., & Patterson, A. S. (2005). Privacy Preserving Decision Trees over Vertically Partitioned Data. *ACM Transactions in Knowledge Discovery from Data, 2*(3), 1–27. doi:10.1145/1409620.1409624

Vaidya, J., Clifton, C. W., & Zhu, Y. M. (2006). Privacy Preserving Data Mining. *Advances in Information Security,* 19.

Verykios, V. S., Elmagarmid, A. K., Bertino, E., Saygin, Y., & Dasseni, E. (2004). Association Rule Hiding. *IEEE Transactions on Knowledge and Data Engineering, 16*(4), 434–447. doi:10.1109/TKDE.2004.1269668

Wang, K., Fung, B. C. M., & Yu, P. S. (2005). Template-Based Privacy Preservation in Classification Problems. In *IEEE International Conference on Data Mining* (pp. 466-473), Houston, TX.

Wang, S. L., & Jafari, A. (2005). Using Unknowns for Hiding Sensitive Predictive Association Rules. In *IEEE International Conference on Information Reuse and Integration* (pp. 223-228), New York.

Willenborg, L., & DeWaal, T. (2001). *Elements of Statistical Disclosure Control.* New York: Springer-Verlag.

Wu, Y. H., Chiang, C. M., & Chen, L. P. (2007). Hiding Sensitive Association Rules with Limited Side Effects. *IEEE Transactions on Knowledge and Data Engineering, 19*(1), 29–42. doi:10.1109/TKDE.2007.250583

Yu, H., Vaidya, J., & Jiang, X. (2006). Privacy Preserving SVM Classification on Vertically Partitioned Data. In *Pacific-Asia Conference on Advances in Knowledge Discovery and Data Mining,* (pp. 647-656), Singapore.

Zhong, S., Yang, Z., & Wright, R. (2005). Privacy Enhancing K-anonymization of Customer Data. In ACM SIGMOD-SIGACT-SIGART Principles of Database Systems, (pp. 139-147), Baltimore, MD.

KEY TERMS AND DEFINITIONS

Privacy Preserving Data Mining: The area of data mining that is concerned with privacy issues related to the course of data mining, and specifically (a) with the protection of privacy in data releases, (b) the preservation of privacy in the mutual mining of data among a set of collaborating parties, and (c) with the protection of sensitive knowledge patterns that can be derived due to the application of data mining tools. Privacy preserving data mining is one of the most challenging research areas within the data mining community, already counting numerous conferences, workshops, and journals.

Sanitization: The process of transforming the original dataset to its privacy-aware counterpart that can be safely released as it protects the sensitive data or shields the sensitive knowledge, from unauthorized exposure.

Rule Hiding Approaches: A category of methodologies that aim at protecting the sensitive knowledge that can be mined from a dataset in the form of sensitive association or classification rules. The rule hiding approaches primarily operate by sanitizing the original dataset such that the significance of the sensitive rules deteriorates in its sanitized counterpart to such an extent that they are no longer mined by the employed rule mining strategy.

Perturbation Techniques: A category of data modification approaches that protect the sensitive data contained in a dataset by modifying a carefully selected portion of attribute-values pairs of its transactions. The employed modification constitutes the released values inaccurate, thus protect the sensitive data, but also achieve to preserve the statistical properties of the dataset (e.g. the first and second order statistics) such that its mining yields accurate results.

Reconstruction Approaches: A category of sensitive knowledge hiding approaches that operate by generating a new dataset based on a portion of the transactions of the original dataset (i.e. those transactions that support the non-sensitive knowledge). This category of approaches has been studied in the context of classification rule hiding. The transactions of the original dataset that support the non-sensitive rules are used to build a classification model from which the transactions of the sanitized dataset are generated.

Secure Multiparty Computation: A research direction within the area of privacy preserving methodologies for the protection of sensitive data. Secure multiparty computation collects distributed privacy preserving methodologies that enable a number of collaborating peers to collectively mine their data without having to reveal their datasets to each other. The approaches of this category operate by employing a family of protocols which allow the peers to exchange data in a secure manner. The security of the protocols is achieved through the application of cryptographic approaches which enable the secure computation of a function based on distributed inputs.

Privacy-Aware Mobility Data Mining: The field of privacy preserving data mining that collects methodologies that offer privacy in the mining of data related to user mobility. The methodologies of this category can be classified along three directions: (a) methodologies that protect the sensitive data that relates to user mobility prior to the course of data mining; (b) methodologies which enable a number of collaborating parties to collectively mine their data in a privacy-aware manner, and (c) knowledge hiding methodologies which conceal sensitive knowledge patterns that summarize user mobility from being identified in the course of mining the dataset.

Chapter 8
Data Mining Challenges in the Context of Data Retention

Konrad Stark
University of Vienna, Austria

Michael Ilger
Vienna University of Technology & University of Vienna, Austria

Wilfried N. Gansterer
University of Vienna, Austria

ABSTRACT

Retaining electronic communication and internet traffic data imposes novel technical and organisational challenges for internet service providers as well as for government authorities. ISP companies are not only burdened by storing extraordinary amounts of data, but also must develop and adhere to data protection and data security policies in order to protect the data against unauthorised access or disclosure and against accidental destruction. The authors present distributed, horizontally partitioned data warehouse architecture for retaining data at each internet service provider separately. Moreover, they elaborate a data warehouse schema for storing e-mail data according to the European data retention directive which facilitate parameterised data retrieval. The authors show how their system allows for applying various types of data mining techniques to both internet access and communication data. Finally, they discuss issues related to data security, cost and performance, and reveal limitations of data retention systems.

INTRODUCTION

The EU Data Retention directive 2006/24/EC ("Data Retention Directive") of the European Parliament, published on 15.03.2006, requires the operators of publicly accessible electronic communication networks to store ("retain") certain data which is generated or processed in their networks to serve the investigation, detection, and prosecution of serious crime (European Parliament, 2007). National service providers are required to implement and maintain the technical means needed to store and provide this data to government authorities upon request. For various categories of electronic communication, including Internet access, Internet e-mail and Internet telephony, the directive defines

DOI: 10.4018/978-1-60566-906-9.ch008

which data has to be retained. Affected are traffic and location data (but not the contents of the communication) for a period of time between six months and two years.

In this chapter, we discuss the application of data mining methods in the context of implementing this EU Directive which has implications for both, public and private sectors. Retaining electronic communication and internet traffic data imposes novel technical and organisational challenges for internet service providers as well as for government authorities. These challenges not only relate to the collection and the management of the data to be retained, but also to the analysis of the data, for example, when having to respond to queries posted by government authorities.

Challenges for the ISP company: A data retention system has to respond to enquiries of competent authorities 'without undue delay' (Elizalde, 2006). That is, instead of storing e-mail communication in log files, data has to be stored in a structured way facilitating *efficient* data retrieval. Although the directive specifies the mandatory information to be stored for each e-mail communication, no technical guidelines are given about how the information may be stored to support parameterised queries.

Challenges for the government authorities: The retained data is distributed among various ISPs which is particularly complicating the analysis of e-mail data. For instance, if an e-mail is sent from person A to person B which are customers of two different providers PV1 and PV2, two separate enquiries are necessary to identify both individuals. If the common social relationships of A and B are surveyed, two result sets are delivered by PV1 and PV2. In order to combine the result sets and perform analyses, standardised data structures are essential.

From the legal point of view, the ISP company is the owner of the customer data and responsible for it. The company must not retain e-mail data externally. Hence, a central data retention system hosted by authorities is not allowed. Further, for competitive reasons companies are usually not interested in storing valuable customer-related data outside their control. An authority may formulate an enquiry for a person as a result of an order of the court. In this case ISPs do have to deliver the communication data for a person timely. Thus, a data retention system is needed allowing distributed, standardized and protected data storage for ISPs and a secure central enquiry interface for the authority. Therefore, we encourage using a distributed data warehouse system to meet all these requirements.

Definitions

'A data warehouse is a subject oriented, integrated, non-volatile and time variant collection of data in support of management decisions' (Kimbal 1996).

Data warehouses (DWH) are designed to facilitate so-called Online Analytic Processing (OLAP) of data. That is, data is analysed interactively based on hypotheses. DWH data is stored in proprietary schemas that are optimised for data analysis.

In the following, we propose a data retention system with standardised data structures, query interfaces, data linkage and data analysis tools. We elaborate a distributed data warehouse that is composed of local data warehouse nodes residing at the ISP companies. We design a data warehouse schema for retaining e-mail and internet access data which satisfies the following requirements:

- store mandatory data according to the EU data retention directive,
- support person, time, and location-related enquiries by appropriate dimensions, and
- store additional information useful for data analysis.

RELATED WORK

Over the past years information technology faced novel demands from data retention requirements (Stampfel et al., 2008; Stampfel, G., &

Gansterer, W. N., & Ilger, M., 2008). Criminals may utilize modern means of communication like phone calls, e-mail, instant messaging, or data sharing to sketch, plan and coordinate their activities. Hence, within the vast amount of data available electronically at phone companies and internet providers, relevant information about interpersonal relationships and ongoing preparation work could be contained. On the one hand, legal and ethical questions concerning violated and deprived civil rights have been raised. Since both communication and internet access data is highly sensitive, privacy-preserving measures are required. Kotzanikolaou (2008) proposes a public-key infrastructure allowing transferring encrypted data between internet service providers, judicious and law enforcement authorities.

On the other hand, efficient and precise data analysis techniques are needed. Much work has been done in context of social network analysis (Menon & Hicks & Larson, 2007; Diesner & Carley, 2005), which strive to reveal social relationships (e.g. communication acts) between individuals. Recently, the National Research Council of the United States released a detailed report on the application of data analysis techniques in counterterrorism activities of the United States (Perry, 2008). Besides describing the limitations of current data analysis techniques, the report recommends a periodic evaluation strategy for these techniques assessing the effectiveness of ongoing programs, evaluating technological advances and ensuring consistency with US Laws.

Various commercial products supporting data retention have been presented recently. Some of them (Teradata Corporation, 2006; DATAllegro, 2008) are based on data warehouse appliances. Others provide server infrastructure together with data appliance in one packet (Sun Microsystems, 2007). These solutions primarily focus on efficient data storing and data integrity issues. Though, no standardised storage schema allowing to query independently of the underlying system has been defined up to now. For instance, one solution

(Hewlett-Packard, 2007) claims to be designed to facilitate integration with law enforcement agency reporting systems. That is, appropriate interfaces to answer enquiries of authorities would have to be implemented. When considering a set of ISP companies, each company may decide to use a different data retention system with proprietary data retrieval and export tools. Therefore, we suggest a standardised data schema allowing well-defined queries and standardised exports to leverage data analyses.

In the following sections we provide a short overview of a possible database implementation which can be used to retain the stored data. Based on the proposed implementation we show how data analysis and queries could work in this situation. Finally we also put a focus on some important limiting factors such as cost aspects related to the creation of a data warehouse, or the security requirements that have to be met to prevent unauthorized access.

DATA STORAGE

Within this section, appropriate data structures for storage and retrieval of e-mail and internet access data are designed. In theory there are many different approaches to store the data. The extreme cases would be to use one single database to store all the data, or to have completely different solutions deployed at each ISP. We propose a distributed data warehouse architecture allowing for retaining sensible customer data inside ISPs. Nevertheless, analyses spanning several ISPs are facilitated by using an identical data warehouse schema in each company and by defining appropriate linkage attributes that may be used to join records across company borders.

Background: Data Warehousing

For building a DWH, relevant data is extracted from various data sources of operational business

Figure 1. Storage schema for e-mail data

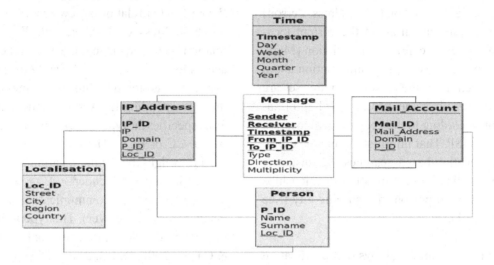

units, transformed, and loaded in the specialised schema. A DWH schema allows viewing data from a multidimensional perspective (Bauer & Guenzel, 2004). That is, data may be viewed from a multitude of views depending on the type and complexity of data analysis requirements. We distinguish entities that are in the centre of analyses and those providing supplementary information for a particular view on the analysed data.

Entities of the former category are called facts while the latter ones are called dimensions. Dimensions of a data warehouse schema are used to aggregate fact table entries and to retrieve summarised data of a subset of interest. Moreover, dimensions may be used to model various granularities of perspectives. Each dimension may be considered as a hierarchical classification allowing access to different levels of granularity. The multidimensional view of data is also considered as a data cube spanned by dimensions and filled by the facts values. A data cube consists of data cells, where every data cell stores a fact value for a certain combination of dimension members.

Email Data Storage Schema

In Figure 1 an adapted star schema illustrates how e-mail data may be stored. In the centre of the schema the fact table Message stores records of e-mail traffic. The fact table is connected with five dimension tables, whereas tables Mail Account and IP Address are connected each with the fact table twice. In the following, the dimension tables are described in detail:

- **Time:** The time dimension stores the date the message was sent or received. Columns Day, Week, Month, Quarter, and Year are used to store the date in different granularities supporting selection, roll-up and drill-down operations.
- **IP Address:** This table is used twice. Once for storing the IP address of the sender and once for storing the address of the recipient However, this information is only available if one or both (sender and receiver) are customers of the same ISP. The idea behind separating the relations between (IP_ Address, Person) and Mail_Account, Person) is that these persons do not have to be identical. Consider a person using his

e-mail account from an internet café. In this case the relation (IP_Address, Person) gives information about the current location (internet café) and the relation (Mail_Account, Person) gives information about the identity of the person. IP addresses are linked with some geographical information according to the geographical location of the ISP. That information may be useful for location-based searches, for instance, for finding communication relationships of a certain person in a specific city (See Figure 1).

Note that this model allows the specification of three different types of location: The person sending or receiving the message has an associated location, the person granting Internet access to the sender or receiver may be assigned a location, and finally the ISP has an associated location.

Like the IP_Address table, Mail_Account is used as dimension table twice: For storing e-mail information of the sender and the receiver. E-mail accounts may be linked with entries of the Person table, if the information is available. This is only the case for customers of the ISP. However, the identity of a person may be detected if records of multiple ISPs are combined for an analysis.

Incoming and outgoing e-mail messages are stored in the same fact table. However, one e-mail may lead to several entries in the Message table, as one e-mail may be sent to multiple recipients. More precisely, one entry in table Message stores a communication act between one sender and one receiver.

Message Storing

An e-mail is sent from one sender (From) to one or more immediate receivers (To). Optionally, one or more persons receive the message as carbon copy (CC) or as blind carbon copy (BCC). For incoming e-mail messages the BCC information is only available for the BCC receiver. For each (From → To) relation a new record is inserted into table Message. Further, each (From → CC) relation is entered in the same way. If the Internet access information of sender and / or receiver is available it is stored by linking the message with the corresponding IP_Address entries. Attribute Type specifies the type of the receiver which could be To, CC or BCC. The message types may be used to weight the communication acts.

For instance, a (sender − TO − receiver) is a more immediate communication act than a (sender − CC − receiver). The type information may be used in social network analysis (Diesner & Carley, 2005; Pathak et al., 2006). We propose to use numerical values to weight the different types, since numerical values may be aggregated in typical OLAP operations. For example, if the top ten communication partners of a certain person have to be determined, an algorithm could calculate a ranking measure out of the frequency and weights of communication acts. The Direction attribute defines if the message is unidirectional or bidirectional. That is, each message containing an In-reply-to entry in its message header is the result of a bidirectional communication.

Further the direction type could be a simple boolean attribute distinguishing between uni- and bidirectional. Attribute Multiplicity specifies the number of addressees of the message. That is, the more addressees receive the message the lower is the degree of privacy of the message. The multiplicity information may be used to filter out private one-to-one communication acts or to weight messages by top-ranking private messages and low-ranking more public messages, for instance, mailing list messages. Outgoing e-mail messages are stored in the same way as incoming messages. The communication partners are extracted from the e-mail message envelopes and corresponding entries are created for all (From → To), (From → CC), (From → BCC) relations.

Figure 2. Storage schema for internet access data

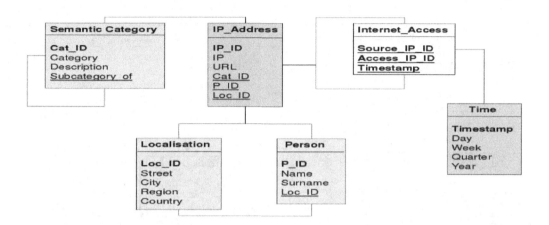

Internet Access Storage Schema

For storing internet access data a similar data warehouse schema may be designed. The fact table Internet_Access stores each visit of a website. That is, each fact corresponds to one website access of a person at a certain time. The fact table is connected to three dimension tables, whereas the table IP_Address is used two times. First, the IP address of the person visiting a certain website is recorded (Source_IP_ID), and second, the IP address of the visited website is stored. If the source IP entries may be related to single persons, they are linked to corresponding Person table entries. Otherwise, they are linked to the localisation of the internet access point (e.g. WLAN hotspot at the airport, internet café) (See Figure 2).

Usually, the access IP entries may be mapped to URLs which are stored in a separate attribute. In order to support elaborated queries, a semantic categorization of websites may be helpful. For example, if the focus of an analysis lies on flight booking, only visits to airline websites, airport websites and flight search engines should be filtered. Semantic categories ease the extraction of meaningful information. Although it's a laborious task to create and maintain semantic an-

notations of websites, the search capabilities are increased significantly.

As semantic categories may be defined for various levels of granularities, we propose to allow a hierarchical classification of categories. A Semantic_Category may be subcategory of another Semantic_Category. For instance, websites of airline and train companies can be generalized to transport websites. Furthermore, as websites may cover several interests or provide a broad range of services, they may be assigned to several categories. Therefore, there is a n:m relationship between IP_Address and Semantic_Category.

The schema allows supporting a multitude of query types. If the focus lies on certain interests or topics, groups of related persons can be identified. On the other hand, if the focus lies on finding common interests or activities of a group of persons, an intersection of all websites visited of all persons of the groups can be determined and common interests may be derived. Further, time and location parameters allow narrowing the result sets. Consider the following example: three persons have been cheated by an unknown criminal trader. Each of them was promised a lucrative profit-sharing of shares for investing several thousand Euros in property funds.

Figure 3. Distributed data warehouse architecture for data retention

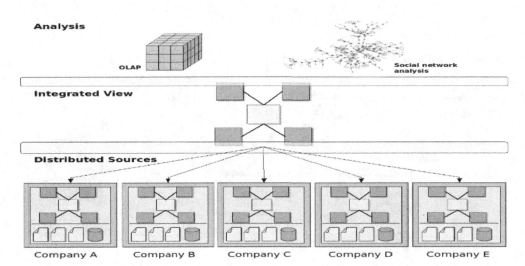

After a personal meeting and handing-over of money, the trader broke the contact. All persons were contacted by email within the same month. As the emails included some personal details (correct profession, place of residence), the trader is assumed to select his victims after a detailed investigation. Hence, a comparative analysis of the internet activities of the cheated persons could shed a light on the investigation activities of the trader. After querying the relevant internet access records of the last month, the common interests are identified. All three persons frequently visited an online gambling casino and were exposing some personal details in associated discussion forums. After investigation of all other participants of the discussion forum and confrontation of the suspicious with the victims, the criminal trader is identified.

Distributed Architecture

Similar to distributed databases, data warehouses may be distributed over various physically separated systems. Much emphasis has been put on distributed architectures (Bellatreche et al., 1999; Noaman & Barker, 1999; Wehrle et al., 2005). Two different types of partitioning may be dis-

tinguished: Horizontal and vertical partitioning. In a vertical partitioning relations are distributed by separating attributes. In a horizontal partitioning, the logical schema remains the same while records are distributed among separate systems. In the context of data retention, we propose a horizontally partitioned data warehouse schema that is distributed over all ISP companies. Thus, sensitive customer-related data is recorded at each ISP and remains at the company's own storage devices.

All ISPs use the same data schema for storing data of the customers and constantly record e-mail and internet traffic. Access to authorities may be granted by exporting and transporting relevant records securely (e. g., by SSH File Transfer Protocol) to analysis software. An illustration of the architecture is given in Figure 3. Each ISP stores its e-mail and internet access data separately as shown in the bottom layer. Data is extracted from log files and written continuously into the predefined relational structures. The fact-dimension schemata illustrated in Figure 1 and Figure 2 are identical for every ISP in order to allow queries and data retrieval across company borders. An integrated view is used to link the distributed data sources together. That is, at least the dimension Person has to be available in a global data repository in order to initiate enquiries.

Each data analysis request is defined on the basis of the global data repository. A set of persons of interest is selected together with parameters for time and location. Then, the data retrieval requests are sent to each data source. Based on the search criteria, all matching entries are filtered out of the local data and returned to the global requester. The result sets may be easily combined because of the identical data structures. The result set is searched for redundant data, and duplicate message entries are eliminated. Finally, data analysis tools – for instance social network analysis tools – may be applied to the retrieved data.

DATA ANALYSIS

Various data analysis techniques exist that may be applied to internet and e-mail data. Generally, these techniques may be assigned to two different categories: subject-based queries and pattern-based queries (DeRosa, 2004). The aim of a subject-based query is to reveal relationships, activities or data of a known subject. A suspected person is observed including its social relationships, financial transactions and planned activities. For example, by querying the credit card transactions, an arranged journey may be identified. Typically, a subject-based query link is answered by searching for data records of an individual in distributed data sources and linking the results. This technique is also referred to as linkage analysis.

Generally, subject-based data mining is likely to enhance traditional police investigations. It allows accessing and analysing large amount of data more comfortably. If one or a few individuals of a communication network are known, entire communication networks can more easily be identified (Perry, 2008). In order to allow correct and exhaustive queries, data records must be unambiguously mapped to individuals, and linkage over various data sources must be supported. In context of data retention standardised query interfaces are required allowing person-centred queries over email and internet access data. Further, queries spanning both kinds of data are possible. For instance, assuming a person is in email contact with a group of people. Then common interests of the group may be deduces by creating an intersection of web access paths of all group members.

DeRosa (2004) specifies data mining as "a process that uses algorithms to discover predictive patterns in data sets". That is, the result of a data mining process is a set of rules, or patterns, or associations revealing knowledge that was previously unknown. While statistical analysis is used to verify or reject predefined hypotheses, data mining algorithms are deployed to generate hypotheses from available data. Data mining may be seen as one processing step in the process of knowledge discovery. After the patterns or relationships are discovered, they are evaluated and transformed in some kind of knowledge representation (Seifert, 2007). One of the most important areas of data mining is the market basket analysis. This analysis focuses on items that are likely to be bought together. A set of association rules reflecting the shopping habits of the consumers is created. For instance, people buying pasta also tend to buy red wine.

Though, the derived patterns do not tell the user anything about the significance or value of the discovered patterns or relationships (Seifert, 2007). That's why the informative value of deduced knowledge should not be overestimated. As described in (Baard, 2002) a federal agency of the United States tried to identify patterns that distinguish the 9/11 hijackers from the rest of the population. By applying data mining techniques to various public and private (e.g. credit card companies) data bases, distinctive patterns should be found. Among some other factors, a high frequency of pizza orders paid by credit cards was detected.

Apart from the questionable relevancy of such patterns there are some other issues concerning data mining that have to be considered.

Taipale (2004) argued that commercial data mining typically operates on homogeneous data sets. Rules or patterns are derived from one type of data. For instance, the consumer buying habits are derived solely from consumers' transactions. Further, the analysis of the navigation behaviour of web users is accomplished by evaluating web logs of a single site. On the contrary, domestic security applications operate on heterogeneous data sets (people, locations, activities). Thus, without modifications established data mining techniques are not applicable to that kind of data. Another problem is the lack of sufficient records that may be used to recognise patterns. Data records of criminal or terrorist activities are rare compared to the vast amount of data that is available for the whole population. As the results of data analysis techniques strongly depend on the quality of data, data records have to be examined carefully. If the internet access data may not related to a single person, because the internet access is shared between two persons, both the data records and the derived patterns are biased.

False Positives and False Negatives

Patterns and rules discovered by data mining techniques are always subject to minor inaccuracies. For instance, a confidence of 98% of a rule specifies that the rule is correct in 98 percent of the analysed data records, but it does not apply in the remaining 2%. Let's assume that a rule is used for fraud detections with credit cards. If the rule applies to the credit card transactions of an honest consumer, he is wrongly assumed to be a criminal. In this case the rule covers a false positive person. Despite of the inconveniences for persons, false positive classifications may impose many costs for the national security because of the employed personal and technical resources (Tapac, 2004). In order to reduce the false positive rate Jensen et

al. (2003) proposed to analyse records of groups simultaneously instead of concentrating single persons. Since the terrorist threat scenarios are based on cooperating individuals, this approach allows concentrating on common interests and communications and may decrease the number of false positive persons.

On the other hand, a rule or pattern may not cover all relevant cases. For instance, the financial transactions of a credit card fraud are unsuspicious and are not covered by any detection rule. The number of false positives and false negatives are complementary. That is, if only the most reliable rules and patterns are selected, the number of false positives will decrease. However, the false negative rate will increase, as fewer relevant cases are discovered. Using less reliable rules hast the contrary effect. Hence, the evaluation and selection of appropriate rules is a challenging task.

Data Analysis Example: Inductive Logic Programming

In the following, we show how inductive logic programming may be leveraged in a pattern-based data analysis of email and internet access data.

Inductive logic programming (ILP) is a *machine learning technique* for synthesising new knowledge from experience. It is used for the construction of first-order clausal theories from examples and background knowledge (Muggleton, 1994). The main idea is to create a knowledge model of a certain domain and to use inductive interference to create hypotheses based on this model. The knowledge model consists of facts and rules, which can be specified in a Prolog notation. Additionally, a set of positive and negative examples is used to support the learning process. The result of ILP is a set of induced hypotheses which are generalised rules that may be used for subsequent classifications. The ILP inference process may be best described by an example. (We are using the syntax of the ILP system Progol (Progol, 2007).

Consider the following scenario: Paul is proven to be involved in illegal weapon export businesses. Though, the group of accomplices has not been identified up to now. There are two other persons – Patrick and Simon – who are suspected to support Paul's activities. In order to identify social relationships and potential common interests the email communication data and internet access data is analysed. Based on Paul's email data and interests, a set of relevant data records (Paul's communication partner and people sharing Paul's interests) is retrieved. These records are transformed into logical facts.

person(paul).
person(patrick).
person(simon).
person(jim).
person(mario).
person(wolf).
person(rudolph).
attends_golf_club(jim).
attends_golf_club(mario).
attends_golf_club(patrick).
attends_golf_club(simon).
communicate(paul,patrick).
communicate(paul,simon).
communicate(simon,paul).
communicate(patrick,paul).
communicate(paul,wolf).
communicate(paul,rudolph).
criminal(paul).

The person facts are type assignments used to classify e.g. the string 'paul' as type *person*. The fact communicate(P1,P2) specifies, that an email was sent from Person P1 to P2 or vice versa. attends_golf_club(Pi) means that the person Pi is a frequent visitor of a certain golf club homepage.

This information was derived by analysing the internet access data. For simplicity, we do not include any other facts regarding the internet access behaviour. However, the fact set may in-

clude much more facts reflecting the interests or participations in organisations of persons. Finally, an artificial fact criminal(paul) is introduced. This fact is some kind of *background knowledge* which should be included in the inference process. Further, we need positive and negative examples to tell the ILP system to filter the relevant rules (hypotheses).

suspicious(patrick).
suspicious(simon).
:-suspicious(jim).
:-suspicious(mario).
:-suspicious(rudolph).
:-suspicious(wolf).

Finally, we need to specify the focus of our analysis. That is, we decide which predicates may appear in the rule heads and which one in rule bodies. In our case, we concentrate on the suspicious predicate and want to generate rules that classify suspicious and not-suspicious persons. The suspicious predicate must be specified as a header (modeh), while all other predicates are only allowed to appear in the rule body (modeb).

:- modeh(2,suspicious(+person))?
:- modeb(1,communicate(-person,+person))?
:- modeb(1,attends_golf_club(+person))?
:- modeb(1,criminal(+person))?

After searching the ILP system finds the following generalised rule:

suspicious(A):- attends_golf_club(A), communicate(B,A), communicate(A,B), criminal(B).

This rule may be interpreted as: all suspicious persons attend the golf club and have bidirectional email contact with a criminal person. As already mentioned, this 'rule' is a hypothesis that be used to distinguish between positive and negative examples and/or find similarities between the positive examples. However, sometimes rules just express tendencies or are only applicable to a small set of learning data. Therefore, an elaborated modelling of the knowledge as well as an evaluation of induced rules are essential tasks.

Let's assume a person 'bill' that has not been assumed to be involved in the weapon businesses. We add some further facts, and query the predicate suspicious:

person(bill).
communicate(paul,bill).
communicate(bill,paul).
attends_golf_club(bill).
:- suspicious(X)?
X = patrick;
X = simon;
X = bill;

Due to the new suspicious rule, bill is classified as a suspicious person and may be eventually related to the criminal weapon circle. Thus, the newly generated rule may be reused as new facts come up. Moreover, the logical representation of relational data allows detecting relationships and links that would have been masked in traditional database systems.

Traditional data mining techniques assume the data is from a single-dimensional table. They have not been designed for analyses of multirelational data. On the other, relational data mining allows to patterns of data from multiple relations that are richly connected (Mooney et al., 2002). Particularly, these techniques seem to be effectively employable in the context of analysis of communication and internet access data. Internet access data is quite complex and hard to analyse. Although, a bulk of site accesses exist for each individual, a high percentage of data may be irrelevant for analysis (e.g. sport news, online newspapers). By enriching site visits with semantic categories, analyses may focus on relevant parts.

Data Analysis Example: Social Network Analysis

Let us assume that the communication acts of a set of persons are to be observed. Either there is a strong indication of social relationships among the persons or they are assumed to communicate with each other. In the latter case, a separate analysis could prove whether there are significant communication acts within the group. In the former case, social relationships between the group and other previously unknown persons could be detected. In the following, the process of extracting common contacts of a group of persons is described. We use the communication network of eight persons illustrated in Figure 4. Each node (P1,.., P8) represents a person whereas each edge models the communication acts between two persons. The weight of edge [w1, w2] summaries the number of messages exchanged between the connected persons. That is, the weights [3, 4] between P2 and P3 indicate that 3 messages were sent from P2 to P3 and 4 messages were sent from P3 to P2.

While the communication between P2 and P3 is bidirectional, unidirectional communication may also occur, for instance, from P1 to P2. We start by globally selecting the persons to be investigated. A group of three persons is defined (P2, P4, P6) and all relevant common contacts between the group and other persons should be detected. Furthermore, a certain period of interest – e.g., two weeks – is specified. Thus, only the message exchange within the last two weeks is considered. In the next step, data requests are created and propagated to all ISPs' data sources. At each ISP a local data extraction is triggered. Hence, for each person of the group, all associated IP_Address and Mail_Account entries are identified and the Message table is searched for related entries.

Furthermore, the result set is filtered according to the time constraint of the last two weeks. After the retrieval has been completed, the data is sent to the global requester who combines all partial

Figure 4. Communication network

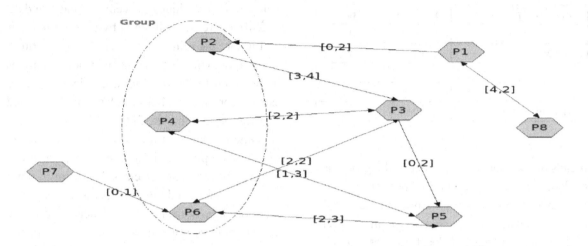

Figure 5. Communication network grouped

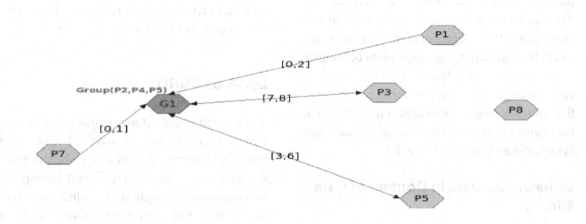

result sets to a global result set. Duplicate entries have to be omitted before the analysis can be started.

In Figure 5 the resulting condensed communication net is shown. As only the communication acts from (P2, P4, P6) are relevant, the edges P1 ←→ P8 and P3 ←→ P5 are omitted. Further, the common edges of (P2, P4, P6) are combined, and weights are accumulated. For instance, P2 ←→ P3, P4 ←→ P3 and P6 ←→ P3 with weights [3, 4], [2, 2], [2, 2] are summed up to one common edge with weight [7, 8]. If we rank all edges we find that persons P3 and P5 are stronger connected to our group than persons P1 and P7. In our example, an edge from a person to our group

Table 1. Message multiplicity

P1 → P2	Mult.	P2 → P3	Mult.
m1	3	m5	1
m2	3	m6	2
m3	5	m7	1
m4	1		
[1.87, 0]		[2.50, 0]	

means that at least one member of the group has exchanged a message with that person.

However, a more conservative approach would be to keep an edge to a person only if all members of the group exchanged at least one message with the person. In our example, all edges except G1 ←→ P3 would disappear. Furthermore, message parameters could be included in the selection and combination process. For instance, if only direct messages sent from one person to exactly one other are examined, all messages having type "TO" as type and a multiplicity value equal to 1 are selected. If the degree of privacy of a message has to be considered, messages might be weighted by multiplying a factor of 1/multiplicity to each message occurrence as Table 1 shows. Although fewer messages were sent from P2 to P3, the degree of privacy of the exchanged messages is higher than between P1 and P2.

Unbalanced Data in Context of Data Mining

Existing learning and classification systems may be significantly influenced by the frequencies of classes (Garcia, 2007). That is, the precision of classifications is reduced if one class is heavily underrepresented (minority class) compared to another (majority class). In the above-mentioned example, the class of suspicious persons may contain significant fewer people than the class of the non-suspicious persons and form a minority class. The suboptimal classification performance was recognized in the machine learning / data

mining research community, who strives to develop new techniques preventing that standard classifiers are overwhelmed by majority classes and ignore the minority classes (Chawla, 2004). Some approaches increase the number of samples in the minority class by adding artificial copies of samples or interpolated samples, which is called oversampling (Chawla, 2002).

Other techniques are based on the concept of undersampling and remove random or noisy samples of the majority class. We want to point out that the retained internet access and communication data is strongly unbalanced due to the vast amount of noisy data. Therefore, appropriate data mining techniques have to be deployed on the retention data. For instance, for applying inductive logic programming on unbalanced data, the Gleaner (Goadrich, 2006) algorithm was developed. However, a detailed experimental evaluation of existing data mining techniques, applied to retention data, is beyond the scope of this chapter and left for future research.

DATA SECURITY ISSUES

The amount of data stored in this scenario combined with the number of involved stakeholders makes it important to think about who can access the data. There are many different scenarios in which somebody might try to gain access to the stored data. These can range from competitors trying to get information about the customers of their competitors, to criminals trying to steal data to steal identities, and use names and user accounts for illegal activities.

Dealing with Distributed Systems

While providing secure access for certain user groups, and monitoring their activities is generally a challenging problem, the level of difficulty increases significantly when dealing with a distributed system. In our scenario we have multiple

ISPs, and each of them has to collect and store data for their own customers. Just by itself this problem seems fairly trivial. It just requires a database, and a set of users who have the rights to access that database. Assigning the required rights to users and maintaining the database is a process that is easily manageable. As mentioned before our scenario includes multiple databases, each maintained by one ISP. This means that each of these companies has not only to make sure that the retained data is stored in its database, but also has to provide means for the authorities to access the data, and also combine the data with the data provided by other ISPs.

Data Access Control

One main problem when it comes to the data access control is that there might be a very large number of people accessing data, and to even more complicate things data is stored in different databases in different locations. There are two main approaches which can be used for data access. Which of the two approaches should be used depends mainly on how easy the actual data retrieval is supposed to be. In a very simple scenario the authorities could ask the ISPs to provide certain information, and one of the ISP's employees queries the data from the database and transmits that data to the authorities. This approach sounds very simple, but requires a lot of manpower on the ISP's side. Furthermore this approach creates a couple of new questions, for example what such a request for data has to look like, or how the data is transmitted to the requester.

The second approach is much more complicated when it comes to the initial setup, but greatly simplifies queries later on. If an architecture is created which allows the authorities to directly pull data from the ISPs' databases (as opposed to a push model in the previous scenario), there is no active data retrieval needed on the ISP's side. The initial setup requires all ISPs to agree on an interface, and a common infrastructure

for authentication and transfer security. This is a challenging problem, as it requires one central point that is trusted by every involved party, and which also has to be willing to take on the work of managing the centralized structure for all parties.

Data Privacy

The aspect of data privacy can be covered by a few basic concepts which have to be considered when designing a system as the one proposed in this chapter. The requirement is to guarantee that the person intended to get some information, is also the only one who gets that information. This means in the first place that each user needs to be identified. This can be achieved by using a public key infrastructure (PKI).

A public key infrastructure is an arrangement in which a user is uniquely identified by a trusted party acting as a certificate authority. This certificate authority then provides that user with a pair of asymmetric keys allowing that user to get encrypted data (which can only be read by the person with the private key), and also allowing the user to sign documents (again, this can only be done by the person with the private key). The counterpart, the public key is published by the certification authority to provide all other involved parties the means to send encrypted information to that user, and to verify that user's signature. This technology provides the means to comply with the most important requirements: Identify the person sending a request, and then when sending the requested data, making sure that this data can only be read by the person who originally requested the data.

Public key infrastructures are quite common today, and there are many initiatives trying to provide people, in some cases for example all citizens of a country, with such certificates. Explaining further details of public key cryptography would by far exceed the scope of this chapter, but there is a plethora of books and scientific articles available on this topic. Right now we only need to know that there are many technologies available that can guarantee the security of data being transmitted to a very large degree.

A second important aspect is to provide means to audit the access to data. A system that is secured against access from people who are not registered as users of a system is not enough. Many attacks of a system could be caused by registered users. For example people could be bribed by criminal organizations, or simply selling the data to whoever is willing to pay most for them. Providing audit trails can greatly reduce the danger of such things happening, and if they still happen despite these precautions, they at least allow the prosecution of the persons who abused the system.

Audit trails are in essence nothing more than a list of chronological events that happened in the system, allowing retracing at a later point which user accessed which data at which time. Of course this does not solve the old problem of users using insecure passwords, leaving workstations logged in to secure systems, or other negligent behaviour of users.

COST AND PERFORMANCE ASPECTS

Two factors that are important for a project such as the one described here are the costs generated by the storage of the data, and also the speed at which requests can be answered. Both of these factors have a strong influence on the general acceptance of a system, and the ease of implementation.

Cost Aspects

Costs can be separated into two different groups. First there are the initial costs to buy all the required hardware and create the system, and then there are the annual costs for keeping the system running and to fulfil all the queries. The first year of service has the highest total costs, as it requires regular operation, just like all other following years, but

also requires initial investments. Besides the purchase of required hardware and software licenses, staff expenses are also significantly higher during that period. Even though the amount of data that has to be stored for each customer per year appears to be relatively small, the requirements of easy access and a good secure infrastructure can generate a relatively high cost per customer.

Expected Query Response Time

A certain level of service has to be guaranteed for all requests. This is especially important in this distributed environment, as many scenarios will require several queries to many different ISPs. To make sure that each request gets a matching reply in a timely manner clear interfaces and processes have to be defined. Additional time might be required to combine the data, if there is no clear interface making sure that the data provided by each of the ISPs matches the format of the others.

In an ideal implementation where a clean architecture is provided that does not require any human interaction, such a query, including the combination of the results provided by the different ISPs, could get a reply in almost real-time. In an architecture that requires a lot of human interaction, in the worst case that would mean that a request is sent to each ISP, and each of them has to verify the request, then prepare the data (each according to their own data structure) and that data has to be combined later on - a workflow that might take a very long time.

LIMITATIONS IN CONTEXT OF DATA RETENTION

There are several circumstances under which an Internet service provider does not possess any personal data about the customer it is serving. In these cases, what is available is information about the equipment used to connect to the provider which depends on the employed type of Internet connection. In the situation of a customer using the free wireless Internet access at a cafe or restaurant for example, the ISP operating this hotspot has no personal data available on which a person is connecting. What he/she does know is the media access control address of the equipment being used to connect to the hotspot. A MAC address is intended to uniquely identify one specific piece of networking hardware. Each equipment vendor has its own address range which can be looked up in certain directories. Although the address is intended to be unique, it is forgeable using readily available software from the Internet which renders the information available to the provider in this case unreliable.

Another possibility of anonymous Internet access is provided by certain dialup providers. Usually a provider asks for a user ID and a password during the authentication process and is able to connect this user ID to an entry in his customer database therefore knowing who it is serving. Because of the different technical possibilities for two parties to communicate via e-mail, there is a difference in the data available for storage depending on the mail server and protocols used and the location of the participating parties. Following is a description of the possible setups and their consequences for data collection. For an Internet service provider there are two possible sites where he/she is able to monitor the e-mail traffic in his/her network and in exchange with other networks at his own mail servers. For the e-mail messages being transmitted and received at person's own mail servers, the data can be collected at these points. If his/her customers are using mail servers outside of his network, the data is being transmitted over the provider's interfaces to other networks, which is where he/she is able to observe this traffic. All the protocols used in the following scenarios may be encrypted or not, which in some cases makes a difference.

Scenario 1: ISP Mail Server only. Scenario one is the situation when two users exchange e-mail messages using the ISP's mail server, independent of the protocols used for mail transmission and receipt. The mail server is controlled by the ISP and the parties are therefore customers of the ISP. This scenario does not specify how the customer is connected to the Internet. The usual case for him would be, as he is using the ISP's mail server, to gain Internet access through this ISP, but it may also be possible for him to be using the mail server from another network. If the communicating users (sender or receiver) are accessing the ISP's mail from inside the network the IP addresses of the corresponding internet accesses are known to the provider and may be immediately related to persons. If another national ISP provides the internet access the identities may be revealed by querying other data retention nodes in the distributed architecture. If the internet access is accomplished by a foreign provider, no information about the persons providing the internet access may be stored. Though, the identities of the communicating users are known, unless the mail accounts are misused by a third or fourth party.

Scenario 2: ISP/Non-ISP Mail Server Mix. In scenario two, again the provider's mail server is used, but this time one party is outside the ISP's network respectively its control. The two mail servers are interconnected by SMTP with the non-ISP mail server communicating with another mail server or directly with the second party. It is both possible that the customer is accessing the mail server either from inside the ISP's network or from the outside. Similar to scenario one the persons providing the internet access for the communicating users may be known or not. Further, the personal data of only one communicating party is known. The personal data of the other party may be available at other national ISP or unknown in case of a foreign communication party.

Scenario 3: Non-ISP Mail Server. As it is the case for people using free mail providers to send their mails, in scenario three an outside mail server, out of the control of the ISP is being used as a mailbox and transmitting server by a provider's customer. This scenario only applies to communications via POP / IMAP and SMTP, therefore excluding web mail access. Opposed to the first two scenarios, this scenario does set the location of the customer. Because of the used mail server not being in control of the ISP, the customer has to be inside of its network for his e-mail traffic to be visible on the network boundary. This scenario is of particular interest because it represents the only circumstances relevant for the EU directive where an encryption, which is possibly applied to the communication, does make a difference: this case is invisible to the provider if the POP, IMAP or SMTP sessions are encrypted.

Scenario 4: Non-ISP Web mail. When using a web mail interface of a mail provider not being the user's ISP, scenario four is the case. The user gains access to his mailbox, residing on a free mail provider's mail server like mail.google.com for example, by using HTTP exclusively. By 'web mail server' the web server hosting the interface for accessing the user's e-mail messages is meant. This web mail server is in some, possible propri- etary way, connected to or is itself the mail server who communicates either directly with the second party or via additional mail servers. This scenario is invisible to the ISP because the communication happens via HTTP. The data is, like in scenario three, being transferred over the provider's lines but not as SMTP but HTTP packets. The e-mail data is therefore embedded in web traffic and may, as it is content of a communication, not be stored according to the EU directive.

CONCLUSION

In March 2006 the European Parliament pub- lished the EU Data Retention directive 2006/24/ EC, requiring operators of publicly accessible electronic communication networks to store data regarding certain activity on their network to help

fighting crime. The directive requires the storage of data describing certain activities, such as who used internet access at which times, or who sent or received e-mail at certain times, but it explic- itly does not allow the storage of any contents of the electronic communication. This directive poses several challenges for authorities, and the affected ISPs alike. A whole new infrastructure has to be created, allowing the easy and efficient retrieval and usage of data that was previously only stored in simple log files, or in many cases not stored at all.

In this chapter we have analyzed the require- ments for a data warehouse that meets the direc- tive's requirements, focusing on two main aspects, the storage of e-mail-related data, and the storage of internet access information. After describing a couple of possible approaches we chose one that we found to be the best. Besides providing an example what the implementation of a database structure might look like, we also showed how a distributed architecture can be used in a scenario like the data retention guideline. In the data analysis chapter we provided examples of how different data mining strategies can be used within the scenario we are faced in this chapter. One of the examples shows how inductive logic programming can be used to derive information from known facts. Another example show how social network analysis can be performed on the data.

Finally we also provided an overview of many factors surrounding the scenario of retaining large amounts of data and later on providing access to the data. To be more precise we described aspects related to data and access security, privacy of sensitive data, as well as cost and performance aspects connected with running such a system. We also provided a short list of examples showing the limitations of data retention in the context of internet related technologies.

REFERENCES

Baard, E. (2002). Buying Trouble: Your Grocery List Could Spark a Terror Probe. *Village Voice.* Retrieved January, 2009, from http://www.villagevoice.com/2002-07-23/news/buying-trouble/

Barandela, R., Rangel, E., Sánchez, J. S., & Ferri, F. J. (2003). *Restricted Decontamination for the Imbalanced Training Sample Problem,* (. *LNCS, 2905,* 424–431.

Bellatreche, L., Karlapalem, K., & Mohania, M. (1999). OLAP query processing for partitioned data warehouses. In *DANTE '99: Proceedings of the 1999 International Symposium on Database Applications in Non-Traditional Environments,* (pp. 35). Washington, DC: IEEE Computer Society.

Chawla, N. V., Bowyer, K. W., Hall, L. O., & Kegelmeyer, W. P. (2002). SMOTE: Synthetic Minority Over-sampling Technique. *Journal of Artificial Intelligence Research, 16,* 321–357.

Chawla, N. V., Japkowicz, N., & Kolcz, A. (2004). Editorial: special issue on learning from imbalanced data sets. *ACM SIGKDD Explorations Newsletter, 6*(1), 1–6. doi:10.1145/1007730.1007733

DATAllegro. (2008). *Datallegro solves telecom data warehouse challenges.* Retrieved May, 2009, from http://www.datallegro.com/data_warehouse_solutions/telecommunications.asp

DeRosa, M. (2004). *Data Mining and Data Analysis for Counterterrorism.* Washington, DC: Center for Strategic & International Studies.

Diesner, J., & Carley, K. (2005) Exploration of communication networks from the Enron email corpus. In *Workshop on Link Analysis, Counterterrorism and Security.*

Elizalde, F. (2006). *EU data retention directive: An onerous burden on service providers.* Retrieved January, 2009, from http://www.frost.com/prod/servlet/market-insight-top.pag?docid=83098430

European Parliament. (2007). *EU data retention directive 2006/24/e.* Retrieved January, 2009, from http://eur-lex.europa.eu/LexUriServ/site/en/oj/2006/l_105/l_10520060413en00540063.pdf

Garcia, V., Sánchez, J. S., Mollineda, R.A., Alejo, R. & Sotoca, J. M. (2007). The class imbalance problem in pattern classification and learning. *CEDI 2007.*

Goadrich, M., Oliphant, L., & Shavlik, J. (2006). Creating Ensembles of First-Order Clauses to Improve Recall-Precision Curves. *Machine Learning, 64*(1-3). doi:10.1007/s10994-006-8958-3

Hewlett-Packard. (2007). *Dragon, data retention and guardian online.* Retrieved May, 2009, from http://h20247.www2.hp.com/enterprise/cache/490843-0-0-82-150.html

Jensen, J., Rattingan, M., & Blau, H. (2003). Information Awareness: a prospective technical assessment. In *Proceedings of the ninth ACM SIGKDD international conference on Knowledge discovery and data mining.*

Jonas, J., & Harper, J. (2006). *Effective Counterterrorism and the limited role of predictive data mining.* Washington, DC: Cato Institute. Retrieved January 2009, from http://www.cato.org/ pub_display.php?pub_id=6784

Kimball, R. (1996). *The data warehouse toolkit: practical techniques for building dimensional data warehouses.* New York: John Wiley & Sons Inc.

Kotzanikolaou, P. (2008). *Data Retention and Privacy in Electronic Communications.* IEEE Security and Privacy.

Memon, N., Hicks, D. L., & Larson, H. L. (2007). *How Investigative Data Mining Can Help Intelligence Agencies to Discover Dependence of Nodes in Terrorist Networks (Vol. 4632).* LNCS.

Mooney, R. J., Melville, P., Shavlik, J., De Castro Dutra, I., & Santos Costa, V. (2002). Relational data mining with inductive logic programming for link discovery. In *Proceedings of the National Science Foundation Workshop on Next Generation Data Mining*.

Muggleton, S. (1995). Inverse Entailment and {P} rogol. *New Generation Computing, 13*.

Muggleton, S., & De Raedt, L. (1994). Inductive logic programming: Theory and methods. *The Journal of Logic Programming*, ▪▪▪, 19.

National Research Council. (2008). Committee on Technical and Privacy Dimensions of Information for Terrorism Prevention and Other National Goals, National Research Council, Protecting Individual Privacy in the Struggle Against Terrorists: A Framework for Assessment.

Noaman, A., & Barker, K. (1999) A horizontal fragmentation algorithm for the fact relation in a distributed data warehouse. In *CIKM '99: Proceedings of the eighth international conference on Information and knowledge management*, (pp. 154–161). New York: ACM Press.

Pathak, N., Mane, S., & Srivastava, J. (2006). Who thinks who knows who? Socio-cognitive analysis of email networks. In *ICDM '06: Proceedings of the Sixth International Conference on Data Mining*, (pp. 466–477). Washington, DC: IEEE Computer Society.

Perry, W. J. (2008). *Protecting Individual Privacy in the Struggle against Terrorists: A Framework for Assessment*. New York: National Academies Press.

Progol. (2007). Retrieved January, 2009, from http://www.doc.ic.ac.uk/~shm/Software/progol5.0/

Seifert, J. W. (2007). *Data Mining and Homeland Security*. Washington, DC: CRS Report for Congress.

Stampfel, G., Gansterer, W. N., & Ilger, M. (2008). *Data Retention - The EU Directive 2006/24/EC from a Technological Perspective*. Vienna, Austria: Medien und Recht Publishing.

Stampfel, G., Gansterer, W. N., & Ilger, M. (2008). *Implications of the EU Data Retention Directive 2006/24/EC. Proceedings of Sicherheit 2008* (pp. 45–58). Gesellschaft für Informatik.

Sun Microsystems. (2007). *Sun Microsystems launches unique data management appliance for communication service providers*. Retrieved, May 2009, from http://www.sun.com/aboutsun/pr/ 2007-06/sunflash.20070607.1.xml

Taipale, K.A. (2004). Technology, Security and Privacy: The Fear of Frankenstein, the Mythology of Privacy and the Lessons of King Ludd. *Yale Journal of Law and Technology, 7*.

Tapac. (2004). *Safeguarding Privacy in the Fight Against Terrorism*. Technology and Privacy Advisory Committee, Department of Defense, Washington, DC: DIANE Publishing.

Teradata Corporation. (2006). *Flexible solution launched by teradata and capgemini to enable compliance with eu data retention directive*. Retrieved, May, 2009, from http://www.teradata.com/t/page/160330/index.html

Wehrle, P., Miquel, M., & Tchounikine, A. (2005). A model for distributing and querying a data warehouse on a computing grid. In *ICPADS '05: Proceedings of the 11th International Conference on Parallel and Distributed Systems*, (pp. 203–209).

Yin, X., & Yang, J. (2006). Efficient Classification across Multiple Database Relations: A CrossMine Approach. *IEEE Transactions on Knowledge and Data Engineering, 18*(6). doi:10.1109/TKDE.2006.94

KEY TERMS AND DEFINITIONS

EU Data Retention Directive 2006/24/EC: Requires that the operators of publicly accessible electronic communication networks to store ("retain") certain data which is generated or processed in their networks to serve the investigation, detection, and prosecution of serious crime.

Data Warehouse (DWH): A specialized data storage technique that facilitates analytic processing of data. That is, data is analyzed interactively based on hypotheses. DWH data is stored in proprietary schemas that are optimized for data analysis.

Data Mining: Is a type of data analysis. The result of a data mining process is a set of rules, or patterns, or associations revealing knowledge that was previously unknown. While statistical analysis is used to verify or reject predefined hypotheses, data mining algorithms are deployed to generate hypotheses from available data.

Social Network Analysis: Is a technique that strives to reveal social relationships (e.g. communication acts) between individuals that have not been known before. It may be applied to communication data such as email traffic data.

Inductive Logic Programming (ILP): Is a pattern-based data analysis technique that may be applied to email and internet access data. The main idea is to create a knowledge model of a certain domain and to use inductive interference to create hypotheses based on this model.

Internet Service Provider (ISP): Is an organization offering internet access to customers. The internet access is provided by servers of the company. Additionally, an ISP may offer email accounts for customers.

Data Privacy: Covers aspects of data protection of person-related information that is collected and stored in information systems of companies and/or authorities. The collected data must be protected from disclosure. That is, authentication and access control policies are used to prevent unauthorized access of person-related data.

Chapter 9
On Data Mining and Knowledge:
Questions of Validity

Oliver Krone
Independent Scholar, Germany

ABSTRACT

Understanding data mining (DM) as part of Information Systems (IS) this contribution investigates the question how this subordination is reasoned in a technological and business logical perspective. For this purpose general characteristics of Enterprise Resources Planning Applications (ERP) and Management Information Systems (MIS; including here Decision Support and Expert Systems) are presented. Based on this evaluation it is examined how knowledge and DM are becoming interdependent for Knowledge Management (KM) in organizations. Knowledge is defined along the Penrose'an dichotomy of information and knowledge in the context of resources and services. Validity of knowledge is analyzed from a methodological (quantitative versus qualitative methods) perspective, probing what key characteristics of both method strands are, and how those fit into the discipline of Organizational Studies. Unveiling a relationship between security and information in Penrose, an alternative account of security originating in Foucault is presented. In this security and knowledge become means for standardization of live in order to allow for continuation of an abstracted, socially generated object. Combining arguments about validity of knowledge claims with that of security, DM based knowledge and security are identified as means abstracting from a human core and attempting constraining variability. Against this background researchers and users of DM based knowledge are asked for awareness of the constructed character of IS, and how much of this constructed character is contained in DM based knowledge.

DOI: 10.4018/978-1-60566-906-9.ch009

INTRODUCTION

The purpose of this paper is examining what grants the special status of data mining (DM), and more general business intelligence (BI), in the dedicated organisation and in organisational sciences. On a conceptional level DM is understood as part of Information systems (IS) research. Furthermore, this paper is interested learning and developing an account of DM and its knowledge creation capabilities. The scope of this paper is limited to intra-organisational and academic development and spread of knowledge to create better "action options". It does not consider actual methods for data mining. The paper is not reporting about DM procedures for generation of data pools originating in different organisations. The author examines the processes of 'knowledge' generation and validity assignment; the paper is of theoretical nature, and rests on interpretative methods.

Two research questions are examined

How does data mining fit into organizations' information system landscape for information (and knowledge) collection and spread?

How validity is attributed to knowledge that is generated by DM, while other methodological approaches are neglected in organisations and organisational sciences?

Based on these research questions in an introduction chapter an overview to information systems (IS) and how DM is related is given. Following this introduction, knowledge/ Knowledge Management and methods for knowledge generation are examined based on an Penrose'an understanding of knowledge. Penrose is chosen here, as she is widely perceived as one "founder" of knowledge management. Taking up the question why DM based knowledge is more valued then qualitative methods originating one, characteristics of knowledge formation in both methodological stances are presented. It is examined how

DM relates to criticism brought forward against knowledge generated outside of academic and research (e.g. Ravetz 1996; Thompson-Klein 1996; Nowotny et al., 2004). Arguments developed there, form the background for identification of Future Trends in knowledge generation via DM. The chapter concludes in consolidating the technical background of DM under the heading of knowledge management and the alleged methodological superiority of DM. This consolidation happens based on Foucault's analysis of security and how IS relate to this understanding.

This paper relates itself to the fields of DM and Information Systems suggesting DM is output from and contributing to Information Systems (IS). The author takes up the offer formulating perspectives on the subject of DM and value creation with knowledge by examining how DM initially was part of the discourse on Knowledge Management with a strong technological emphasis (IT technologies). Questioning the validity of knowledge generated with DM the relation between DM and decision making in organizations is analysed. This contribution explores implications of DM and its social (and network) impact. In the author's account, the paper relates itself to the handbook by highlighting features of DM in organisations and the discipline of Organisational Sciences under the perspective of knowledge creation and validity of DM based knowledge.

Societal effects of technological advancement as enabler for DM, and their impact on globalization (e.g. Castells, 1996), are taken for granted. Reason being that the author is not interested in technologies and their contribution to globalisation, but on the process by which validity is attached to the outcomes from DM (cp. Floyd, 1992 a/b; D'Adderio, 2002; Kallinikos, 2004).

This contribution does not consider data quality, while acknowledging data qualities eminent important role in the process of DM. This omission is justified by noting that the author explicitly refers in course of the paper to notation differences on what is important for whom when the generation of data-marts is described (Markus, 2001).

BACKGROUND: DATA MINING AND INFORMATION SYSTEMS

In this part, terminological clarifications are given and the theoretical questions inspiring this article are unveiled.

Information Systems

The definition of IS used rests on the distinction between technical- and human-systems, and their interaction in socio-technical systems. IS are "[..] system[s] of communication between people. Information systems are systems involved in the gathering, processing, distribution and use of information. Information systems support human activity systems" (Beynon-Davies, 2002, p.4). Human activity systems are any kind of human interaction that is happening for a given purpose; public and private organisations represent human activity systems. Based on this perspective IS are divided into infrastructure and instruments (applications) built onto this infrastructure (Beynon-Davies, 2002, p. 66). Applying this definition Management Information Systems (MIS) and Enterprise Resources Planning Applications (ERP), and applications utilised for the administration of databases themselves are of interest.

MIS are information-oriented applications. Their purpose is structuring and controlling different processes in organisations (Turban, McLean, and Wetherbe, 2002, p. G-7). MIS are employed for standard operations and decision-making in organisations (ibid., p. 52). Beynon-Davies (2002) stipulates a close link between data used for MIS and Expert Systems (ES). Latter, are employed for non-routine activities with high levels of insecurity, as less knowledge is existent about the impacts and potential outcomes of actions (Beynon-Davies 2002, v p. 92). ES (cp. Stahlknecht & Hasenkamp,

2002) attempt structuring information available to managers. ES are based on a multi-layered technical architecture using ontologies, represented by semantic means (natural language), of a certain field of examination (Stahlknecht and Hasenkamp, 2002, pp. 435-439). ES's automate the process of decision-making in order to allow management refocusing on managerial activities. During the late nineties of the last century, these expert systems became subject to strict scrutiny. With the social movement of knowledge management, it became apparent that ES are limited in their capabilities describing in unitary ways the universes' of examination among experts from different domains (e.g. Pipek, Hinrichs & Wulf, 2003; cp. Markus, 2001).

Enterprise Resources Planning Applications (ERP) are similar to MIS. They emerged during the 1980s' and extended the view of MIS by combining data collected for each domain (functional area of an organisation) into overall organisational data. Allowing, and facilitating, for the generation of ever more abstract data, senior-management ideally anticipates based on data the direction organisations are heading too. During the nineties of the last century ERP were enriched with workflow (process) steering elements (e.g. Kallinikos, 2004).

A dedicated class of applications directly associated with the creation of the data repositories are databases. Those exist in different varieties. According to Beynon-Davies (2002, p. 139; cp. Stahlknecht and Hasenkamp, 2002) a database is a logical description of a given object in line with the attributes that describe the object in question (Stahlknecht and Hasenkamp, 2002, p. 139-140). A database is an "[..] organised repository for data having similar properties" (Beynon-Davies, 2002, p. 139). Given this functional task description, high technological efforts are required to maintain the functions of data a) sharing, b) integration, c) integrity maintenance, d) security, e) abstraction, f) independence (ibid., p. 140). For data mining in particular the properties of data sharing, integration, abstraction and independence are important; they allow for new knowledge generation (cp. Blackwell and Ravda, w/o year, chapter 2).

Database management systems (DBMS) facilitate these functions, and ensure structural maintenance, transaction processing, information retrieval, and finally data administration of databases. DBMS are the interface between the actual data storing and the data model with the normalised data description (Beynon-Davies 2002, 140-141).

DATA GENERATION FOR DATABASES

Data normalisation is the process of stripping a given focal object of all its features and define thereby the properties (attributes, and tables) describing and defining the objects characteristics (Stahlknecht and Hasenkamp, 2002, pp. 177-179; Beaulieu, 2005, pp. 4-6). Information systems and databases involve descriptions of real-life objects. In addition, a question rises how developers and users understand them.

In the relevant IS literature, there exists criticism to this process of abstraction. Authors are disturbed with the process by which scientific computing develops and applies without questioning conceptional models underlying software design (e.g. Floyd, 1992 b; Capurro, 2008; Stahl and Brooke 2008). Some of this criticism is directed to the form of software design (Floyd, 1992 a), while others refer to the involvement and apprehension of the uninvolved users into system design (Markus, 1983; Curtis, Krasner and Iscoe, 1988; more recent Capurro, 2008; Stahl and Brooke, 2008). Another stream of criticism relates to the reality shaping forces inherent to IS (e.g. Orlikowski and Gash, 1994). IS are not only technological objects representing a translation of social reality into code, but become part of a reality construction - IS and social reality are interdependent objects. This interdependency is validated and controlled for

side effects (cp. Flyod, 1992 a; Orlikowski and Gash, 1994; Adler and Borys, 1996). Kallinikos (2004) and Isomäki (2002) show how much IS are based on rationalistic accounts humans by software designers.

Data Mining

Data mining has many different definitions, of which here two are given. First it is "[..] described as 'the nontrivial extraction of implicit, previously unknown, and potentially useful information from data' [Witten and Frank, 2005, XXIII] and 'the science of extracting useful information from large data sets or databases. 'Data mining in relation to enterprise resource planning is the statistical and logical analysis of large sets of transaction data, looking for patterns that can aid decision making."

The first definition of DM is guiding this paper. This is achieved is by applications that

[..] sift through databases automatically, seeking regularities or patterns. Strong patterns, if found, will likely generalize to make accurate predictions on future data (Witten & Frank 2005).

DM's focus is unfolding of patterns in information contained in databases – or data warehouses –that are not immediately open to human perception; it helps humans generating new knowledge from information in order to take decisions. DM is a method for information conversion in a triadic relationship of "data-information-knowledge" (Luft, 1994; Tuomi, 1999; Lee and Yang, 2000; Alavi and Leidner, 2001). For Witten and Frank (2005) DM is the process of "abstraction: taking the data, warts and all, and inferring whatever structure underlies it" (Witten and Frank, 2005, XXIII). Given this scope, it is not surprising that they focus on the process

[..] in which the result of "learning" is an actual description of a structure that can be used to classify examples. This structural description supports

explanation, understanding and prediction (Witten & Frank 2005).

This is interestingly a very formal and close description of the term theory as it is maintained in many conceptions of scientific knowledge (e.g. Stacey, 2001). With this focus on information generation from existent data, the author takes databases as representations of normalised objects contained in reality allowing for their machine based manipulation. Against this background, a clarification is required how data used in DM are generated for automated data analysis. Keeping the abstraction process in mind (normalization), it is necessary outlining characteristics of data warehouses in the field of data mining.

Data Warehouses and Data Marts

"A data warehouse is a subject oriented, integrated, non-volatile, and time-variant collection of data in support of management's decision-making process" (Immon, 2002). A vendor defines data-warehouses as

[..] a relational database that is designed for query and analysis rather than for transaction processing. It usually contains historical data derived from transaction data, but it can include data from other sources. It separates analysis workload from transaction workload and enables an organization to consolidate data from several sources. (Oracle 2008, 321).

Quite often data warehouses are either filled by transactional data (originating in ERP and MIS systems; Online transaction processing - OLTP) or fed by inputs for Decisions Support Systems (DSS; for more generalised description of data warehouses and interactions with DM Beynon-Davies, 2002, pp. 456-457). Data warehouses' content originates in OLTP. Data are more history oriented making it common referring to data warehouses' content as a predecessor for online

analytical processing (OLAP). OLTP data have to be condensated and normalised in order to be usable for OLAP.

An OLAP is dependent on results from the different departmental OLTP, and the conversion/normalisation of these data for the data warehouse. If this does not happen data inconsistencies occur that lead to skewed and wrong results (Chaudhuri & Dayal, 1997, chapter 2; see also Markus, 2001 op cit).

In particular during data cleansing for importing data into warehouses issues of data quality are of eminent importance. This is also the stage were organisational departments begin battling for the power describing overall organisational internal reality, and the environment in which it is acting (e.g. D'Adderio, 2002).

In the field of Business Intelligence OLTP, data are referred too as data marts. Latter are extracts from the overall data warehouse. Data marts are repositories of a given domain and data utilisation can be restricted in an organisation, but data are subject to the same data purification methods as those for data warehousing (Chaudhuri & Dayal 1997). In Figure 1 the process of data extraction, normalisation, and upload to the warehouse is described in a schematic description.

KNOWLEDGE AND VALIDITY: A METHODOLOGICAL ORIENTATION FOR DM

In this chapter, the task is deciphering what knowledge is in the field of KM and what the relation between data mining and knowledge is. In order to do so the author sketches some of the arguments forwarded by Penrose. These arguments form the basis for the strategic management idea of Knowledge Management (Grant, 1996 a / b). The publication of Nonaka and Takeuchi (1995) and Leonard-Barton (1995) can be interpreted as the final stages in the process of the emergence of Knowledge Management as a dedicated field

Figure 1. Architecture of a data warehouse (Oracle, 2008, p. 324)

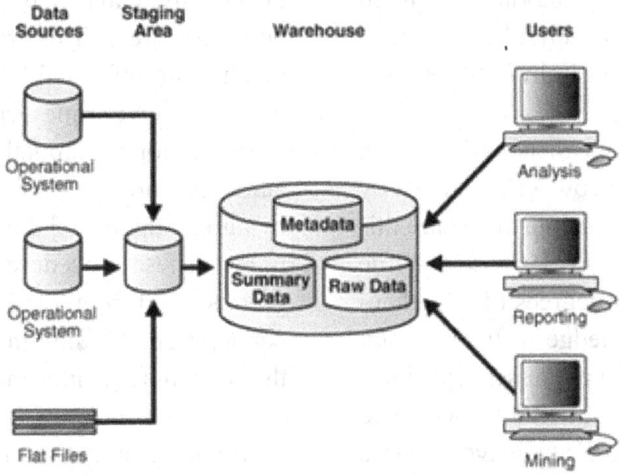

of research in Business Administration and / or Information System research. The task is checking whether Penrose sets the groundwork for Knowledge Management as it is regularly suggested.

Penrose and the Knowledge Term

Penrose's understanding of knowledge cannot be isolated from the organisational form in which knowledge is dealt with. For her the firm is the "[..] 'flesh and blood' organizations that business-men call firms"(Penrose 1995, 13).

Firms execute economic activities in accordance with plans defining the utilisation of resources as contributions to the provisioning of services and goods to the economy in general. Behaviour of, and within, the firm is determined by these plans devised by an independent unit within the firm which is part of the overall bureaucracy of the corporation. This bureaucracy entails policies, decisions rights and the work distribution (ibid., pp. 15 – 17). Furthermore, the firm is described by the existence of "[..] productive resources" (Penrose 1995, 24) and their utilisation in line with plans. Resources are capable rendering services to the production process. For the analysis here the pair of terms of services and resources

is enlightening, as 'knowledge's' character is subsumed into this dichotomy.

Penrose (1995) argues that

[..] resources consists of a bundle of potential services and can [..] be defined independently of their use, while services cannot be so defined, the very word 'service' implying a function, an activity.

Services inherent to a resource are exposed while utilising latter. Resource utilisation defines the value to the firm, which relate to other characteristics of resources. Resources can be bought in the market, produced in the firm, sold to the market, or produced and used by the firm (Penrose 1995, 24-25).

She does not give a terminological definition of knowledge, but there is an alleged affinity to constructionist understandings of knowledge. This definitional lapse arises from the fact that Penrose is not concerned with the concept of knowledge per se. Rather, she attempts understanding how the application of resources and services rendered from them, is dependent on each other.

In this analysis information gathering relates to uncertainty minimisation, while knowledge is contextualised with resources and services and their development and utilisation. She differentiates two kinds of knowledge. One kind is acquired during formal education ("objective knowledge"), while a second results from individual learning processes ("experiences").

Objective knowledge is characterised by a level of specify that is not to narrow and is shared by a sufficient large group of people that share this objective knowledge (Penrose 1995, 53). While people can have different degrees of apprehension of this objective knowledge, differences of it result from communication processes (cp. Hinds & Pfeffer, 2003) they do not lead to dedicated different sets of knowledge. Knowledge acquired by the individual as result of learning processes is experience. Experience and knowledge are different for two reasons: first experience is bound to individuals "[..] it produces a change – frequently a subtle change – in individuals and [second, it] cannot be separated from them" (Penrose, 1995, p.53). Second, experiences are results of actions taken. Due to this action-orientation, experiences lead to an enhanced understanding of where and how objective knowledge is employable. Consequently, Penrose speaks of experiences of individuals if they have acquired new knowledge, and they employ objective knowledge in different ways (ibid.).

Subjective uncertainty is defined by Penrose as a "[..] feeling that one has too little information [that] leads to a lack of confidence in the soundness of the judgments that lie behind any given plan of action" (Penrose 1995, 59). In this understanding information collected are means obtaining a better view on the potential sequences of activities taken during plan implementation. The acquisition of information

[..] requires an input of resources, and to evaluate information requires the services of existing management. Therefore one of the important effects of subjective uncertainty is to induce a firm to devote resources to what might be termed 'managerial research' (ibid.).

The amount of information gathered will wary on an individual firm basis. Even after a comprehensive search, firms are taking risks - but on a much more informed basis and are thereby less uncertain. Over time firms become used to this type of information gathering. In turn specified amounts, and types, of information are selected by agreed upon "[..] defined procedures" (ibid., p. 60). These procedures satisfy the managerial groups' need for information gathering; they become part in decision-making. The fulfilment of the procedure of information collection thereby ensures the validity of the information generated.

Looking at data mining from this angle it becomes apparent that information aggregation in data warehouses and data normalisation is seemingly a predecessor activities to information processing via OLAP; and thus knowledge generation. It can be uncovered that DM has a relationship to knowledge whereby latter becomes operationally more 'secure', and plan implementation more risk resilient.

According to Castells (2002), we are living in a global and network world that increases the amount of insecurity (cp. Dornier et al. 1998 for the field of operational and logistic planning). Under these conditions, DM becomes a "natural process" for the evaluation of potential negative impacts on organisations action plan realisation. Paradoxically DM, and the information technologies used by it, contributes to the process of globalisation (cp. Castells; Dillon 2008 for the field of globalised securities markets). The question remains why in particular DM is so favourable evaluated for its knowledge generating capabilities, while other means are omitted from the evaluation of valuable inputs to decision making in the individual organisation.

First Generation Knowledge Management

In this section main threads of the first phase of knowledge management endeavours are examined and contrasted with the understanding of knowledge and information coming from Penrose. For Penrose knowledge in the first instance is available, and used, on an individual level. Knowledge is conceived as a property of individual and belonging to a given group to which a given set of 'objective knowledge' is available; knowledge is not the central object of the analysis. That knowledge is a device for the realisation of other things needs to be emphasised, as this clearly sets her off from later proponents of KM, who treat knowledge as an asset (cp. Leonard-Barton, 1995, Nonaka & Takeuchi, 1995; Grant, 1996 a/b). Penrose is concerned with the capability of how knowledge is employed generating further services.

Knowledge management, as elaborated by Nonaka and Takeuchi (1995) and Leonard-Barton (1995), rests on the assumption that knowledge brought to the organisational level is immediately accessible for taking actions. Often technical means are perceived sufficient to provide options for innovations. Pfeffer and Sutton (2000) take issue with the very consequence of the attitude that often corporations use Knowledge Management in the explicit/ tacit understanding (Nonaka and Takeuchi, 1995) leading to

[...] to build stock[s] of knowledge [and information], acquiring or developing intellectual property (note the use of the term property) under the presumption that knowledge, once possessed, will be used appropriately and efficiently (Pfeffer & Sutton 2000, 16).

Wilson (2002) argues that during the initial phases KM was examined in fields of computing and information systems, information science-information management and management. Most papers were publicised in journals about Decisions Support Systems. Often knowledge and information were used synonymous. Knowledge was conceived as a deeply individual, personalised item, referring to either action, in the meaning of executing a task, or to the human capacity

to draw conclusions from information via the contextualisation - referring to the knowledge triade described above (Wilson, 2002 and Penrose op.cit.). Examining consecutively the definitions of KM offered by consulting corporations in the early 21st century many of the technological frameworks for data mining were treated as instances of KM. It seems that during the early days KM was set synonymous with DM and information distribution in organisations. Both activities are here discussed here with a critical eye to their reality content in terms of knowledge validity. Given the lack of terminological rigour as to what knowledge is, how practices look like that guide KM, and the heavy emphasis on IT, Wilson (2002) concludes that KM can described by a strong practical impetus.

A hermeneutical reading of Penrose suggests a very different picture on a number of topics. In the first instance it becomes apparent that the social embedding of knowledge is recognised, and that seldom two people share exactly the same knowledge. This is due to the character of knowledge in its tripartite understanding (cp. Luft, 1994; Tuomi, 1999; Lee & Yang, 2000; Alavi and Leidner, 2001). It seems that proponents of Knowledge Management work on the assumption originating in Penrose's understanding that there is a set of objective knowledge available to all; a view to which Wilson has nothing to say except that it is a highly dubious conception. Furthermore this perspective on KM is wrong when observing that other means are required allowing for Knowledge Sharing.

Knowledge Sharing in its own right is as well short in explanatory power on how new knowledge comes into the world. Reason being: it is rarely taken into consideration which effects knowledge differences, based on socialisation, have on Knowledge Sharing (e.g. Pfeffer and Sutton, 2000, Hinds and Pfeffer, 2003; Huysman and de Wit, 2003). Authors taking up the problem of information understanding, defined as conversion of information into knowledge, argue much more based on information exchanges. Information exchanged are treated in data mining as inputs for the computation of knowledge (Witten and Frank, 2004). This holds in particular true for the works of Lichtenstein and Hunter (2005) and Markus (2001). It seems that authors arguing in the field of Knowledge Sharing employ the data-information-knowledge hierarchy.

Organisational Knowledge, as another field that has an enormous interest in IS, and thus the data mining, shows in a much more pronounced way some of the difficulties. In particular it is the indecisiveness whether organisations have knowledge of their own, or whether employees, as representatives of the organisation, exchange their knowledge that is in turn taken as organisational knowledge (e.g. Nelson and Winter, 1982; Jones, 1995; Robey, Boudreau and Rose, 2000; Stacey, 2001; Lehesvirta, 2004).

This admittedly cursory overview of KM indicates that DM based knowledge generation has problematic features (cp. Dennis et al., 1998 for the example of knowledge conveyance capacities of different media; Markus, 2001; Mulder, 2004). Referring back the definition of IS, it becomes apparent that IS and knowledge are seemingly dependent on each other in the light if data mining. Moving a step further it is argued that data stored in the data marts or data warehouses, of organisations represent very different, point of view dependent, interpretations of organisations themselves and their environment.

At this stage it becomes apparent that this chapter contributes to the content of this Handbook by developing a genealogy on the emergence of DM based knowledge generation as result of the availability of different technologies, and how those are used to develop accounts of reality in which organisations (be those private or public) act. Furthermore, this chapter attempts showing where and whether classical organisational theories (here Penrose, but also Nelson and Winter, 1982 could be taken), can be considered possible

ancestors to DM based KM – and thus knowledge generation and assigning validity to it.

METHODS FOR KNOWLEDGE GENERATION FROM 'OPERATIONS'

Under this heading it is attempted understanding why in organisational sciences data mining has received so much attention, and as important, why knowledge created by non-quantitative methods is somewhat neglected.

The Rational-Empirical Legacy

Science has followed, according to Toulmin (1990) and Nowotny et al. (2004), a very long time the depersonalised and rational conception of knowledge creation with an emphasis on the general (Toulmin, 1990). If looking into the field of organisational sciences the same holds true and there even more prominent (e.g. Mintzberg 1978; and the whole classic economics oriented school of Principal – Agent theory and the related field of Transaction Cost Economics – e.g. Eisenhardt 1989b; Holmstrom & Tirole 1989; Willimason 1991; Tsoukas & Cummings 1997).

Tsoukas and Cummings (1997) refer to this development in, and of, organisational studies as the desire of management sciences being treated as a science based discipline. In an academic strict understanding of sciences, organisational studies begin during the 19th century. Tsoukas and Cummings suggest that the rather strict formalistic approach toward knowledge and science was selected to achieve recognition of the discipline towards the end of the 19th century (cp. Turner, 2001, pp. 47-51 for a discussion of methodological choices during the development of the academic sector during the 19th century). It is suggested that the field of organisational sciences begins considering management as 'management sciences' only after the full implementation of rationalism as way of doing sciences in the wake of the Industrial Revolutions.

This phase represents historically the combination of technology and 'management methods' (Tsoukas & Cummings, 1997). Toulmin (1990) argues that many of the main tenants of rational knowledge (sciences) - written form, universal scope and search for appliance, a temporal validity (Toulmin 1990, 30-35) - are reflections of the attempt to minimise humans' fallacies. Formalism is a mean overcoming and dealing with fallacies of humans' cognition and ambitions as exposed during the Thirty Year War (Toulmin 1990, 54-56).

Thus, a first hint on the supremacy of rational arguments relates back to the time of the beginning 18th century and the academic endeavour looking for eternal truth (cp. Tsoukas & Cummings 1997; Foucault 2006a, 394-400). How does DM fit into organisational sciences when it is based on the particular data sets of the individual organisation– a move that represents almost a turnaround of the rational ethos? In the wider discourse on rationality information are referred to as a resource minimising risk, and thus to the concept of security. This resembles Penrose's understanding of information as a source for taking action on a more informed way by gaining better understanding of the consequences of actions taken. Security, in line with Foucault (2006 a/b), is one of the main tenants of the modern way of thinking in liberal democratic states - but security takes for Foucault a very different form that is elaborated below in more detail.

One of the main properties of knowledge generated during the 18th and 19th century is its foundation in an academic setting under conditions of academic peer review. This review, and the methods employed for knowledge generation, established the validity. There were no, or little, external locations that engaged in the production of knowledge.

As result of the industrial revolution, and latest after World War II, Nowotny et al. (2004) observe that knowledge generation moved out of the traditional, state-sanctioned, predominant field of academic research into the individual (industrial-)organisation (Nowotny et al. 2004, pp. 66-75 and pp. 80-84). In particular the commercial oriented production of knowledge, while adhering to procedures resting on rational-methodological empirical methods, has led to a re-orientation to the particular organisation (ibid. pp. 88-90). Knowledge becomes particular, and validity - results of research conducted – is assigned to the outcomes of research by their fit to the purpose for which solutions were looked for (Nelson & Winter, 1982 have labelled this process "search"). "Knowledge" generation becomes temporal, oriented to the particular, and "personalised" to the employee working in a given process and conducting the inquiry – and mediated by this process knowledge becomes organisational (cp. Nelson & Winter, 1982, 247-250).

In line with the overall move towards constructionist bases, it starts with Kuhn (1996) and then reaches the late 20th and early 21st century management sciences (e.g. Von Krogh, Roos & Slocum, 1994; Leonhard-Barton, 1995; Nonaka & Takeuchi, 1995). Thus, the discipline of organisational sciences begins re-appropriating qualitative methods by its interdisciplinary character (for a discussion of different disciplinarily understandings, Thompson Klein 1996; Krone 2007, 23-24). Simultaneously, internal to organisations, the old 'rationalistic-empirical' mode of knowledge generation is favoured – in particular in the mathematics and formulae oriented way (e.g. Tsoukas & Cummings, 1997). So, where is DM situated in this dialogue between technological inspired knowledge creation and the quest for the general?

DM and the Particular: Methodology for the General

Data mining is oriented to individual organisation's knowledge creation. This does not happen consciously. Rather, this 'individualised' form of knowledge creation is part of the appropriation of IS in due course of their implementation in the organisation (cp. Swanson, 1994; Krone, 2007). Due to the character of IS, being based on 'Best Practice' from a wide array of industries and many implementations, they have a general appeal, layout and organisational model included (Kallinikos, 2004, 22). From a practitioners perspective DM is seemingly oriented to the creation of general valid, a-temporal knowledge. This dualism is identified when recognising ERP's foundation on software engineers idiosyncratic understanding of humans and the task at hand in the individual organisation where ERP are implemented (Isomäki 2002, 184-187; Kallinkos 2004, 9-11). Based on Penrose's idea that information minimise reluctance in taking actions the rise of DM becomes explainable in line with the traditional self-understanding of economics and the field of organisational sciences as a very much-related field of studies.

Economics as a discipline is about the most efficient allocation of resources in a given setting under constrains of scarcity. In line with this understanding, DM's property of allowing developing new modes of conducting business make it attractive planning resources deployment in operations (Luan, 2002 for the academic field; Sartipi, Yarmand and Down, 2007 for the field of Electronic Health Provision; Blackwell and Ravada, w/o). With the aid of DM organisations develop and improve their internal procedures by 'technological' task execution based on data originating in OLTP. For scholars conducting research in the field of organisational sciences, the question to be asked is: why there is no outcry about the return to the particular?

It shall suffice suggesting that insofar as data mining, and the infrastructural applications leading to raw data used for machine learning, is constructed with a rational impetus it reinforces a rationale world perspective (Floyd, 1992; Tsoukas and Cummings 1997; Kallinikos 2004). Results gained from the particular organisation are perceived generally valid, since methods used in DM are generally valid ones. Knowledge creation

becomes an activity isolated from the general discourse of knowledge validity; or rather, the methods assure validity as such (cp. Penrose, op. cit.). Knowledge created in commercial settings adheres to the same principles as that generated for scientific purposes, so one could argue: It is rational science with the general in focus, so why bother (Nowotny et al., 2004, pp. 198-200 and p. 223). The remaining question to be asked becomes: if the particular results from data mining are not challenged in their validity, why the same status is not granted to knowledge that is created by non-quantitative methods?

UNCOVERING THE RATIONAL IN QUALITATIVE METHODS

Following Toulmin (1990), Kvale (1995), Czarniawska(-Joerges) (1998, 2001), Sandberg (2005) qualitative methods, and thus as "weak" perceived information, are critisised for failing minimising impacts of human accounts of organisational reality in the knowledge creation process.

When later engaged in qualitative research I encountered the positivist trinity [...] used by mainstream researchers to disqualify qualitative research. [..,]"The results are not reliable, they are produced by leading interview questions"; "The results are not to be generalized, there are too few interview subjects"; and "The interview findings are not valid, how can you know if you find out what the person really means? (Kvale 2005).

Kvale shows that these weaknesses are endemic to knowledge creation with qualitative methods (Kvale, 1995). For him qualitative and quantitative oriented methods are not per se right or wrong. They deviate in their scope of application and intentions of explanation. Following Kuhn (1996) there is not so much difference in respect to the ways in which knowledge is generated, but rather how relevant others are convinced that a dedicated set of knowledge is valid (understood as reality description that is shared in a given social setting; cp. Berger & Luckmann 1990; Barnes 1995; Stacey 2001).

Peculiarities of Qualitative Research

For Kvale (1995) quantitative and qualitative forms of knowledge creation have their subjective influences. Under conditions of constructionist knowledge generation, here exemplified on the example of theories, knowledge sets are considered valid if they recognise:

Validity as Quality of Craftsmanship

The validity of research result arises from the capacity of the researcher to remain within the limits of his/ her original research. This includes a constant process of self-reflection by the researcher. He/she is asking him-/herself whether methods used are correctly applied, and whether potentially other methods might be of benefit. Researcher become part of their findings in that these reflect the integrity of the researcher. Knowledge claims generated by qualitative research are valid if they expose the representativity of object researched. The research process, and the presentation of findings, is characterised by a constant questioning of what and why should be presented as studies content (Kvale 1995).

Communicative Validity

This criterion for validity involves the requirement for dialogue among researchers and the social environment into which he/she is integrated. A discussion about the reality in which the dialogue partners live ideally takes place. Valid knowledge is generated when knowledge claims are weighted against each other and author's results are considered trustworthy by peers. The trustworthiness of knowledge is evaluated by asking about the character of the discourse – the how of the argu-

mentation. When considering the criteria under which the discourse is held and when something is considered true - the why- Kvale refers to elements like e.g. "[..] conssousseurship and criticism, accepting the personal, literary and even poetic as valid sources of knowledge" (Kvale 1995). The dialogue itself – the who – is held among researchers, but should include the wider audience. Under conditions of postmodernity valid knowledge is produced by an inter-subjective validation of the content of knowledge claims.

Pragmatic Validity

In line with the pragmatists' view that knowledge is there to obtain better action options, knowledge validity is achieved in allowing for better actions. The audience of the results of researchers' work assigns validity to a knowledge claim. Applying the criterion of pragmatic validity, communicative validity becomes obsolete. The pragmatic validity criteria include ethical aspects of knowledge utilisation. Under these conditions the how of the validity is established by different measures, pending on the expected outcome. Knowledge claims can be valid if they are accompanied by actions taken in line with the claim. In a second form, a knowledge claim is valid when guiding to different action options by the knowledge applicant. The cause of actions – the why – is whether knowledge can lead to better, and ethical, actions. Given the process of defining validity, the why on the knowledge set, leads to the question whether this allows for change. Validity of knowledge in line with pragmatic criteria is established by a dialogue among the researcher and users of it – the who of its establishment.

Positivistic Sciences and the Personal Element

Reconsidering knowledge generation in organisational sciences Tsoukas and Cummings (1997; similar Toulmin, 1990 on a more general perspective) show that in lockstep with the emergence of rational sciences the art of story telling in personalised - human oriented - ways vanished. However, these forms of knowledge did not vanish as such, but they became subject to strong criticism for their 'unscientific character' in the eyes of rationalists.

Following Kuhn, Barnes and other authors in the constructionistic 'camp', qualitative methods imply and embody as strict rules as quantitative rules. Often these qualitative methods are used masking personal opinions. Implicitly researchers act thereby less ethical, in respect to the research field at hand (Bridges 2003; Sandberg 2005). Bridges (2003) uncovers that there is no inferiority of educational science knowledge (as both fields are concerned with humans the author stipulates here an analogy between organisational sciences and educational sciences) created by qualitative methods (Bridges, 2003). Scientists employing these methods regularly tend to work less ethical by not complying too standards of scientific work, a point that was made a long time ago by Ravetz (1996). He argues that with the increasing necessary investments in the field of (natural) sciences ethical issues increase. Reason is that research investments exceed individual researchers' budgets, opening the avenue to industrial oriented research. This form of research, according to Nowotny et al. (2003, 15-20), adheres to the logic of commercialisation and demands for different rules then academic for research (Ravetz 1996; and for the ethical conditions that lead to 'good research', see pp. 37-44).

When the topic of (organisational) knowledge in organisations is added to the discourse of methodology, and the discussion is confined to the field of qualitative or quantitative methods themselves, the background description of data mining should be recalled. The argument was that knowledge generation by means of machine learning happens based on human defined pre-rules (Witten & Frank, 2005, pp. 4-6, 30-35). As the rules developed by machines are human

made in respect to the search algorithms to be looked for, and the data collected and captured for DM, Witten and Frank argue that knowledge sets resulting from machine learning have to be subject to words of attention. Reason being, that those are based on language and search biases ('overfitting-avoidance bias' exists but these are less relevant for the paper at hand; Witten and Frank, 2005, pp. 32-4).

The language bias takes its origin in the question whether natural language methods should be used in order to describe findings, and whether there are limits in what should be accepted as knowledge sets originating in the machine learning process. Included in this bias is the question how, and whether, results from machine learning can be expressed in a natural language, or not, due to knowledge deficits about the domain and language used in the domain (ibid. p. 32-33; Krone, 2007). Thus, as a side note one comes back questioning whether and how Expert Systems can produce general understandable and applicable solutions for managerial decision-making.

Search bias refers to the problem that data (knowledge sets) gathered via data mining are, in a statistical sense, attempts fitting data collected to the problem at hand. Data are not assessed in their breadth of potential applications and available different readings, but in line with a human inspired maximum range of potential solutions. This process confines the heuristic of the machine learning processes. Potentially not all possible interpretations of the data are obtained. Problems like this are avoided when rechecking data after initial results were used. Manually reshaping results in order to prevent narrow results can happen. Search regimes (general to specific, or vice versa) can lead to skewed data that later have to be reconsidered (Witten & Frank, pp. 33-34).

Considering data mining under this perspective not only the understanding of social environment as embedded in Information Systems (cp. Floyd 1992 a/b; D'Adderio 2002; Isomäki 2002; Kallinikos 2004) is problematic, but also the form of knowledge generation and the principles the knowledge output adhere too. The eminent question is again: Why using quantitative methods that are resting on individuals' understanding of a given field? Hence, as related to the aspect of organisational learning the question is: why these mechanised procedure for knowledge generation in organisational settings?

TRENDS OF DM AND KNOWLEDGE: SECURITY AND ORGANISATIONS

First technical and organisational boundary conditions for data mining were presented. Emphasised was developing an understanding that the data mining rests on different sources of data derived from human made Information Systems, and is thus necessarily subjective in many respects. Data mining can be defined as the process of using data generated from different sources in order to produce forward-looking predictions of causes of events during plan execution in any organisation.

Knowledge is described in Penrose (1995) perspective as principally shared in a given community (objective knowledge), but due to work experience giving rise to different application fields of it (experience). Knowledge becomes a resource rendering different services to different people. Information represents means for taking decisions under conditions of uncertainty, by collecting new/additional information. The load of information gathered by organisational staff will vary, but whichever amount of information will suffice when collected by means defined by the organisation to be methodological sound in order to overcome uncertainty.

On the methodological diversity element, the argument is made that not necessarily qualitative methods are inferior to quantitative ones. Science, and scientific knowledge creation, can deal with different approaches for knowledge generation. Problems of knowledge generation, and thus validity, are not inherent to methods, but rather

to the process and intentions when using a given meta-methodological choice. With Nowotny et al. (2004) and Ravetz (1996) the two extremes of this continuum are presented. Common thread of these authors is showing that humans conduct research, and therefore deficits in the utilisation of both methodological stance are relating back to scientific practices of the host setting in which they are embedded –the cutting line between 'science' and commercial oriented 'applied science' (Ravetz 1996).

What can then explain the strong drive in more and more organisations to create knowledge by means of the data mining? Going a step back to the understanding of information as minimising insecurity in taking actions for organisation an important term is given namely security.

Economising and Normalising for Security

Security understood with Penrose is about the anticipations of the consequences of a given course of actions (Penrose, 1995, pp. 58-60). A different understanding of security is available in the social sciences and re-emerging only recently as important. It is the understanding developed by Michel Foucault.

In his account security as an action, guiding category coincides with the emergence of the modern rational science discourse (cp. Foucault 2006a/b; cp. Toulmin 1990). It is necessary to trace some of elements of security in the Foucault's understanding, as this allows answering the second research question. Toulmin (1990) makes the compelling argument that rationality and security have to be thought together when describing Descarte's and other rationalists view that the firm principles of rationality are expressions of nature like laws that should be discovered by scientific ways (Toulmin, 1990, pp. 129-131; Foucault, 1996 a, pp. 428-431). In this view, natures like laws are expressions of strict and strong hierarchies that hold true for societies (Toulmin, pp. 132-135).

This argument nicely matches with the institutionalisation of the "rationalisation" of life as a form to comply with, and to, the emergent market order that swept away the old middle-aged feudal form of government (Foucault 2006a, 332-339). This kind of life goes beyond the individual market participant (cp. Foucault, 2006 a, pp 93-96; Foucault, 2006 b, pp. 390-2; Dillon, 2008, 317). For Foucault the market, and the way it was becoming ubiquitous in the western-world, is a mechanism by which the state attempts to secure its own society on the one side, and on the other delimits its own action options in order to ensure security (Foucault 2006a, 105-108, 394-402; cp. Dillon 2008, 310). Dillon (2008) extrapolates this Foucault's idea and suggests that nowadays life has become unsecurable against the contingencies of its own development.

[..B]iopolitically speaking, contingency is constitutive of what it is to be a living thing, the referent of object of biopolitics – life – cannot be secured against contingency. Biopolitically, it is instead secured through contingency (Dillon, 2008, 310).

Life is secured by gambling on contingencies of events that may occur at some point in time. By this means life is virtualised as a variable in the overall calculation of probabilities that form the motor of today's derivative oriented financial economics (Dillon, 2008, 311, 326-329). Given that these derivative oriented financial economics are based on data mining, and the development of rules of statistics (Foucault, 2006 a, 90-8, in particular p. 95-98), it is due rethinking the security and the data mining as interdependent objects.

According to Foucault (2006), the success of the statistical method relies on the definition of objects – cities, citizens, states – as abstracted 'normalised' neutral objects circulating in a given territory. Similarly, Witten and Frank (2005) argue to some extent that the results of data mining are matched like statistical results against a given description of reality. For Foucault, by initially

applying the statistical method, research was concentrated on those measures allowing minimising deviations from the declared normalised status (Foucault, 1996 a, p. 96-97). Thus, the re-interpretation of data mining in line with such an understanding of security, and further the creation of knowledge resting on normalised data from OLAP, can be taken for understanding the emphasis given to machine learned knowledge sets.

A Security Oriented Genealogy of Organisations

When overseeing the literature on organisational design and management (cp. Mintzberg, 1978; Eisenhardt 1989a; Ghoshal & Moran, 1996; Gibson et al. 2003) it is no exaggeration suggesting that much emphasis is on the topic of normalising the operations and procedures, and maintain a status of optimised flow through of products, or service provision. Insofar as the focus is on the optimised flow-through (the double-edged perspective of this word when remembering Foucault is interesting) there is a strong impetus cutting down on variability in task execution on the side of employees (March & Simon 1958, 29; Mintzberg 1978; Gibson et al. 357–362). Adler and Borys (1996), Sia et al. (2002) and Kallinikos (2004) argue that in particular ERP and MIS are means dramatically cutting-down on employees' autonomy in task execution- even if declared otherwise.

Furthermore, the management science principal – agent model can be used showing that in management sciences there is a constant thrive to detect and apply models allowing minimising risks of individual autarkic behaviour by enframing it 'technologically' (e.g. Eisenhardt 1989b; Holmstrome & Tirole, 1989). When this admittedly short overview is considered valid, the role of IS in organisations also can be read in the light of security in Foucault'ian terms, which answers the second research question.

CONCLUSION: DM AND SECURITY OR PREDICTABILITY AND IGNORANCE

Extending the argument of the previous sub-chapter IS are means that ensure organisational security by allowing for predictability by cutting-down in variability of actions carried out by employees. The data mining is then the automated process by which information from the IS are converted into knowledge and valid "per se".

Qualitative- human oriented modes of knowledge creation are suspect to fallacies, and subjectivities, in line with the rational emphasis of organisational sciences that goes hand in hand with security concerns (Foucault 2006a/b; Floyd 1992a/b; Capurro 2008 for the critical analysis of dehumanised and unreflective IS design; Tsoukas & Cumming, 1997 in organisational sciences). In more abstract terms, this leads to a process, in which the human element is squashed in order to allow for smooth operations. Interesting aspect in this de-humanisation process of IS in organisations is the emphasis and strictness. This, on the one-hand side the market element (customer focus in organisations for better action options – the Penrose'an interpretation of information), is favoured while on the other hand results of data mining are not questioned (Witt & Frank 2005, 35-37; Floyd 1992 a with her call for a reflective-discursive approach toward IS).

Adding a further step on this sceptical account on the autonomy of data mining based knowledge, Capurro (2008) stresses the ethical problems of IT in more general. One part of these ethics is

[..T]o learn not just to store, retrieve, and manage information but to become aware that what we do is handle with biased knowledge, i.e. that our basic ability in an information society should be a hermeneutical one, which includes such critical arts as the interpretation, aesthetic or creative design, and responsibility towards our lives (Capurro, 2008).

Consequently, the 'self', understood as a mediator between the "ego" and the environment, has to be strengthened and recaptured against and with IT. Taking a step back, it becomes apparent that the exclusion of qualitative methods within the field of organisational sciences leads to an extended securitisation and abstraction from the human element. By these means, consumers of data mining based knowledge become subject to self-deception in respect to the validity and neutral character of knowledge generated. Reason is that ERP, MIS, and their respective data pools, are mediated representations of designers' understanding of the world we are living in.

The challenge is that even knowledge generated from machine learning has a human core –mediated by the IS design and the DM in particular- of which users should be aware. In data mining, the level of normalisation of lives is biggest, and the alleged level of neutrality of knowledge sets most given. Witt and Frank (2005) have shown, even if data warehouses and machine learning are means by which knowledge is gathered, some inference and/ or deductive means are to be borne - humans define the universe of inquiry about which they want to learn something.

REFERENCES

Adler, P. S., & Borys, B. (1996). Two Types of Bureaucracy: Enabling and Coercive. *Administrative Science Quarterly*, *41*(1), 61–89. doi:10.2307/2393986

Alavi, M., & Leidner, D. (2001). Review: Knowledge Management and Knowledge Management Systems: Conceptual Foundations and Research Issues. *Management Information Systems Quarterly*, *25*(1), 107–136. doi:10.2307/3250961

Barnes, B. (1995). *The Elements of Social Theory*. Princeton, NJ: Princeton University Press.

Beaulieu, A. (2005). Learning SQL. Sebastopol, CA: O'Reilly Inc.

Berger, P. L., & Luckmann, T. (1999). *Die gesellschaftliche Konstruktion der Wirklichkeit. Frankfurt/Main*. Germany: Fischer.

Beynon-Davies, P. (2002). *Information Systems: An Introduction to Informatics in Organisations*. Basingstoke, UK: Palgrave Macmillan.

Blackwell, B., & Ravda, S. (n.d.). Oracle's Technology for Bioinformatics and Future Directions. In Y.-P. Chen, (ed.), *First Asia – Pacific Bioinformatics Conference, Adelaide, Australia. Conferences in Research and Practice in Information Technology*.

Bridges, D. (2003). *Fiction written under Oath? Essays in Philosophy and Educational Research*. Dordrecht, The Netherlands: Kluwer Academic Publishers.

Capurro, R. (2008). Information Technology as an Ethical Challenge.19-28. *Journal of Information Ethics, 5* (2). Retrieved 09.08.2009 from http://www.acm.org/ubiquity/volume_9/v9i22_capurro.html

Castells, M. (2000). *The Rise of the Network Society* (*Vol. 1*). Oxford, UK: Blackwell Publisher.

Chaudhuri, S., & Dayal, U. (1997). An Overview of Data warehousing and OLAP Technology. *SIGMOD Record, 26*(1), 65–74. doi:10.1145/248603.248616

Curtis, B., Krasner, H., & Iscoe, N. (1988). A field study of the software Design process for large Systems. *Communications of the ACM, 31*(11), 1268–1287. doi:10.1145/50087.50089

Czarniawska, B. (2001). Narrative, Interviews, and Organizations. In Gubrium, J. F., & Holstein, J. A. (Eds.), *Handbook of Interview Research; Context & Method* (pp. 733–749). London, New Delhi: Sage Publications.

Czarniawska-Joerges, B. (1998). *A narrative Approach to organizations Studies*. London: Sage Publications.

D'Adderio, L. (2002). Configuring Software, reconfiguring memories: the influence of integrated systems on knowledge storage, retrieval and reuse. In *Proceedings of the 2002 ACM symposium on Applied computing*, (pp. 726–731), Madrid, Spain.

Dennis, A. R., Valacich, J. S., Speier, C., & Morris, M. G. (1998). Beyond Media Richness: An Empirical Test for Media Synchronicity Theory. In *Proceedings of the 31st Hawaii International Conference on Systems Sciences (HICSS '98)"*, Los Alamitos, CA: IEEE Computer Society.

Dillon, M. (2008). Underwriting Security. *Security Dialogue, 39*(2-3), 309–332. doi:10.1177/0967010608088780

Dornier, P.-P., Ernst, R., Fender, M., & Kouvelis, P. (1998). *Global Operations and Logistics Text and Cases*. Chichester, UK: Wiley & Sons.

Eisenhardt, K. M. (1989a). Agency Theory: An Assessment and Review. *Academy of Management Review, 14*(1), 57–74. doi:10.2307/258191

Eisenhardt, K. M. (1989b). Building Theories from Case Study Research. *Academy of Management Review, 14*(4), 532–550. doi:10.2307/258557

Floyd, C. (1992a). Human Questions in Computer Science. In Floyd, C., Züllighoven, R., Budde, R., & Keil-Slawik, R. (Eds.), *Software Development and Reality Construction* (pp. 15–27). Berlin: Springer.

Floyd, C. (1992b). Software Development and Reality Construction. In Floyd, C., Züllighoven, R., Budde, R., & Keil-Slawik, R. (Eds.), *Software Development and Reality Construction* (pp. 86–100). Berlin: Springer.

Foucault, M. (2006a). Sicherheit, Terretorium, Bevölkerung Geschichte der Gouvernementalität I. Frankfurt/ Main, Germany: suhrkamp taschenbuch wissenschaft.

Foucault, M. (2006b). Die Geburt der Biopolitik Geschichte der Gouvernementaltiät II. Frankfurt/ Main, Germany: suhrkamp taschenbuch wissenschaft.

Ghoshal, S., & Moran, P. (1996). Bad for Practice: A critique of the Transaction Cost Theory. *Academy of Management Review, 21*(1), 13–47. doi:10.2307/258627

Gibson, J. L., Ivancevich, J. M., Donnelly, J. H., & Konopaske, R. (2003). *Organizations: Behavior Structure Processes*. New York: McGraw-Hill Irwin.

Grant, R. M. (1996 a). Prospering in Dynamically-competitive Environments: Organizational Capability as Knowledge Integration. *Organization Science, 7*(4), 375–387. doi:10.1287/orsc.7.4.375

Grant, R.M. (1996 b). Toward a Knowledge-based Theory of the firm. *Strategic Management Journal*, (Winter Special Issue), 109– 122.

Hinds, P. J., & Pfeffer, J. (2003). Why Organizations Don't "Know What They Know": Cognitive and Motivational Factors Affecting the Transfer of Expertise. In Ackerman, M., Pipek, V., & Wulf, V. (Eds.), *Sharing Expertise Beyond Knowledge Management* (pp. 3–26). Cambridge, MA: The MIT Press.

Holmstrom, B., & Tirole, J. (1989). The Theory of the Firm. In R. Schmalensee & R. Willig (Eds.), Handbook of Industrial Organization, (pp. 63–131). North-Holland: Elsevier Science Pub Co.

Hoopes, D. G., & Postrel, S. (1999). Shared Knowledge, "Glitches" and Product Development Performance. *Strategic Management Journal, 20*(9), 837–865. doi:10.1002/(SICI)1097-0266(199909)20:9<837::AID-SMJ54>3.0.CO;2-I

Huysman, M., & de Wit, D. (2003). A Critical Evaluation of Knowledge Management Practices. In Ackerman, M., Pipek, V., & Wulf, V. (Eds.), *Sharing Expertise Beyond Knowledge Management* (pp. 27–55). Cambridge, MA: The MIT Press.

Immon, W. H. (2002). *Building the data warehouse*. New York: John Wiley & Sons, Inc.

Isomäki, H. (2002). *The Prevailing Conceptions of the Human Being in Information Systems Development: Systems Designer's Reflections*. Tampere, Finland: Tampere University Press.

Jones, M. (1995). Organisational Learning: Collective Mind or Cognitive Metaphor? *Accounting. Management and Information Technology, 5*(1), 61–77. doi:10.1016/0959-8022(95)90014-4

Kallinikos, J. (2004). Deconstructing information packages: Organizational and behavioural implications of ERP systems. *Information Technology & People, 17*(1), 8–30. doi:10.1108/09593840410522152

Krone, O. (2007). *The Interaction of Organisational Structure and Humans in Knowledge Integration*. Rovaniemi, Finland: University of Lapland, Lapland University Press.

Kuhn, T. S. (1996). *The Structure of Scientific Revolutions*. Chicago: Chicago University Press.

Kvale, S. (1995). The Social Construction of Validity. *Qualitative Inquiry, 1*(1), 19–40. doi:10.1177/107780049500100103

Lee, C. C., & Yang, J. (2000). Knowledge value chain. *Journal of Management Development, 19*(9), 783–793. doi:10.1108/02621710010378228

Lehesvirta, T. (2004). Learning processes in a work organization: From individual to collective and/or vice versa? *Journal of Workplace Learning, 16* (1, 2), 92–100.

Leonard-Barton, D. (1995). *Wellsprings of Knowledge Building and Sustaining the sources of Innovation*. Boston: Harvard Business School Press.

Lichtenstein, S., & Hunter, A. (2005). *Receiver Influences on Knowledge Sharing.* Retrieved 09.07.2009 from http://is.lse.ac.uk/asp/aspecis/20050103.pdf

Luan, J. (2002). *Data Mining and Knowledge Management in Higher Education – Potential Applications; Presentation at AIR Forum, Toronto Canada.* Retrieved 09.05.2009 from www.cabrillo.edu/services/pro/oir_reports/DM_KM2002AIR.pdf

Luft, A. L. (1994). Zur begrifflichen Unterscheidung von 'Wissen', 'Information' und 'Daten'. R. Wille & M. Zickwolff (eds.), Begriffliche Wissensverarbeitung / Grundfragen und Aufgaben, (pp. 61–79). Mannheim, Germany: BI Wissenschaftsverlag.

March, J. G., & Simon, H. A. (1958). *Organizations.* New York: Wiley & Sons.

Markus, M. L. (1983). Power, Politics, and MIS Implementation. Association for Computing Machinery. *Communications of the ACM, 26*(6), 430–445. doi:10.1145/358141.358148

Markus, M. L. (2001). Toward a Theory of Knowledge Reuse: Types of Knowledge Reuse Situations and Factors in Reuse Success. *Journal of Management Information Systems, 18*(1), 57–93.

Mintzberg, H. (1978). *The structuring of Organizations.* Englewood Cliffs, NJ: Prentice Hall.

Mulder, I. (2004). *Understanding Designers Designing for Understanding,* (Telematica Instituut Fundamental Research Series, vol. 010). Enschede, the Netherlands. Retrieved 30/12/2008 from https://doc.telin.nl/dsweb/Get/File-41827/mulder4.0.pdf

Nelson, R. R., & Winter, S. R. (1982). *An Evolutionary Theory of Economic Change.* Cambridge, MA: Belknap Harvard.

Nonaka, I., & Takeuchi, H. (1995). *The Knowledge creating Company How Japanese Companies create the Dynamics of Innovation.* New York: Oxford University Press.

Nowotny, H., Scott, P., & Gibbons, M. (2004). *Re-Thinking Science Knowledge and the Public in an Age of Uncertainty.* Cambridge, UK: Polity Press.

Oracle (2008). *Oracle Database Concepts 11g Release (11.1) B28318-05.* Retrieved 09.01.2009 from http://download.oracle.com/docs/cd/B28359_01/server.111/b28318.pdf

Orlikowski, W. J., & Gash, D. C. (1994). Technological frames: Making Sense of Information Technology in Organzations. *ACM Transactions on Information Systems, 12*(2), 174–207. doi:10.1145/196734.196745

Penrose, E. (1995). *The Theory of the growth of the Firm.* New York: Oxford University Press. doi:10.1093/0198289774.001.0001

Pfeffer, J., & Sutton, R. I. (2000). *The Knowing Doing Gap: how smarts companies turn knowledge into knowledge.* Boston: Harvard Business School Press.

Pipek, V., Hinrichs, J., & Wulf, V. (2003). Sharing Expterise: Challenges for Technical Support. In Ackerman, M., Pipek, V., & Wulf, V. (Eds.), *Sharing Expertise Beyond Knowledge Management* (pp. 111–136). Cambridge, MA: The MIT Press.

Ravetz, J. R. (1996). *Scientific Knowledge and Its Social Problems.* New Brunswick, NJ: Transaction Publishers.

Robey, D., Boudreau, M.-C., & Rose, G. M. (2000). Information technology and organizational learning: a review and assessment of research. *Accounting. Management and Information Technology, 10*(2), 125–155. doi:10.1016/S0959-8022(99)00017-X

Sandberg, J. (2005). How do we justify Knowledge Produced within Interpretative Approaches. *Organizational Research Methods, 8*(1), 41–68. doi:10.1177/1094428104272000

Sartipi, K., Yarmand, M. H., & Down, D. G. (2007). Mined-knowledge and Decision Support Services in Electronic Health. In *IEEE International Workshop on Systems Development in SOA Environments (SDSOA'07)*. Retrieved 09.08.2009 from http://portal.acm.org/citation.cfm?id=1270307

Sia, S. K., Tang, M., Soh, C., & Boh, W. F. (2002). Enterprise Resource Planning (ERP) Systems as a Technology of Power: Empowerment or Panoptic Control? *The Data Base for Advances in Information Systems, 33*(1), 23–37.

Stacey, R. A. (2001). *Complex responsive processes in organizations: learning and knowledge creation*. New York: Routledge.

Stahl, B. C., & Brooke, C. (2008). The contribution of critical IS research. *Communications of the ACM, 51*(3), 51–55. doi:10.1145/1325555.1325566

Stahlknecht, P., & Hasenkamp, U. (2002). *Einführung in die Wirtschaftsinformatik*. Berlin: Springer.

Thompson-Klein, J. (1996). *Crossing Boundaries Knowledge, Disciplinarities, and Interdisciplinarities*. London: Virginia University Press.

Toulmin, S. (1990). *Cosmpolis the Hidden Agenda of Modernity*. Chicago: The University of Chicago Press.

Tsoukas, H., & Cummings, S. (1997). Marginalization and recovery: the emergence of Aristotelian themes in organizational studies. *Organization Studies*. http://findarticles.com/p/articles/mi_m4339/is_/ai_n27518846, last accessed 09.08. 2009

Tuomi, I. (1999). Data is More Than Knowledge: Implications of the Reversed Knowledge Hierarchy for Knowledge Management and Organizational Memory. *Journal of Management Information Systems, 16*(3), 103–118.

Turban, E., McLean, E., & Wetherbe, J. (2002). *Information technology for management: transforming the business in the digital economy*. New York: John Wiley & Sons, Inc.

Von Krogh, G., Roos, J., & Slocum, K. (1994). An Essay on Corporate Epistemology. *Strategic Management Journal, 15*(1), 53–71.

Williamson, O. E. (1991). Comparative Economic Organization: The Analysis of Discrete Structural Analysis. *Administrative Science Quarterly, 36*(2), 269–296. doi:10.2307/2393356

Wilson, T. D. (2002). The non-sense of 'knowledge management'. *Information Research, 8* (1). Retrieved 09.01.2009 from http://informationr.net/ir/8-1/paper144.html

Witten, I. H., & Frank, E. (2005). *Data Mining: practical machine learning tools and techniques*. San Francisco: Elsevier.

KEY TERMS AND DEFINITIONS

Data Mining: Process of collecting and analysing data originating from IS for underlying structures that can inform about patterns invisible to human perception; predominantly applied against abstracted data

Information Systems: Combination of technological and human systems in order to facilitate for the exchange of information; different forms exist, e.g. DSS, ERP, MIS

Knowledge Creation & Methodology: Process by which a given sequences of procedures is taken in order to interpret data or information for the creation of new insight

Organisation: Human generated and enacted social object, serving a given purpose for a not defined amount of time with an internally defined structure

Qualitative Methods: A given set of procedures for the generation of knowledge attempting minimising human impact on knowledge outcomes; formal oriented uses abstractions

Security: Taking actions in an informed way and being aware of the consequences these actions will have.

Validity: An outcome of knowledge operations representing reality in an uncontested way when humans using different knowledge creation methodologies engage in dialogue

Section 3
Data Mining in Organizational Situations to Prepare and Forecast

Chapter 10
Data Mining Methods for Crude Oil Market Analysis and Forecast

Jue Wang
Chinese Academy of Sciences, China

Wei Xu
Renmin University, China

Xun Zhang
Chinese Academy of Sciences, China

Yejing Bao
Beijing University of Technology, China

Ye Pang
The People's Insurance Company (Group) of China, China

Shouyang Wang
Chinese Academy of Sciences, China

ABSTRACT

In this study, two data mining based models are proposed for crude oil price analysis and forecasting, one of which is a hybrid wavelet decomposition and support vector Machine (SVM) model and the other is an OECD petroleum inventory levels based wavelet neural network model (WNN). These models utilize support vector regression (SVR) and artificial neural network (ANN) technique for crude oil prediction and are made comparison with other forecasting models, respectively. Empirical results show that the proposed nonlinear models can improve the performance of oil price forecasting. The findings of this research are useful for private organizations and governmental agencies to take either preventive or corrective actions to reduce the impact of large fluctuation in crude oil markets, and demonstrate that the implications of data mining in public and private sectors and government agencies are promising for analyzing and predicting on the basis of data.

DOI: 10.4018/978-1-60566-906-9.ch010

INTRODUCTION

The need for both private organizations and government agencies to utilize data in public and private sector activities is increasing in recent years, including collecting and managing the data, analyzing and predicting on the basis of data. For example, the manager of an energy sector, in order to make the right decisions, must know the expectation of international crude oil price, energy supply and demand. Simultaneously, he should know the main factors affecting oil fluctuation, demand and the supply capacity. Both the strategic and operational decisions of an organization or government agencies require the exploration of the current relationship among all the factors and construction of forecast models.

As a source of energy and chemical raw materials, crude oil plays an important role in the development of world economy. In recent years, the fluctuation of crude oil price becomes larger and larger, which not only directly affect global economic activities, but also bring risk to the oil-related enterprises and investors. Crude oil price is emerging as one of the hottest topics in the world. Influenced by many complicated factors, however, oil prices appear highly nonlinear and even chaotic (Panas and Ninni, 2000; Adrangi et al., 2001), which makes it rather difficult to forecast the future oil prices.

Although oil price forecasting is very difficult, it has fascinated many academic researchers and business practitioners in the past few decades. There have been substantial literatures on analysis and forecast of crude oil prices including qualitative and quantitative methods, on the basis of which many decisions with regard to oil prices have to be made (Fan et al. 2008). Among the qualitative methods, Nelson et al. (1994) used the Delphi method to predict oil prices for the California Energy Commission. Abramson and Finizza (1991) used belief networks, a class of knowledge-based models, to forecast crude oil prices.

Besides these qualitative methods, a large number of quantitative methods and models are developed to analyze and forecast crude oil prices. According to Zhang et al. (2008), the quantitative methods can be grouped into two categories: structure models and data-driven methods. Standard structure models outline the world oil market and then analyze the oil price volatility in terms of a supply-demand equilibrium schedule (Zhang et al. 2008). For example, Bacon (1991) discussed the factors determining the demand of oil, the supply of oil by OPEC and non-OPEC countries, and gave the forecast of crude oil prices. Al Faris (1991) analyzed the determinants of crude oil price adjustment in the world petroleum market. Data-driven methods include various models and approaches, such as traditional time series methods, econometric models and data mining techniques.

There are abundant studies on crude oil price prediction using time series and econometric methods. Huntington (1994) applied a sophisticated econometric model to predict crude oil prices in the 1980s. Abramson and Finizza (1995) utilized a probabilistic model for predicting oil prices. Gulen (1998) used co-integration analysis to predict the West Texas Intermediate (WTI) price. Barone-Adesi et al. (1998) suggested a semi-parametric approach for oil price prediction. Similarly, Morana (2001) offered a semi-parametric method for short-term oil price forecasting based on the GARCH properties of crude oil price. In a more recent study by Ye et al. (2002, 2005 and 2006), some short-term forecasting models of monthly WTI crude oil spot prices using OECD petroleum inventory levels are proposed. Lanza et al. (2005) investigated crude oil and oil products' prices using error correction models (ECM). Sadorsky (2006) used several different univariate and multivariate models such as TGARCH and GARCH to estimate forecasts of daily volatility in petroleum futures price returns.

As mentioned in Yu et al. (2008), the traditional time series and econometric models can provide good prediction results when the time series is linear or near linear. However, a great deal of nonlinearity and irregularity exists in crude oil price series and numerous experiments have demonstrated the poor performance of traditional statistical and econometric models. Hence, the exploration of forecasting model based on data mining techniques attracts much attention from researchers. Recent work by a number of study (Kaboudan, 2001; Mirmirani and Li, 2004; Xie et al. 2006; Shambora and Rossiter, 2007; Yu et al. 2007) has shown that data mining techniques may provide potential solutions to crude oil price prediction. Kaboudan (2001) employed GP and ANN to forecast crude oil price. Similarly, Mirmirani and Li (2004) offered the ANN model with genetic algorithm (GA) to predict crude oil price and compared the results with the VAR model. Xie et al. (2006) presented a support vector regression (SVR) model to predict crude oil price. Shambora and Rossiter (2007) suggested the ANN model to predict crude oil price, and Yu et al. (2007) also used the ANN ensemble model to predict crude oil price. Meanwhile, some hybrid methods using data mining have been used to predict crude oil price and obtain the satisfied performances. For example, Wang et al. (2004) developed a hybrid approach by means of a systematic integration of ANN and rule-based expert system, with web text mining, to predict crude oil price. Wang et al. (2005) proposed a TEI@I methodology for crude oil price forecasting and obtained good prediction performance.

Although some data mining techniques including ANN (e.g., Shambora and Rossiter 2007) and SVM (e.g., Xie et al. 2006) have been used to forecast crude oil prices, there are still some difficulties in data mining forecasting. First of all, most of forecasting models failed to produce the consistently good results due to the nonlinear mechanism and intrinsic complexity of crude oil market. In the past, the crude oil price was usually treated as a single series, the intrinsic complex modes involved in the price series are mixed and

can not be deep explored. Secondly, as petroleum inventory levels provide a good market barometer of crude oil price fluctuation in the short run, the relationship between petroleum inventory levels and crude oil prices has been studied by many researchers and been found nonlinear (Ye et al. 2002). However, the nonlinear relationships between inventory and crude oil prices may be more complicated than that suggested by Ye et al (2002). Moreover, it is also known that some main geopolitical events like 9-11 in USA affects crude oil prices significantly with variable length of influence or impulse functions.

Based upon the above two aspects, it is necessary to introduce new data mining forecasting models for crude oil prediction. For this reason, this chapter will formulate two data mining forecasting models in an attempt to overcome the two main difficulties mentioned above. One is a hybrid wavelet decomposition and SVM model and the other is an OECD petroleum inventory levels based wavelet neural network model. These models utilize support vector regression (SVR) and artificial neural network (ANN) technique for crude oil prediction. The main objectives of this chapter are as follows: (1) to show how to construct the forecasting models using data mining technique; and (2) to display how to predict crude oil prices using the proposed models. In view of the two objectives, this chapter mainly describes the building process of two data mining forecasting approaches and the application of these forecasting methods in crude oil price prediction, while comparing the forecasting performance with different evaluation criteria.

In this chapter, we highlight data mining techniques for crude oil price prediction. The rest of this chapter is organized as follows. Next we describe data mining techniques for crude oil prediction. The building process of monthly crude oil prices forecasting models using data mining methods are then proposed. After that experimental analysis and comparison are given in details. Finally some concluding remarks and future work are presented.

DATA MINING METHODS AS A CRUDE OIL PRICE FORECASTING TOOL

With the complexity of organizational and governmental growing, it is more and more important how to pick out relevant or evident information for organizational and governmental purposes. To support the corporate decisions, we should create systems and procedures to explore scenarios based on quantitative and/or qualitative information. For crude oil price forecasting, the traditional time series models and econometric models can not satisfy the practical need. The main reason is that these models are based on linear assumptions, but oil prices appear highly nonlinear and even chaotic. Hence it is emerging as an important problem to explore more efficient methods and models for crude oil price forecasting. Data mining techniques provide an immediate alternative to construct reasonable oil price forecasting model, which can analyze and forecast crude oil price efficiently and accurately by capturing the nonlinear patterns hidden in the crude oil price series. Data mining also plays an important role in improving the forecast accuracy.

Data mining is the exploration analysis of large quantities of data in order to discover implicit, previously unknown, and potentially useful information (Berry and Linoff, 2004). The main idea is to build computer programs that sift through databases automatically, seeking regularities or patterns. Strong patterns, if found, will likely generalize to make accurate predictions on future data (Witten and Frank, 1999). Data mining is a multidisciplinary field drawing works from statistics, database technology, artificial intelligence, pattern recognition, machine learning, information and data visualization, and it has been used to implement the tasks of classification, estimation, clustering, profiling and prediction.

Among the numerous data mining techniques, the ANN and SVM have been widely used in the field of forecasting. ANN is often regarded as a class of reliable and cost-effective methods for crude oil price prediction. The neural net work model can be trained to approximate any smooth and measurable nonlinear function without prior assumptions on the original data (Yu et al., 2007b); it has produced many promising results in this field of crude oil price prediction (Kaboudan, 2001; Mirmirani and Li, 2004; Wang et al., 2004, 2005; Shambora and Rossiter, 2007; Yu et al., 2007a, 2008). These studies show that ANN models are very effective in simulating and describing the dynamics of non-stationary time series due to its unique non-parametric, noise-tolerant and highly adaptive characteristics.

However, the inherent drawbacks of ANN models, e.g., local minima, over-fitting, poor generalization performance and the difficulty of determining appropriate network architectures, hinder practical applications of ANN models. Support vector machine (SVM), first proposed by Vapnik (1995), provides a class of competitive learning algorithms to improve generalization performance of neural networks and achieve global optimum solutions simultaneously. SVM is a very specific type of learning algorithm characterized by the capacity control of the decision function, use of kernel functions, and sparsity of the solution (Vapnik, 1995, 1999; Cristianini and Taylor, 2000). Established on the unique theory of the structural risk minimization (SRM) principle to estimate a function by minimizing an upper bound of the generalization error, SVM is resistant to the over-fitting problem and can simulate nonlinear relations in an efficient and stable way. This property leads to a better generalization than conventional methods. Furthermore, SVM is trained as a convex optimization problem, result-

Figure 1. A procedure of ANN/SVM-based time series forecasting

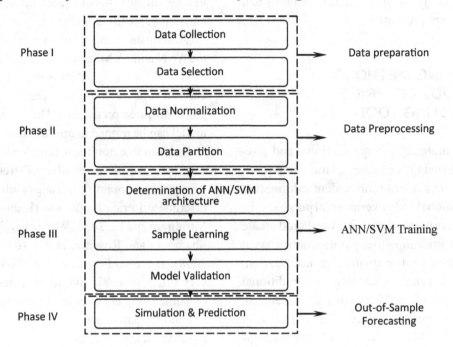

ing in a global solution that in many cases yields unique solutions.

When time series prediction is conducted by ANNs or SVMs, input vector {x} to the ANN/SVM is a finite set of consecutive measurements of the series $x = (x(t), x(t-1), ..., x(t-s))$, with time-delays, which is a sliding window for the input vector. The output of the model is $x(t+h)$ where h is the prediction horizon and it is a user-specified parameter. The procedure of developing an ANN/SVM-based time series prediction is illustrated in Figure 1.

As can be seen from Figure 1, the procedure of ANN/SVM-based time series prediction model can be divided into four phases, briefly described as following phases:

Phase I: Data Sampling. In situations where there are vast volumes of data to sift through, a process called data sampling can help minimize data processing and significantly reduce computational costs. Data sampling is a process whereby a statistically representative portion of the information is examined to determine if it

contains responsive data. Using data sampling can help narrow the research focus, for example, by determining whether there are time periods in which relevant events do not exist; this makes it unnecessary to process or review that particular part of the data set. To develop a SVM-based model for forecasting, different data should be collected, and data collected from various sources must be selected in terms of some specific criteria.

For crude oil price, there are a variety of data used for this research. West Texas Intermediate (WTI) and Brent crude oil prices are two main crude oil price benchmarks. From the viewpoint of data type, spot prices and futures prices are available. From the point of data frequency, daily, weekly, monthly, quarterly, and yearly data can be used. The main purpose of data sampling is to select a representative data for further processing and analysis.

Phase II: Data Preprocessing. After data sampling, the next task is data preprocessing. It includes two steps: data normalization and data division. In any model development process, familiarity with the available data is of the utmost importance. ANN models and SVM models are no exception. Data normalization can have a significant effect on models' performances. After that, normalized data should be divided into two subsets: in-sample data and out-of-sample data, to be used for model estimation and model evaluation and verification respectively.

Phase III: ANN/SVM Training. After the data is preprocessed, ANN/SVM training can be performed using the processed data. In this phase, there are three main tasks: determination of ANN structure/SVM input vector, sample learning, and model validation. For ANN models, the architecture and parameters: i.e., learning rate, momentum, and architecture, must be decided firstly. There are no criteria in deciding the parameters other than a trial-and-error basis. Then all weights should be initialized randomly. The training for ANN model will be ended where the stopping criterion is either the number of iterations reached or when the total sum of squares of error is lower than a predetermined value. Usually, the SVM input vector is determined by time-delay s via the trial and error method. In sample learning, regularization constant C, suitable kernel functions K(.), and associated kernel parameters in kernel functions should be determined. Often they are determined by trial and error because there are no universal criteria for deciding the parameters. As an alternative, some search-based methods, such as grid search and direct search methods can also be used to determine the ANN or SVM parameters. After training, model validation must be performed so as to guarantee the generalizability of models. After validation, an ANN or SVM predictor with optimal parameters can be obtained.

Phase IV: Out-of-Sample Forecasting. Using the optimal ANN/SVM predictor, the trained ANN/SVM can be used for out-of-sample time series prediction.

BUILDING PROCESS OF MONTHLY CRUDE OIL PRICE FORECASTING MODELS

Model A: A Hybrid Wavelet Decomposition and LSSVM Model for Crude Oil Price Forecasting

In this section, a hybrid model (W-LSSVM) for crude oil price forecasting is proposed by integrating the wavelet and LSSVM. The formulation of this proposed model is composed of three stages. In the first stage, original crude oil price series is decomposed into several sub-series (approximated series and several detailed series) by Haar à trous wavelet transform, each of which has distinct contributions to the original series. In the second stage, each sub-series is predicted with LSSVM individually. In the final stage, crude oil price forecast is obtained by reconstructing the sub-series' forecasts.

Wavelet Decomposition of Original Time Series

In wavelet decomposition, a redundant Haar à trous algorithm, which is un-decimated wavelet transform, can get more complete characteristics of the analyzed series. Thus it produces more precise information for localization (Shensa, 1992). The non-decimated Haar algorithm with the low-pass filter $h(\frac{1}{2}, \frac{1}{2})$, provides a convincing solution to troublesome time series boundary effects at the time point t. Since $h(\frac{1}{2}, \frac{1}{2})$ is non-symmetric, calculation of scaling coefficients and wavelet coefficients at time t uses information before time t only. This is a very desirable feature in time series prediction.

The non-decimated Haar wavelet is presented as follows:

First, the original time series C_0 is decomposed into an approximation component C_1 and an accompanying detail component W_1. C_1 may be created from C_0 by convolving the latter with $h(\frac{1}{2}, \frac{1}{2})$,

$$C_1(k) = \frac{1}{2}[C_0(k) + C_0(k-1)] \qquad (1)$$

Wavelet coefficients W_1 are obtained from the difference between approximate coefficients C_1 and C_0, which can capture small features in the data.

$$W_1(k) = C_0(k) - C_1(k) \qquad (2)$$

The decomposition process is then iterated with successive approximation C_j (j=1, 2, ...,N-1) being decomposed in turns, until the approximation C_N is smooth, where N is the decomposed level.

$$C_{j+1}(k) = \frac{1}{2}[C_j(k) + C_j(k-1)] \qquad (3)$$

$$W_{j+1}(k) = C_j(k) - C_{j+1}(k) \qquad (4)$$

Thus, the original series is decomposed into N detail series W_j, j=1,2,..., N, and an approximation series C_N. The original time series $P(t) = C_0(t)$ can be reconstructed by summing up all the decomposed sub-series on multiple scales.

Sub-Series Forecasting with LSSVM

Suppose x_t, the value of a time series at time t, is related to its historical data, and the relation can be expressed by an unknown function $f(X)$. The time series is converted into a state-vector representation $\{(X_t, y_t), X \in R^k, y \in R\}$, using the embedding dimension k (Cao, 1997), here $X_t = [x_{t-1}, x_{t-2}, ..., x_{t-k}]$.

Suykens et al. presented the LSSVM approach, in which the following function is used to approximate the unknown function $f(X)$.

$$y(X) = w^T \phi(X) + b \qquad (5)$$

where φ is a nonlinear function which maps the input space into a higher dimension feature space.

Given training data, LSSVM defines an optimization problem as follows:

$$\min_{w,b,e} J(w,e) = \frac{1}{2} w^T w + \gamma \frac{1}{2} \sum_{k=1}^{N} e_k^2, \, (\gamma > 0) \qquad (6)$$

Subject to the equality constrains

$$y_k = w^T \phi(X_k) + b + e_k, \, k=1, ..., N \qquad (7)$$

Having solved this optimization problem, the resulting LS-SVM model for regression can be expressed as follows:

$$y(X) = \sum_{k=1}^{N} \alpha_k K(X, X_k) + b \qquad (8)$$

$$K(X, X_k) = \phi(X)^T \phi(X_k) \qquad (9)$$

Where, $K(X, X_k)$ is defined as kernel function, which can be any symmetric function satisfying Mercer's condition.

Each sub-series are predicted with LSSVM model individually. Considering the strong nonlinearity, the Radial Basis Function kernel is selected as the kernel function for LSSVM in this chapter.

Time Series Forecasting Reconstruction

The predicted values for each detail series are expressed as $\hat{W}_j(t)$, j=1,2,..., N, and the predicted values for the approximation series is expressed as $\hat{C}_N(t)$. The time series forecasting is obtained by reconstructing the results of these

Figure 2. The typical structure of WNN

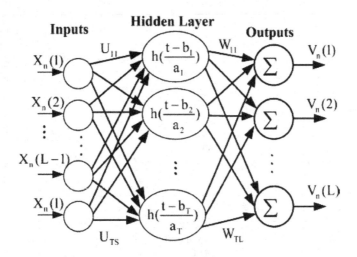

sub-series forecasts in the form of an additive manner.

$$\hat{P}(t) = a\hat{C}_N(t) + \sum_{j=1}^{N} b_j \hat{W}_j(t) \qquad (10)$$

Parameters a and b_j are obtained by least square regression with training sample set.

$$P(t) = aC_N(t) + \sum_{j=1}^{N} b_j W_j(t) \qquad (11)$$

Although many other reconstruction techniques, such as nonlinear reconstruction by an ANN, or SVM, are also available, here we just use the linear additive reconstruction for simplicity.

Model B: Forecasting Crude Oil Spot Price by Wavelet Neural Network Using OECD Petroleum Inventory Levels

In this section, a wavelet neural network (WNN) based forecasting model is proposed to predict crude oil price, which can depict the nonlinear relationships among variables. WNN, which combines the wavelet analysis and feed-forward neural networks, shows surprising effectiveness in solving the conventional problems of poor convergence, or even divergence, encountered in other kinds of neural networks (Zhang et al., 1992 and Khayamian et al., 2005). The WNN consists of three layers: input layer, hidden layer and output layer, as illustrated in Figure 2.

Selection of Model Variables

A number of factors were considered for crude oil price forecasting model. The first one is inventory. Petroleum inventory levels are a measure of the balance or imbalance between petroleum production and demand, which can reflect volatile market pressures on crude oil prices, and thus provide a good market barometer of crude oil price fluctuation in the short run. Relationship between petroleum inventory levels and crude oil price has been studied by many researchers and be found nonlinear (Dale, 1997; Timothy, 2000 and Saif Ghouri, 2006). More specifically, Ye et al. (2005) built a linear forecasting model, using relative inventories, to forecast the WTI crude oil price. At the same time, since inventories have a lower bound or a minimum operating level, some

Figure 3. Crude oil spot price and total OECD inventory

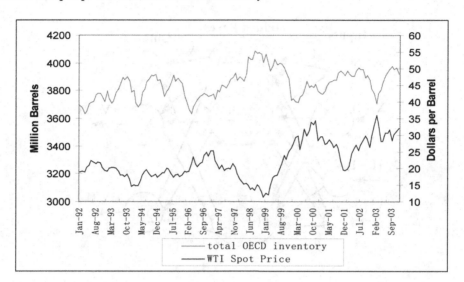

economic literature, such as Deaton and Larque (1992), Miranda and Glauber (1993), Chambers and Bailey (1996), Michaelides and Ng (2000), and Routledge et al. (2000) suggest a relationship between inventory levels and commodity prices.

The proposed model focuses the research on the nonlinear relation between OECD inventory and WTI crude oil spot prices. The Figure 2 shows the correlation between the behavior of WTI crude oil spot price and the total OECD inventories from 1992 to 2003. As is shown in Figure. 3, the large swings in WTI spot price during the late 1990s are coupled with counter-swings in inventory. During this period, when the total inventory dropped from 3991 to 3943 million barrels in March 1999, WTI spot prices rose from $14.68 to $17.31 per barrel in the next month. The same situation also occurred in February 2003. It is obvious that inventory can reflect the change of petroleum production and demand to some extent. Hence OECD industrial petroleum inventory levels is involved in the model.

We also found that WTI price is influenced by its former value, consistent with those findings in other researchers' papers. So in order forecast

the WTI price better, we can include the lags of WTI in the model.

Besides inventory and the lag of WTI, we should consider some dummy variables in out model, such as events that significantly impacted crude oil markets which may lead to structural change or market disequilibrium.

The variables and their lags which will be used in nonlinear model can be confirmed by multivariable linear model, as shown in the following equation,

$$WTI_t = a + \sum_{i=1}^{n} b_i INVENTORY_{t-i} + \sum_{j=1}^{m} c_j WTI_{t-j} + \sum_{k=1}^{q} d_k Dummy_k + \varepsilon_t$$

(12)

From model estimation results we can get the variables which are significant and then use them in a nonlinear model.

WNN Approach for Oil Price Series Modeling

The detailed steps of the new WNN-based model are as follows:

First, analyzed the variables which could influence the variable being forecasted, then build multivariable linear models to adjust and confirm the variables which can be used in nonlinear model and determine the number of lag variables at the same time based on the model estimation results.

Then, initialize network parameters, determine the parameters of the WNN-based model including WNN step size for learning, neurons in a single hidden layer, generalized delta learning rule, wavelet transfer function and the number of iterations. Initialization of network parameters is an important issue during WNN modeling which contributes on the convergence of the model. In this study, an appropriate initialization is selected which is presented by Oussar et al (1998). Supposing the input vectors ranges in the domain $[x_{j,min}, x_{j,max}]$, then the initial values of the *ith* neuron for translation and scaling parameters are set to $b_{ij} = 0.5(x_{j,min} + x_{j,max})$ and $a_{ij} = 0.2(x_{j,min} + x_{j,max})$, to guarantee that wavelets will not concentrate on localities of the input universe in a certain extent. Selection of the number of nodes in the hidden layer of WNN is another important issue. If the number is too small, WNN may not reflect the complex function relationship between input data and output value. By contrary, a larger one may result in so complex a network with a very large output error caused by overfitting of the training sample set. Usually, the selection of the number of neurons in the hidden layer was made according to the previous experience; it was shown that the increase of the number of neurons in the hidden layer did not improve performance and generalization of the WNN. In the study, we select the network with 8 neurons in the hidden layer after checking various options.

Throughout the training, step size for learning is 0.01, and the Morlet wavelet transfer function is considered. The number of iterations is 1000. All the parameters are listed in Table 1.

Third, set the training samples and testing samples. Get WNN-based training and testing

Table 1. Parameters setting in WNN model

Variables	Description
Transfer function	Morlet
The number of layers	3
Output neuron	1
neurons in hidden layer	8
Step size	0.01
Iteration	1000

results using the final variables and parameters. We train the model with data of training samples to forecast the $WTIt+1$, then actual value of $t+1$ was added, and the model was re-fitted to forecast the price of $WTIt+2$. The results are averages of value of experiments repeated certain times such as twenty. In the WNN, the following steps are carried out:

1. Initializing the dilation parameter a_t, translation parameter b_t and node connection weights u_{ti}, w_t to some random values. All those random values are limited in the interval (0, 1).

2. Inputting data $x_n(i)$ and corresponding output values v_n^T, where the superscript T represents the target output state.

3. Propagating the initial signal forward through the network:

$$v_n^T = \sum_{t=1}^{T} w_t h \left(\frac{\sum_{i=1}^{s} u_{ti} x_n(i) - b_t}{a_t} \right) \qquad (13)$$

where h is taken as a Morlet wavelet

$$h(t) = \cos(1.75t) \exp\left(-\frac{t^2}{2}\right) \qquad (14)$$

4. Calculating the WNN parameter:

$$\Delta w_t = -\eta \frac{\partial E}{\partial w_t} + \alpha \Delta w_t$$

$$\Delta u_{ti} = -\eta \frac{\partial E}{\partial u_{ti}} + \alpha \Delta u_{ti}$$

$$\Delta a_t = -\eta \frac{\partial E}{\partial a_t} + \alpha \Delta a_t$$

$$\Delta b_t = -\eta \frac{\partial E}{\partial b_t} + \alpha \Delta b_t \text{, the error function}$$

E is taken as $E = \sqrt{\sum_{n=1}^{N} (v_n^T - v_n)^2}$, and v_n^T

v_n are the experimental and calculated values, respectively. N stands for the data number of training sets, and η and α are the learning rate and the momentum term, respectively.

5. The WNN parameters are changed until the network output satisfies the error criteria.

EXPERIMENTAL ANALYSIS

In this section, the experimental results of the proposed Model A and Model B are presented. First of all, we describe the data source and the evaluation criteria used in this study and then report the experimental results, respectively.

In this study, we select monthly nominal West Texas Intermediate (WTI) crude oil spot prices in our experiments, which plays a significant role and are usually considered as a world benchmark price in the international crude oil markets. All the data comes from Energy Information Administration (EIA).

Two typical criteria are employed to assess and compare the in-sample and out-of-sample forecasting ability of the proposed forecasting models and others in this study, which are root mean squared error (*RMSE*) and directional statistics (D_{stat}), respectively. Given N pairs of the

actual values (or targets, x_t) and predicted values ($\hat{x}_t$), the *RMSE* can be defined as

$$RMSE = \sqrt{\frac{1}{N} \sum_{t=T+1}^{T+N} (x_t - \hat{x}_t)^2} \qquad (15)$$

Clearly, the RMSE is a quadratic scoring rule which measures the average magnitude of the error. Since the errors are squared before they are averaged, the *RMSE* gives a relatively high weight to large errors. This means the *RMSE* is most useful when large errors are particularly undesirable. But in oil price forecasting, correct forecast of movement directions or turning points between the actual and predicted values, x_t and $\hat{x}_t$, is also of great importance. The ability to predict movement direction or turning points can be measured by a statistic developed by Yao and Tan (2000). Directional change statistics (D_{stat}) can be expressed as

$$D_{stat} = \frac{1}{N} \sum_{t=1}^{N} a_t \times 100\% \qquad (16)$$

where $a_t=1$ if $(y_{t+1} - y_t)(\hat{y}_{t+1} - y_t) \geq 0$, and $a_t=0$ otherwise, and N is the number of the testing samples.

Experimental Results of Model A

Data Description and Structural Breaks Test

The available WTI data covers the period from January 1986 to July 2007. In order to make a good prediction, a structural break testing is performed with the iterated cumulative sums of squares algorithm (ICSS) (Inclan, Carla, and Tiao, 1994).

Structural break is a kind of nonstationarity. It is often caused by changes in the structure of the economy, industry, and events that change the dynamics of specific industries or firm related quantities, such as inventories, sales, and production, etc. The breaks often lead to a misleading inference or forecasting if they are neglected in the models used. Therefore, the structure break testing is to help restrict the training and testing sample to the same structure period. In this study, the BP multiple structure break point test method, developed by Bai and Perron (2003) based on sum of squared residuals minimization criterion, is used to detect the number and timing of breaks for oil price series.

Four breaks including 1987.01, 1990.08, 1991.02, 1998.09, are found in the WTI oil price from January 1986 to July 2007. Based on these breaks, the whole WTI oil price data can be divided into five sections: 1986/01-1986/12 (12 months), 1987/01-1990/07 (43 months), 1990/08-1991/01 (6 months), 1991/02-1998/08 (91 months) and 1998/09-2007/07 (107 months).

Because the former three sections are too short to be suitable for model training, we select the latest two sections for the sample sets in the experiment.

Sample set 1: 1991/02-1998/08. The training set is from 1991/02 to 1995/12 with 59 data points, and the testing set is from 1996/01 to 1998/08 with 32 data points.

Sample set 2: 1998/09-2007/07. The training set is from 1998/09 to 2004/12 with 76 data points, and the testing set is from 2005/01 to 2007/07 with 31 data points.

Crude Oil Price Series Decomposition

The Haar à trous transform provides a convincing and computationally straightforward solution to troublesome time series boundary effects at the time point t. The calculation of scaling coefficients and wavelet coefficients at time t uses information before time t only. So it is not necessary to repeat the decomposition process for each prediction,

but select the whole sample data, Sample set 1 or Sample set 2, to decompose only once. Both the Figure 4 and Figure 5 illustrate the decomposition results of sample set 1 and sample set 2, respectively. As can be seen that there are one approximation and four detail components for each oil price series.

Training and Testing Results

To evaluate the performance of W-LSSVM, wavelet-based multi-scale ARIMA (W-ARIMA) model and two single-scale models, ARIMA and LSSVM, are used for the comparison analysis. For testing sets of Sample set 1 and Sample set 2, the Figure 6 and Figure 7 present the forecasting results. In order to compare the multi-scale model and the single-scale model clearly, four models are shown in two sub-figures separately, for each test sample.

For example, as can be seen from Figure 6, the curve of the crude oil price forecast of W-LSSVM is closer to the curve of the actual time series than that of LSSVM. By comparing W-ARIMA and ARIMA, the same result is obtained. It is shown that the multi-scale models outperform single-scale models.

The final results are summarized in Table 2 and Table 3. MAPE, *RMSE* of multi-scale models are smaller than relevant single-scale models. In additional, the hit rate D_{stat} is heightened obviously. It proves that multi-scale decomposition improves prediction accuracy. By comparing the performance of linear and nonlinear models, it is found that nonlinear models behave generally better than linear models in most cases. So the multi-scale model W-LSSVM is the best among all the models among the four models.

To fully integrate the advantages of several models, a simple combination forecasting is presented as follows,

Figure 4. Decomposition of sample set 1

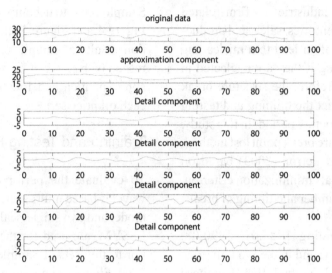

Figure 5. Decomposition of sample set 2

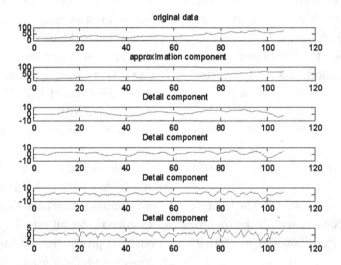

$$\hat{p}(t) = \frac{1}{n} \sum_{i=1}^{n} \hat{p}_i(t) \qquad (17)$$

The performance of the combination forecast model is also included in Table 3. The study shows the combination model is better than any individual model, for crude oil price forecasting.

Experimental Results of Model B

Data Preparation and Statistical Analysis

Because OECD inventory data are only available monthly, we use monthly WTI crude oil spot prices and OECD inventories in this study. All the data

Figure 6. Comparison for testing set 1

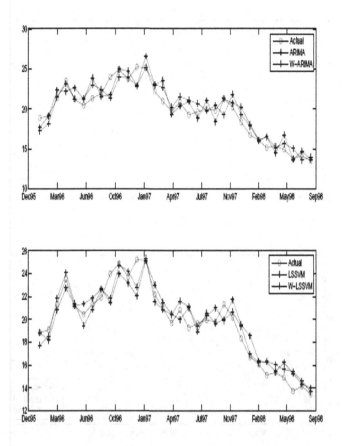

comes from Energy Information Administration (EIA).

In order to compare the performance of the proposed model with other similar ones and test the stability of the new model, two sample sets are selected from WTI data:

Sample set 1: January 1992 ~ September 2003, the training set is January 1992 ~ September 2002 and testing set is October 2002 ~ September 2003.

Sample set 2: January 1992 ~ September 2006, the training set is January 1992 ~ September 2003 and testing set is October 2003 ~ August 2006.

Between 1992 and 2003, there were two significant events which had made a great impact on crude oil market. One was "OPEC quota tightening" at the beginning of April 1999, which

resulted in the deviation and mean value of the WTI price changing, as a whole. The other was "911 terrorist attacks" in USA in 2001, which also lead to violent market disequilibrium. Both events are considered in the existed model of Ye et al., the same case with this chapter.

First, we present a multivariable linear model to confirm the variables which can be involved in a nonlinear model. The model is shown in Eq. (18). Note that subscript t in the model is for the tth month; subscript i is for ith month prior to the tth month; a, b_i, c_j, d and e_k are coefficients to be estimated; $k = 0$, 1, 2,..., 5 refer to six months from October 2001 to March 2002; M_k and *LAPR* are variables to account for market disequilibrium

Figure 7. Comparison for testing set 2

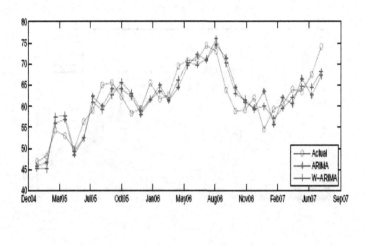

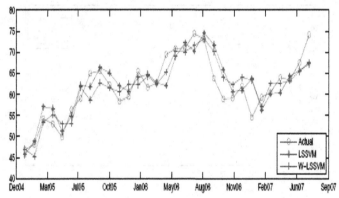

Table 2. The RMSE comparison with different forecasting models

Models	Sample set 1		Sample set 2	
	RMSE	Rank	RMSE	Rank
ARIMA	1.28	4	4.12	4
LSSVM	1.27	3	4.06	3
W-ARIMA	1.23	2	3.67	2
W-LSSVM	1.05	1	3.44	1

Table 3. The D_{stat} comparison with different forecasting models

Models	Sample set 1		Sample set 2	
	D_{stat} (%)	Rank	D_{stat} (%)	Rank
ARIMA	65	4	58	3
LSSVM	74	2	58	3
W-ARIMA	71	3	71	2
W-LSSVM	81	1	74	1

and shifting caused by the two events mentioned in the previous paragraph.

$$WTI_t = a + \sum_{i=1}^{4} b_i INVENTORY_{t-i} + \sum_{j=1}^{2} c_j WTI_{t-j} + dLAPR + \sum_{k=0}^{5} e_k M_k + \varepsilon_t$$

(18)

From the estimation results for Eq. (18), we can see that only inventory with one-order lag, WTI with one-order lag, *LAPR* and M_k (dummy variables of "911 terrorist attacks") are significant. But according to the data, we found that different inventory changes lead to significantly different movements in price in the next month and even similar changes in inventory can result in diverse changes in price. For example, inventory increased from 3651 to 3704 million barrels in May 1992, and WTI price increased by $1.4 per barrel in June 1992. While in November 2004, inventory increased from 4012 to 4065 million barrels which also rises 53 million barrels, but WTI price decreased by $5.32 per barrel in the next month. So we use the following model to explore a more consistent relationship between WTI_t and $\Delta INVENTORY_{t-i}$,

$$WTI_t = a + \sum_{i=1}^{4} b_i \Delta INVENTORY_{t-i} + cWTI_{t-1} + \varepsilon$$

(19)

where $\Delta INVENTORY_{t-i} = INVENTORY_{t-i} - INVENTORY_{t-i-1}$. From the estimation results for Eq. (19), it is easy to find that the results support the above findings about the relationship between changes in inventory and oil price. According to the results of the second multivariable linear model, we formulate model variables to one-order lag of WTI, one-order lag of Inventory, $\Delta INVENTORY_{t-1}$, and dummy variables of the two events as the input variables of our WNN-based nonlinear model.

In the process of modeling, however, we found that the dummy variable of "911 terrorist attacks" can not improve forecasting accuracy and slow down the constringency velocity of the WNN program. So it is eliminated from the set of variables. The input variables of our WNN-based nonlinear model are shown in Table 4.

Training and Testing Results

We take $INVENTORY_{t-1}$, $INVENTORY_{t-2}$, WTI_{t-1} and *APR99* as input nodes of the WNN model. The WNN forecast program is run on Matlab 7.0. Specially, *APR99* is represented by a binary form,

Table 4. Variables of the forecasting model

Variables	Description
$INVENTORY_{t-1}$	One lag of Inventory
$INVENTORY_{t-2}$	Two lag of Inventory
WTI_{t-1}	One lag of WTI monthly spot price
APR99	Dummy variable capturing a structural change in April 1999

i.e. the values before April 1999 are set to 0, and the others are 1.

The performance of the proposed model is compared with Ye's linear model (Ye et. al. 2005) and nonlinear model (Ye et al. 2006). For the training sets of Sample set 1 and Sample set 2, Table 5 shows the *RMSE* comparison results with different forecasting models. Meanwhile, Directional change statistics (D_{stat}) of the proposed method is given in Table 6. As can be seen from Table 5, WNN model performs the best among three models, which has the lowest *RMSE*, not only on Sample set 1, but also Sample set 2. The new model can also get higher Directional change statistics, which is over 70% for both sample sets and shown in Table 6. It is noted that two statistics of WNN model (*RMSE* and D_{stat}) are average of experiments results run 20 times with different initial parameters.

The evaluations of testing results for Sample set 1 are shown in Table 7. For consistent comparison with Ye's models, *Mean, MAE* (Mean Absolute Error) and *St. Dev* (standard deviation) are involved in the following comparison. The testing procedure of sample set 1 begins by training the model with data from January 1992 to September 2002, and forecasting the value of October 2002. Then actual value of October 2002 was added, and the model was re-fitted to forecast the price for November 2002. The process is repeated until the value of September 2003 is predicted.

From the performance comparisons of various models shown in Table 7, the prediction perfor-

Table 5. The RMSE of training results for two sample sets

Models	Sample set 1		Sample set 2	
	RMSE	Rank	RMSE	Rank
Linear RI	1.5352	3	1.5352	3
Nonlinear RI	1.2611	2	1.2611	2
WNN	1.0662	1	1.0605	1

Table 6. D_{stat} of training results for two sample sets

	Sample Set1	Sample Set 2
$D_{stat (\%)}$	71.2%	71.8%

Table 7. Testing results comparisons of Sample set 1

Models	WNN	Nonlinear RI	Linear RI
Mean	-0.4476	0.2687	-0,2874
St. Dev	0.7701	1.8412	2.2657
RMSE	0.8785	1.7892	2.1952
MAE	0.6189	1.4006	1.9494

Table 8. Testing results of Sample set 2

Statistics	Value
Mean	-0.8394
St. Dev	1.2444
RMSE	1.4862
MAE	1.0735

Table 9. D_{stat} of testing results of the two sample sets

	Sample Set1	Sample Set 2
$D_{stat (\%)}$	75%	82.3%

mance of the WNN-based nonlinear forecasting model is better than those of other models. *RMSE, MAE, St. Dev* and *Mean* indicators of prediction errors are all decreased for testing results. Specially, *RMSE* for WNN is almost half of nonlinear RI model. The decreased standard deviation of prediction error can also prove the great stability of the proposed model. This demonstrates that the WNN model performs very well for oil price forecasting even with sharp fluctuation, like in February 2003.

The evaluations of testing results for Sample set 2 are shown in Table 8 and the D_{stat} for two samples shown in Table 9. As can be seen from Table 8, *RMSE* of sample set 2 is higher than one of sample set 1. The main reason is that the oil price rose from $34.31 in Jan. 2004 to $74.41 per barrel in July 2006, which has a 217% increase in the short two years. In this period, there are 11 months in which oil price rose more than 8%. Specially, the price rose more than 13% in October 2004, March 2005, and June 2005. Hence, such a violent fluctuation leads to a relative higher prediction error. The D_{stat} value in Table 9 proves that our model can depict the direction of the WTI price changes very well, especially for Sample set 2.

From the experiments presented in this study, we can draw the following conclusions: the rela-

tionship between oil price and inventory is nonlinear, and WNN can reveal this nonlinear relationship. In terms of the empirical results, we conclude that a nonlinear model can be used as an alternative tool for oil price forecasting, to obtain higher forecasting accuracy and improve the prediction quality further.

CONCLUSION AND FUTURE DIRECTIONS

This chapter proposes two data mining based models for crude oil price analysis and forecasting to obtain accurate prediction results and improve prediction quality further. Specially, we have demonstrated that the relationship between oil price and inventory is nonlinear and WNN can reveal this nonlinear relationship. Also, SVM can capture the nonlinear structure of each decomposed subseries of oil price. The experiments show that nonlinear models based on WNN and SVM are more effective for forecasting crude oil price compared with other models like ARIMA.

As can be seen from this study, data mining based technologies show more promising performance than the time series model and econometric methods, which can be used as an alternative tool for crude oil price analysis and forecasting. Meanwhile, some other data mining techniques can also be introduced to this field, for example, cluster analysis and association rules mining. The high volatility and irregularity of crude oil market creates uncertainty, mainly because of the interaction of many factors in crude oil markets.

Further, how to analyze and use these factors to forecast the crude oil price has attracted increasing attention from academics and practitioners. Cluster analysis can be used to study all kinds of factors affecting crude oil price, like war, climate, speculation, foreign exchange, and so on. Meanwhile, association rules mining can be introduced to extract decision rules about oil price and these factors. Such rules can help the decision maker have a good knowledge of the reason of great volatility and contribute their important investment decisions. Other data mining techniques for crude oil market can be worth exploring further in the future.

ACKNOWLEDGMENT

This work is supported by the National Natural Science Foundation of China (NSFC No. 70801058).

REFERENCES

Abramson, B., & Finizza, A. (1991). Using belief networks to forecast oil prices. *International Journal of Forecasting*, *7*(3), 299–315. doi:10.1016/0169-2070(91)90004-F

Abramson, B., & Finizza, A. (1995). Probabilistic forecasts from probabilistic models: a case study in the oil market. *International Journal of Forecasting*, *11*(1), 63–72. doi:10.1016/0169-2070(94)02004-9

Adrangi, B., Chatrath, A., Dhanda, K. K., & Raffiee, K. (2001). Chaos in oil prices? Evidence from futures markets. *Energy Economics*, *23*, 405–425. doi:10.1016/S0140-9883(00)00079-7

Al Faris, A. (1991). The determinants of crude oil price adjustment in the world petroleum market. *OPEC Review*, 15.

Bacon, R. (1991). Modelling the price of oil. *Oxford Review of Economic Policy*, *7*(2), 17–34. doi:10.1093/oxrep/7.2.17

Barone-Adesi, G., Bourgoin, F., & Giannopoulos, K. (1998). Don't look back. *Risk (Concord, NH)*, (August): 100–107.

Chambers, M. J., & Bailey, R. J. (1996). A theory of commodity price fluctuations. *The Journal of Political Economy*, *104*(5), 924–957. doi:10.1086/262047

Dale, C., & Zyren, J. (1997). Petroleum futures markets: volatile prices, controversial functions, stagnant volumes. In Petroleum 1996: Issues and Trends, (pp. 92-100). Washington, DC: DOE/EIA-0615.

Deaton, A., & Larque, G. (1992). On the behavior of commodity prices. *The Review of Economic Studies*, *59*(198), 1–23. doi:10.2307/2297923

Fan, Y., Liang, Q., & Wei, Y. M. (2008). A generalized pattern matching approach for multi-step prediction of crude oil price. *Energy Economics*, *30*, 889–904. doi:10.1016/j.eneco.2006.10.012

Gulen, S. G. (1998). Efficiency in the crude oil futures markets. *Journal of Energy Finance & Development*, *3*(1), 13–21. doi:10.1016/S1085-7443(99)80065-9

Huntington, H. G. (1994). Oil price forecasting in the 1980s: what went wrong? *The Energy Journal (Cambridge, Mass.)*, *15*(2), 1–22.

Kaboudan, M. A. (2001). Compumetric forecasting of crude oil prices. In *The Proceedings of IEEE Congress on Evolutionary Computation*, (pp. 283–287).

Lanza, A., Manera, M., & Giovannini, M. (2005). Modeling and forecasting cointegrated relationships among heavy oil and product prices. *Energy Economics*, *27*, 831–848. doi:10.1016/j.eneco.2005.07.001

Michaelides, A., & Ng, S. (2000). Estimating the rational expectations model of speculative storage: a Monte Carlo comparison of three simulation estimators. *Journal of Econometrics*, *96*(2), 231–266. doi:10.1016/S0304-4076(99)00058-5

Miranda, M. J., & Glauber, J. W. (1993). Estimation of dynamic nonlinear rational expectations models of primary commodity markets with private and government stockholding. *The Review of Economics and Statistics*, *75*(3), 463–470. doi:10.2307/2109460

Mirmirani, S., & Li, H. C. (2004). A comparison of VAR and neural networks with genetic algorithm in forecasting price of oil. *Advances in Econometrics*, *19*, 203–223. doi:10.1016/S0731-9053(04)19008-7

Morana, C. (2001). A semiparametric approach to short-term oil price forecasting. *Energy Economics*, *23*(3), 325–338. doi:10.1016/S0140-9883(00)00075-X

Nelson, Y. S., Stoner, G., & Gemis, H. D. (1994). *Nix: Results of Delphi VIII survey of oil price forecasts*. Energy Report, California Energy Commission.

Panas, E., & Ninni, V. (2000). Are oil markets chaotic? A non-linear dynamic analysis. *Energy Economics*, *22*, 549–568. doi:10.1016/S0140-9883(00)00049-9

Routledge, B., Seppi, D., & Spatt, C. (2000). Equilibrium Forward Curves for Commodities. *The Journal of Finance*, *55*(3), 1297–1338. doi:10.1111/0022-1082.00248

Sadorsky, P. (2006). Modeling and forecasting petroleum futures volatility. *Energy Economics*, *28*, 467–488. doi:10.1016/j.eneco.2006.04.005

Saif Ghouri, S. (2006). Assessment of the relationship between oil prices and US oil stocks. *Energy Policy*, *34*(17), 3327–3333. doi:10.1016/j.enpol.2005.07.007

Shambora, W. E., & Rossiter, R. (2007). Are there exploitable inefficiencies in the futures market for oil? *Energy Economics*, *29*, 18–27. doi:10.1016/j.eneco.2005.09.004

Timothy, J. C., & Eunnyeong, H. (2000). Price and inventory dynamics in petroleum product markets. *Energy Economics*, *22*(5), 527–548. doi:10.1016/S0140-9883(00)00056-6

Xie, W., Yu, L., Xu, S. Y., & Wang, S. Y. (2006). *A new method for crude oil price forecasting based on support vector machines*, (. *LNCS*, *3994*, 441–451.

Ye, M., Zyren, J., & Shore, J. (2002). Forecasting crude oil spot price using OECD petroleum inventory levels. *International Advances in Economic Research*, *8*, 324–334. doi:10.1007/BF02295507

Ye, M., Zyren, J., & Shore, J. (2005). A monthly crude oil spot price forecasting model using relative inventories. *International Journal of Forecasting*, *21*, 491–501. doi:10.1016/j.ijforecast.2005.01.001

Ye, M., Zyren, J., & Shore, J. (2006). Forecasting short-run crude oil price using high and low-inventory variables. *Energy Policy, 34*, 2736–2743. doi:10.1016/j.enpol.2005.03.017

Yu, L., Lai, K. K., Wang, S. Y., & He, K. J. (2007). *Oil price forecasting with an EMD-based multiscale neural network learning paradigm, (LNCS), 4489*, 925–932.

Yu, L., Wang, S. Y., & Lai, K. K. (2005). A novel nonlinear ensemble forecasting model incorporating GLAR and ANN for foreign exchange rates. *Computers & Operations Research, 32*(10), 2523–2541. doi:10.1016/j.cor.2004.06.024

Yu, L., Wang, S. Y., & Lai, K. K. (2008). Forecasting crude oil price with an EMD-based neural network ensemble learning paradigm. *Energy Economics, 30*, 2623–2635. doi:10.1016/j.eneco.2008.05.003

Zhang, X., Lai, K. K., & Wang, S. Y. (2008). A new approach for crude oil price analysis based on Empirical Mode Decomposition. *Energy Economics, 30*, 905–918. doi:10.1016/j.eneco.2007.02.012

KEY TERMS AND DEFINITIONS

Data Mining: Data mining is the process of extracting hidden patterns from data. Data mining is becoming an increasingly important tool to transform this data into information.

Crude Oil Price Forecasting: Crude oil price forecasting is the process of judge the trend of crude oil price by analyzing the factors affecting oil price fluctuation.

Least Square Support Vector Regression: Least squares support vector machines (LSSVM) are reformulations to the standard SVMs which lead to solving linear KKT systems.

Neural Network: Traditionally, the term neural network (NN) had been used to refer to a network or circuit of biological neurons. The modern usage of the term often refers to artificial neural networks, which are composed of artificial neurons or nodes, which can be used for classification, forecast and regression and so on.

Support Vector Machine: Support vector machines (SVM) are a set of related supervised learning methods used for classification and regression.

Wavelet Neural Network: Wavelet neural network (WNN) is a novel approach towards the learning function. Wavelet networks, which combine the wavelet theory and feed-forward neural networks, utilize wavelets as the basic function to construct a network.

Chapter 11
Correlation Analysis in Classifiers

Vincent Lemaire
France Télécom, France

Carine Hue
GFI Informatique, France

Olivier Bernier
France Télécom, France

ABSTRACT

This chapter presents a new method to analyze the link between the probabilities produced by a classification model and the variation of its input values. The goal is to increase the predictive probability of a given class by exploring the possible values of the input variables taken independently. The proposed method is presented in a general framework, and then detailed for naive Bayesian classifiers. We also demonstrate the importance of "lever variables", variables which can conceivably be acted upon to obtain specific results as represented by class probabilities, and consequently can be the target of specific policies. The application of the proposed method to several data sets shows that such an approach can lead to useful indicators.

INTRODUCTION

Given a database, one common task in data analysis is to find the relationships or correlations between a set of input or explanatory variables and one target variable. This knowledge extraction often goes through the building of a model which represents these relationships (Han & Kamber, 2006). Faced with a classification problem, a probabilist model allows, for all the instances of the database and

given the values of the explanatory variables, the estimation of the probabilities of occurrence of each class target.

These probabilities, or scores, can be used to evaluate existing policies and practices in organizations and governments. They are not always directly usable, however, as they do not give any indication of what action can be decided upon to change this evaluation. Consequently, it seems useful to propose a methodology which would, for every instance in the database, (i) identify the importance of the explanatory variables; (ii) identify

DOI: 10.4018/978-1-60566-906-9.ch011

the position of the values of these explanatory variables; and (iii) propose an action in order to change the probability of the desired class. We propose to deal with the third point by exploring the model relationship between each explanatory variable independently from each other and the target variable. The proposed method presented in this chapter is completely automatic.

This chapter is organized as follows: the first section positions the approach in relation to the state of the art; the second section describes the method at first from a generic point of view and then for the naive Bayes classifier. Through three illustrative examples the third section allows a discussion and a progressive interpretation of the obtained results. In each illustrative example different practical details of the proposed method are explored. Finally we shall conclude.

BACKGROUND

Machine learning abounds with methods for supervised analysis in regression and/ or classification. Generally these methods propose algorithms to build a model from a training database made up of a finite number of examples. The output vector gives the predicted probability of the occurrence of each class label. In general, however, this probability of occurrence is not sufficient and an interpretation and analysis of the result in terms of correlations or relationships between input and output variables is needed.

Furthermore, the interpretation of the model is often based on the parameters and the structure of the model. One can cite, for example: geometrical interpretations (Brennan & Seiford, 1987), interpretations based on rules (Thrun, 1995) or fuzzy rules (Benitez, Castro, & Requena, 1997), statistical tests on the coefficient's model (Nakache & Confais, 2003). Such interpretations are often based on averages for several instances, for a given model, or for a given task (regression or classification).

Another approach, called sensitivity analysis, consists in analyzing the model as a black box by varying its input variables. In such "what if" simulations, the structure and the parameters of the model are important only as far as they allow accurate computations of dependant variables using explanatory variables. Such an approach works whatever the model. A large survey of "what if" methods, often used for artificial neural network, are available in (Leray & Gallinari, 1998; Lemaire, Féraud, & Voisine, 2006).

VARIABLE IMPORTANCE

Whatever the method and the model, the goal is often to analyze the behavior of the model in the absence of one input variable, or a set of input variables, and to deduce the importance of the input variables, for all examples. The reader can find a large survey in (Guyon, 2005). The measure of the importance of the input variables allows the selection of a subset of relevant variables for a given problem. This selection increases the robustness of models and simplifies the understanding of the results delivered by the model. The variety of supervised learning methods, coming from the statistical or artificial intelligence communities often implies importance indicators specific to each model (linear regression, artificial neural network...).

Another possibility is to try to study the importance of a variable for a given example and not in average for all the examples. Given a variable and an example, the purpose is to obtain the variable importance only for this example: for additive classifiers see (Poulin et al., 2006), for Probabilistic RBF Classification Network see (Robnik-Sikonja, Likas, Constantinopoulos, & Kononenko, 2009), and for a general methodology see (Lemaire & Féraud, 2008). If the model is restricted to a naive Bayes Classifier, a state of art is presented in (Možina, Demšar, Kattan, & Zupan, 2004; Robnik-Sikonja & Kononenko,

2008). This importance gives a specific piece of information linked to one example instead of an aggregate piece of information for all examples.

IMPORTANCE OF THE VALUE OF AN INPUT VARIABLE

To complete the importance of a variable, the analysis of the value of the considered variable, for a given example, is interesting. For example Féraud et al. (2002) propose to cluster examples and then to characterize each cluster using the variables importance and importance of the values inside every cluster. Framling (1996) uses a "what if" simulation to place the value of the variable and the associated output of the model among all the potential values of the model outputs. This method which uses extremums and an assumption of monotonous variations of the output model versus the variations of the input variable has been improved in (Lemaire & Féraud 2008).

INSTANCE CORRELATION BETWEEN AN EXPLANATORY VARIABLE AND THE TARGET CLASS

This chapter proposes to complete the two aspects presented above, namely the importance of a variable and the importance of the value of a variable. We propose1 to study the correlation, for one instance and one variable, between the input and the output of the model.

For a given instance, the distinct values of a given input variable can pull up (higher value) or pull down (lower value) the model output. The proposed idea is to analyze the relationship between the values of an input variable and the probability of occurrence of a given target class. The goal is to increase (or decrease) the model output, the target class probability, by exploring the different values taken by the input variable. For

instance for medical data one tries to decrease the probability of a disease; in case of cross-selling one tries to increase the appetency to a product; and in government data cases one tries to define a policy to reach specific goals in terms of specific indicators (for example decrease the unemployment rate).

This method does not explore causalities, only correlations, and can be viewed as a method between:

- selective sampling (Roy & McCallum, 2001) or adaptive sampling (Singh, Nowak, & Ramanathan, 2006): the model observes a restricted part of the universe materialized by examples but can "ask" to explore the variation space of the descriptors one by one separately, to find interesting zones and causality exploration (Kramer, Leventhal, Hutchinson, & Feinstein, 1979; Guyon, Constantin Aliferis, & Elisseeff, 2007): as example D. Choudat (Choudat, 2003) propose the imputability approach to specify the probability of the professional origin of a disease. The causality probability is, for an individual, the probability that his disease arose from exposures to professional elements. The increase of the risk has to be computed versus the respective role of each possible type exposures. In medical applications, the models used are often additive models or multiplicative models.

LEVER VARIABLES

In this chapter we also advocate the definition of a subset of the explanatory variables, the "lever variables". These lever variables are defined as the explanatory variables for which it is conceivable to change their value. In most cases, changing the values of some explanatory variables (such a sex, age...) is indeed impossible. The exploration of instance correlation between the target class and the explanatory variables can be limited in practice to variables which can effectively be changed.

The definition of these lever variables will allow a faster exploration by reducing the number of variable to explore, and will give more intelligible and relevant results. Lever variables are the natural target for policies and actions designed to induce changes of occurrence of the desired class in the real world.

CORRELATION EXPLORATION - METHOD DESCRIPTION

In this section, the proposed method is first described in the general case, for any type of predictive model, and then tested on naive Bayes classifiers

General Case

Let C_z be the target class among T target classes. Let f_z be the function which models the predicted probability of the target class $f_z(X=x) = P(C_z \mid X=x)$, given the equality of the vector X of the J explanatory variables to a given vector x of J values. Let v_{jn} be all the n different possible values of the variable X_j.

The Algorithm 1 describes the proposed method. This algorithm tries to increase the value of $P(C_z \mid X = x_k)$ successively for each of the K examples of the considered sample set using the set of values of all the explanatory variables or lever variables. This method is halfway between selective sampling (Roy & McCallum, 2001) and adaptive sampling (Singh et al., 2006). The model observes a restricted part of the universe materialized by examples but can "ask" to explore the variation space of the descriptors one by one separately, to find interesting zones. The next subsections describe the algorithm in more details.

Exploration of Input Values

For the instance x_k, $P(C_z \mid x_k)$ is the "natural" value of the model output. We propose to modify the values of the explanatory variables or lever variables in order to study the variation of the model output for this example. In practice, we propose to explore the values independently for each explanatory variable. Let $P_j(C_z \mid x_k, b)$ be the output model f_z given the example x_k but for which the value of its jth component has been replaced with the value b. For example, the third explanatory variable is modified among five variables: $P_3(C_z \mid x_k, b) = f_z(x_k^1, x_k^2, b, x_k^4, x_k^5)$. By scanning all the variables and for each of them all the set of their possible values, an exploration of "potential" values of the model output is computed for the example x_k.

Domain of Exploration of Each Variable

The advantage of choosing the empirical probability distribution of the data as domain of exploration has been showed experimentally in (Breiman, 2001; Lemaire et al., 2006; Lemaire & Féraud, 2008). A theoretical proof is also available for linear regression in (Diagne, 2006) and for naive Bayes classifiers in (Robnik-Sikonja & Kononenko, 2008). Consequently the values used for the J explanatory variables will be the values of the K examples available in the training database. This set can also be reduced using only the distinct values: let N_j be the number of distinct values of the variable X_j.

Results Ranking

The exploration of the explanatory variables or of the lever variables is done by scanning all the possible values taken by the examples in the training set. When the modification of the value of the variable leads to an improvement of the-

Figure 1. Algorithm 1: Exploration and ranking of the score improvements

```
For the example (the customer) x_k do
    w=0;
    For all the explanatory variables X_j from j = 1 to j = J do
        For all the n, different values (v_jn) of the variable X_j from n = 1 to n = N_j do
            If P_j(C_z|x_k, b = v_jn) > P(C_z|x_k) then
                Ca[w] = v_jn;
                PCa[w] = P_j(C_z|x_k, v_jn)
                XCa[w] = j
            else
                Ca[w] = 0.0;
                PCa[w] = 0.0;
                XCa[w] = j
            end If
            w=w+1;
        end For
    end For
    Decreasing sort, using the values of PCa[w], Ca[w], XCa[w].
end For
```

probability predicted by the model, three pieces of data are kept (i) the value which leads to this improvement (*Ca*); (ii) the associated improved probability (*PCa*); and (iii) the variable associated to this improvement (*XCa*). These triplets are then sorted according to the improvement obtained on the predicted probability. Note: if no improvement is found, the tables *CA* and *PCa* only contain null values.

It should also be possible (i) to explore jointly two or more explanatory variables; (ii) or to use the value (*Ca*[0]) which best improves the output of the model ($P(C_z | X = x)$) (this value *Ca*[0] is available at the end of the Algorithm) and then to repeat again the exploration on the example x_k on its others explanatory variables. These other versions are not presented in this chapter but will be the focus of future works.

Cases with Class Changes

When using Algorithm 1 (Figure 1), the predicted class can change. Indeed it is customary to use the following formulation to designate the predicted class of the example x_k:

$$\arg \max_z P(C_z | x_k)$$

Using Algorithm 1 for x_k belonging to the class t ($t \neq z$) could produce $P(C_z | x_k, b) > P(C_t | x_k)$. In this case the corresponding value (*Ca*) carries important information which can be exploited.

The use of Algorithm 1 can exhibit three types of values (*Ca*):

- values which do not increase the target class probability;

- values which increase the target class probability but without class change (the probability increase is not sufficient);
- values which increase the target class probability with class change (the probability increase is sufficient).

The examples whose predicted class changes from another class to the target class are the primary target for specific actions or policies designed to increase the occurrence of this class in the real world.

Case of a Naive Bayesian Classifier

A naive Bayes classifier assumes that all the explanatory variables are independent knowing the target class. This assumption drastically reduces the necessary computations. Using the Bayes theorem, the expression of the obtained estimator for the conditional probability of a class C_z is:

$$P(C_z \mid x_k) = \frac{P(C_z) \prod_{j=1}^{J} P(X_j = v_{jk} \mid C_z)}{\sum_{t=1}^{T} P(C_t) \prod_{j=1}^{J} P(X_j = v_{jk} \mid C_t)}$$

(1)

The predicted class is the one which maximizes the conditional probabilities. Despite the independence assumption, this kind of classifier generally shows satisfactory results (Hand & Yu, 2001). Moreover, its formulation allows an exploration of the values of the variables one by one independently.

The probabilities $P(X_j = v_{jk} \mid C_z)$ ($\forall j, k, z$) are estimated using counts after discretization for numerical variables or grouping for categorical variables (Boullé, 2008). The denominator of the equation above normalizes the result so that $\sum_z P(C_z \mid x_k) = 1$.

The use of the Algorithm 1 requires to compute $P(C_z \mid X = x_k)$, and $P_j(C_z \mid X = x, b)$ which can be written in the form of Equations 2 and 3:

$$P(C_z \mid x_k) = \frac{\overbrace{P(C_z) \prod_{j=1}^{J} P(X_j = v_{jk} \mid C_z)}^{e^{Lz}}}{\sum_{t=1}^{T} P(C_t) \prod_{j=1}^{J} P(X_j = v_{jk} \mid C_t)}$$

(2)

$$P_j(C_z \mid x_k, b) = \frac{\overbrace{P(C_z) \prod_{j=1, j \neq q}^{J} P(X_j = v_{jk} \mid C_z) P(X_q = b \mid C_z)}^{e^{Lz'}}}{\sum_{t=1}^{T} \left[P(C_t) \prod_{j=1}^{J} P(X_j = v_{jk} \mid C_t) \right] P(X_q = b \mid C_t)}$$

(3)

In Equations 2 and 3 numerators can be written as e^{Lz} and $e^{Lz'}$ with:

$$L_z = \log(P(C_z)) + \sum_{j=1}^{J} \log(P(X_j = v_{jk} \mid C_z))$$

and

$$L_{z'} = \log(P(C_z)) + \sum_{j=1, j \neq q}^{J} \left[\log(P(X_j = v_{jk} \mid C_z)) + \log(P(X_q = b \mid C_z)) \right]$$

This formulation will be used below.

Implementation Details on Very Large Databases

To measure the reliability of our approach, we tested it on marketing campaigns of France Telecom (results not allowed for publication until now). Tests have been performed using the PAC platform (Féraud, Boullé, Clérot, & Fessant, 2008) on different databases coming from decision-making applications. The databases used for testing had more than 1 million of customers, each one represented by a vector including several thousands of explanatory variables. These tests raise several implementation points enumerated below:

- To avoid numerical problems when comparing the "true" output model $P(C_z \mid x_k)$ and the "explored" output $P_j(C_z \mid x_k, b)$, $P(C_x \mid x_k)$ is computed as:

$$P(C_x \Big| x_k) = \frac{1}{\sum_{t=1}^{T} e^{L_t - L_x}}$$

where

$$L_t = \log(P(C_t)) + \sum_{j=1}^{J} \log(P(X_j = v_{jk} \Big| C_t))$$

- To reduce the computation time: the modified output of the classifier can be computed using only several additions or subtractions since the difference between L_z (used in Equation 2) and $L_{z'}$ (used in Equation 3) is:

$$L_{z'} = L_z - \log(P(x_q = v_{jk} \mid C_z)) + \log(P(X_q = b \mid C_z))$$

- Complexity: For a given example x_k, the computation of tables presented in Algorithm 1 is of complexity $O(\sum_{j=1}^{d} N_j)$.

This implementation is "real-time" and can be used by an operator who asks the application what actions to do, for example to keep a customer.

EXPERIMENTATIONS

In this section we describe the application of our proposed method to three illustrative examples. This first example, the Titanic database, illustrates the importance of lever variables. The second example illustrates the results of our method on the dataset used for the PAKDD 2007 challenge. Finally, we present the results obtained by our method on a government data problem, the analysis of the type of contraceptive used by married women in Indonesia.

The Titanic Database – Data and Experimental Conditions

In this first experiment the Titanic (www.ics.uci.edu/~mlearn/) database is used. This database consists of four explanatory variables on 2201 instances (passengers and crew members). The first attribute represents the class trip (status) of the passenger or if he was a crew member, with values: 1st, 2nd, 3rd, crew. The second (age) gives an age indication: adult, child. The third (sex) indicates the sex of the passenger or crew: female or male. The last attribute (survived) is the target class attribute with values: no or yes. Readers can find for each instance the variable importance and the value importance for a naive Bayes classifier in (Robnik-Sikonja & Kononenko, 2008).

Among the 2201 examples in this database, a training set of 1100 examples randomly chosen has been extracted to train a naive Bayes classifier using the method presented in (Boullé, 2008). The remaining examples constitute a test set. As the interpretation of a model with low performance would not be consistent, a prerequisite is to check if this naive Bayes classifier is correct. The model used here (Guyon, Saffari, Dror, & Bumann, 2007) gives satisfactory results:

- Accuracy on Classification (ACC) on the train set: 77.0%; on the test set: 75.0%;
- Area under the ROC curve (AUC) (Fawcett, 2003) on the train set: 73.0%; on the test set: 72.0%.

The purpose here is to the see another side of the knowledge produced by the classifier: we want to find the characteristics of the instances (people) which would have allowed them to survive.

Input Values Exploration

Algorithm 1 has been applied on the test set to reinforce the probability to survive. Table 1 shows an abstract of the results: (i) it is not possible to

Table 1. Ranking of explanatory variables

	Size	Status / Age / Sex
Predicted 'yes'	343	118 / 125 / 100
Predicted 'no'	758	0 / 0 / 758

increase the probability for only one passenger or crew; (ii) the last column indicates that, for persons predicted as surviving by the model (343 people), the first explanatory variable (status) is the most important to reinforce the probability to survive for 118 cases; then the second explanatory variable (age) for 125 cases; and at last the third one (sex) for 100 cases. (iii) For people predicted as dead by the model (758) the third explanatory variable (sex) is always the variable which is the most important to reinforce the probability to survive.

These 758 cases predicted as dead are men and if they were women their probability to survive would increase sufficiently to survive (in the sense that their probability to survive would be greater than their probability to die). Let us examine then, for these cases, additional results obtained by exploring the others variables using the algorithm 1:

- the second best variable to reinforce the probability to survive is (and in this case they survive):
- for 82 of them (adult + men + 2nd class) the second explanatory variable (age);
- for 676 of them (adult + men + (crew or 3rd class)) the first explanatory variable (status);
- the third best variable to reinforce the probability to survive is (and in this case nevertheless they are dead):
- for 82 of them (adult + men + 2nd class) the first explanatory variable (status);
- for 676 of them (adult + men + (crew or 3rd class)) the second explanatory variable (age).

Of course, in this case, most explanatory variables are not in fact lever variables, as they cannot be changed (age or sex). The only variable that can be changed is status, and even in this case, only for passengers, not for crew members. The change of status for passengers means in fact buying a first class ticket, which would have allowed them a better chance to survive. The other explanatory variables enable us to interpret the obtained survival probability in terms of priority given to women and first class passengers during the evacuation.

APPLICATION TO SALE: RESULTS ON THE PAKDD 2007 CHALLENGE

Data and Experimental Conditions

The PAKDD 2007 challenge data is used (http://lamda.nju.edu.cn/conf/pakdd07/dmc07/): The data are not on-line any more but data descriptions and analysis results are still available. Thanks to Mingjun Wei (participant referenced P049) for the data (version 3).

The company, which gave the database, has currently a customer base of credit card customers as well as a customer base of home loan (mortgage) customers. Both of these products have been on the market for many years, although for some reasons the overlap between these two customer bases is currently very small. The company would like to make use of this opportunity to cross-sell home loans to its credit card customers, but the small size of the overlap presents a challenge when trying to develop an effective scoring model to predict potential cross-sell take-ups.

A modeling dataset of 40,700 customers with 40 explanatory variables, plus a target variable, had been provided to the participants (the list of the 40 explanatory variables is available at http://perso.rd.francetelecom.fr/lemaire/data_pakdd.zip). This is a sample of customers who opened a new credit card with the company within a

Table 2. PAKDD 2007 challenge: the first three best results

id participant	AUC for test set	Rank	Modeling Technique
P049	70.01%	1	TreeNet + Logistic Regression
P085	69.99%	2	Probit Regression
P212	69.62%	3	MLP + n-Tuple Classifier

specific 2-year period and who did not have an existing home loan with the company. The target categorical variable "Target_Flag" has a value of 1 if the customer then opened a home loan with the company within 12 months after opening the credit card (700 random samples), and has a value of 0 otherwise (40,000 random samples).

A prediction dataset (8,000 sampled cases) has also been provided to the participants with similar variables but withholding the target variable. The data mining task is to produce a score for each customer in the prediction dataset, indicating a credit card customer's propensity to take up a home loan with the company (the higher the score, the higher the propensity).

The challenge being ended it was not possible to evaluate our classifier on the prediction dataset (the submission site is closed). Therefore we decide to elaborate a model using the 40 000 samples in a 5-fold cross validation process. In this case each 'test' fold contains approximately the same number of samples as the initial prediction dataset. The model used is again a naive Bayes classifier (Boullé, 2008; Guyon, Saffari, et al., 2007). The results obtained on the test sets are:

- Accuracy on Classification (ACC): 98.29% ± 0.01% on the train sets and 98.20% ± 0.06% on the test sets.
- Area under the ROC curve (AUC): 67.98% ± 0.74% on the train sets and 67.79% ± 2.18% on the test sets.

- Best results obtained on one of the folds: Train set AUC=68.82%, Test set AUC=70.11%.

Table 2 shows the first three best results and corresponding method of winners of the challenge. Results obtained here by our model are coherent with those of the participants of the challenge.

Input Values Exploration

The best classifier obtained on the test sets in the previous section is used. This naive Bayes classifier (Boullé, 2007) uses 8 variables out of 40 (the naïve Bayes classifier takes into account only input variables which have been discretized (or grouped) in more than one interval (or group) see (Boullé, 2006)). These 8 variables and their intervals of discretization (or groups) are presented in Table 3. All variable are numerical except for the variable "RENT_BUY_CODE" which is symbolic with possible values of 'O' (Owner), 'P' (Parents), 'M' (Mortgage), 'R' (Rent), 'B' (Board), 'X' (Other).

The lever variables were carefully chosen by using their specification (see http://lamda.nju.edu.cn/conf/pakdd07/dmc07/ or the appendix A). These lever variables are those for which a commercial offer to a customer can change the value. We define another type of variable which we will explore using our algorithm, the observable variables. These variables are susceptible to change during a life of a customer and this change may augment the probability of the target class, the propensity to take up a home loan.

In this case, the customers for which this variable has changed can be the target of a specific campaign. For example the variable "RENT_BUY_CODE" can not be changed by any offer but is still observable. The customer can move from the group of values [O,P] ('O' Owner, 'P' Parents) to [M,R,B,X] ('M' Mortgage, 'R' Rent, 'B' Board, 'X' Other). Among the eight variables (see Table

Table 3. Selected explanatory variables (there is no reason in (Boullé, 2006) to have two intervals for each variable, it is here blind chance)

Explanatory Variables	Interval 1 or Group 1	Interval 2 or Group 2
RENT_BUY_CODE	M,R,B,X	O,P
PREV_RES_MTHS	]-∞,3.5[	[3.5,+∞ [
CURR_RES_MTHS	]-∞,40.5[	[40.5,+∞ [
B_ENQ_L6M_GR3	]-∞,0.5[	[0.5,+∞ [
B_ENQ_L3M	]-∞,0.5[	[3.5,+∞ [
B_ENQ_L12M_GR3	]-∞,1.5[	[1.5,+∞ [
B_ENQ_L12M_GR2	]-∞,0.5[	[0.5,+∞ [
AGE_AT_APPLICATION	]-∞,45.5[	[45.5,+∞ [

Table 4. Best $P(C_z)$='yes' obtained

C1: explored variable	C2	C3	C4	C5
RENT_BUY_CODE	0.6	0.26	[O,P]	[M,R,B,X]
CURR_RES_MTHS	0.36	0.21	[40.5,+∞[	]-∞,40.5[
B_ENQ_L6M_GR3	0.25	0.10	]-∞,0.5[	[0.5,+∞[
B_ENQ_L3M	0.12	0.12	]-∞,1.5[	[1.5,+ ∞[
B_ENQ_L12M_GR3	0.36	0.16	]-∞,0.5[	[1.5,+∞[
B_ENQ_L12M_GR2	0.36	0.24	[0.5,+∞[	]- ∞,0.5[

3) chosen by the training method of the naive Bayes classifier, two are not considered as 'lever' variables or observable variables ("AGE_AT_AP-PLICATION" and "PREV_RES_MTHS") and will not be explored.

Algorithm 1 has been applied on the 40700 instances in the modeling data set. The 'yes' class of the target variable is chosen as target class (C_z = 'yes'). This class is very weakly represented (700 positive instances out of 40700). The AUC values presented in Table 2 or on the challenge website does not show if customers are classified as 'yes' by the classifier. Exploration of lever variables does not allow in this case a modification of the predicted class. Nevertheless Table 4 and Figure 2 show that a large improvement of the 'yes' probability (the probability of cross-selling) is possible.

In Table 4 the second column (C2) presents the best $P_j(C_z \mid x_k, b)$ obtained, the third column (C3) the initial corresponding $P(C_z \mid x_k, b)$, the fourth column (C4) the initial interval used in the naive Bayes formulation (used to compute $P(C_z \mid x_k, b)$) and the last column (C5) the interval which gives the best improvement (used to compute $P_j(C_z \mid x_k, b)$). This table shows that:

- for all lever or observable variables, there exists a value change that increases the posterior probability of occurrences of the target class;
- the variable that leads to the greatest probability improvement is B_ENQ_L3M (The number of Bureau Enquiries in the last 3 months), for a value in [1.5,+∞[rather than in]- ∞,1.5[; This variable is an observable variable, not a lever variable, and means that a marketing campaign should be focused on customers who contacted the bureau more than once in the last three months
- nevertheless, none of those changes leads to a class change as the obtained probability ($P_j(C_z \mid x_k, b)$) stays smaller than $P(C_z \mid x_k)$.

In Figure 2 the six dotted vertical axis represent the six lever or observable variables as indicated on top or bottom axis. On the left hand size of each vertical axis, the distribution of $P(C_z \mid x_k)$ is plotted (□) and on the right hand size the distribution of $P_j(C_z \mid x_k, b)$ is plotted (v). Probability values are indicated on the y-axis. In this Figure only the best $P_j(C_z \mid x_k, b)$ ($PCa[0]$ in Algorithm 1) is plotted. This figure illustrates in more details the same conclusions as given above.

Figure 2. Obtained results on $P_j(C_z \mid x_k, b)$

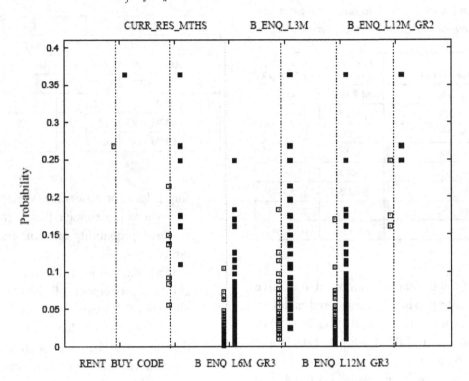

APPLICATION TO GOVERNMENT DATA: RESULTS FOR THE CONTRACEPTIVE METHOD CHOICE DATA SET

Data and Experimental Conditions

The Contraceptive Method Choice Data Set is an available data set in the UCI Machine Learning Repository. This data set is a subset of the 1987 National Indonesia Contraceptive Prevalence Survey. It consists of 1473 instances, corresponding to married women either not pregnant or who did not know if they were at the time of the survey. The problem is to predict, from 9 explanatory variables (age, education, husband's education, number of children ever born, religion, working or not, husband's occupation, standard of living index, good media exposure or not) the type of contraceptive method used (no contraceptive method, short-term contraceptive method or long-

term contraceptive method). Three explanatory variables are binary (religion either Islam or not, working or not, and good media exposure or not), two are numerical (age and number of children ever born) and the others are categorical.

The model used is a selective naive Bayes classifier (Boullé, 2007), trained on 75 percent of the dataset (1108 instances), the rest of the dataset being used for testing purposes. On the training subset, we obtained an AUC (Area Under ROC Curve) of 0.74, and an AUC of 0.73 for the test subset.

Input Values Exploration

The selective naive Bayes classifier (Boullé, 2007) uses 8 of the 9 explanatory variables, discarding the binary variable working or not. Among these variables, only two are chosen as lever variables, education and good media exposure or not. The other variables are not considered as possible

Table 5. Number of instances for each predicted class and level of education

	No contraceptive	Short term	Long term
Low education	137	0	15
Middle education	387	19	338
High education	67	211	299
Total	591	230	652

targets for policies. Education is a categorical variable with four values from 1 (low education) to 4 (high education), partitioned into three groups by the classification algorithm: low education (value 1), middle education (values 2 or 3) and high education (value 4). Algorithm 1 has been applied on the 1473 instances. The target variable is in this case a three class variable (no contraceptive, short-term contraceptive, and long-term contraceptive). As the proposed algorithm can only try to increase the probability of one class, it was applied twice, once to try to increase the probability of using a short-term contraceptive, once to try to increase the probability of using a long-term contraceptive.

Applying our method to increase the probability of using a long-term contraceptive showed that the most significant lever variable is the education level. Table 5 indicates the number of instances for each predicted class and each level of education.

Out of 1473 instances, 577 instances are already at a high education level. Out of the remaining 895 instances, 99 were predicted to switch from no contraceptive to a long term contraceptive if the education level was changed from whatever value (low or middle) to a high value, and 30 instances were predicted to switch from short term contraceptive to long term contraceptive with the same change in education level. Media exposure do not seem to have any significant impact (only 2 instances of 'class changes' to long term con-

traceptive, by changing the media exposure to good media exposure).

Applying our current method to increase the probability of using a short term contraceptive, 157 instances were predicted to switch from no contraceptive to short term contraceptive with a higher education, and 18 with change to good media exposure. This example illustrates the great importance of education level for the choice of contraceptive in developing countries.

CONCLUSION AND FUTURE TRENDS

In this chapter we proposed a method to study the influence of the input values on the output scores of a probabilistic model. The method has first been defined in a general case valid for any model, and then been detailed for naive Bayes classifier. We also demonstrate the importance of "lever variables", explanatory variables which can conceivably be changed. Our method has first been illustrated on the simple Titanic database in order to show the need to define lever variables. Then, on the PAKDD 2007 challenge databases, a difficult problem of cross-selling, the results obtained show that it is possible to create efficient indicators that could increase sells. Finally we demonstrated the applicability of our method to a government data case, the choice of contraceptive for Indonesian women.

The case study presented on the Titanic dataset illustrates the point of applying the proposed method to accident research. It could be used for example to analyze road accidents or air accidents. In the case of the air accidents any new plane crash is thoroughly analyzed to improve the security of air flights. Despite the increasing number of plane crashes, the relative frequency of those in relation to the volume of traffic is decreasing and air security is globally improving. Analyzing the correlations between the occurrence of a crash and several explanatory variables could lead to a new approach to the prevention of plane crashes.

This type of relationship analysis method has also great potential for medicine applications, in particular to analyze the link between vaccination and mortality. The estimated 50% reduced overall mortality currently associated with influenza vaccination among the elderly is based on studies neither fully taking into account systematic differences between individuals who accept or decline vaccination nor encompassing the entire general population. The proposed method in this paper could find interesting data for infectious diseases research units. Another potential area of application is the analysis of the factors causing a disease, by investigating the link between the occurrence of the disease and the potential factors.

The proposed method is very simple but efficient. It is now implemented in an add-on of the Khiops software (see http://www.khiops.com), and its user guide is available at: http://perso.rd.francetelecom.fr/lemaire/understanding/Guide.pdf

This tool could be useful for companies or research centers who want to analyze classification results with input values exploration.

REFERENCES

Benitez, J. M., Castro, J. L., & Requena, I. (1997, September). Are artificial neural networks black boxes? *IEEE Transactions on Neural Networks*, 8(5), 1156–1164. doi:10.1109/72.623216

Boullé, M. (2006). MODL: a Bayes optimal discretization method for continuous attributes. *Machine Learning*, 65(1), 131–165. doi:10.1007/s10994-006-8364-x

Boullé, M. (2007). Compression-based averaging of selective naive Bayes classifiers. [JMLR]. *Journal of Machine Learning Research*, 8, 1659–1685.

Boullé, M. (2008). Khiops: outil de préparation et modélisation des données pour la fouille des grandes bases de données. In Extraction et gestion des connaissances (EGC), (pp. 229-230).

Breiman, L. (2001). Random forest. *Machine Learning, 45.* Retrieved from www.berkeley.edu/users/breiman/Breiman.

Brennan, J. J., & Seiford, L. M. (1987). *Linear programming and l1 regression: A geometric interpretation.* Computational Statistics & Data Analysis.

Choudat, D. (2003). Risque, fraction étiologique et probabilité de causalité en cas d'expositions multiples, i: l'approche théorique. *Archives des Maladies Professionnelles et de l'Environnement, 64*(3), 129–140.

Diagne, G. (2006). *Sélection de variables et méthodes d'interprétation des résultats obtenus par un modèle boite noire.* Unpublished master's thesis, UVSQ-TRIED.

Fawcett, T. (2003). *Roc graphs: Notes and practical considerations for data mining researchers.* Technical Report HPL-2003-4, HP Labs, 2003. Retrieved from citeseer.ist.psu.edu/fawcett03roc.html

Féraud, R., Boullé, M., Clérot, F., & Fessant, F. (2008). Vers l'exploitation de grandes masses de données. In *Extraction et gestion des connaissances* (pp. 241–252). EGC.

Féraud, R., & Clérot, F. (2002). A methodology to explain neural network classification. *Neural Networks, 15*(2), 237–246. doi:10.1016/S0893-6080(01)00127-7

Fern, X. Z., & Brodley, C. (2003). Boosting lazy decision trees. In *International conference on machine learning* (pp. 178–185). ICML.

Framling, K. (1996). *Modélisation et apprentissage des préférences par réseaux de neurones pour l'aide à la décision multicritère.* Unpublished doctoral dissertation, Institut National des Sciences Appliquées de Lyon, France.

Guyon, I. (2005). *Feature extraction, foundations and applications.* New York: Elsevier.

Guyon, I., Constantin Aliferis, C., & Elisseeff, A. (2007). In Liu, H., & Motoda, H. (Eds.), *Computational methods of feature selection* (pp. 63–86). Boca Raton, FL: Chapman and Hall/CRC.

Guyon, I., Saffari, A., Dror, G., & Bumann, J. (2007). Report on preliminary experiments with data grid models in the agnostic learning vs. prior knowledge challenge. In *International Joint Conference on Neural Networks (IJCNN).*

Han, J., & Kamber, M. (2006). *Data mining: concepts and techniques.* San Francisco: Morgan Kaufmann.

Hand, D., & Yu, K. (2001). Idiot's Bayes - not so stupid after all? *International Statistical Review, 69*(3), 385–399.

Kramer, M. S., Leventhal, J. M., Hutchinson, T. A., & Feinstein, A. R. (1979). An algorithm for the operational assessment of adverse drug reactions. i. background, description, and instructions for use. *Journal of the American Medical Association, 242*(7), 623–632. doi:10.1001/jama.242.7.623

Lemaire, V. Féraud, R., & Voisine, N. (2006, October). Contact personalization using a score understanding method. In *International Joint Conference on Neural Networks (IJCNN),* Hong-Kong.

Lemaire, V., & Féraud, R. (2008). Driven forward features selection: a comparative study on neural networks. In *International Joint Conference on Neural Network (IJCNN).*

Leray, P., & Gallinari, P. (1998). *Variable selection.* Tech. Rep. No. ENV4-CT96-0314, University Paris 6, France.

Lichtsteiner, S., & Schibler, U. (1989). *A glycosylated liver-specific transcription factor stimulates transcription of the albumin gene.* CELL.

Možina, M., Demšar, J., Kattan, M., & Zupan, B. (2004). Nomograms for visualization of naive Bayesian classifier. In *Proceedings of the 8th european conference on principles and practice of knowledge discovery in databases (PAKDD),* (pp. 337–348). New York: Springer-Verlag, Inc.

Nakache, J., & Confais, J. (2003). *Statistique explicative appliquée.* TECHNIP.

Poulin, B., Eisner, R., Szafron, D., Lu, P., Greiner, R., & Wishart, D. S. (2006). *Visual explanation of evidence with additive classifiers.* IAAI.

Raymer, M. L., Doom, T. E., A., K. L. & Punch, W. L. (2003). Knowledge discovery in medical and biological datasets using a hybrid Bayes classifier/evolutionary algorithm. *IEEE Transactions on Systems, Man, and Cybernetics, Part B.*

Robnik-Sikonja, M. & Kononenko, I. (2008). *Explaining classifications for individual instances,* (to appear in IEEE TKDE).

Robnik-Sikonja, M., Likas, A., Constantinopoulos, C., & Kononenko, I. (2009). *An efficient method for explaining the decisions of the probabilistic RBF classification network.* (currently under review, partially available as TR, http://lkm.fri.uni-lj.si/rmarko)

Roy, N., & McCallum, A. (2001). Toward optimal active learning through sampling estimation of error reduction. In *Proc. 18th international conf. on machine learning* (pp. 441-448). San Francisco, CA: Morgan Kaufmann.

Singh, A., Nowak, R., & Ramanathan, P. (2006). Active learning for adaptive mobile sensing networks. In *Proceedings of the fifth international conference on information processing in sensor networks* (IPSN), (p. 60-68). New York: ACM Press.

Thrun, S. (1995). Extracting rules from artificial neural networks with distributed representations. In Tesauro, G., Touretzky, D., & Leen, T. (Eds.), *Advances in neural information processing systems (NIPS)* (*Vol. 7*). Cambridge, MA: M. Press.

KEY TERMS AND DEFINITIONS

Classifier: A mapping from a (discrete or continuous) feature space X to a discrete set of labels Y.

Probabilistic Classifier: A classifier with the probability of each label (class) as output.

Exploration: Attempt to develop an initial, rough understanding of some phenomenon.

Correlation: The strength and direction of a linear relationship between two variables.

Supervised Learning: Supervised learning is a technique for learning a function (a mapping) from training data.

Variable Importance: Measure of the importance of a variable for the output of a classifier.

Sensibility Analysis: Analysis of the influence of a change in input variable on the output of the classifier.

ENDNOTE

[1] The description of the proposed method is done only for classification problems but the method is easily adaptable for regression problems

Chapter 12
Forecast Analysis for Sales in Large–Scale Retail Trade

Mirco Nanni
ISTI Institute of CNR, Italy

Laura Spinsanti
Ecole Polytechnique Fédérale de Lausanne, Switzerland

ABSTRACT

In large-scale retail trade, a very significant problem consists in analyzing the response of clients to product promotions. The aim of the project described in this work is the extraction of forecasting models able to estimate the volume of sales involving a product under promotion, together with a prediction of the risk of out of stock events, in which case the sales forecast should be considered potentially underestimated. Our approach consists in developing a multi-class classifier with ordinal classes (lower classes represent smaller numbers of items sold) as opposed to more traditional approaches that translate the problem to a binary-class classification. In order to do that, a proper discretization of sales values is studied, and ad hoc quality measures are provided in order to evaluate the accuracy of forecast models taking into consideration the order of classes. Finally, an overall system for end users is sketched, where the forecasting functionalities are organized in an integrated dashboard.

INTRODUCTION

Important business decisions and organization require a scientific framework to make systematic analysis of alternatives, as recognized since Taylor's classic work "The Principles of Scientific Management" (Taylor, 1911), that essentially marks the beginning of the Decision Science field.

A fundamental task in decision science is forecasting, involved in most decision making processes, sometimes even at an unconscious level. The basic idea is that the known history of the market (global or limited to a single company organization) can help to induce reasonable guesses of the effects of an action, therefore providing a valuable support in evaluating the several alternatives business managers typically have to sift through, and in choosing the most promising one.

DOI: 10.4018/978-1-60566-906-9.ch012

Forecasting in the business context, and sales forecasting in particular, can be studied and applied at several different levels:

- in global market analysis, also called the macro level, where offers and demands are studied in the general context of global market without a specific focus on single products or services;
- in sector- or product-specific market analysis, also called the micro level, where the above analysis is focused on single or families of products/services;
- in within-company market analysis, where the focus is in ascertaining the health status of the company activities, mainly in a evolution perspective that allows to recognize trends and possible weak points (actual or future), and in evaluating the future overall effects of actions to be taken within the company;
- in within-company product-specific sales analysis, where a single product is put under the lens of a microscope and analyzed in detail, highlighting its performances and its reactions to various kinds of inter-company stimuli (e.g., promotions or change of exposition level) and external ones (e.g., the introduction in the market of a new competitor product).

The aim of this work is to analyze a real case study in the latter context, focusing on the effects of promotions on the sales of a single product, mainly aimed at optimizing its stoking. The closed world context of such analysis, on one hand simplifies the forecasting problem by omitting external factors that are difficult to handle and that, in some cases, might have a large uncertainty; on the other hand, it allows to work with a complete and detailed history of previous sales, precise measures directly collected by the company, and even permits (to an economically-limited extent) to empirically evaluate models and

strategies on the ground, by replicating situations and later measuring the effects.

This chapter contributes to two main topics covered by this book, namely the role and impact of data mining in the management and in the decision making tasks within private organizations. In particular, the chapter provides a view of both methodological aspects of the problem, technical solutions adopted, and empirical results on the field.

Coop Italia is today the largest holding of large retailers and the largest organization of consumers of Italy. Overall, Coop Italia includes 163 consumer cooperatives with approximately 1261 stores, 6 million members and over 52,000 employees. As part of this large organization, Unicoop Tirreno is a great reality of organized distribution that is present in Tuscany, Lazio, Umbria and Campania with 112 stores (in 3 different size store), more than 770,000 members and approximately 6,300 employees. In 2007 it exceeded 1.16 billion euro of total sales.

In this context Unicoop Tirreno decided to develop Business Intelligence solutions, reactive to market changes, and start the project Business Intelligence and Data Warehouse (BI-Coop). The objectives of the BI-Coop project can be summarized as follows: (one) to create and populate a data warehouse from the operational data and to create interactive data reports (two) to develop forecasting models through the use of data mining technologies. In particular, data mining is used to predict customer defection and promotion sales previsions.

In this paper we describe the methodology and results obtained on models for promotion sales. This forecasting task can use only promotion features and sales data over the recent past. Moreover, in order to face this problem, we need to consider a side effect of promotions: the so-called "out of stock" phenomenon, i.e. the event a store is found out of products to sell before the promotion is finished, a signal of an incorrect storage estimate and a cause of lost income. Out of stocks (OOS) are not currently tracked in the operational database, making it difficult to quantify the extent of the phenomenon.

The forecast models described in this work have been developed using SPSS Clementine (Clementine, 2009), and they will be used by Coop in marketing planning to optimize the storage of goods in shops and to develop new promotions.

BACKGROUND

Forecasting is the process of estimation in unknown situations and Sales Forecasting is used in the practice of Customer Demand Planning in everyday business forecasting for manufacturing companies. It is a complex problem that has to take into account many different factors, not always easy to model and to control (new competitors, economic changes, and social events). Many approaches were developed to capture all these aspects, from statistical to machine learning ones, to develop decision support systems aimed to help managers.

Data mining identifies trends within data that go beyond simple data analysis, through the use of sophisticated algorithms: it could be described as the process of extracting hidden patterns from data. One of the first examples of data mining application to retail system was the market baskets analysis to understand the purchase behavior of groups of customers, and use it to increase sales, and for cross-selling, store design, discount plans and promotions. Developing data mining techniques for marketing is an ongoing tasks as recent books can confirm (Berry, 2004) and (Ohsawa, 2009).

In this context, predictive data mining models for sales data are classification models. Classification is a procedure in which individual items are placed into groups based on quantitative information on one or more characteristics inherent in the items (referred to as traits, variables, characters,

etc) and based on a training set of previously labeled items.

Promotions analysis could not be separate from OOS phenomenon. In our scenario, OOS is the event a store is found out of products to sell before the promotion is finished. In some cases this event is referred as Out Of Shelf, if referred only to shelf availability analysis. Anyway, the corporate data warehouse does not have data about the quantity of goods in storage, so the occurrence of the OOS event has been derived from an analysis of sales data. The definition was made in conjunction with experts, essentially by identifying sharp decreasing in sales quantity over each promotion day.

Related Works

Sales Forecasting

There exists a wide literature regarding sales forecasting. However, most approaches focus on time series analysis and prediction (for a survey, see for instance (Arsham, 1994)), which present two big drawbacks in our context:

- time series analysis is based on the extraction of trends and other behavioral models that are then matched to the current situation to forecast future values, implicitly assuming that a model that captured the past behavior of the system is applicable to the present situation. However, in our context, we aim to predict what happens in response to an external event – a promotion – that naturally creates a discontinuity with the past behavior of the series, therefore compromising the above mentioned regular evolution assumption;
- time series represent only part of the information we need to handle. In particular, in addition to the sales history of the promoted product, each promotion has its own characteristics which include, among the

others, the promotion type, its size, its duration, and various descriptors of the conditions under which the promotion takes place. An approach purely based on time series might not be able to take advantage of this important knowledge.

Other complex approaches like neural networks and regression-based models (linear and non-linear), can be appealing for what concerns potential accuracy, yet they usually yield models that are hard to inspect and interpret. On the opposite, in practice, the domain expert (which also plays the role of end user) requires that the resulting models can be understood, and possibly also amended, and therefore simplicity is a must. Moreover, another Coop requirement about the model is twofold: on one side, they wish to be able to quickly modify it in order to satisfy market department requests, and on the other side, they wish to be able to quickly recalculate it on order to consider new trends.

The most natural candidate satisfying all the requirements listed above is classification by means of decision trees, for instance computed by the standard C4.5 algorithm (Quinlan, 1992) or its variants. In particular, decision trees allow to:

- obtain a simple-to-read model, suitable for interaction with the domain expert analyst;
- take as input both the history of sales (for instance in the form of monthly, quarterly and yearly aggregates) and the context descriptors, whatever their nature (numerical, categorical);
- provide as output a set of classes, representing the sales bands that are forecast by the model. Determining the optimal number and size of such bands is a problem that is also tackled in this work.

Multi-Class Classification with Ordinal Classes

In this scenario, from the market department point of view, the goal is to predict a meaningful interval of sales, not just a number. Sales, in fact, are influenced also by largely unpredictable factors, such as social events, weather, traffic, and so on, making precise numeric predictions not meaningful. Hence, we have decided to discretize the objective function (sales amount) into a set of classes.

This step is critical and needs a good *trade-off* among:

- low number of classes (useful for classification algorithms and also for easy model evaluation)
- significance of the predicted value compared to storage choices
- distribution as uniform as possible between classes.

The particular contribution of our approach was to work directly with multi-class ordinals classifiers. In addition, the measures generally used, accuracy and standard deviation, do not perfectly fit our problem. Therefore, a specific measure for classifiers with ordinal classes is defined.

An ordinal quantity differs from a nominal one because it exhibits an order among the different values it can assume. An ordinal attribute could be, for example, a temperature measure represented by the values Hot, Mild and Cool. It is clear that there is an order among those values: Hot > Mild > Cool. Standard classification algorithms map a set of attribute values to a categorical target value. These algorithms generally are unable to use ordering information during the classification process and treat an ordinal target class attribute like a nominal class. However, some information is lost when this is done, information that can potentially improve the predictive performance of a classifier.

Real circumstances frequently involve situations exhibiting an order among different categories represented by the class attribute. There are many statistical approaches to this problem, but they are generally based on specific distributional assumptions for the class values (Herbrich, Graepel, & Obermayer, 1999). In recent years different approaches for ordinal classification were proposed using different approaches: decision trees (Potharst & Bioch, 2000; Frank & Hall, 2001), regression (Herbrich, Graepel, & Obermayer, 1999; Lin & Li, 2007; Rennie & Srebro, 2005), regression trees (Kramer et al., 2001), boosting (Freund, 2003), decision rules (Dembczyński, Kotłowski, & Słowiński, 2007). In each of these cases, the proposed algorithms or methodologies improve ordinary results by a marginal-to-moderate amount, usually not greater than a 5% gain in accuracy. Moreover, this is obtained through implementation costs and loss in flexibility or comprehension of results. In our applicative experience this kind of improvement is not critical – nor very significant – for the end user. Therefore, in this work we choose to use well know algorithm C4.5 (Quinlan, 1992), and define new measures of accuracy for evaluating the output models.

Out of Stock

The stock-out problem has been investigated in the area of Inventory Management for over 30 years and several models have been presented W. Hopp and M. Spearman, Factory Physics (International edition), McGraw Hill (2000) and (Hopp, 2000). On the other hand, the problem is mainly discussed in the marketing literature from the consumer reaction perspective (Campo, 2000) and (Emmelhainz, 1991). The focus of our investigation is the automatic detection of OOS events using rules approaches. For the best of our knowledge, the only paper we can compare with is (Papakiriakopoulos, 2009).

The most important difference is that our approach is completely automatic: in fact we define a model of the OOS event only using data of sales. Moreover we extract data from the data warehouse: these results in a quick and efficient process that can lead to refine experiments at low time and resource costs. The data results of the two analyses cannot be compared: their data consider all the possible goods existing in the stores, instead our data are focused only to promotional items.

DATA MINING ON PROMOTIONAL SALES

Data Exploration

The analysis focused on promotional sales of stores using only promotions on food products. A first distribution analysis of volumes sales, through a discretization in 25 equidistant (i.e., equal-size) bins, exhibits the following behavior: 20.53% of the promotions in a single store sold between 0 and 24 items, the 12.89% sold between 25 and 49 items, and so on. The distribution shows a large number of promotions with a low volume of sales: in fact over 50% of the promoted products sold less than 125 pieces. This is an entirely unexpected result since these sales are calculated over a period of sales promotion for 15 days and for a large store.

A deeper analysis shows that there are many products with zero sales. Regardless of the possible reasons (incomplete population of the database, promotions never started in some store), for the purposes of our analysis it was decided to disregard promotions with less than 5 pieces sold. These promotions have been eliminated from the tables, obtaining the distribution in Figure 1.

The classification models were built as ad hoc models for each store: this solution requires to develop more models, nevertheless it produces closer previsions of actual sales for each store that is the real interest of Coop.

Figure 1. Sales volume distribution of promotions with at least 5 items sold

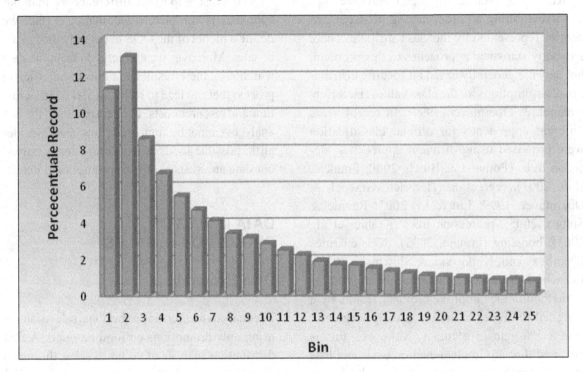

Figure 2. Structure of relevant portion of the data warehouse

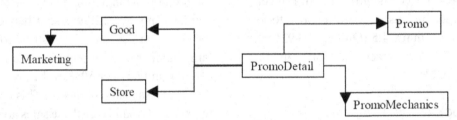

Data Preprocessing Issues

The starting point for this work was the use of a corporate data warehouse: among the several tables available, the most interesting for our purpose was the sales data table, characterized by a very large number of lines (926,774,117), since each line of each cash receipt is a record. The tables interest are 6 and are structured as in Figure 2.

The selected information include the promotions, their type (or mechanics) and details, the goods involved, their position in the product clas-

sification taxonomy and, finally, the stores where promotions are performed.

Mining Table

Creating the *mining table,* i.e., the table that collects the information used in the model mining phase needs to define the level of detail of the individual records and then determine the appropriate data aggregation. We have evaluated different strategies: the final choice was for one row for each promo detail. A promo detail identifies an item that belongs to a promotion in a store.

Table 1. Derived attributes and their description

Field name	Description
Sold_Art_3_1	Sales of the article from 3 months to 1 month before the promotion
Sold_Seg_3_1	Sales of the segment from 3 months to 1 month before the promotion
Sold_Art_1_0	Sales of the article in the last month before the promotion
Sold_Seg_1_0	Sales of the segment in the last month before the promotion
Days_Promotion	Duration of the promotion in days

In this way we can get a detailed response to the promotion for every article in all the different shops where the same promotion was active.

We used data sales of 16 months in 134 stores (522,541,764 records). The data were aggregated into 4 time slots, collecting total sales information of an item for each store in a single row of the table. The use of aggregation creates a mining table of 240,059 rows. The fields of the table are the union of the fields present in the 6 separate tables shown in Figure 1, for a total of 62 fields, with the addition of 5 calculated fields that are described in Table 1.

These attributes are meant to capture the recent variations in sales from two different prospective: the singe good under promotion and the all segment it belongs to. The latter, in particular, allows taking in consideration possible sales fluctuations that involve the all market segment. Moreover, the history of sales is divided in two time slot, in order to detect general trends. The target variables used to train the models are: (1) the sales amount of the promoted item and (2) the number of *OOS* that occurred during the promotion.

Discretization

The target variable is continuous and to be able to use many classification algorithms it is necessary a discretization. Moreover, it is strongly skewed to low values and the distribution of sales volume is very sparse: the values range between 0 and 105,650, yet 80% of promotions sold less than 500 items.

Table 2. Sample discretization with equal-size bins

Bin width	Resulting no. of classes	Population within first 3 classes
10	965	18,38%
25	572	32,63%
50	382	47,28%
100	249	64,28%

A first attempt to discretize the target variable has been an equal-size binning produces too many classes. Even increasing the size of the bin, the number of classes remains large (unless we adopt extremely large intervals) and data are heavily unbalanced: this leads to a decrease of prediction accuracy. What follows are some examples of discretization (See Table 2).

Classification algorithms are unable to generate high accuracy models over such a great number of classes. As alternative, we tried to performed an equal-frequency binning, but with not satisfactory result. For instance, using 20 bins the result is not particularly significant: first, it is non interesting for market analysis to know whether a product will sell between 6 and 14 items or between 14 and 23, and it is an extremely useless knowledge to know that it will sell more than 1600 items.

We manually refined the discretization trying to satisfy the following issue:

- Low number of classes (maximum 20)

Figure 3. Discretization through equal-frequency binning (top) and its manual refinement (bottom)

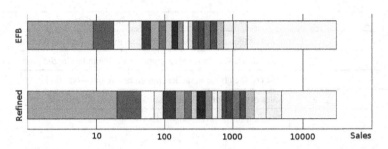

- Significance of the predicted value with respect to subsequent storage choices
- Uniform distribution among classes

The chosen discretization, which will be used for the forecast model construction, is shown in Figure 3 compared to the result of an equal-frequency binning.

The each bar represents the whole dataset, divided into 20 bins. The horizontal axis is in logarithmic scale, for better emphasizing lower value bins. As we can see, the refined discretization "moves" the bins towards higher values, thus providing a more detailed division for middle-high sales values. The same refined discretization is shown in Figure 4 as a bar plot.

Predicting the Percentage Variation of Sales

In this work, we developed two separate models that differ on the variable to predict: *intervals in volume sales*, which used the discretization previously defined; and *response to the promotion*, which provides the change percentage in sales with respect to the previous time period. In both cases we are dealing with the creation of multi-class classifiers with ordinal classes. Both the classifiers generated, respectively aimed to predict the sales volume and its percentage variation w.r.t. recent past, have their pros and cons.

In the first case, it is easy to find a satisfactory granularity of the classification classes, but, on the other hand, the resulting classes are strongly unbalanced. In the second case, the opposite happens, yielding balanced classes that, however, might gather largely different absolute values. Anyway a comparison of the two models was performed, aimed to measure the level of coherence of their predictions. The results could be summarized as follow: almost half the records yield coherent results (i.e., they show a null distance, so they make the same prevision), and moreover the distance distribution decreases very quickly (percentage is under 5% from class distance equal to 5 forward), showing that the two classifiers are strongly coherent. For this reason, we only refer of the second of the two approaches.

In order to cope with the unbalancing of the sales data, we defined a new target function, aimed to forecast the percentage variation of sales during the promotion w.r.t. sales in the 15 days that preceded the promotion. This variation is able to effectively express the real response of customers to the promotions.

A first rough summary of the distribution of sales variation during promotions – promotions where the promoted article was not sold at all during the preceding 15 days were not considered in the analysis – shows a largely significant increase during promotions: for 91% of goods the percentage variation of sales under promotion is larger than 20%. Further explorations of the data led to the definition of a set of percentage variation intervals that reaches a trade-off among the following common properties:

Figure 4. Distribution of sales volume discretized in 20 bins – refined discretization

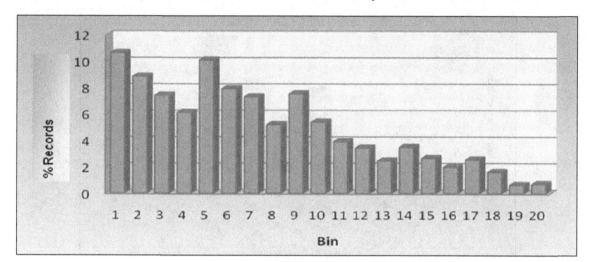

Table 3.Classes for percentage variations of sales

Class	Contents and interpretation
1	Drop of sales (sales variation ≤ -20/%)
2	No variations (variation between +20% and -20%)
3	Small increase 1 (variation between + 20% and +100%)
4	Small increase 2 (variation between +100% and 200%)
5	Small increase 3 (variation between +200% and 300%)
6	Large increase 1 (variation between +300% and 500%)
7	Large increase 2 (variation between +500% and 1000%)
8	Large increase 3 (variation between +1000% and 1500%)
9	Extreme increase 1 (variation between +1500% and 2500%)
10	Extreme increase 2 (variation ≥ 2500%)

- yield a precise information about the sales volume of each article, by means of small intervals;
- adopt a small number of classes, in order to ease the task of classification algorithms and to make the resulting predictive models easier to evaluate and to understand;
- obtain a class distribution as even as possible.

The discretized classes adopted in the successive model extraction phases were the result of both data inspection, consideration of the algorithms to be used, and the indications and practical requirements of the domain experts. The result consists of ten intervals of percentage sales variations, indicated in the Table 3.

Using the classes defined above, the distribution is the one in Figure 5.

The figure shows peaks on classes 7 and 10, thus indicating that several promotions lead to a large or extreme increase of sales. A representative insight is depicted in the following graph (Figure 6), that represents the percentage coverage of the

Figure 5. Distribution of promotions along the percentage variation classes defined in Table 3

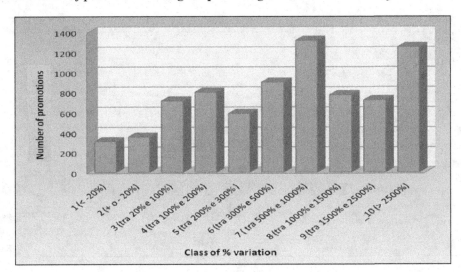

Figure 6. Sector distribution with classes of sales variations

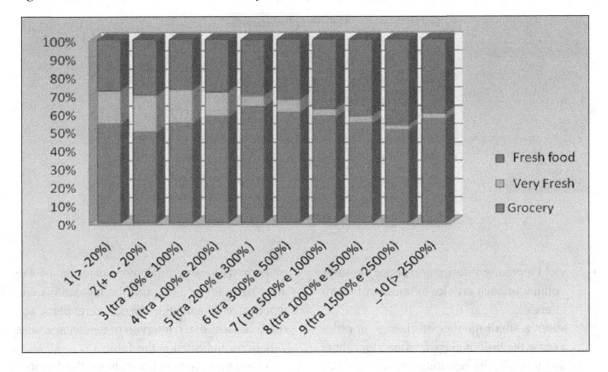

variation classes by the three sectors of the food category.

This graph highlights some interesting facts. For instance, we can infer that promotions for the *very fresh* sector (highly perishable products) have a relatively low response, since they are mostly concentrated over the first 4 classes, where the sales show only a small increase or even a drop. An opposite behaviour is that of the *fresh* sector (fresh products), whose promotions tend to fall in higher classes, in some cases reaching the same

Figure 7. Distribution of class prediction error

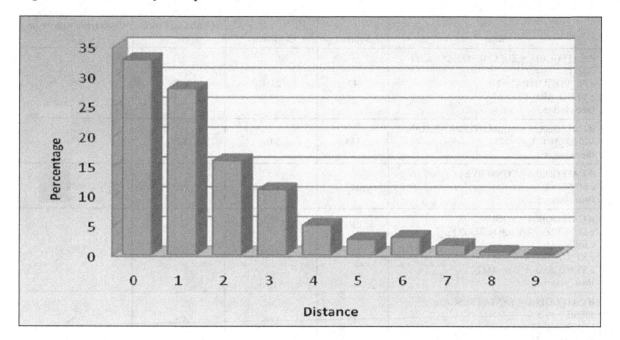

coverage of the (larger, in terms of promotions) *grocery* sector – e.g., in class 9.

Following a standard procedure, the input dataset was randomly partitioned into a *training set*, containing the 70% of available promotions, and a *test set*, containing the remaining 30%. The records of the former are used to build the classifier, while the records of the latter are exclusively used to validate the classifier.

The classification model was extracted by means of C4.5, a standard decision tree construction algorithm, applied with several different parameter settings, including various pruning strengths, minimum number of records that fall in each leaf of the tree, usage of boosting techniques, etc. The best performing model, which is described in the following, had moderate settings: a small pruning factor (45) and a small minimum population for each leaf (3). The output model was produced without any kind of boosting, in the form of classification rules.

Accuracy reaches the 49.99% on the training set and 32.67% on the test set. Such apparently low percentages are much larger than what a purely

random classifier can achieve, due to the relatively high number of classes (10). The confusion matrix has a strongly diagonal structure that attests the good quality of the output model. Anticipating the more exhaustive discussion provided in Section 5, a useful summary of the confusion matrix is given in Figure 7, where the corresponding distribution of class prediction errors (i.e., the distances between predicted and actual classes) is plotted. As we can see, the distribution quickly drops after the first values, and indeed, ca. 76% of the records falls in the first three groups, i.e., 76% of predictions have error equal to or smaller than 2.

Classification Rules

Inspecting the rules that constitute the classification model obtained above, we can highlight some behaviour generally common to all shops. In particular, in Table 4 we provide a sample of such rules, also characterized by:

- support – number of cases where the rule applied

Table 4. Classification rules with support and confidence, including limited tolerance to errors

Rule	Support	Confidence	Confidence with error ≤ 1	Confidence with error ≤ 2
if CATEGORIA = ZUCCHERO E DOLCIFICANTI e FL_VOLANTINO = No e VEND_ART_1_0 > 37 **then** class = 2	47	23%	82%	93%
if CATEGORIA = 'ALIMENTI INFANZIA' e VEND_ART_1_0 > 275 **then** class = 3	138	50%	82%	97%
if CATEGORIA = CONSERVE DI FRUTTA e MESE = 8 **then** class = 5	113	24%	65%	86%
if CATEGORIA = YOGURT e DESCRIZ. = TAGLIO PREZZO e MESE = 9 e VEND_ART_1_0 > 54 e VEND_SEG_1_0 <= 4487 **then** class = 6	110	35%	65%	82%
if CATEGORIA = 'PASTA FRESCA' e MESE = 10 e VEND_ART_1_0 > 51 **then** class = 7	42	38%	57%	78%
if FL_COOP = Si e CATEGORIA = BISCOTTI e FL_VOLANTINO = Si e VEND_ART_1_0 <= 275 **then** class = 8	52	25%	61%	78%

- confidence – accuracy of the rule

Beside the basic confidence of rules, Table 4 reports the confidence values we obtain when a prediction error not larger than 1 (column 4) or 2 (column 5) is tolerated. In general, we can see that such small error tolerance increases the confidence considerably. Some of the rules above (which make use of the original names, in Italian) can be explained as follows:

- Rule 1: if more than 37 articles were sold in the last month before the promotion (vent_art_1_0 > 37) in the category "sugar" (categoria = zucchero e dolcificanti), and the promotion was not advertised in the advertising leaflets, the promoted item will sell the same or just a slightly higher amount than before the promotion (class = 2).

- Rule 2: similar to Rule 1, but for food for children and with an higher threshold (275) and a slightly higher gain in sales (class = 3).

- Rule 6: biscuits of the Coop brand that sold less than 25 pieces in the last month before the promotion and that was advertised in the leaflets will dramatically increase their sales (class = 8, corresponding to a gain up to 1500%).

EVALUATION OF MULTI-CLASS CLASSIFIERS

Problem Definition

Evaluating the quality of the classifiers generated so far by means of a synthetic measure is a challenging problem. Indeed, most of them are defined over several *ordinal* classes, that is to say there is a natural order between classes, that should be considered in evaluating predictions. That is a direct consequence of the fact that such classes were obtain through discretization of a continuous variable.

Accuracy, the most commonly used quality measure in model evaluation, only considers perfect matches between predicted and actual classes, counting all other cases simply as generic *misclassification errors*. On the contrary, our context suggests that the distance between the predicted class and the actual one should be part of the evaluation function, thus considering trade-offs between perfect matches and perfect mismatches. In the literature on classification models validation, there is a substantial lack of quality measures that solve these problems. Therefore, in the following we discuss some approaches that provide more precise evaluations of the quality of multi-class models with ordinal classes.

Distance from the Diagonal

The basic step, already mentioned in the previous sections, consists in computing the distance between the predicted class and the actual class of each promotion in the dataset. Then, we plot the distribution of these values, which provides the means for easily checking the *diagonality* of the confusion matrix, and therefore to obtain a first qualitative assessment of the model under analysis.

Example 1

In Figure 8 three sample distributions are plotted, corresponding to three fictitious classification models. In the following we present an analysis of how these distributions can help to infer the quality of the corresponding classifiers.

With classifier (a) a large number of records falls in the first categories, corresponding to low distance values, and the distribution quickly drops

for larger distances. That means that most records are correctly or quasi-correctly classified, and only a small number of them is associated to classes that are very different from the correct one. Therefore, (a) appears to be a good classifier.

Classifier (b) was built in such a way that its value for the traditional accuracy measure is the same as classifier (a). Indeed, leftmost bar on both the plots, corresponding to perfectly classified elements, show the same length. However, it is clear that classifier (a) should be preferred to (b), since the latter has an almost uniform error distribution for errors greater than zero, meaning that small and large errors are equally probable.

Finally, classifier (c) presents the same problems of (b) and, moreover, the peak on the zero-error bar is missing, meaning that the classifier does not guarantee a good accuracy (in the standard sense) or a good percentage of quasi-correct classifications. This is a clear case of bad classifier.

Quantitative Measures

In order to provide an objective means for evaluating models or for comparing two of them, a quantitative measure should be defined that revises the traditional notion of accuracy. This measure had to take into consideration the overall class errors distribution. In this section we provide two improvements of the standard definition of accuracy, that essentially compute an aggregate count of errors of the model, weighted on the basis of the gravity of each error.

Weights Vector-Based Approach

In this approach, we assume the user provides a vector *weights* of N positive (possibly null) values, where N is the number of classes in the classification problem, and such that each value *weights[i]* ($i=0,...,N-1$) represents the weight associated to the errors of size i. For instance, *weights[3]* represents the weight associated to er-

Figure 8. Distribution of class error for three sample classifiers

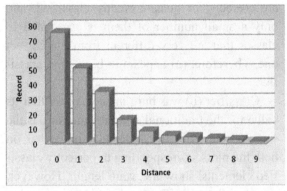

8a. A good classifier

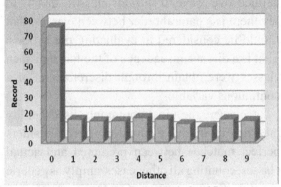

8b. A not so good classifier

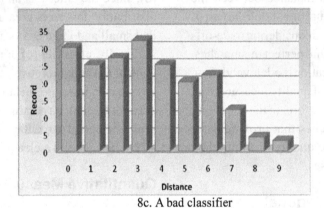

8c. A bad classifier

rors where the predicted class has a displacement of 3 classes w.r.t. the correct one, whichever is the direction of the displacement. Then, a vector *freq* of *N* elements is computed, each value *freq[i]* (*i=0,..., N-1*) representing the number of promotions whose predicted class has distance *i* from the correct class. Then, we define the *vector-based accuracy* of the model as follows:

$$Accuracy^{vector} = \frac{\sum_{i=1}^{N} \left(freq[i] \cdot weights[i] \right)}{\sum_{i=1}^{N} freq[i]}$$

In principle, the values of *weights* should fall in the range *[0,1]*, in order to preserve the statistical meaning of accuracy, however, small negative values might be used to *penalize* some particular

errors. Table 5 reports three examples of weight vectors, each putting a different emphasis to the different types of errors.

In *Weights 1*, only the records that are correctly classified are considered (distance zero). In this case *Accuracy^vector = Accuracy*, since the computed aggregate has the same value as the traditional accuracy. *Weights 2* consider as partially correct also the records that are classified *close* to the correct class. While a perfect prediction has weight 1, quasi-correct ones have a smaller one. *Weights 3* differs from the previous one because negative weights are associated to predictions that are very distant from the correct class. That strongly penalizes large errors.

The effects of these three different weight settings are reported in Table 6.

Table 5. Three sample weight vectors over 10 classes

Distance	Weights 1	Weights 2	Weights 3
0	1	1	1
1	0	0,7	0,7
2	0	0,5	0,5
3	0	0,2	0,2
4	0	0	0
5	0	0	0
6	0	0	0
7	0	0	-0,2
8	0	0	-0,3
9	0	0	-0,5

Table 6. Vector-based accuracy over distributions of Figure 8 and with weights of Table 7

	Distribution (a)	Distribution (b)	Distribution (c)
Weights 1	37,5%	37,5%	15,0%
Weights 2	65,7%	47,6%	33,7%
Weights 3	64,8%	40,9%	31,1%

The values obtained are coherent with the qualitative results discussed above:

- classifier (c) has a value of *Accuracy^vector* smaller than classifiers (a) and (b), independently of the weights adopted;
- classifiers (a) and (b) have the same value of standard accuracy (equal to *Accuracy^vector* computed with *Weights 1*) yet they differ significantly on the new accuracy measure. In particular, classifier (a) performs better and classifier (b), especially with *Weights 3,* which penalizes the significant amount of large errors yielded by classifier (b).

Limits of the Vector-Based Approach

The simplicity of the vector-based model causes a few drawbacks that might limit its usefulness in some contexts:

- *there is no distinction between approximations by excess and by defect.* In some contexts it can be useful to stress the importance of one error against the other. For instance, in the case of stocking of articles, it might be convenient to prefer overestimates that correspond to the risk of having

stock on hand after the end of a promotion, against underestimates, that would correspond to the risk of getting OOS during the promotion.

- *the weight of an error does not directly depend on the actual class to be predicted.* Indeed, only the distance between the predicted class and the actual one is considered. In some cases, it might be useful to discriminate also w.r.t. the actual class. For instances, when the classes (as in our classification approach) are obtained through a discretization process that can yield discretization intervals of highly variable width, the gravity of an error could be dependant on such interval width, penalizing errors performed around larger bins.

Empirical experimentation on the field tells us that *Accuracy^vector* yields a precise evaluation of the model quality in most practical cases. However, when the above mentioned limitations play a too strong role to be neglected, a generalization of the approach can be followed, which will be described later in this section.

Vector-Based Accuracy of the Generated Models

Following the procedure described above, we choose vectors of weights, in order to decide how important should be each classification mistake. In our experiments, we selected two vectors, shown in Table 7, that mainly differ on the severity of

Table 7. Weights for vector-based accuracy of the percentage variation model

Distance	Weights 1	Weights 2
0	1	1
1	0,8	0,8
2	0,5	0,5
3	0,3	0,3
4	0	0
5	0	0
6	0	-0,5
7	0	-0,8
8	0	-1
9	0	-1

Table 8. Accuracies for the percentage variation model, using weights in Table 7

Traditional accuracy	Vector-based accuracy Weights 1	Vector-based accuracy Weights 2
32,70%	66,10%	62,60%

penalties for errors of large extent. Both vectors assign an almost linearly decreasing weight to errors from zero to 3. However, while in the first vector all other cases have a null weight, in the second one larger errors receive further penalties.

Both vector-based accuracies are relatively high, therefore attesting the good quality of the model extracted. We can observe that the second measure, that penalizes large errors, yields a drop w.r.t. the first one, meaning stressing more importance of errors of large extent. Anyway, the performances are *stable*. Indeed, the accuracy over *Weights 2* is very close to the one obtained over *Weights 1*, meaning that there were not many large errors to be penalized, and therefore the predicted classes are generally close to the true ones.

The corresponding vector-based accuracies are shown in Table 8, together with the value of traditional accuracy.

Matrix Vector-Based Approach

This solution is a generalization of the vector-based accuracy that starts directly from the confusion matrix of a model and takes into consideration each single error type. In particular, a *NxN* matrix of weights, *mat_weights*, is provided by the user,

such that each *mat_weights[i,j]* represents the weight associated with the cases (promotions, in our context) where the true class was *i* and the predicted class is *j*. The definition of the new accuracy is then computed by combining such matrix of weights with the confusion matrix (*mat_confusion*):

$$Accuracy^{matrix} = \frac{\sum_{i=1}^{N}\sum_{i=1}^{N}\left(mat\_confusion[i,j] \cdot mat\_weights[i,j]\right)}{\sum_{i=1}^{N}\sum_{i=1}^{N} mat\_confusion[i,j]}$$

Example 2

Table 9 shows a sample confusion matrix that generated the first distribution discussed in Example 1.

As we can see, the matrix has a predominance of values along the diagonal, and moreover there is a higher density right below the diagonal, meaning that the model tends to predict values lower than the real ones. We apply the approach with two, slightly different matrices of weights, shown respectively in Table 10 and in Table 11.

The first matrix penalizes more the errors of larger extent, since the weights decrease as the distance from the main diagonal increases. Moreover, the extreme cells of the matrix (lower left and upper right corners) contain negative values, since these cases of very large errors highly degrade the usability of a predictive model. The second matrix presents a similar structure, but the records below the main diagonal are given stronger penalties, meaning that overestimates of the predicted class are preferred to underestimates. In the context of sales forecasting for stocking

Table 9. Sample confusion matrix

	\multicolumn{10}{c}{Predicted class}									
	1	**2**	**3**	**4**	**5**	**6**	**7**	**8**	**9**	**10**
1	15	6	3	3	2	2	1	1	0	0
2	8	14	4	3	1	1	0	0	1	0
3	7	9	15	5	4	1	2	1	0	0
4	3	4	6	16	3	4	2	3	2	2
5	2	4	4	9	15	4	3	2	2	1
6	4	3	2	5	8	19	3	4	0	1
7	3	0	2	2	3	7	15	4	2	2
8	1	0	4	3	3	5	8	18	2	1
9	0	0	1	2	2	3	6	4	9	4
10	1	0	1	0	1	2	3	7	6	14

purposes, that corresponds to prefer avoiding OOS situations that might compromise the effectiveness of a promotion.

The matrix-based accuracy values corresponding to the two weight matrices presented above are summarized in Table 12. The results show that the second set of weights introduces a loss of accuracy, due to the fact that the classification model analyzed, as mentioned above, tends to predict values lower than the actual classes, which are particularly penalized by the weight matrix.

Table 10. Matrix of weights 1

	\multicolumn{10}{c}{Predicted Class}									
	1	**2**	**3**	**4**	**5**	**6**	**7**	**8**	**9**	**10**
1	1,00	0,85	0,70	0,50	0,40	0,00	0,00	-0,50	-0,75	-1,00
2	0,85	1,00	0,85	0,70	0,50	0,30	0,00	0,00	-0,50	-0,75
3	0,70	0,85	1,00	0,80	0,65	0,40	0,20	0,00	0,00	-0,50
4	0,50	0,70	0,80	1,00	0,80	0,65	0,30	0,10	0,00	0,00
5	0,40	0,50	0,65	0,80	1,00	0,80	0,65	0,20	0,00	0,00
6	0,00	0,30	0,40	0,65	0,80	1,00	0,75	0,60	0,20	0,00
7	0,00	0,00	0,20	0,30	0,65	0,75	1,00	0,75	0,60	0,15
8	-0,50	0,00	0,00	0,10	0,20	0,60	0,75	1,00	0,70	0,55
9	-0,75	-0,50	0,00	0,00	0,00	0,20	0,60	0,70	1,00	0,70
10	-1,00	-0,75	-0,50	0,00	0,00	0,00	0,15	0,55	0,70	1,00

Table 11. Matrix of weights 2

	\multicolumn{10}{c}{Predicted Class}									
	1	**2**	**3**	**4**	**5**	**6**	**7**	**8**	**9**	**10**
1	1,00	0,85	0,70	0,50	0,40	0,00	0,00	-0,50	-0,75	-1,00
2	0,75	1,00	0,85	0,70	0,50	0,30	0,00	0,00	-0,50	-0,75
3	0,60	0,75	1,00	0,80	0,65	0,40	0,20	0,00	0,00	-0,50
4	0,40	0,60	0,70	1,00	0,80	0,65	0,30	0,10	0,00	0,00
5	0,40	0,40	0,55	0,70	1,00	0,80	0,65	0,20	0,00	0,00
6	0,00	0,20	0,30	0,55	0,70	1,00	0,75	0,60	0,20	0,00
7	0,00	0,00	0,10	0,20	0,55	0,65	1,00	0,75	0,60	0,15
8	-0,50	0,00	0,00	0,00	0,10	0,50	0,65	1,00	0,70	0,55
9	-0,75	-0,50	0,00	0,00	0,00	0,10	0,50	0,60	1,00	0,70
10	-1,00	-0,75	-0,50	0,00	0,00	0,00	0,05	0,45	0,60	1,00

Table 12. Accuracies for the sales prediction model, using weights in Table 10 and Table 11

Traditional accuracy	Matrix-based accuracy Weights 1	Matrix-based accuracy Weights 2
37,50%	70,38%	66,50%

Table 13. Out of stock scenario

Morning	Lunch	Afternoon	Evening
40	30	2	1

DATA MINING FOR 'OUT OF STOCK' EVENT

Every time the number of items available in a shop is less than its customer request, an OOS event occurs. A consequence is that the good is not on shelf. Each OOS is an income failure and sometimes it could be for significant amount. More, this could be a source of customer discontent that could lead to the shop abandonment.

This event is often connected to promotional occurrence and could be derived from different causes. Most frequent cause is a wrong esteem of future sells that have, as consequence, a lower stoking number of items with respect to customer needs. Others causes could be a delay delivery from general warehouse to the shop or could be a delay delivery from the local warehouse to the shelves. For these reasons is it possible to define two different OOS typology: warehouse level or shop level. In the first case the warehouse can not delivery items to the shop during the promotion days. This case could be treated only using stock data and is not possible in our scenario. In the second case, the shop is not furnished during a single day and OOS could be happen. It is also possible to have more than one OOS during promotions period. This second scenario could be treated starting from sell data and it is the analysis we propose. A model ad hoc is required.

Out of Stock Model Definition

The model was made trying to capture all possible scenarios in which OOS could occur. We model this phenomenon at the shop granularity using a division of a single day into four time slots: morning, lunch, afternoon and evening.

The model, at first approximation, is directed towards the detection of abrupt declines in sales between two contiguous time slots. The percentage change between contiguous time slots is analyzed and if this change exceeds a fixed threshold (default -90%) we assume an OOS event took place (Condition 1). In the sample table an OOS occurs between *Lunch* and *Afternoon*.

Considering only the percentage changes between the time slots, however, this first formulation of the model does not capture two possible anomalies: the resumption of sales and the existence of products with very low sales.

(Condition 2) If there is a sharp fall in sales in a intermediate slot (such as in condition 1), but then the sales increase, it is clear that this is not an OOS event. To take in account this aspect, we need to verify that the sales at the time slot right after the fall stops below a threshold, in other words there is not a significant upturn in sales. In order to provide greater flexibility, this threshold value is calculated dynamically using the following formula:

Table 14. Scenario with gradually decreasing sales

Morning	Lunch	Afternoon	Evening
25	4	0	0

$$OutOfStock^{threshold} = \min\left(\max\left(2, criticalValue\right), 10\right)$$

The *critical value* is the sales value that caused the OOS.

(Condition 3) The model with only the percentage changes (condition 1) recognizes an OOS if a product sells 1 unit in all time slots except one in which it sells 0 (there is a percentage change of -100%). This is clearly a product that has very low sales and therefore not a case of rupture of stock. To properly handle such situations we introduce a new threshold that determines the minimum number of units sold which must precede an OOS (Default value is 5).

(Condition 4) Condition 3 could mask some cases. In the scenario of Table 14 there is a strong decrease percentage between lunch and afternoon which satisfies the condition 1, but would not be regarded as OOS as it has not checked the condition 3. In these cases the percentage decline is gradual and involves several time slots. To consider this case, too, a second threshold of percentage variation is introduced in the model and it is set to a lower value with respect of Condition 1 (default -70%).

Now, in case there is a high percentage change that checks the condition 1 but not condition 3, the lowest threshold it is used, to identify decline in sales spanning several time slots. Choices and parameters for the thresholds were validated by a Coop marketing manager.

Model Construction

Data Analysis of food sector in the *super* stores produces the following distribution for the number of OOS events calculated as previously defined (See Figure 9).

The OOS event occurs in 44% of cases. Moreover, for half of these cases it happens more than once. Whereas a promotion extends during 15 days and since the OOS is a daily event, these numbers are surprising. Because of the strong unbalance of the distribution, it is not difficult to build a classifier using the number of OOS in the promotion as objective function. Also in this case, it is necessary to use a discretization to allow the classifier to achieve good results. Two possible discretizations of the variable representing the number of OOSs are possible: (1) in three classes (zero vs. one vs. more than one) or (2) in two classes (zero vs. at least one). The class distribution for both cases is provided in Figure 10.

The first solution choice is certainly more convenient for the significance of the forecast: we have three different values that identify the degree of risk of OOS event. The second solution, on the other hand, has a more balanced distribution (56% - 44%) and therefore it is more suitable for classification.

Both as regards the division of records between training set and test set, both for the choice of predictors used, the same considerations outlined in the previous chapter in connection with the construction of models for forecasting sales volumes are applied. The main parameters chosen for the construction of this model are similar to those used for sales forecast: pruning severity = 45, min. number of cases per leaf = 3, no boosting, and output model in form of rules. The accuracy on the training set is found to be 75.14% and on the test set of 72.61%.

Figure 9. Distribution of out of stocks in the Super stores

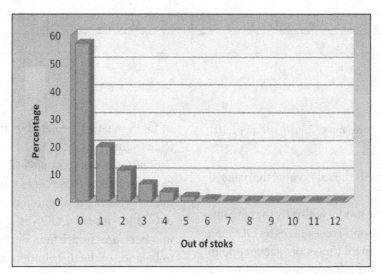

Figure 10. Discretization for out of stock events with three (left) and two classes (right)

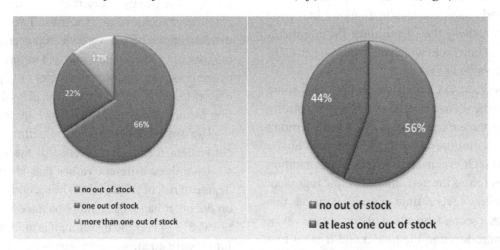

Generalizing the analysis of data for the food sector in the *hyper* stores, the distribution that results is very similar to the previous one. OOS are 65.9% and the number decreases with the same trend, even if more quickly. In this case too, the discretization was binary. The parameters used for the construction were the same as for the previous case, excepted for the pruning severity, set to 75 instead of 45. The accuracy found on the training set is 71.65% and on the test set of 67.58%. This accuracy decrease is an expected result, given the greater variety of goods and promotions taking place in *hypermarket* stores.

Creating the classifier as a set of association rules permits to verify the existence of some interesting phenomena. The following table shows some general rules that fit well, in which support and confidence values are calculated on all stores data.

- Rule 3 states that promotions involving food for children that were advertised in

Table 15. Classification rules for out of stock prediction

Rule	Support	Confidence
if PRES_MKT = LEADER **and** VendSeg_1_0 > 479 **and** CATEGORIA = CAFFE' **then** class = 1	560	86%
if FL_VOLANTINO = Si **and** CATEGORIA = ACQUE **and** VEND_SEG_1_0 <= 78583 **then** class = 1	219	58%
if FL_VOLANTINO = Si **and** CATEGORIA = ALIMENTI INFANZIA **and** VEND_ART_3_1 > 142 **and** VEND_ART_1_0 > 96 **then** class = 1	677	65%
if FL_VOLANTINO = Si **and** CATEGORIA = ALIMENTI PER GATTI **and** VEND_SEG_1_0 > 4369 **then** class = 1	121	76%
if MESE = 12 **and** FL_VOLANTINO = Si **then** class = 1	3671	64%
if MESE = 12 **and** CATEGORIA = GELATI **then** class = 0	379	95%
if RILEVANZA = IGIENE **and** CATEGORIA = ALIMENTI INFANZIA **and** VEND_ART_1_0 <= 45 **then** class = 0	1509	73%

the leaflets, such that the product sold more than 96 pieces in the last month and more than 142 in the last three months before the promotion, are likely to go OOS. We can notice that when the conditions of this rule are satisfied, also Rule 2 of Table 6 is, in which case we can expect that the sales prediction of the latter rule represents an underestimate of the real need of stocking for the promotion.

• Rule 1 states that promoted coffee of a leader brand that sold more than 479 pieces in the last month will most likely go OOS. Therefore, the estimates provided by the sales forecast models should generally be interpreted as underestimates.

• Rule 6 states that ice creams promoted during December almost never (95% of confidence) go OOS, which was expected since

the consumption and request of this kind of food is usually very limited during the winter season.

DEPLOYMENT AND FUTURE TRENDS

The project ends with a first deployment of the system for end users, generally marketing staff managers. The application offers them a dedicated area for forecast sales analysis and for consulting historic promotions trend.

Users can connect to a *prevision* web page, shown in Figure 11 through an example, in which they can query the system about a sales forecast. They can choose the good to promote, the store, starting date, the duration and the mechanics of the promotion, and then launch the prediction step

Figure 11. Prevision Web page

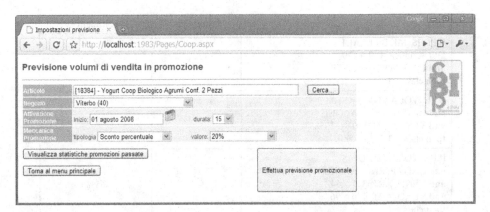

(bottom right button in Figure 11). The sample parameters in our example are the following:

- Good = yogurt [product id 18384]
- Store = Viterbo (near Rome) [id store 40]
- Starting date = 2008, August, 1st
- Duration of promotion = 15 days
- Promotion mechanics = 20% discount

At the end of the computation, results are shown in a trend of sales graph, as in Figure 12. The time period analyzed covers several months proceeding the promotion. Forecasting of sales is expressed in terms of number and percentage range change over the previous period. It gives also an estimate of possible OOS in the promotion time period.

The example output shows that the promoted yogurt will sell from 240 to 360 items (sales forecasting model), or it will increase its sell from 100% to 200% (percentage variation model). Moreover, the item results positive to OOS prevision. This additional information could lead to understand that the forecast is underestimated.

Users can also access a statistical trend page in which to choose a the store, a time period and a good. The output is the good sales trend per month (in blue in the Figure 13). Using the *compare* button a new trend is drawn (the red on the right side of the figure), representing the average sell of other goods in the same marketing segment.

In this way, marketing end users could browse the promotion data warehouse in a convenient analysis.

Evaluation and Future Trends

Although an exhaustive analysis of the economic impact of the proposed approach is difficult and requires ad hoc investigation, a rough estimation can be easily computed by exploiting Gruen's work (Gruen, 2002). The latter established that in a retail context, the direct loss caused by OOS attests around 4% of the potential sales of promoted articles. On the other hand, our predictive models estimate that around 50% of promotions result in an increase of sales to over 500% of the normal amount, i.e., the amount of sales obtained when the article is not under promotion. That means that our model can potentially avoid an economic loss estimated as: promotions evaluated x Percentage of sales loss = 50% x (500% x 4%) = 10% i.e., a correct stocking can help avoiding around 10% of loss due to OOS.

The methodological and empirical results obtained in this work provide the basis for several improvements and refinements of the approach adopted. Among them, we mention the following:

Figure 12. Web page – forecast prevision

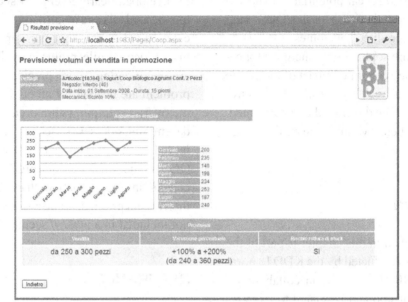

Figure 13. Web page – statistics (left) and comparison (right)

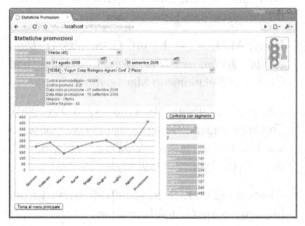 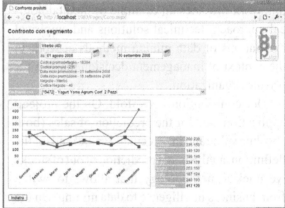

- The two models proposed, one for sales forecasting and the other for OOS prediction, might integrated, in order to obtain a more sophisticated sales forecasting model that does not suffer of under-estimation problems.
- The kind on analysis and models produced so far might be extended and adapted to the case of the articles that are not directly involved by promotions,

comparing the results with those obtained by Papakiriakopoulos (2009)
- Similarly, the behaviours of promoted and non-promoted articles might be analysed in a comparative way, and thus allowing to understand both effects and side effects of promotions.
- A deeper analysis might be performed for checking the predictive value of the variables that the models selected as important.

The goal is to reveal potential unexpected dependencies between sales/OOS and some "less credited" attributes.

- Finally, more sophisticated methods for estimating the economic impact of the whole approach, as well as empirical measurements, might be developed and performed, in order to better validate the methodology proposed.

CONCLUSION

The work described in this chapter is part of the BI-Coop project conducted by the KDD Laboratory at ISTI-CNR (Pisa, Italy) in collaboration with Unicoop Tirreno and is related to large retails. The goal was to analyze the trends in sales of articles offered for promotion to improve the quality of storage of such products. As such, this work provides an example of methodological approach, technical solutions and empirical evaluations of data mining methods at work in the context of management/decision making for private organization.

Our contribution is twofold. On the project/application side for the prediction of sales (both absolute value and in percentage value) and for the definition, analysis and prediction of out of stocks we track a methodology that allows to switch from business intelligence to data mining. On the research side, we defined a methodology for the qualitative and quantitative analysis of multi-class classifiers with ordinal classes. This seems to be essentially an open problem: literature does not explore convincing and consolidated solutions, although such cases are particularly frequent in the analysis of social phenomena, in which discretization of continuous values if often applied.

Despite the difficulty of the problem in terms of quantity and quality of data, excellent results were achieved both regarding the prevision of promotional sales, and the analysis of the OOS phenomenon. Beside positive results several lines

of developed clearly emerged. Especially concerning the analysis and quantitative evaluation of the economical impact that our approach can have in practice. While preliminary basic estimates are encouraging, more precise solutions to the problem are needed for an effective usability of the overall solution within organizations. On the data mining side, several technical issues emerged, including the integration of sales forecasting and OOS prediction in a unique predictive model, and considering the correlations that may exist between the various products in promotion and the others not included in a *what-if* scenario.

REFERENCES

Arsham, H. (1994). *Time-Critical Decision Making for Business Administration.* (Web site checked on February 2nd, 2009) http://home.ubalt.edu/ntsbarsh/stat-data/Forecast.htm

Berry, M. J. A., & Linoff, G. S. (2004). *Data Mining Techniques: For Marketing.* Sales, and Customer Relationship Management.

Campo, K., Gijsbrechts, E., & Nisol, P. (2000). Towards understanding consumer response to stock-outs. *Journal of Retailing, 76*(2), 65–78. doi:10.1016/S0022-4359(00)00026-9

Clementine, S. P. S. S. (2009). Retrieved from http://www.spss.com/clementine/

CRISP-DM. (2009). Retrieved from http://www.crisp-dm.org/

Dembczyński, K., Kotłowski, W., & Słowiński, R. (2007). Ordinal Classification with Decision Rules. *Mining Complex Data – ECML/PKDD Third International Workshop, MCD 2007*, Warsaw, Poland, September 17-21, *Revised Selected Papers* (LNCS 4944). Berlin: Springer.

Emmelhainz, M., Emmelhainz, L., & Stock, J. (1991). Consumer responses to retail Stock-outs. *Journal of Retailing, 67*(2), 32–49.

Frank, E., & Hall, M. (2001). A simple approach to ordinal classification. In *12th European Conference on Machine Learning,* Freiburg, Germany, September 5–7, (LNCS 2167). Berlin: Springer.

Freund, Y., Iyer, R., Schapire, R., & Singer, Y. (2003). An efficient boosting algorithm for combining preferences. *Journal of Machine Learning Research, 4,* 933–969. doi:10.1162/jmlr.2003.4.6.933

Gruen, T. W., Corsten, D., & Bharadwaj, S. (2002). *Retail Out-of-Stocks: A Worldwide Examination of Causes, Rates, and Consumer Responses.* Washington, DC: Grocery Manufacturers of America.

Herbrich, R., Graepel, T., & Obermayer, K. (1999). *Regression models for ordinal data: A machine learning approach. Technical Report.* Germany: TU Berlin.

Hopp, W., & Spearman, M. (2000). *Factory Physics* (International edition). New York: McGraw Hill.

Kramer, S., Widmer, G., Pfahringer, B., & De-Groeve, M. (2001). *Prediction of ordinal classes using regression trees.* Fundamenta Informaticae.

Larose, D. T. (2006). *Discovering Knowledge in Data: An Introduction to Data Mining.* New York: Wiley.

Lin, H. T., & Li, L. (2007). Ordinal regression by extended binary classifications. *Advances in Neural Information Processing Systems, 19,* 865–872.

Ohsawa, Y., & Yada, K. (2009). *Data Mining for Design and Marketing.* Boca Raton, FL: Chapman & Hall/Crc Data Mining and Knowledge Discovery.

Oracle Sql Developer. (2009). Retrieved from Web site (checked on March 4, 2009): http://www.oracle.com/technology/products/database/sql_developer/index.html

Oracle Warehouse Builder. (2009). Retrieved from http://www.oracle.com/technology/products/warehouse/index.html

Papakiriakopoulos, D., Pramatari, K., & Doukidis, G. (2009). A decision support system for detecting products missing from the shelf based on heuristic rules. *Decision Support Systems, 46*(3), 685–694. doi:10.1016/j.dss.2008.11.004

Potharst, R., & Bioch, J. C. (2000). Decision trees for ordinal classification. *Intelligent Data Analysis, 4*(2), 97–112.

Quinlan, J. R. (1992). *C4.5 Programs for Machine Learning.* San Francisco: Morgan Kaufmann.

Rennie, J., & Srebro, N. (2005). Loss functions for preference levels: Regression with discrete ordered labels. In *Proc. of the IJCAI Multidisciplinary Workshop on Advances in Preference Handling.*

Tan, P.-N., Steinbach, M., & Kumar, V. (2006). *Introduction to Data Mining.* Reading, MA: Addison-Wesley.

Taylor, F. W. (1911). *The Principles of Scientific Management.* New York: Harper. Digital version available on http://melbecon.unimelb.edu.au/het/taylor/sciman.htm (link checked on February 22nd, 2009).

KEY TERMS AND DEFINITIONS

Classification Model: Classification is a procedure in which individual items are placed into groups based on quantitative information on one or more characteristics inherent in the items (referred to as traits, variables, characters, etc) and based on a training set of previously labeled items.

Classification Rule: Classification Rule is a popular and well researched method for discovering interesting relations between variables in large databases.

Data Mining: Data mining is the process of extracting hidden patterns from data. Data mining identifies trends within data that go beyond simple data analysis, through the use of sophisticated algorithms.

Discretization: Discretization concerns the process of transferring continuous models and equations into discrete counterparts.

Multi-Class Classification: Multi-class Classification is a kind of Classification in which there are strictly more than two groups.

Out of Stock: Out of Stock is the event a store is found out of products to sell before the promotion is finished.

Sales Forecasting: Forecasting is the process of estimation in unknown situations. Sales Forecasting is used in the practice of Customer Demand Planning in everyday business forecasting for manufacturing companies.

Chapter 13
Preparing for New Competition in the Retail Industry

Goran Klepac
Raiffeisen Bank Austria, Croatia

ABSTRACT

A business case presents a retail company facing new competitors and consequently preparing a customer retention strategy. The business environment in which the company was operating prior to the arrival of new competitors can be described as a stable market. Bearing in mind the plans and marketing activities of a competitor retail chain and making use of the data mining methods a system is being devised for the purpose of preventing or at least buffering the churn trend. Development of an early warning indicator system based on data mining methods is also being described as a support to the management in early detection of both market opportunities and threats. Research in data mining could also be concentrated on applying existing data mining techniques to find the best solution regarding practical business problems in the public or private sector. Knowledge regarding how some business cases were solved using data mining techniques could contribute in a better understanding of the nature or data mining nature and help solve specific business issues.

INTRODUCTION

In a turbulent business environment with fierce competition, getting new customers on board and selling a product or a service is more than a challenge (Berry 1997, Berry 2000, Giudici 2003). Companies usually resort to intense campaigns, which along with campaign costs sometimes include price reduc-

tions below the current market prices and/or quality improvements Klepac (2006).

Once the sales goals have been achieved and marketing and product development costs covered, a new battle geared towards keeping existing users of products and services starts. Reasons for customer churn are diverse. They range from the unexpected moves of competitors trying to gain a bigger piece of market share by using swift campaigns (possibly directly endangering your company's market

DOI: 10.4018/978-1-60566-906-9.ch013

position) to unsatisfied clients suddenly starting to churn (Berry,2000). High initial costs of new products development as well as campaign expenses are seen as investments with the aim of gaining bigger market share. In some cases, the success can be measured by the time-span of usage of the advertised product by the customer, which eventually decreases the unit investment cost per product Berry (2000).

BACKGROUND

There are numerous case studies regarding how to recognise and reduce churn in retail business (Berry 2000, Berry 2003, Giudici 2003). Data mining methods which could be of use for this purpose could be logistic regression (Larose, 2005; Larose, 2006), survival models Berry (2003), Neural networks Alexander (1995), and self-organizing maps by Kohonen (2001).

If we review case studies for churn recognition (Berry 2000, Berry 2003, Giudici 2003, Namid 2004) there are numerous different solutions regarding business environment, market conditions, industry, dominant customer segments etc. Sometimes the source of data or data organization has an influence on the final data mining solution Agosta (2000). The business case presented in this chapter gives a potential solution of a business case related to wholesale and retail business in the situation where incoming competitors enter into a relatively peaceful market environment. In such a case, the following temporal market chapter provides a solution applied in practice which demonstrates good results after implementation.

How to Fight Competition

Trgovina is a wholesale and retail business, owning approximately thirty retail stores (supermarkets) across Croatia, as well as three wholesale stores whose main purpose is to provide goods to the retail stores, but also to

sell goods to other legal persons in the retail and wholesale business.

Trgovina deals in consumer goods and it owns a central transactional database (Oracle) system, integrating all stores. The main transactional data stored in the information system consist of data sets from each filled out invoice related to codes of goods sold (categorised in the system), quantities bought, time of issuing the invoice and all other legally relevant elements necessary for creating a turnover book. Two years ago, the aforementioned company started a loyalty cards program. Within the program, customers collected points and, having collected a certain number of points, they earned the right to buy products at discount prices and periodically they were awarded gifts depending on the number of points collected.

The customers were obliged to provide the following data into the loyalty card application form:

- Name and surname
- Full address
- Year of birth
- Family status (married or not)
- Number of children
- Education level
- Categorised hobbies (sport, arts, etc.).

As a response to one competitor's plans to increase the number of its retail stores in a substantial number of regions where Trgovina's retail stores are present, the company has to increase the loyalty of existing customers and acquire new ones with the tendency of keeping them even in conditions when competition starts operating in the neighbourhood of some of the existing Trgovina retail stores.

The company is well aware of the fact that the initial strategy of its competitors to acquire business in a certain region involves attracting as many customers as possible and ensuring their long-term loyalty. It is expected that, in order to achieve this goal, the competition will be willing to invest a certain amount of money, resulting in very low and competitive prices, other benefits and a strategy aimed at targeted market segments. Based on the previous analyses, Trgovina has segmented its market and performed an analysis of typical profiles and behaviour models for each market segment at the regional level.

Since the onset of fierce market competition is inevitable, during which the competition will try to acquire and keep as many customers of other retail stores as possible, it is necessary to devise a strategy for keeping as many existing customers in given circumstances. On the one hand, it is obvious that Trgovina will have certain costs related to accomplishing this goal. In all probability, a number of customers will defect to the competition. It is of vital importance to distinguish which customers will go to the competition, i.e. it is crucial that the resources spent in keeping the existing customers are invested to keep the most important customers. The competition probably counts on the attractiveness factor which, multiplied by curiosity, is certainly on their side. Regardless of the loyalty level, it is very probable that a great number of customers loyal to Trgovina will make a certain number of purchases in the competitors store, but the aim is to bring back as many customers as possible. This fact will probably significantly decrease Trgovina's income during the estimated maximum period of two months where competitors stake their ground in a new region. After the two months, a period of stabilisation is expected mostly due to the planned analysis.

An additional latent danger present in the described situation is the threat of potential long-term loss of customers; in this kind of a new market situation there is a continued danger of customer attrition. Such loss may be caused by well positioned competitors campaigns geared towards acquiring customers from the other retailers. On the other hand, the loss may be caused by the increase in the numbers of existing customers which are dissatisfied with service provided or the extreme differences in prices of some or most of the products offered on the shelves.

Due to this reason, it is necessary to develop a monitoring system primarily responsible for recording customer churn or stagnation of sales amount. Furthermore, it is necessary to make an estimated profile of a typical customer prone to buying Trgovina goods and to conduct the analysis prior to the opening of the competitors store as well as two months after the competitors store had been opened. With regard to the comparatively stable situation in the market over the last five years, the estimation of churn based on data from the previous period may be questionable, especially given that in most of the regions where Trgovina stores are located, no other large stores opened, with the exception of small shops which posed no competitive danger. In order to make a precise estimation of churn probability, it is possible to conduct classical market research on a sample of Trgovina's customers with the purpose of getting a clearer picture of possible churns after the opening of a competitor store.

GOALS OF THE ANALYSIS

The goals of the analysis have to be in line with the strategic goals. The main strategic goal is to retain existing customers, primarily the high quality ones. In accordance with this objective, certain activities will be planned with the purpose of motivating all customers (especially the highest quality customers) to increase their loyalty level and continue buying in the Trgovina store. A further strategic goal, observed from the defensive point of view, is to monitor the customers with the purpose of preventing long-term churn trends. These goals are common for data mining projects Dresner (2008), Berry (2000), Berry (1997), Faulkner (2003).

In accordance with the strategic goals, the first step of the analysis should encompass the evaluation of customers and their classification in a number of categories, in order to estimate the importance of customer to the company by segment. It was decided that only customers with loyalty cards will be included in the evaluation model, because they comprise 85% of all customers. Customers having no loyalty card are impossible to identify based on past transactions only.

The obtained results shall yield the customer structure classified on the basis of their importance for the company. Taking into account the results, the following steps will be considering further analytical procedures with the aim of increasing customer loyalty and monitoring the customers during the period of entry of competition into the region with the purpose of maintaining the market share. The monitoring should serve as a decision support system for the decision makers in conditions when the competition exercises a more aggressive market approach.

Since retail stores are dispersed throughout Croatia, the analyses shall encompass microsegments, i.e. the market shall be analysed from the regional perspective. The idea is to keep as many existing customers, especially those who are of vital importance for the company, to acquire new customers if possible, and to prepare for the first wave of competitive campaigns using customer-related monitoring systems with the possibility of ad hoc analyses in case of massive customer churn that would serve as means of preventing those trends. Once the market has stabilised, the aims of analysis may have a proactive structure and be aimed at acquiring competitor's customers.

DEVELOPMENT OF THE CONCEPTUAL SOLUTION MODEL

In literature there are numerous solution regarding churn analysis (Berry 2000, Berry 1997, Namid 2004). The presented case is specific because of expected churn trends, and the fact that it describes a different approach to problem solution.

Firstly we need to recognize customers with high perceived customer value, and after that we should develop a churn monitoring system. The conceptual solution model consists of two basic segments. The first segment should evaluate customers on a regional basis using the scoring model. Customers from each region should be evaluated in several categories based on expert knowledge. In this manner better insight into customer behaviour based on their importance to the company should be gained. Since the goal of the company is to retain as many clients as possible (especially the most important ones) a strategy shall be devised based on the results of the analysis with the purpose of increasing customer loyalty.

The competition will inevitably attract a certain number of customers, so the second segment of the solution model will focus on monitoring customer churn or stagnation of sales Trgovina retail stores. With regard to the stable market conditions in the past and almost negligible percentage of customer churn, which makes the analysis more difficult, a classical market research should be performed in the beginning with the aid of a market research agency. This research should provide answers to questions such as which market segments of existing customers of Trgovina stores on a regional basis would be prone to start buying from competition and under which conditions. As well as what would be their prime reasons for continuous buying in competitor's stores, and what would motivate them to continue buying from the Trgovina retail stores.

All the aforementioned information could serve as a basis for devising a strategy for successful resistance during the period of competitor's intense and aggressive advertising campaigns at the time of their entering the market and to their attempts to win over the customers. Since it is almost certain that the competition shall constantly and suddenly undertake advertising activities with the aim of taking over a number of customers, a system of permanent monitoring should be developed with the purpose of early diagnosis of churn trends in certain market segments, with the possibility

Table 1. A proposition of table for monitoring the promotional activities

Date of the campaign	Character of the campaign	Accent is on:	Duration of the campaign
05.05.2006	Discount Sale	Consumer goods	7 days
10.06.2006	Regular campaign	Gardening tools	14 days
10.07.2006	Promotion of new products	Tools	14 days
...	...	...	...

of analysing their dominant characteristics. To this aim, the so-called survival models would be implemented.

Having in mind that each future aggressive advertising campaign of the competition poses a threat of losing a number of customers, one should also note that this present an opportunity for conducting additional analyses which would help the Trgovina company to recognise the behaviour of its customers and promptly react to reduce the consequences of future market actions of the competition. For example, if a sudden competitor's advertising campaign manages to win over a portion of customers having a common attribute, it is an outcome which Trgovina may use to its advantage in order to aim its own campaign towards winning those customers back (with respect to motivating factors of that market segment) and, if possible, attract competitor's customers. For the purposes of future analyses, it is possible to store the data related to competitor's campaigns and their main attributes, as shown in Table 1.

If the data from such tables are paired with the results obtained using the survival models, which can provide us with common attributes of customers who churned or decreased the cooperation, it is possible to obtain additional information related to the character of competitor's campaigns. Based on the accumulated knowledge of possible motivators of a certain market segment, Trgovina may plan its own campaigns at a regional level. For instance, if a decrease is observed in purchases made by male clients (data known from loyalty cards), which are regular customers with relatively high turnover per invoice in previous

transactions, and if that stagnation of sales amount correlates with the period of competitor's promotion of new assortment of tools, this data can be very useful for planning a campaign aimed at returning the customers and attracting new ones.

First of all, it is important to conduct the analysis of the new tool selection. Is buying those tools a matter of prestige, or are the tools sold at a very good price but their quality is not guaranteed, or are these the high quality tools, with good price, but their purchasing is not a matter of prestige... Taking into account all the variables, it is possible to launch a campaign with the goal of returning churned customers. One must always bear in mind that it is much cheaper to prevent situations of possible customer churn, than to try and win customers back. Concerning fierce market competition, it is advisable to develop an action plan for such situations as well.

Conceptual solution models are idea generators and present a beginning of any serious analysis. They also serve as a recapitulation of goals, primarily from the perspective of available methodology and data. Conceptual solution models mostly do not represent the final model solutions which may be considered as a finished project task, because the flow of analysis itself and the obtained results guide further analytical processes, while the goals of the analysis are clearly defined. Having developed the conceptual solution model, where the methodology of conducting the analysis is clearly profiled, the following step is to select software for performing the needed analyses and creating the analytical models.

THE DEVELOPMENT OF SCORING MODEL

There are two dominant planned types of analysis in this case – the scoring analysis and the customer churn analysis. The scoring model may be developed with the aid of fuzzy expert systems, based on the rules resulting from expert knowledge.

Since the goal of the first step of the analysis is the evaluation of customers based on the scoring model at the level of each region, it is necessary to define the possible sub-goals of analysis which are defined, in this business case, as measuring the level of client loyalty. In the development of scoring models based on fuzzy logic, it is crucial to hire business experts as team members who are active in the development (Aracil, 2000; Pedrycz,1998;Siler, 2005). The work of the team is coordinated by an analyst or consultant who is at the same time in charge of the entire project. The Trgovina team consisted of a consultant, sales executive and his assistant, marketing executive and chief information system architect.

The consultant's task was to coordinate and lead the team and to develop the scoring model. The sales executive and his assistant worked with the marketing executive and they were in charge of creating business rules and defining the key indicators for scoring (with the help of the consultant). The chief information system architect of Trgovina gave suggestions and opinions related to the existence of the data in the database based on the defined key indicators. He was also in charge of creating the documentation used for subsequent pre-processing of the data for the needs of the scoring model. During the final stage of the project, the chief information system architect worked with the consultant to create the solution for the integration of the scoring model into the existing information system. Alongside the mentioned team members, a certain number of programmers also worked on the project. They developed the ETL solutions for the scoring model based on the specification and took part in the operative segment of the integration of the scoring model into the existing information system based on the documentation created.

Interviewing the Users

Successful interviewing of users is one of the crucial factors on which the overall success of scoring projects based on fuzzy expert systems depends. During the user interviews it is essential to have in mind the desired goal of scoring. In the case of Trgovina, it is the evaluation of customers in retail stores. The interviews are conducted by the consultant, or the person in charge of the development of the model itself.

It is crucial to ask the questions that will be used to recognize the key indicators and categories relevant for scoring. Based on the interviews, we obtain a clearer picture of the users' perception of a problem we want to solve, i.e. in this case to model it using the fuzzy expert systems. Some of the questions put to the Trgovina were:

- Name at least three categories (e.g. promising, profitable, loyal…) based on which you can evaluate each of your customers.
- Is loyalty as category relevant for the evaluation of customers (scoring) in your company?
- On which grounds (which procedures, behaviour models) may loyalty of a customer be evaluated within your company?
- Which indicators (e.g. turnover, difference in turnover per invoice, campaign costs…) are relevant for estimation of customer profitability within your company?

The questions listed here are just an example of questions put to the auditorium during the brainstorming process, the goal of which was to recognize the key categories and indicators for building a scoring model. In this business case, as well as in all other business cases where scoring models are developed, the consultant (or person in charge of the development of the scoring model) plays a key role in conducting the interview in the right manner. During the interview, this person obtains key information relevant for establishing a basic version of the model.

The described business case defines a situation typical in cases where some team members belong to a business and other to a technical sector. Team members belonging to the business sector made their suggestions disregarding the fact that some suggested indicators would take a long time to pre-process regarding the scope of the data and complexity of the procedure of algorithm processing. The presence of the chief information system architect was very useful here, since he suggested considering other solution modalities. On the other hand, the chief information system architect questioned the suggestions made by team members belonging to the business sector related to using indicators which were important in their opinion but were stored in databases other than the main one. The consultant had a prominent role in the motivation of team members to reach a compromise acceptable from the perspective of model development which does not diminish its plausibility, at the same time having respect of the technical limitations and difficulties resulting from the database architecture.

Defining Key Indicators

The primary goal of the interviewing process was to define key indicators and basic categories as structural elements of a fuzzy expert system. Key indicators may be defined as basic variables, which provide input to a fuzzy expert system (Aracil, 2000; Pedrycz,1998;Siler, 2005). The categories consist of more abstract notions defined using the key indicators. For example, key indicators are sales revenue, campaign costs, duration of business relationship. Based on these key indicators, a category of profitability is defined and limited with a set of rules.

Based on business experience and with the help of the consultant, Trgovina recognised during the interview the three main categories which had an immediate influence on the client scoring:

- Client profitability
- Client loyalty
- Client outlook

Each of the categories should be defined using key indicators, developed on the grounds of available databases. These indicators are input parameters for a fuzzy expert system model. As a result of brainstorming during the interview, the key indicators for each category (at the customer level) are defined as illustrated in Table 2.

Having finished the brainstorming session, the expert team agreed that the selected indicators best describe the chosen categories. Since the internal company experts know their customers the best, based on their expert knowledge, they estimate which indicators in the databases are the best to describe the chosen categories further used for evaluation of scoring. The consultant's task during the brainstorming (as it was the case in this example) is to guide the experts to select the most significant indicators describing the chosen categories. During this process, the number of key indicators defining a category must be taken into account. Sometimes this involves the additional selection of the most important indicators among the important ones in order to keep a number of indicators allocated to a category under four or five. The reason for such a reduction of indicators stems from limited human perception. Each indicator comprises a body of a rule.

When more than five indicators comprising the rule conditions are present (and each indicator may have a number of subcategories), the process of defining rules is often burdened with more than five conditions in addition to the inevitable, often large number of rules. Under such circumstances, it is extremely hard to define the rules. If more

Table 2. The definition of key indicators

Client profitability
Total sales price difference in the last six months
Total promotion expenses based on the loyalty card program (gifts) within the last six months
Total expenses based on the advertising campaigns within the last six months
Client loyalty
Frequency of purchasing within the last six months (number of visits)
Response to campaigns aimed at loyalty card holders within last six months
Number of points on the loyalty card
Client outlook
Purchasing trends within the last two quarters
Tendency of purchasing new brands in the store within the last year
Cross selling trends within the last two quarters

Table 3. A process of key indicator calculation

Category: Client profitability	
Indicators	Calculation process
Total sales price difference in the last six months	Market value – (purchase value + rebate + dependent costs) summed for all invoices within last six months per each customer. Unit – Croatian kuna.
Total promotion expenses based on the loyalty card program (gifts) within the last six months	Total sum of distributed promotional materials and gifts obtained based on the loyalty card data for the period of last six months per each customer. Unit – Croatian kuna.
Total expenses based on the advertising campaigns within the last six months	Total sum of expenses based on each campaign executed during the last six months estimated per each customer (global campaigns on regional level promoted in the press and on the television + targeted campaigns in the form of direct mailing to selected market segments containing product samples). Unit – Croatian kuna.

than five indicators must inevitably be used, it is possible to introduce more categories into the system. This simplifies the process of defining the rules by the experts, and the expert system itself becomes more transparent and easier-to-survey.

Defining the Preprocessing Algorithms

In most cases, it is necessary to deduce the defined key indicators serving as an entrance to the fuzzy expert system model on the basis of the available data, because they do not exist in the transactional database in a form defined as entry into a fuzzy

expert system. For example, in order to obtain a key indicator number of visits within the last six months, which is an element used in the estimation of loyalty to the mentioned company, an algorithmic procedure for reconstruction of number of visits within the last six months based on the invoice numbers had to be defined.

After discovering the key indicators, the consultant and the chief information system architect created the documentation for the preprocessing of the data, encompassing all defined categories and their key indicators. Documentation pertaining to the profitability category is shown in Table 3.

Figure 1. Fuzzy scoring model

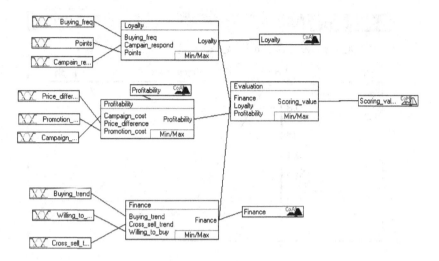

Using the documentation in such a form, the chief information system architect developed detailed algorithms for each indicator. Based on these algorithms the team of programmers created the application for data pre-processing. The data pre-processing is much easier to perform when a data warehouse exists. In the described case, PL/SQL was used for the data pre-processing, which resulted in the creation of a table of key indicators for each customer.

Structural Model Development

After defining the key indicators and the categories and subcategories during the interview, the basis of a fuzzy scoring model was defined. Having defined the categories, it was necessary to unite them in the form of a model depicted in Figure 1.

The depicted model was developed using the FuzzyTech program package. The key indicators in the model comprise the input variables for rule blocks. Each rules block estimates the output value of a category based on the defined rules. These output category values enter the block of rules for final scoring, where the final scoring is estimated on the basis of a defined set of rules. The rules were defined by the experts, and the consultant entered the so defined rules into the fuzzy model. As it can be observed in the figure, the method used for the defuzzification is the so-called Mean-of-Maximum Method (MoM). The reason why it was used originates from the fact that the output results obtained using this defuzzification method are very easy to interpret, especially when such models are integrated in the form of an applicative solution.

Defining the Key Indicator Range

Classical logic, allowing only strict limits among classes, is much further from human perception mechanisms that it is the case with fuzzy logic. For example, if we define the key indicator 'number of visits' resorting to classical logic, we would categorize a small number of visits in the class of 0 to 20 visits during the last six months. Of course, we can ask ourselves what happens with a customer who visited the retail store 21 times during the last six months. If we apply the mechanisms of classical logic, he would be placed in the subsequent class. Human perception mechanisms function on significantly different premises, and are more liberal when it comes to such classification. The limit of a small number of visits

Figure 2. Defining the range of key indicator frequency of purchasing

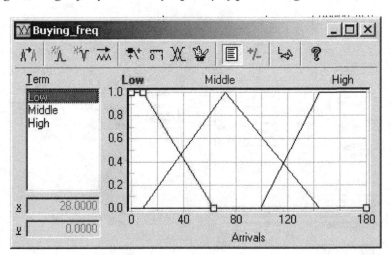

observed through the eyes of human perception mechanisms is subject to tolerance and deviation which are often subjective in nature.

In order to make categorization systems (or scoring systems, as it is the case here) as similar to the human process of making decisions and having in mind the limitations arising from the classical logic and its application, fuzzy expert systems were used in the development of scoring models for the Trgovina. These systems enable defining the range of key indicators on the premise of fuzzy logic, which is very close to the human way of thinking and categorizing. Figure 2 illustrates a manner of defining the range of key indicator frequency of purchasing within the last six months calculated by counting the number of visits during the last six months.

The frequency of purchasing is defined as low, medium or high based on the input parameters. The calculated values are further processed using the defined expert rules. The expert team defined a number of fuzzy classes for each key indicator, as well as their titles and ranges. After that step, they were defined in FuzzyTech as it is shown in the example of key indicator frequency of purchasing within the last six months. The key indicators were defined in such a manner as were the

ranges of output variables in the model and became the basic elements for forming the rules.

Defining the Rule System

One common error present during the implementation of the scoring system using fuzzy expert systems is neglecting the role of the number of indicators describing a category and number of fuzzy classes defined by the expert team. The same happened during the development of such a system in the mentioned company. During the early phases of system development, in the interviewing process, the expert team often emphasized the importance of a large number of indicators for describing a certain category. The consultant played a key role here, since he had to limit the expert team to define a maximum of four or five key indicators best describing a category. Otherwise, a combinatory explosion of a number of rules may occur. The following formula is used for the prediction of total number of rules in a system Klepac (2006):

$$p_j = \prod_{i=1}^{n} r_i \, , \text{n>1,}$$

Table 4. Illustration of rule number growth

Number of fuzzy categories of the first key indicator	Number of fuzzy categories of the second key indicator	Number of fuzzy categories of the third key indicator	Number of fuzzy categories of the fourth key indicator	Number of rules in a block
3	3	3	3	81
3	4	4	4	192
4	4	4	4	256

Table 5. Creating expert rules

IF			THEN	
No_points_card	Campaign_resp	Purchase_freq	DoS	Loyalty
Small	Low	Low	1.00	Low
Small	Low	Medium	1.00	Low
Small	Low	High	1.00	Medium
Small	Medium	Low	1.00	Low
Small	Medium	Medium	1.00	Medium
Small	Medium	High	1.00	Medium
Small	High	Low	1.00	Medium
Small	High	Medium	1.00	Medium
...	...	...	1.00	...

where p_j denotes a number of rules in block j, and is calculated as a product of a number of fuzzy categories of each i-th key indicator r. Based on that, the total number of rules in a system is calculated using the following formula:

$$P = \sum_{j=1}^{m} p_j,$$

where P denotes a total number of rules in a system, calculated as a sum of number of rules in all rules blocks of the system. Table 4 illustrates the relation of number of rules in a block, with four key indicators and different number of fuzzy categories defined within the key indicators.

In the table, we can observe a tendency towards growth in the number of rules in rule blocks with the increase in number of fuzzy categories. In addition to that, we can observe that the increase in number of rules is also influenced by the increase in number of key indicators. The control of the total number of rules in a fuzzy expert system may be exercised through reduction of the number of key indicators or reduction of the number of fuzzy categories within key indicators. Such methodology helped Trgovina to optimize the number of expert rules within their system.

After reaching a consensus regarding the number of rules, the experts created the rules for the system, using the form in Table 5 depicting the key indicator loyalty.

In this manner, the experts defined the rules, for each category defined, as well as for the final scoring.

Scoring

Having created the model and performed the data pre-processing, as well as having defined the rules,

Table 6. Relation table containing the results of the performed analysis

Customer code	Customer loyalty	Customer profitability	Customer outlook	Scoring
28121998	High	High	High	Very high
34909332	High	High	Medium	High
67482875	Low	Medium	Medium	Low
...	...	...	...	...

Table 7. Relative structure of customer shares based on the scoring categories

Scoring category	%
Very low	12
Low	16
Medium	23
High	30
Very high	19

the scoring of pre-processed data followed. The analysis was performed in three main stages. The first stage was characterized by conducting scoring using the created fuzzy expert system model, from which a sampling of obtained results was performed with the purpose of diagnosing the errors in the model. After several cycles of running the data through the model and controlling its reliability, the model has been declared reliable. The following stage, scoring and accepting the results obtained from the model, was performed. Based on the scoring results for each region, a relation table (Table 6) was created.

Further analysis at the level of each region was aimed at finding the relative structure of customer shares based on scoring. As a result of the analysis within one of the regions, the data in Table 7 was obtained.

The client structure shows that 49% of customers were classified in the high and very high scoring ranges. These customers are of great importance for the company. Further analyses established that 80% of the customers belonging to scoring category High obtained the value based on the high profitability and bright outlook, but their loyalty is Medium. This fact placed them in scoring category High instead of Very high.

Speaking from the business point of view, this is a very important segment of clients and it is crucial to significantly increase their loyalty level in the future in order to successfully overcome the new situation on the market. Further analysis of the data using decision trees pointed out the fact that this category primarily consist of customers who rarely come to the store and rarely respond to campaigns that help them collect a large number of points on loyalty cards if they buy products advertised in the campaigns aimed at loyalty card holders. It was also noticed that this category of customers prefers a smaller number of visits to the store during one month, but the amounts on their invoices are higher than average for every purchase. Market basket analysis and clustering were performed using the data related to that group of customers. Based on the analyses, two main customer segments were defined.

"Healthy Life" Segment

Customers who belong to this segment usually buy large amounts of fruit and vegetables, wines of better quality and ingredients related to specific cuisines (Chinese, Japanese, Indian). They rarely buy meat and meat products (even then in small quantities), but they buy more milk and milk products than usual. Based on the data from loyalty cards, this segment mostly consists of members of younger age groups and higher education.

"Cleanliness is Next to Godliness" Segment

Customers who belong to this segment usually buy home cleaning products and detergents. Some 70% of articles in their basket are related to the mentioned category and the remaining 30% is food. The representatives of this segment do not exhibit any regularity in buying foodstuffs. Based on the data from loyalty cards, this segment mostly consists of middle aged persons, who are married with children. Further analyses showed that both segments mostly shop at the end of the week or during the weekends.

All these data were used in planning of further promotional activities in the region. Based on the information, a certain number of promotional activities were directed towards the mentioned market segments. There were more promotional activities offering fruit and vegetables at reduced prices and an extra discount was given for buying certain wines with fruit and vegetables or milk. Such purchases were rewarded with more points on loyalty cards. Customers who took part in a certain number of promotional purchases of this type entered a competition for a vacation in an exotic destination. A number of promotional activities were directed to the second market segment, and these included buying home cleaning products and detergents at discount prices. This type of promotional purchase also included getting more points on loyalty cards. Customers who took part in a certain number of promotional purchases of this type entered a competition for complete child-size furniture for a nursery.

After conducting the described promotional activities, 60% of clients who scored as High increased their loyalty level and scored as Very high during the following five months. Such analyses were conducted for each region. Each region exhibited its own specificities partially discovered after scoring and partially after additional analyses.

The conducted analysis gains extra value if the results are observed in different time intervals. Based on that, we can obtain information on market differentiation and the success of past campaigns, the goal of which was to increase the number of customers with specified scoring values. This data may serve as basis for calculating the amount of resources invested per client in order to upgrade his scoring value from High to Very high. Monitoring of customers in this manner may also serve as a tool for monitoring customers' activities across different segments. It can yield very transparent information on a potential decrease in customers' activities on the market segment level

Monitoring the market segments over time provides us with a new dimension of analytical data overview. General trends of decreasing or increasing the volume of market structure provide us with guidelines for performing further analytical procedures. These analytical procedures should answer questions such as why these trends occur, what are their causes, how to prevent the trends if they are bad for business, or how to strengthen them if they are good for business. For example, if we observe a 30% increase in the number of customers who acquired scoring value "Very high" between two quarters, and if their scoring value was "High" during the previous period, it is necessary to discover the reason that lead to the change in their status. Besides that, it is necessary to conduct further analysis and discover potential regularities within the population of such customers. These insights can be used to motivate other customers from "High" scoring category who are the most similar to this population to achieve the scoring value "Very high" in a certain period of time.

The insights regarding the regularities within a population which can be recognized using data mining techniques can be useful in developing a strategy for promotional activities with the aim of increasing the value of clients from the perspective of a sales-oriented company.

Integration of Scoring Models into the Existing Information System

The implementation of a scoring model based on a fuzzy expert system is mostly performed in two main steps. The first step consists of scoring based on the basic model. In such a model there is no applicative solution based on the designed fuzzy expert system, but the analyst performs most of the scoring based on the created model. This step is also characterized by the procedures for evaluation of the model, so the model is subject to frequent changes in this phase.

The second step, characterized by stability of the created model is oriented towards finding and developing a more permanent applicative solution, which is based on the created model.

The same happened during the implementation of the model to Trgovina. After a period of intensive testing and analysis of the scoring, an applicative solution which should be integrated into the existing information system was needed. Such a solution had to meet some basic criteria in its final phase:

- The possibility of viewing scoring results for each client with explanation why of the client was allocated to a certain scoring category
- The possibility of running an automated scoring procedure over the entire customer database, with the possibility of saving the scoring values
- The possibility of retrieving historical scoring results for each customer.

The integration of the fuzzy model and the existing information system was performed with the aid of ActiveX objects. Figure 3 depicts a part of that solution related to the evaluation of customer loyalty.

Besides monitoring the individual categories (the figure illustrates the example of loyalty category), the scoring problem is also solved in a

Figure 3. Application used for evaluation of customer loyalty

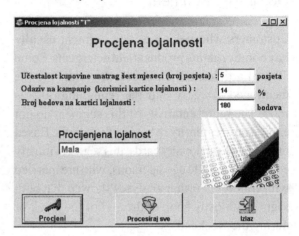

manner that encompasses the values of all categories, together with the score value. The applicative solution with such a concept provides the end user with the derived information that resulted from the estimation made by the expert system. Applicative solutions designed in this manner may be a part of a CRM system, or even a central module of a CRM system.

DEVELOPMENT OF CUSTOMER CHURN ANALYSIS MODEL

Definition of Customer Churn Analysis Strategy in the Trgovina Company

Having performed the scoring of its customers with respect to the expected activities of its competition, Trgovina has to establish a system for permanent monitoring of customer churn and a decrease in the purchase activities of existing customers. Since the market was stable prior to the arrival of the competition when it comes to the intensity and volume of purchase, the first step of evaluation of possible customer churn encompassed market research performed before the competition started its business on the representative sample of customers using telephone interviewing method. This research roughly indicated that the existing Trgovina customers would be strongly motivated to defect to the competition if the competition offered significantly lower prices. The results of the research suggest that more than 60% of Trgovina customers in almost all regions had the intent to make at least one purchase in competitor store once it opened. Although troublesome, this information was expected and it was used in developing a strategy for retaining the existing population of customers. After they perform the initial purchase in the competitor's store, the customers must stay loyal to Trgovina. During the last eight years the market was stable and the customer churn in Trgovina was negligible.

Based on data from the company it is very difficult, almost impossible, to build a transparent prediction model of customer churn, especially if the expected market turbulences are taken into account. One segment of the strategy aimed at retaining the existing customers was to add extra points to loyalty cards in accordance with their scoring category and to inform the customers of the number of points based on which they can buy products at cheaper prices. The points were added based on the scoring category. For example, the customers labelled "Very high "were given more points than the customers with the "High" scoring category. The final goal is to keep as many existing customers, especially those labelled as desirable for the company. As opposed to e.g. the telecommunication sector, where customer churn is clearly defined through the moment of breaking a contract, the moment of ending cooperation in retail is not clearly defined. Thus the expert team had to define the moment of customer churn in retail.

Based on the market research results the management expected a decrease in turnover and number of customers in stores during the first month after opening the competition retail stores in regions where they were opened. This was partially due to the curiosity of customers

and partially to the aggressive campaign of the competition. The customer churn in Trgovina was defined for each region as the absence of an existing customer from the store within two months after competitor retail store was opened in the region or if an existing customer decreased the amount of monthly purchase by an average 60% within two months in comparison to the previous three months. It was decided that the customer churn analysis will be conducted on a monthly basis even before the end of the two month period with the aim of predicting the customer churn in future period. After two months, a comprehensive analysis of customer churn will be conducted, which should provide the guidelines for further strategic planning. Based on the mentioned analyses and competition's moves, precise actions aimed at retaining customers will be defined.

In order to achieve market advantage over the competition even before they enter the market, the plan is to increase the loyalty of existing customers by adding points to their loyalty cards so that they can buy products at discount prices. As a measure of precaution, a couple of weeks before the competition opens the stores promotional campaigns based on the reduction of prices of some products will be intensified as well as advertising in local media. From the perspective of Trgovina, the fact that the competition will not open stores in all regions simultaneously, but within intervals of several months is good news. This will make the development of the strategy for retaining customers in regions where the competition will open stores later on easier, based on the strategic patterns discovered in other regions.

Preprocessing of the Data for Survival Models

In order to analyze customer churn in Trgovina, Cox regression was used Berry (2003). The advantage of this method is the possibility to include predictive variables (covariance) into the model. The goal of the analysis was to discover not only

Figure 4. Different periods of beginning and ending the business cooperation

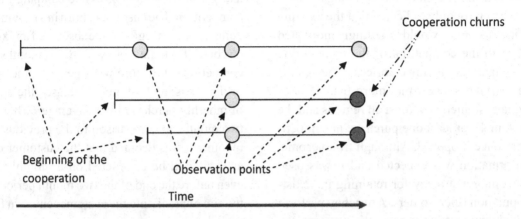

the trend of the customer churn curve, but also to estimate the probability of customer churn with regard to different customer characteristics, which is possible using this model. It is important to notice that customers can begin and end their cooperation lifecycle with Trgovina during different periods of time, as it is illustrated in Figure 4.

For the purpose of the evaluation of customer churn, it is necessary to define discrete time intervals (days, months, years…). The basic idea of a survival model boils down to the estimation of probability that someone who has "survived" as a Trgovina customer during a certain period of time will either stop or continue purchasing during the following period. Cox regression answered the question regarding the probability of customer churn with respect to their different attributes.

For the purpose of creating the model, it is important to define the notion of customer churn as absence of an existing customer during the last two months after the competition opened a retail store in the region or if an existing customer decreased the amount of monthly purchase by an average of 60% within two months in comparison to the previous three months. Based on the definition, a pre-processing of the data for the status variable was performed. A status designation of 1 denotes a churned customer, while a status designation of 0 denotes an existing customer.

Another important variables important for the model is the number of months of continuous purchase. This variable is defined as the number of months since the date of customer churn minus number of months since the date of issuing the loyalty card. Having in mind the nature of the Cox regression, the model includes other attributes (predictive variables). Continuous variables, such as age variable are made discrete. Data pre-processing resulted in the table of the structure in Table 8.

Based on such table, it is possible to perform the analysis using Cox regression.

Performing the Analysis

Unlike businesses such as telecommunications, retail business is characterized by a range of specificities, which guide the data adjustment in order to build a customer churn model. Besides the specificities related to the definition of the moment of customer churn, retail business does not have the privilege of receiving transparent information on a daily basis regarding the relationship of a customer and the company defined by a contract. Due to that reason, it is much easier to monitor the client structure in telecommunications with regard to breaking the contracts.

If we observe the situation from the competition's point of view for a moment, we can notice

Table 8. Structure of the data for performing Cox regression

Customer code	Number of purchasing months	Status	Age	Gender	No of complaints	...
23345342	18	1	<25	M	1	...
54336564	20	0	46+	Z	1	...
34566334	19	0	36-45	M	3	...
...	...	...	...	...	...	...

that they lack usable data for performing a deeper analysis of the structure of clients who decided to make a purchase in their store during the first month, since they will not issue loyalty cards during the first couple of months and having in mind the specificities of retail business.

At the moment of closing the contract, the telecommunication companies obtain much more information from the client, which may be used for analysis. At the same time, client of a retail company provides only the data on past transactions, so he can not be uniquely identified. From this point of view, Trgovina has a certain analytical advantage, because they own data more suitable for analysis acquired from loyalty cards, which is important for analyzing the customer churn. Currently as entering to the market, telecommunication companies and similar businesses that base their operation on contracts closed with clients count on a certain percentage of customer churn which is manifested in the form of breaking the contracts. Such companies do not have a problem with conducting the analysis of reasons and profiles of clients who churn based on the collected data.

From the point of view of a competition retail company, the analogy of customer churn can be compared with the arrival of a customer who makes a purchase during the first month after acquisition motivated by an aggressive advertising campaign, and gives up purchasing in the competition store after that. It is very difficult to uniquely identify a group of such customers. This fact almost disables the

Figure 5. Survival curve for the Trgovina company customers

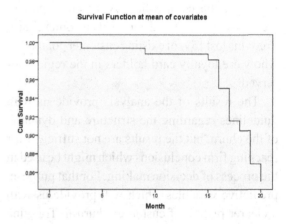

competition company to perform the analytical procedures in order to influence those trends with the purpose of motivating this group of customers to further purchasing. In such cases, the competition company has to rely on market research results obtained through performing surveys on samples of customers, which are a rather big investment.

Trgovina performed the analysis of customer churn based on pre-processed data using Cox regression. In regards to market stability during the previous period, the focus of the analysis was on the last twenty months of operations. The competition started its operation in the region since the sixteenth month observed within the model. After the analysis was performed, the survival curve for Trgovina customers was obtained, as illustrated in Figure 5.

The figure clearly indicates that with regard to the population of customer after the sixteenth observed month, in a relatively stable market, there is a decrease in Trgovina customer population. Translated to model jargon, the probability of survival of the customer population is decreasing. The curve shows that the decrease in promotional activities of the competition had influence on the decrease of customer churn in Trgovina (seventeenth and eighteenth month in the model on Figure 5. With the intensification of promotional activities, the trend again started to shift in favour of the competition. After the twentieth week, using the defined notion of customer churn, Trgovina lost 15% of existing customer population who were loyalty card holders in the region observed.

The results of the analysis provide us with guidelines regarding the structure and dynamic of the churn, but the results are not sufficient for reaching firm conclusions which might be used in the process of decision making. For that purpose, predictive variables which will provide us with a clearer picture of customer churn in Trgovina need to be included in the model. Predictive variables are included in the table made on the basis of data pre-processing. These variables were selected based on the attribute relevance analysis. A certain number of variables for which it was proved that they best describe the variable end of churning status based on the calculated gini index were included in the data model which was further analyzed.

After the analysis was performed on the pre-processed data using Cox regression, it was found that certain categories of age structure and customers with a defined number of complaints filed through the call centre have the biggest influence on churn trends. It was also noticed that there are no significant differences in churn trends among customers classified in different scoring categories.

The results of the analysis are shown in Figure 6 and Figure 7.

Figure 6. Survival function with regard to "complaints" variable

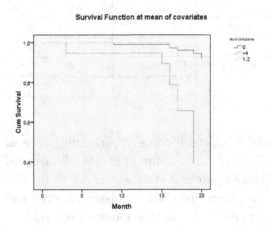

Figure 7. Survival function with regard to "age" variable

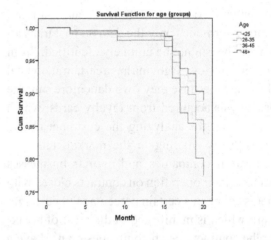

If we pay closer attention to the graphs and compare the intensities of competition advertising campaigns that were less intense during the seventeenth and eighteenth month observed, we can notice that during this period customer churn decreased in comparison to the following periods and that it increased in the following months observed. It can also be noticed that the highest probability of churn is connected with younger customers, as well as customers who filed more than four complaints through the call centre. Based on the analysis, it was concluded that the risk of customer churn grows with younger age groups as well as with the number of complaints via the call centre.

The probable reason of more frequent churn when it comes to younger population stems from the fact that the competition advertising campaign targets that exact group – their strategic market segment. Regarding the more frequent customer churn related to clients who filed more than four complaints through the call centre, further analysis was conducted on that customer population with the aim of finding common attributes of customers belonging to that population. The analysis did not yield results that would enable recognizing the dominant significant attributes in that population.

Business Decisions Based on the Analysis

Diagnosed risky categories for the observed region exhibiting a greater tendency towards customer churn are younger customers and customers who had more that four filed complaints in the call centre. Generally speaking, the risk of customer churn grows with the diminishing age of customer and with the increase in number of complaints. Regarding the competition campaign aimed at younger customers, Trgovina decided to pay special attention to that market segment through the advertising campaigns in order to prevent as much churn related to younger customers. Special attention will be paid to younger customers who were categorized based on the performed scoring in the "High" and "Very high" scoring categories. These groups will be targeted by special promotional activities in order to additionally motivate them to continue purchasing in Trgovina stores.

Regarding the discovered regularities related to customer complaints, the decision was made to further analyze the reasons of dissatisfaction and contact each client who had filed more than two complaints through the call centre with the intent of solving them. This is another strategy for increasing client loyalty which will also influence the reduction of customer churns.

FUTURE TRENDS IN CHURN PREDICTION AND CONCLUSIONS

A relatively stable market takes on a significantly different character after the arrival of competition to certain regions. Trgovina discovered the structure of its customers according to their value to the company using scoring techniques. This knowledge resulted in focusing on the most valuable customers from the perspective of the company, with the purpose of retention and increasing their loyalty. Based on the scoring results, an even more flexible policy of discount prices was developed for purchasing products from recognized categories obtained during the scoring procedure. The period immediately before the arrival of the competition was used for conducting activities for increasing client loyalty with the aim of their long-term retention. Trgovina was aware of the fact that they will inevitably lose a portion of their customers, so their goal was to diminish those trends as much as possible. Although their final goal was to keep as many of existing customers as possible, the main emphasis was on the customers who were most valuable for the company.

A further step was aimed at the creation of an early warning system in the shape of a customer churn analysis model, based on which it is possible to recognize basic regularities within the population of customers who either churn or decrease the intensity of purchase according to the specified criteria.

The analyses conducted and business decisions made based on that analyses resulted in a significant reduction of customer churn, especially in the younger customers segment, which was targeted by the competition. Trends of customer churn related to customers with higher number of complaints were also diminished with the help of call centre operators who contacted customers who had filed complaints trying to solve their problems and alleviate the consequences related to the complaints. In the long run, this approach resulted in an increase in customer satisfaction and consequently in growth of sales revenue.

Trgovina managed to keep a satisfactory number of customers who were ranked high in the scoring procedure, which was one of the goals. Regarding the new market conditions of fierce competition, Trgovina had to constantly monitor the development of the market and analyze market trends on a global and regional level, especially the population of its customers. Mandatory scoring on a monthly basis initiated the analysis of market segments differentiation and its causes on the level of the Croatian market and on regional levels. Such an approach enabled establishing an early warning system which is of vital importance in conditions where the competition continually undertakes targeted promotional actions with the aim of winning clients. The system of conducted analyses proved to be very effective concerning the situation on the market and it served as a basis for the development of further analytical systems that contributed to the success of Trgovina decision support at all management levels.

The presented case represents one of the possible solutions in given circumstances. The developed model shows good performance in practice. Churn is specific to a given area and there is no cookbook data mining solution which could be applied in each case (Berry, 2000; Berry, 2003; Giudici, 2003; Namid, 2004). The existing model could be extended with an early warning system, and segmentation model which takes into consideration the customer prospective value as a part of customer relationship model.

Churn analyzes will certainly use more than several common data mining models. As the market condition becomes complicated, and that fact leads us to combine a variety of data mining techniques to achieve better results. Customer relationship management systems will play a more important role in churn prediction, as churn

prevention system. Recognizing customer needs and behavior is first and most important step in churn prevention.

REFERENCES

Agosta, L. (2000). *The Essential Guide to Data Warehousing*. Upper Saddle River, NJ: Prentice Hall.

Aleksander, I., & Morton, H. (1995). *An introduction to neural computing*. New York: International Thompson Computer Press.

Aracil, J., & Gordillo, F. (Eds.). (2000). *Stability Issues in Fuzzy Control*. Heidelberg, Germany: Physica-Verlag.

Berry, J. A., & Linoff, G. (1997). *Data mining techniques for marketing sales and customer support*. New York: John Wiley &Sons Inc.

Berry, J. A., & Linoff, G. (2000). *Mastering data mining*. New York: John Wiley &Sons, Inc.

Berry, J. A., & Linoff, G. (2003). *Mining the web*. New York: John Wiley &Sons Inc.

Dresner, H. (2008). *Performance management revolution*. New York: John Wiley &Sons Inc.

Faulkner, M. (2003). *Customer management excellence*. New York: John Wiley &Sons Inc.

Giudici, P. (2003). *Applied Data Mining: Statistical Methods for Business and Industry*. New York: John Wiley &Sons Inc.

Hampel, R., Wagenknecht, M., & Chaker, N. (Eds.). (2000). *Fuzzy Control: Theory and Practice*. Heidelberg, Germany: Physica-Verlag.

Han, J., & Kamber, M. (2000). *Data Mining: Concepts and Techniques*. San Francisco: Morgan Kaufmann.

Klepac, G., & Mršić, L. (2006). *Poslovna inteligencija kroz poslovne slučajeve*. Zagreb, Croatia: Liderpress.

Klepac, G., & Panian, Ž. (2003). *Poslovna inteligencija*. Zagreb, Croatia: Masmedia.

Kohonen, T. (2001). *Self-organizing maps*. Berlin: Springer.

Larose, D. T. (2005). *Discovering Knowledge in Data: An Introduction to Data Mining*. New York: John Wiley &Sons Inc.

Larose, D. T. (2006). *Data mining methods and models*. New York: John Wiley &Sons Inc.

Mannila, H., & Hand, D. (2001). *Principles of Data Mining*. Cambridge, MA: The MIT press.

Namid, R. N., & Christopher, D. B. (Eds.). (2004). *Organizational Data Mining: Leveraging Enterprise Data Resources for Optimal Performance*. Hershey, PA: Idea Group.

Pedrycz, W., & Gomide, F. (1998). *An Introduction to Fuzzy Sets: Analysis and Design of Complex Adaptive Systems*. Cambridge, MA: MIT Press.

Pyle, D. (1999). *Data preparation for Data Mining*. San Francisco: Morgan Kaufmann.

Siler, W., & Buckley, J. J. (2005). *Fuzzy expert systems and fuzzy reasoning*. New York: John Wiley &Sons, Inc.

Vose, D. (2000). *Quantitative Risk Analysis*. New York: John Wiley & Sons Inc.

KEY TERMS AND DEFINITIONS

Data Mining: Discovering hidden useful knowledge in large amount of data (databases)

Fuzzy Logic: Logic which presumes possible membership to more than one category with degree of membership, and which is opposite to (exact) crisp logic

Fuzzy Expert System: Expert system based on fuzzy logic

Scoring: Process of assigning some value (usually numeric) as a grade to represent the performance of an observed case/object

Churn: Interruption of the contract or using product or services

Survival Analysis: Analysis which shows survival rate (example: from population of customers) in a defined period of time

Cox Regression: One of the methods for survival analysis.

Section 4
Data Mining as Applications and Approaches Related to Organizational Scene

Chapter 14
An Exposition of CaRBS Based Data Mining:
Investigating Intra Organization Strategic Consensus

Malcolm J. Beynon
Cardiff University, UK

Rhys Andrews
Cardiff Business School, UK

ABSTRACT

The non-trivial extraction of implicit, previously unknown, interesting, and potentially useful information is at the heart of efforts to solve real-world problems; perhaps nowhere more so than in the field of organization studies. This chapter aims to describe the ability of a nascent data mining technique, Classification and Ranking Belief Simplex (CaRBS), to undertake analysis in the area of organization research in the public sector. The rudiments of CaRBS, and the RCaRBS development also employed, are based on the general methodology of Dempster-Shafer theory (DST), as such, the data mining analysis undertaken with CaRBS is associated with uncertain modelling. Throughout this chapter, a real application is considered, namely, using survey data drawn from a large multipurpose public organization, to examine the argument that consensus on strategic priorities is, at least partly, determined by an organization's structure, process and environment.

INTRODUCTION

Deriving predictions from hidden patterns amongst large amounts of data is the cornerstone of data mining (Chen, 2001). The non-trivial extraction of implicit, previously unknown, interesting, and potentially useful information is at the heart of efforts to solve real-world problems (see Berry and Linoff, 1997; Westphal and Blaxton, 1998); perhaps nowhere more so than in the field of organization studies. This chapter aims to describe the ability of a nascent data mining technique, based on uncertain modelling, to undertake analysis in the area of organization research in the public sector. Further, the chapter also demonstrates how such a technique itself can be developed to perform more pertinent analysis in this area.

DOI: 10.4018/978-1-60566-906-9.ch014

The Classification and Ranking Belief Simplex (CaRBS) non-parametric technique, introduced in Beynon (2005a, 2005b), was presented as a novel approach to undertake data mining. The rudiments of CaRBS are based on the general methodology of Dempster-Shafer theory (DST), introduced in Dempster (1967) and Shafer (1976). As such, the data mining analysis undertaken with CaRBS is associated with uncertain modelling. Indeed, DST is considered one of the three key mathematical approaches to uncertainty modeling (Roesmer, 2000), along with the probabilistic and fuzzy logic approaches (see Mantores, 1990; Zadeh, 1975; Yang *et al.*, 2006). Further, it is often described as a generalisation of the well-known Bayesian theory (Shafer and Srivastava, 1990).

One consequence of the association of the non-parametric technique CaRBS with DST, is the ability to undertake analysis in the presence of a form of mathematical based ignorance (Safranek *et al.*, 1990; Beynon, 2005b). The original CaRBS technique is employed in the classification-type analysis of strategic consensus in a public organization (see later), plus a development, termed RCaRBS, which affords the ability to undertake regression-type analysis on the same problem. The RCaRBS analysis presented here illustrates, at the technical level, how a data mining technique based on uncertain modelling, such as CaRBS, can be developed to undertake more general types of analysis pertinent to the types of continuous data generally used by organizational researchers (using RCaRBS). Indeed, uncertain modelling is uniquely able to accommodate the ambiguity that surrounds the subjective measures of organizational characteristics that are often used in studies of strategic management (see Dutton *et al.*, 1983).

Throughout this chapter, a real application is considered, namely, using survey data drawn from a large multipurpose public organization, to examine the argument that consensus on strategic priorities is, at least partly, determined by an organization's structure, process and environment (Dess and Origer, 1987). This is a pertinent ap-

plication, since management theory suggests that strategic consensus has important implications for organizational performance (Bourgeois, 1980). Despite widespread speculation on the veracity of these propositions on consensus (see Bowman and Ambrosini, 1997), few studies have systematically examined the antecedents of strategic consensus in public, private or non-profit organizations (see Kellermanns *et al.*, 2005). Moreover, there has been a relative dearth of studies employing non-parametric techniques, such as the well known neural networks (and the CaRBS here in particular), in research on this and related issues in organizational research (see for example De-Tienne *et al.*, 2003).

Amongst the technical expositions given in this chapter, the binary classification based data mining presented, using the original CaRBS technique, is operationalised in terms of a constrained optimisation problem. This problem is solved here using the evolutionary computation technique Trigonometric Differential Evolution (TDE - Fan and Lampinen, 2003), which employs an objective function which confers the minimisation of ambiguity, in the classification of vertical consensus based on managers' perceptions of strategic priorities, but not concomitant ignorance (Beynon, 2005b). The second analysis exposited, using the RCaRBS development on CaRBS, demonstrates regression-type analysis in the presence of ignorance (again using TDE and an objective function based on the minimisation of the level of predictive fit 'sum of squares error' of the degree to which vertical consensus exist on perceived strategic priorities). This latter analysis is pertinent since the majority of quantitative organizational research is regression oriented (DeTienne *et al.*, 2003).

Throughout the analysis presented in this chapter, there is emphasis on the graphical representation of results, primarily using the simplex plot method of data representation, an intrinsic part of the CaRBS technique (and RCaRBS), explicitly referred to in its introduction (see Beynon, 2005a).

The intention of the chapter is to exposit the workings and potential application of a data mining technique based on uncertain modeling (CaRBS and RCaRBS) for organizational research, in this case through the general methodology of DST. With respect to the considered intra-organizational consensus problem, how the CaRBS based data mining modelling of strategic consensus fits with the considered organization characteristics investigated is of theoretical and practical interest, with the graphical inferences produced offering a novel clear perspective on how organizations can adapt their internal characteristics to increase levels of strategic consensus.

The structure of the rest of the book chapter is as follows: The background section discusses the general methodology of DST, including a small example, followed by an exposition of the CaRBS technique and its development with RCaRBS. The main thrust of the chapter describes the strategic consensus problem considered, before presenting the CaRBS and RCaRBS analyses. Finally, conclusions are drawn and the implications of the content of the chapter are discussed.

BACKGROUND

The background discussed here surrounds the concomitant technical issues, namely an exposition of the CaRBS technique (and the associated RCaRBS development), and before it, the general methodology of Dempster-Shafer theory is described, upon which the CaRBS technique is grounded.

Dempster-Shafer Theory

The methodology underwriting the technique described in this section is Dempster-Shafer theory (DST), introduced in Dempster (1967) and Shafer (1976), and generally acknowledged to be a mathematical approach to uncertainty modelling (Roesmer, 2000). As a technique viewed in terms of probabilistic reasoning, DST is also considered one of the fundamental methodologies making up the notion of soft computing (*ibid.*).

Fundamentally, DST is based on the idea of obtaining degrees of belief for one question (the equivalent of a dependent variable), from subjective probabilities describing the evidence from others (the equivalent of independent variables), and that the concordance of pieces of evidence reinforce each other. This evidential reasoning methodology, it has been argued, is a generalization of the well-known Bayesian probability calculus (Shafer and Srivastava, 1990; Schubert, 1994), see also Dempster (2008) for a contempory reflection of DST.

With DST a general methodology, its fundamentals consider a finite set of p hypotheses $\Theta = \{o_1, o_2,..., o_p\}$, called a frame of discernment. A *mass value* is a function $m: 2^\Theta \rightarrow [0, 1]$ such that $m(\emptyset) = 0$ ($\emptyset$ - the empty set) and $\sum_{s \in 2^\Theta} m(s) = 1$ (2^Θ - the power set on Θ). Any proper subset s of the frame of discernment Θ, for which $m(s)$ is non-zero, is called a focal element and the $m(s)$ value represents the exact belief in the proposition depicted by s. The collection of mass values (and focal elements) associated with a single piece of evidence is called a *body of evidence* (BOE). The mass value $m(\Theta)$ assigned to the frame of discernment Θ is considered the amount of mathematical ignorance within the BOE, since it represents the level of exact belief that cannot be discerned to any proper subsets of Θ.

DST also provides a method to combine the BOEs from different pieces of evidence, using Dempster's rule of combination. This rule assumes these pieces of evidence are independent, then the function $[m_1 \oplus m_2]: 2^\Theta \rightarrow [0, 1]$, acting on two BOEs, is defined by (on a focal element s);

$$[m_1 \oplus m_2](s) =
\begin{cases}
0 & s = \varnothing \\[2ex]
\dfrac{\displaystyle\sum_{s_1 \cap s_2 = x} m_1(s_1)m_2(s_2)}{1 - \displaystyle\sum_{s_1 \cap s_2 = \varnothing} m_1(s_1)m_2(s_2)} & s \neq \varnothing
\end{cases}$$

and is a mass value, where s_1 and s_2 are focal elements from the BOEs, $m_1(\cdot)$ and $m_2(\cdot)$, respectively.

The combination rule can be considered over all the elements in the power set of Θ ($s \in 2^\Theta$), to formulate the new BOE. Further, the combination rule can be used iteratively to combine the evidence contained in a number of BOEs. The denominator part of the combination rule includes $\sum_{s_1 \cap s_2 = \varnothing} m_1(s_1)m_2(s_2)$, considered to measure the level of conflict in the combination process between BOEs (Murphy, 2000), and is based on the sum of the products of mass values associated with focal elements from the different BOE, which have empty intersection.

To clarify a reader's understanding of the fundamentals of DST, a small example is next presented. Commonly called the "assassins problem", it has previously been presented to elucidate the fundamental of DST and its own development (see for example, Smets, 1990). Let us say there are three individuals (assassins), Henry, Tom and Sarah, who are suspects for the murder of Mr. White. Within DST, these three suspects make up a frame of discernment, $\Theta = \{\text{Henry, Tom, Sarah}\}$. Two witnesses (W1 and W2), have information regarding the murder of Mr. White:

Witness W1: is 80% sure that the murderer was a man.

Witness W2: is 60% confident that Henry was leaving on a jet plane when the murder occurred.

Each of these pieces of evidence (information) are converted, in DST, into concomitant BOEs, defined $m_{W1}(\cdot)$ and $m_{W2}(\cdot)$.

Witness W1's evidence furnishes belief on the murderer being a man, which pertains specifically to Henry and Tom (the male suspects). Thus, in the respective BOE $m_{W1}(\cdot)$, the focal element $\{\text{Henry, Tom}\}$ exists, with associated mass value 0.8, namely $m_{W1}(\{\text{Henry, Tom}\}) = 0.8$. This mass value is assigned to the set $\{\text{Henry, Tom}\}$ and not the individual elements in the set, indeed, central to DST is that the distribution of this mass value amongst the elements of such a set is unknown (Srivastava and Liu, 2003). Since there is no information regarding the remaining mass value $(1.0 - 0.8 = 0.2)$, it is considered ignorance (mathematical), and allocated to Θ (all the suspected assassins), hence $m_{W1}(\{\text{Henry, Tom, Sarah}\}) = 0.2 \; (= m_{W1}(\Theta))$.

Following a similar argument, the BOE constructed from the evidence of witness W2, the respective BOE $m_{W2}(\cdot)$ is made up of the two focal elements and mass values, $m_{W2}(\{\text{Tom, Sarah}\}) = 0.6$ and $m_{W2}(\{\text{Henry, Tom, Sarah}\}) = 0.4$. Within the two BOEs, $m_{W1}(\cdot)$ and $m_{W2}(\cdot)$, each mass value represents the exact belief in that focal element (of suspects), including the murderer of Mr. White.

Having established the mathematical evidences from the two witnesses (two sources of information), its combination (aggregation) is next carried out using Dempster's combination rule, presuming the witnesses are giving independent evidence. At the technical level, the combination process is based on the intersection and multiplication of the focal elements and mass values from the previously constructed BOEs, $m_{W1}(\cdot)$ and $m_{W2}(\cdot)$, see Table 1, for intermediate findings of the combination process.

In Table 1, the intersection and multiplication of the focal elements and mass values included in the BOEs, $m_{W1}(\cdot)$ (first column) and $m_{W2}(\cdot)$ (first row), are presented (bottom right hand of table). Amongst the findings, the new focal elements found are all non-empty, it follows, the level of conflict $\sum_{s_1 \cap s_2 = \varnothing} m_{W1}(s_1)m_{W2}(s_2) = 0$ (part of the denominator of the combination rule – see

Table 1. Intermediate findings from the combination of the BOEs, $m_{W1}(\cdot)$ and $m_{W2}(\cdot)$

$m_{w1}(\cdot) \setminus m_{w2}(\cdot)$	{Tom, Sarah}, 0.6	Θ, 0.4
{Henry, Tom}, 0.8	{Tom}, 0.48	{Henry, Tom}, 0.32
Θ, 0.2	{Tom, Sarah}, 0.12	Θ, 0.08

previously), then the resultant BOE, defined $m_{w}(\cdot)$, can be taken directly from the results in Table 1 (since denominator part of combination rule equals 1), namely;

$m_{w}(\{Tom\}) = 0.48$, $m_{w}(\{Henry, Tom\}) = 0.32$,

$m_{w}(\{Tom, Sarah\}) = 0.12$ and $m_{w}(\{Henry, Tom, Sarah\}) = 0.08$.

Amongst this combination of evidence, in the BOE $m_{w}(\cdot)$, the mass value assigned to ignorance ($m_{w}(\Theta) = m_{w}(\{Henry, Tom, Sarah\}) = 0.08$), is less than that present in the original individual witness based BOEs ($m_{W1}(\cdot)$ and $m_{W2}(\cdot)$), as expected when combining evidence using DST. In summary, the combined evidence, in terms of mass values, is spread over a number of focal elements of suspects (more focal elements than present in any of the individual witness BOEs). The newly formed BOE $m_{w}(\cdot)$, could then be used to exposit the evidence supporting the individual suspects association with being the murderer of Mr. White (see later in the context of the CaRBS based analyses undertaken).

The Classification and Ranking Belief Simplex (CaRBS) and RCaRBS

The CaRBS technique was originally devised as a tool to undertake the binary classification and ranking of objects in the presence of ignorance (see Beynon, 2005a). Alongside its description (and subsequent employment), here it is developed to perform regression-type analysis (termed RCaRBS).

The technical details of the CaRBS technique are next briefly described (see Beynon, 2005a; 2005b, for further details), with its subsequent development to undertake regression-type analyses then exposited (using RCaRBS). To aid in the clarity of the presentation, the given description will be undertaken using terminology, where appropriate, associated with the regression models conventionally used in strategic management research (see Meilich, 2006), whereby objects (in this case survey respondents - see later) are associated with a dependent variable (e.g. strategic consensus) and described by a number of independent variables (e.g. respondents' perceived organizational characteristics).

Within CaRBS, the information from a respondent's perceivance of an organization's characteristic on a specific issue (see later), termed here a characteristic value, is quantified in a BOE, generally denoted by $m(\cdot)$, where all assigned mass values sum to unity and there is no belief in the empty set (as stated earlier in the technical description of DST). Moreover, for a respondent R_{j} ($1 \leq j \leq n_{O}$) and the ith characteristic C_{i} ($1 \leq i \leq n_{C}$) describing it, a *characteristic* BOE, defined $m_{j,i}(\cdot)$, is made up of the mass values, $m_{j,i}(\{x\})$ and $m_{j,i}(\{\neg x\})$, which denote levels of exact belief in the association of the object to a hypothesis x (strategic consensus) and not-the-hypothesis $\neg x$ (strategic not-consensus), and $m_{j,i}(\{x, \neg x\})$ the level of concomitant ignorance. In the case of $m_{j,i}(\{x, \neg x\})$, its association with the term ignorance is because this mass value is unable to be assigned specifically to either x or $\neg x$.

The characteristic BOE represents the evidence from one of a respondent's characteristic values (responses). From Safranek *et al.* (1990), used in

CaRBS, the mass values in a characteristic BOE are given by the expressions (for a characteristic value v);

$$m_{j,i}(\{x\}) = \frac{B_i}{1 - A_i} cf_i(v) - \frac{A_i B_i}{1 - A_i}, \; m_{j,i}(\{\neg x\}) =$$

$$\frac{-B_i}{1 - A_i} cf_i(v) + B_i$$

and $m_{j,i}(\{x, \neg x\}) = 1 - m_{j,i}(\{x\}) - m_{j,i}(\{\neg x\})$, where $cf_i(v) = 1/(1 + \exp(-k_i(v - \theta_i)))$ (a sigmoid function similar to that used in neural networks - see later), and k_i, θ_i, A_i and B_i are control variables incumbent in CaRBS (for its configuration). Importantly, if either $m_{j,i}(\{x\})$ or $m_{j,i}(\{\neg x\})$ are negative they are set to zero, and the respective $m_{j,i}(\{x, \neg x\})$ then calculated.

Figure 1 presents, with respect to the CaRBS technique, a graphical presentation of the process from a characteristic value v to a characteristic BOE, and its subsequent representation as a single simplex coordinate in a simplex plot (and then its "regression" to a single predicted strategic consensus value as part of the RCaRBS development - discussed later).

In Figure 1, one of a respondent's characteristic values v is first transformed into a confidence value ($1a$), from which it is de-constructed into its associated characteristic BOE ($1b$), made up of the triplet of mass values, $m_{j,i}(\{x\})$, $m_{j,i}(\{\neg x\})$ and $m_{j,i}(\{x, \neg x\})$, using the expressions given previously. Stage ($1c$) then shows a characteristic BOE $m_{j,i}(\cdot)$; $m_{j,i}(\{x\}) = v_{j,i,1}$, $m_{j,i}(\{\neg x\}) = v_{j,i,2}$ and $m_{j,i}(\{x, \neg x\}) = v_{j,i,3}$, can be represented as a simplex coordinate ($p_{j,i,v}$) in a simplex plot (equilateral triangle), labeled $p_{j,i,v}$ in this case. That is, a point $p_{j,i,v}$ exists within an equilateral triangle such that the least distance from $p_{j,i,v}$ to each of the sides of the equilateral triangle are in the same proportions (ratios) to the values, $v_{j,i,1}$, $v_{j,i,2}$ and $v_{j,i,3}$ (see for example, Canongia Lopes, 2004). In the case of a simplex plot with unit side, with vertices $(0, 0)$, $(1, 0)$ and $(0.5, 0.5\sqrt{3})$, the $p_{j,i,v}$ simplex coordinate (x_p, y_p) is given by $x_p = v_{j,i,1} + 0.5 v_{j,i,3}$ and $y_p = 0.5\sqrt{3} v_{j,i,3}$.

The set of characteristic BOEs $\{m_{j,i}(\cdot), i = 1, ..., n_C\}$, associated with a respondent R_j, found from its characteristic values, can be combined using Dempster's combination rule into a *respondent* BOE, defined $m_j(\cdot)$. Moreover, considering $m_{j,i}(\cdot)$ and $m_{j,k}(\cdot)$ as two independent characteristic BOEs, $[m_{j,i} \oplus m_{j,k}](\cdot)$ defines their combination (on a single focal element), and is given here by (in terms of a newly created BOE made up of three mass values): (see Box 1)

The ability to explicitly write out the combination of two characteristic BOEs (rather than the original combination rule), is due to a binary frame of discernment being considered (the hypotheses x and $\neg x$ only). This process is then used iteratively to combine all the characteristic BOEs describing the evidence in a respondent's characteristic

Box 1.

$$[m_{j,i} \oplus m_{j,k}](\{x\}) = \frac{m_{j,i}(\{x\})m_{j,k}(\{x\}) + m_{j,k}(\{x\})m_{j,i}(\{x, \neg x\}) + m_{j,i}(\{x\})m_{j,k}(\{x, \neg x\})}{1 - (m_{j,i}(\{\neg x\})m_{j,k}(\{x\}) + m_{j,i}(\{x\})m_{j,k}(\{\neg x\}))},$$

$$[m_{j,i} \oplus m_{j,k}](\{\neg x\}) = \frac{m_{j,i}(\{\neg x\})m_{j,k}(\{\neg x\}) + m_{j,k}(\{x, \neg x\})m_{j,i}(\{\neg x\}) + m_{j,k}(\{\neg x\})m_{j,i}(\{x, \neg x\})}{1 - (m_{j,i}(\{\neg x\})m_{j,k}(\{x\}) + m_{j,i}(\{x\})m_{j,k}(\{\neg x\}))},$$

$$[m_{j,i} \oplus m_{j,k}](\{x, \neg x\}) = 1 - [m_{j,i} \oplus m_{j,k}](\{x\}) - [m_{j,i} \oplus m_{j,k}](\{\neg x\}).$$

values, into its associated respondent BOE. In the original CaRBS technique, the respondent BOE contained the evidence that described a respondent's association to the considered, hypothesis, not-the-hypothesis and concomitant ignorance (viewed here as binary classification with ignorance).

To illustrate this method of combination (illustration given because of its novelty), the two example BOEs, $m_1(\cdot)$ and $m_2(\cdot)$, shown in Figure 1c, are considered. Their combination to a BOE, denoted $m_C(\cdot)(- [m_1 \oplus m_2](\cdot))$, is evaluated to be $m_C(\{x\}) = 0.467$, $m_C(\{\neg x\}) = 0.224$ and $m_C(\{x, \neg x\}) = 0.309$. This combination process is graphically shown within the simplex coordinate representation of the combined BOE $m_C(\cdot)$ presented in Figure 1c (with evaluated simplex coordinate (0.622, 0.268)).

The relative position of $m_C(\cdot)$ to the simplex coordinates of $m_1(\cdot)$ and $m_2(\cdot)$ shows it is nearer the base line of the equilateral triangle (furthest away from the $\{x, \neg x\}$ vertex of the presented BOEs), so has less associated ignorance than each of the pieces of evidence that combined to create it (as is the case). Further, the horizontal position of $m_C(\cdot)$, nearer to the $\{x\}$ vertex that the $\{\neg x\}$ vertex, indicates the evidence in $m_C(\cdot)$ supports more the association to x than $\neg x$.

The CaRBS technique is governed by the values assigned to the incumbent control variables k_i, θ_i, A_i and B_i, evaluated through a configuration process. Where these control variables contribute directly to the construction of the characteristic BOEs $m_{j,i}(\cdot)$, which are combined to produce the respective respondent BOEs $m_j(\cdot)$. A CaRBS configuration is considered a constrained optimi-

Figure 1. Stages in CaRBS for a single characteristic value v to formulate a characteristic BOE and its representation in a simplex plot

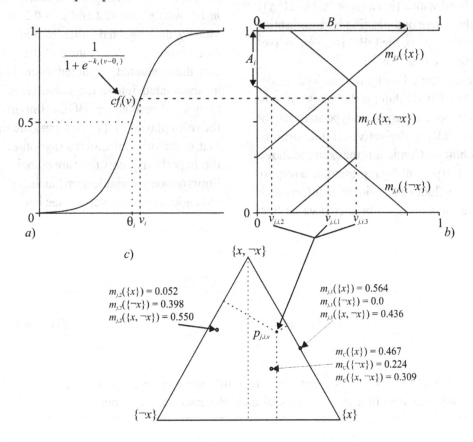

sation problem (see later), able to be solved using an evolutionary algorithm such as Trigonometric Differential Evolution (TDE - Storn & Price 1997, Fan & Lampinen 2003). In summary, TDE is an evolutionary algorithm that iteratively generates improved solutions to an optimization problem through the marginal changes in previous solutions with the differences in pairs of other previous solutions.

The effectiveness of a configured CaRBS system is measured by a defined objective function (used in the TDE process), whether for classification-type or regression-type analyses. With CaRBS (classification-type analyses), an objective function, defined OBC, uses the equivalence classes, $E(x)$ and $E(\neg x)$, the groups of respondents known to be associated with x and $\neg x$, respectively. The optimum solution, based on the respondent BOEs $m_j(\cdot)$ here, is to maximise the difference values $(m_j(\{x\}) - m_j(\{\neg x\}))$ and $(m_j(\{\neg x\}) - m_j(\{x\}))$ depending on where the considered respondent R_j is associated with x (in $E(x)$) or $\neg x$ (in $E(\neg x)$), respectively, where optimisation is minimisation with lower limit zero, the OBC is given by (see Beynon, 2005b): (see Box 2)

Also demonstrated in Figure 1c is the development of the CaRBS technique that allows it to be considered a tool for regression-type analysis, the proposed RCaRBS derivative of the original CaRBS technique. Continuing the example above, the BOE $m_C(\cdot)$ (potentially representing a respondent BOE), includes the evidential information to calculate the associated predicted value over the domain ranging from $\neg x$ to x (as would be found from a regression analysis), where each respondent R_j has an actual known value in this domain. Returning to Figure 1c, this predicted value is found by projecting the associated simplex coordinate for $m_C(\cdot)$ onto the base line of the simplex plot (projected using a line from the $\{x, \neg x\}$ vertex through the simplex coordinate of $m_C(\cdot)$). Representing the simplex coordinate of $m_C(\cdot)$ as (x_C, y_C), and considering an equilateral triangle of unit side (as previously), the projected value is given by $(\sqrt{3} x_C - y_C)/(\sqrt{3} - 2y_C)$, over a domain 0 to 1.

The projected value evaluated for each respondent, found this way, is considered their respective predicted value, defined Rp_j (in keeping with the use of the equilateral triangle with unit side in RCaRBS, the original strategic consensus values (see later), are *a priori* formatted into the same 0 to 1 domain - through normalization, see Kim, 1999). For the example considered here, using $m_C(\cdot)$, with $x_C = 0.622$ and $y_C = 0.268$ found previously, the projected value from $m_C(\cdot)$ is 0.6758 (see Figure 1c). One feature of this projection is that the evaluated predicted value is devoid of an associated ignorance value (existing in the associated respondent BOE). Importantly also, the roles played by $\{x\}$ and $\{\neg x\}$ are different to that in the original CaRBS (hypothesis and not-the-hypothesis), now they are associated with the limits on some variable term (such as a continuous strategic consensus value - see later).

Box 2.

$$\text{OBC} = \frac{1}{4}\left(\frac{1}{|E(x)|}\sum_{R_j \in E(x)}(1 - m_j(\{x\}) + m_j(\{\neg x\})) + \frac{1}{|E(\neg x)|}\sum_{R_j \in E(\neg x)}(1 + m_j(\{x\}) - m_j(\{\neg x\}))\right),$$

in the limit, $0 \leq OB \leq 1$. It is noted, maximising a difference value such as $(m_j(\{x\}) - m_j(\{\neg x\}))$ minimises classification ambiguity but only indirectly the associated ignorance.

As with the original CaRBS, the required configuration of a RCaRBS model depends on the assignment of values to the incumbent control variables $(k_i, \theta_i, A_i$ and $B_i, i = 1, \ldots, n_C)$. In RCaRBS, this configuration is defined by minimizing the error between the respective actual and predicted strategic consensus values (through its objective function - defined OBR). The specific measure (OBR) employed will focus on using the well known sum of squares error term, see Radhakrishnan and Nandan (2005). With the respondents' actual strategic consensus values Rv_j $(j = 1, \ldots, n_O)$, and respective predicted values Rp_j from a RCaRBS configured model, the fit is measured by OBR $= \sum_j (Rv_j - Rp_j)^2$.

With closed domains also defined on the individual control variables present in RCaRBS, the minimization of OBR similarly becomes a constrained optimization problem, solved here again using the evolutionary computation algorithm TDE. The necessary operating parameters used throughout this chapter with TDE, were (*ibid.*): amplification control $F = 0.99$, crossover constant $CR = 0.85$ and number of parameter vectors $NP = 200$.

MAIN THRUST

This section outlines the main thrust of this chapter, namely the exposition of the CaRBS (and RCaRBS) technique in the data mining analysis of an organization research problem, in this case the antecedents of intra-organizational consensus on strategic priorities.

Strategic consensus is a key issue within the literature on strategic management (see Kellermanns *et al.*, 2005). Intra-organizational agreement on strategic priorities is a vital resource for senior managers seeking to reap the benefits of cooperation and coordination for organizational performance (Bourgeois, 1980, 1985; Dess, 1987;

Homburg *et al.*, 1999). The benefits of consensus may be especially significant for government organizations, since they are often required to meet multiple and often conflicting goals that place great demands on the need for close collaborative working relationships (Moore, 1995). Indeed, theory and evidence has grown on the role of intra-organizational behaviour and strategic planning and management in public organizations (see for example, Boyne and Walker, 2004; Bryson, 2004). However, although much has been written about the hypothesised benefits of intra-organizational consensus in the private sector, little is yet known about its antecedents or how it might best be analysed in either the public or private sectors. In particular, few researchers have systematically evaluated the correlates of "vertical" consensus across different managerial levels, rather than "horizontal" consensus within top management teams, and to date none have drawn upon uncertain modelling techniques.

Principal agent models of managerial decision-making indicate that top management is likely to seek agents who share the same values and priorities. In other words, senior managers in public organizations will seek to establish alignment on strategic priorities across the organization to minimize the potential for shirking amongst middle managers. To achieve consensus on strategic priorities, the most effective managerial choices might be to centralize the decision-making of the organization, formalize the role and responsibilities of staff and introduce systematic planning processes thereby obviating the need to expend significant time and resources to gain a high level of alignment. These choices may be even more important when organizations confront a high degree of environmental uncertainty, as they can reduce the transaction costs associated with generating a coordinated response to difficult operating conditions. Indeed, contingency theory also suggests that the degree of consensus on strategic priorities, present within organizations, is likely to be positively related to centralization and formal planning processes, while perceived environmental uncertainty is associated with dissensus on strategic priorities (Dess and Origer, 1987).

Evidence on this issue is so far sparse and has been restricted to studies of "horizontal" consensus amongst top management teams within private firms, principally in North America (e.g. Priem, 1990). By applying an uncertain modelling approach, such as CaRBS and RCaRBS, to the issue of "vertical" consensus between senior and middle managers within the public sector, we therefore seek to introduce a novel technique for data mining within organizational research, and provide initial exploratory findings on an important but under-researched topic within the field.

Consensus Data Set

The consensus data set is drawn from a questionnaire survey gauging managers' views on strategic management within a large urban local government in Wales. Welsh local governments are governed by elected bodies with a Westminster-style cabinet system of political management, in which the cabinet represents the *de facto* executive branch of government, and is usually made up of senior members of the ruling political party. They operate in specific geographical areas, employ professional career staff, and receive approximately two-thirds of their income from the central government. The local government analysed here is a multipurpose authority providing education, social care, environmental services (such as land use planning and waste management), housing, and leisure and cultural services. By focusing on a single local government, we are able to draw on a more comprehensive coverage of managers throughout an organization than would be possible using a sample of several governments. In doing so, we follow Meyer *et al.*' (1993) argument that researchers should pay more serious attention to the micro-level determinants of intra-organizational behaviour.

Data on strategic management in our sample organization are derived from an electronic survey of top and middle managers within the local government conducted in autumn 2002. The survey explored informants' perceptions of organization, management and performance (a copy of the full questionnaire is available on request from the authors). Survey respondents were asked a series of questions assessing strategy, structure, process and environment in the organization. For each question, informants placed the organization on a seven-point Likert scale ranging from 1 (strongly disagree with the statement) to 7 (strongly agree with the statement). The sampling frame consisted of 82 informants within five major service departments and the top management team of the organization. Responses were received from 49 per cent of individual informants (40 – 2 members of the top management team and 38 middle managers).

In this study, the priority accorded to Miles and Snow's (1978) defending strategy is investigated. Empirical studies have indicated that defending is often a successful strategy in the public sector (e.g. Andrews *et al.*, 2009; Meier *et al.*, 2007). Defending organizations typically take a conservative view of innovation, focusing on service quality and devoting 'primary attention to improving the efficiency of their existing operations' (Miles and Snow 1978, p. 29). To explore the extent to which our study organization displayed defender characteristics, informants were asked three questions: "we seek to maintain stable service priorities"; "the service emphasizes efficiency of provision"; and "we focus on our core activities". These questions were all based on prior work (Snow and Hrebiniak, 1980; Miller, 1986). To capture the complex multi-dimensional nature of strategic management, a single defending index was then created for the purposes of our analysis (from the three questions).

To gauge the relative degree of consensus on a strategy of defending within the study organization we take the absolute value of the distance between

Table 2. Descriptive statistics for defending and consensus on defending

Description	Mean	Std dev
We seek to maintain stable service priorities	2.9211	1.1942
The service emphasizes efficiency of provision	3.0263	1.5680
We focus on our core activities	2.6842	1.1415
Consensus on defending	8.8435	.7392

each middle manager's perceptions of defending within the organization from that held by the two top managers. The resulting consensus measure for the middle managers was subtracted from 10 to ensure that a higher score indicated greater consensus with the priority accorded to defending by top management. Even though the decision variable of consensus on a defending strategy is continuous in nature, here, it is also considered as a binary variable, through the discretisation of the variable. This discretisation is created by assigning the value of 0 where a respondent's strategy value is below the organizational mean and 1 where it is above the mean. Descriptive statistics for middle managers' perceptions of defending and their score on the measure of defending consensus are shown in Table 2.

In this study, eight organization characteristics are hypothesised to influence relative degree of consensus between middle and top management on a defending strategy, described here as respondents (middle managers) perceived organization characteristics. To control for the possibility that strategic priorities varied by service department within the local government, four dichotomous variables were included, coded 1 for each of the service departments in which respondents worked (education, social services, environment and leisure) and 0 otherwise (with housing the omitted category).

Centralized decision-making is arguably associated with higher levels of consensus. The relative degree of centralization within the organization was gauged by asking middle manager respondents whether: "strategy for our service is usually made by the head of service". Similarly, highly formalized job specifications are likely to tighten the link between the priorities of senior and middle managers. By contrast, if middle managers enjoy significant levels of job autonomy it is conceivable that consensus is more difficult to achieve. This was evaluated by simply asking middle manager respondents if they experienced: "a great deal of autonomy". Systematic step-by-step procedures for the formulation of strategic decisions can reduce the potential for divergent views to emerge, thereby bolstering levels of intra-organizational consensus. To assess the presence of rational planning processes, the following question was posed to middle managers: "targets in the service are matched to specifically identified citizen needs". Finally, to assess the extent to which perceived environmental uncertainty influenced consensus, middle manager respondents were asked if: "the socio-economic context is unpredictable". Table 3 presents a brief description of the respondent (middle manager) perceived organization characteristics and concomitant descriptive statistics (used later in the CaRBS and RCaRBS analyses).

CaRBS Analysis

This section undertakes a CaRBS analysis of the previously described strategic consensus data set. The CaRBS analysis is to undertake binary classification optimisation using the defined objective function OBC (previously defined). The utilisation of the objective function OBC in the configuration of the CaRBS system is to directly minimize the level of ambiguity present in the classification of managers (respondents) within the organization to their association to strategic consensus and not-consensus, but not the concomitant ignorance (binary classification with ignorance using CaRBS).

To configure a CaRBS system through the minimization of the respective OBC, the respon-

Table 3. Description of respondents (middle manager) perceived organization characteristics and concomitant descriptive statistics

Characteristic	Description	Mean	Std dev
C1	Education dummy variable	0.2368	0.4251
C2	Social services dummy variable	0.1579	0.3646
C3	Environment dummy variable	0.1842	0.3877
C4	Leisure dummy variable	0.2368	0.4251
C5	HoS makes strategy	3.3421	1.5774
C6	Great deal of autonomy	3.2368	1.3462
C7	Targets matched to citizen needs	3.5789	1.5497
C8	Environmental uncertainty	5.1053	1.5354

Table 4. Control variables values associated with respondent perceived organization characteristics, using OBC in configuration of CaRBS system

Char.	C1	C2	C3	C4	C5	C6	C7	C8
k_i	−2.869	−3.000	−3.000	3.000	3.000	3.000	3.000	−3.000
θ_i	0.760	−1.476	−1.801	−1.557	0.454	−0.451	0.153	−0.441
A_i	0.252	0.958	0.982	0.953	0.954	0.331	0.776	0.247
B_i	0.596	0.600	0.600	0.600	0.600	0.600	0.600	0.600

dent perceived organization characteristic values were standardized (using the descriptive statistics in Table 3), prior to the employment of TDE (see later), allowing consistent domains over the control variables incumbent in CaRBS, set as; $-3 \le k_i \le 3$, $-2 \le \theta_i \le 2$, $0 \le A_i < 1$ and $B_i < 0.6$ (see Beynon, 2005b). The upper bound on the B_i control variables ensured a predominance of ignorance in the evidence from individual characteristic values (in the concomitant characteristic BOEs), so reduced over-conflict during the combination of the pieces of evidence (combination of characteristic BOEs).

The TDE method was employed, based on the previously defined TDE-based parameters, and run five times, each time converging to an optimum value, the best out of the five runs being OBC = 0.304. A reason for this value being away from its lower bound of zero is related to the implicit minimum levels of ignorance associated with each characteristic BOE (fixing of the upper

bounds of B_i control variables), possibly also due to the presence of conflicting evidence from the characteristics. The resultant CaRBS associated control variables found from the best TDE run are reported in Table 4.

A brief inspection of these results shows the near uniformity in the k_i control variables, with the majority of the absolute values near the limit of 3.000 (positive and negative), the exception being with C1. This exhibits the attempt to offer most discernment between the hypothesis (strategy consensus) and its complement (strategy not-consensus), in the evidence from the respondent perceived organization characteristics (see Figure 1 and definition of confidence factor $cf_i(\cdot)$). The role of these defined control variable values is to allow the construction of characteristic BOEs and their subsequent combination to formulate a series of respondent BOEs for the 38 respondents considered.

Table 5. Characteristic values and characteristic BOEs for the respondents, R_1 and R_{31}, using OBC in configuration of CaRBS system

BOE	C1	C2	C3	C4	C5	C6	C7	C8
R_1 (actual)	1	0	0	0	7	6	7	7
R_1 (standardized)	1.795	−0.433	−0.475	−0.557	2.319	2.053	2.208	1.234
$m_{1,i}(\{C\})$	0.000	0.000	0.000	0.000	0.600	0.591	0.533	0.000
$m_{1,i}(\{\neg C\})$	0.557	0.000	0.000	0.000	0.000	0.000	0.000	0.595
$m_{1,i}(\{C, \neg C\})$	0.443	1.000	1.000	1.000	0.400	0.409	0.467	0.405
R_{31} (actual)	0	1	0	0	3	3	2	6
R_{31} (standardized)	−0.557	2.309	−0.475	−0.557	−0.217	−0.175	−1.019	0.583
$m_{31,i}(\{C\})$	0.578	0.000	0.000	0.000	0.303	0.000	0.000	0.000
$m_{31,i}(\{\neg C\})$	0.000	0.600	0.000	0.000	0.000	0.000	0.444	0.565
$m_{31,i}(\{C, \neg C\})$	0.422	0.400	1.000	1.000	0.697	1.000	0.556	0.435

The construction of a characteristic BOE is next demonstrated, considering the respondent R_1 and the organization characteristic C1. Starting with the evaluation of the confidence factor $cf_{C1}(\cdot)$ (see Figure 1a), for the respondent R_1, C1 = 1.000, when standardised, it is $v = 1.795$ (see Table 5 presented later), then;

$$cf_{C1}(1.795) = \frac{1}{1 + e^{2.869(1.795 - 0.760)}} = \frac{1}{1 + 19.505}$$
$$= 0.049,$$

using the control variables in Table 4. This confidence value is used in the expressions making up the mass values in the characteristic BOE $m_{1,C1}(\cdot)$, namely; $m_{1,C1}(\{C\})$, $m_{1,C1}(\{\neg C\})$ and $m_{1,C1}(\{C, \neg C\})$, found to be;

$$m_{1,C1}(\{C\}) = \frac{0.596}{1 - 0.252}0.049 - \frac{0.252 \times 0.596}{1 - 0.252}$$
$$= 0.039 - 0.201 = -0.162 < 0.000 \text{ so} = 0.000,$$

$$m_{1,C1}(\{\neg C\}) = \frac{-0.596}{1 - 0.252}0.049 + 0.596 =$$
$$-0.039 + 0.596 = 0.557,$$

$$m_{1,C1}(\{C, \neg C\}) = 1 - 0.000 - 0.557 = 0.443.$$

For the respondent R_1, this characteristic BOE is representative of all the associated characteristic BOEs $m_{1,i}(\cdot)$, presented in Table 5 (using standardised characteristic values), along with those for the respondent R_{31}. These characteristic BOEs describe the evidential support from all the perceived organization characteristic values, associated with a respondent, to the overall intra-organizational strategic consensus or strategic not-consensus classification (R_1 and R_{31}, are known to exhibit consensus and not-consensus with the top management team's perspective on defending, respectively).

In Table 5, for the evidence from the characteristics to support correct classification of the respondent R_1, in this case to strategic consensus ($\{C\}$), it would be expected for the $m_{1,i}(\{C\})$ mass values to be larger than their respective $m_{1,i}(\{\neg C\})$ mass values, which is the case for the characteristics, C5, C6 and C7. Whereas, C1 and C8, offer more evidence towards the respondent having not-consensus, and C2, C3 and C4 only total ignorance. The predominance of characteristic BOEs supporting correct classification (of those giving evidence), is reflected in the final

Figure 2. Simplex coordinates of characteristic and respondent BOEs for R_1 and R_{31}, using OBC in configuration of CaRBS system

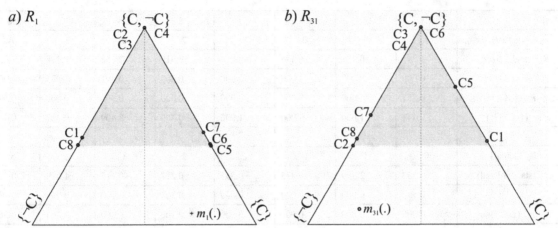

respondent BOE $m_1(\cdot)$ produced (through the combination of all the characteristic BOEs), which has mass values $m_1(\{C\}) = 0.684$, $m_1(\{\neg C\}) = 0.259$ and $m_1(\{C, \neg C\}) = 0.057$. This respondent BOE, with $m_1(\{C\}) = 0.684 > 0.259 = m_1(\{\neg C\})$, suggests the respondent R_1 is more associated with strategic consensus, which is the correct classification in this case.

For the respondent R_{31}, the evidence from the characteristics is more towards their strategic not-consensus (in particular C2, C7 and C8). The combination of the concomitant characteristic BOEs produces a respondent BOE $m_{31}(\cdot)$, with $m_{31}(\{C\}) = 0.189$, $m_{31}(\{\neg C\}) = 0.733$ and $m_{31}(\{C, \neg C\}) = 0.079$, which indicates majority association to strategic not-consensus ($\{\neg C\}$), which is correct in this case. For further interpretation of the characteristic and respondent BOEs associated with the respondents, R_1 and R_{31}, their representations as simplex coordinates in a simplex plot are reported in Figure 2.

Figures 2a and 2b, offer a visual representation of the evidence from the eight perceived organization characteristics to the classification of the respondents, R_1 and R_{31}, as to whether they approximate strategic consensus (C) or not-consensus (¬C). In each simplex plot the dashed vertical line partitions the regions in a simplex plot where either of the mass values assigned to $\{\neg C\}$ (to the left) and $\{C\}$ (to the right) is the larger in a BOE. The grey shaded sub-regions show the domains where the characteristic BOEs can exist (due to the bounds on B_i control variables).

In both presented simplex plots, the simplex coordinates of the final respondent BOEs, $m_1(\cdot)$ and $m_{31}(\cdot)$, are nearer their base lines than those of the associated characteristic BOEs. This is solely due to the reduction of ignorance from the combination of evidence present in the characteristic BOEs (see also Table 5). The positions of the simplex coordinates of the characteristic BOEs allow their possibly supporting and conflicting support for correct (or incorrect) classification of the respondents to be clearly identified (compare with discussion of characteristic BOEs associated with respondent R_1).

The process of positioning the classification of a respondent, in a simplex plot, on the strategic consensus, can be undertaken for each of the 38 respondents considered, see Figure 3.

Figures 3a and 3b partition the presentation of the respondents' respondent BOEs between those known to be more associated with being strategic not-consensus (3a) and consensus (3b),

Figure 3. Simplex plot based representation of final respondent BOEs, using OBC in configuration of CaRBS system

a) Not-Consensus {C, ¬C}   b) Consensus   {C, ¬C}

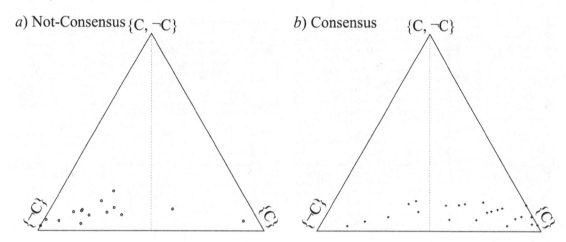

where each respondent BOE is labelled with a circle and cross, respectively. Based on their simplex coordinate respondent BOE positions either side of the vertical dashed lines in the simplex plots in Figure 3, it was found 13 out of 15 (86.666%) and 17 out of 23 (73.913%) respondents were correctly classified as strategic not-consensus (¬C) and consensus (C), respectively. This combines to a total of 78.947% classification accuracy.

Consideration of the contribution of the individual respondent perceived organization characteristics can be graphically gauged from combining stages *a* and *b* in Figure 1, for the individual characteristics C1, ..., C8, see Figure 4.

In Figure 4, each graph shows the explicit mass values which make up a characteristic BOE, based on the individual characteristic values from respondents. From the description of the respondent perceived organization characteristics considered, see Table 3, C1 to C4 are dummy variables (denoted here by 0 and 1 values - see later), C5 to C8 are based on Likert values, here shown over the minimum and maximum values shown in the strategic consensus data set (of respondents).

For the characteristic C1 (Education dummy variable), the interpretation is that a respondent value of 0 or 1 offers evidence towards strategic consensus and not-consensus respectively (as well as a level of ignorance). The thin lines show the actual continuous movements of the underlying functional forms of the mass values (see Figure 1). For the characteristics, C2, C3 and C4, the functional forms towards the evaluation of the mass values are the same, with a value 0 offering only ignorance, and a 1 value offering more evidential support to being strategic not-consensus from C2 and C3 and strategic consensus from C4. These findings suggest that the priority attached to defending by middle managers in education, social services and environmental services is more likely to diverge from the top management team than their counterparts in housing and leisure services. More detailed investigation of the management strategies in each service department could reveal whether this reflects service-specific considerations.

For the characteristics described by Likert-based valued responses (C5 to C8), the graphs range over the domains of response values given amongst the 38 respondents. For C5, as the value goes from 1 up to 2 there is decreasing evidence towards strategic not-consensus, and for the values 3 up to 7 there is increasing evidence towards

Figure 4. Contribution graphs for organization characteristic values in terms of their characteristic BOEs, for, C1, ..., C8 (using OBC in configuration of CaRBS system)

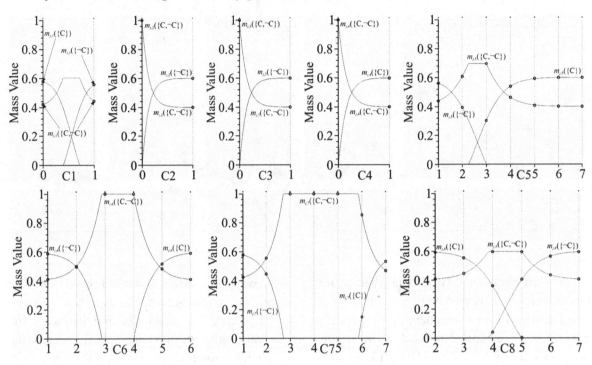

strategic consensus (with the concomitant level of ignorance changing accordingly). This confirms our hypotheses that centralization is positively associated with strategic consensus. Similarly, the graphs for C7 and C8 confirm the arguments that planning is positively related to consensus, but that environmental uncertainty has the opposite relationship. However, the graph for C6 suggests that managerial autonomy may be positively rather than negatively related to consensus as expected. It is conceivable that middle managers in government organizations may have an in-built tendency to share top managers' views on the significance of a defending strategy. Investigation of the relationship between managerial autonomy and consensus on alternative strategic priorities (e.g. an innovative strategy of prospecting) could therefore throw further light on this important topic. In summary, the directions of contributions of the characteristics, follow the signs of the k_i values in Table 4.

RCaRBS Analysis

This section undertakes an RCaRBS analysis of the strategic consensus data set. Rather than thinking in terms of the binary classification of respondents to strategic consensus and not-consensus, the continuous consensus values associated with the respondents are normalised over the domain 0 to 1, signifying a level of strategic consensus (now from not-consensus (0) up to consensus (1)). This highlights how CaRBS can be adapted for use with the continuous variables most commonly found in organizational research.

The utilisation of the objective function OBR in the configuration of the RCaRBS system is to minimise the predictive error ('sums of squares error') between the predicted and actual levels of strategic consensus of the respondents. The same consistent domains over the control variables incumbent in CaRBS were used, set as; $-3 \leq k_i \leq 3$, $-2 \leq \theta_i \leq 2$, $0 \leq A_i < 1$ and $B_i < 0.6$ (see Beynon,

Table 6. Control variable values associated with respondent perceived organization characteristics, using OBR in configuration of RCaRBS system

Char.	C1	C2	C3	C4	C5	C6	C7	C8
k_i	−2.128	2.238	−2.001	2.598	3.000	3.000	2.975	−3.000
θ_i	−0.350	−1.779	1.783	0.206	−0.556	0.937	0.482	−0.317
A_i	0.721	0.648	0.777	0.912	0.689	0.247	0.988	0.444
B_i	0.568	0.128	0.363	0.306	0.461	0.380	0.600	0.281

Figure 5. Simplex coordinates of characteristic and respondent BOEs for R_1 and R_{31}, using OBR in configuration of RCaRBS system

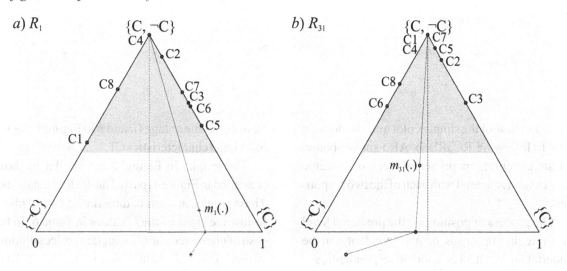

2005b). The TDE method was again employed based on the previously defined parameters and run five times, each time converging to an optimum value, the best out of the five runs being OBR = 1.444. The resultant control variable values found from the best TDE run, using OBR, are reported in Table 6.

A brief inspection of these results shows a lack of consistency in any of the sets of parameters across the different characteristics. In the case of the k_i variable values, this is in contrast to the same absolute values consistently found in the initial CaRBS analysis. The variations in the other control variable values (again those in the CaRBS analysus), are most appropriately considered in the resultant characteristic BOEs found for the respondents.

The characteristic BOEs describe the evidential support from all the organization characteristics to a respondent's level of consensus (respondents, R_1 and R_{31}, are known to have 0.683 and 0.137 levels of strategic consensus (normalised values), respectively). The interpretation of the characteristic and respondent BOEs associated with the respondents, R_1 and R_{31}, is undertaken here only through their representation as simplex coordinates in a simplex plot, and subsequent mapping to single predicted values, see Figure 5.

Figures 5a and 5b, offer a visual representation of the evidence from the characteristics to the regression-type analysis of the respondents, R_1 and R_{31}. In each simplex plot the contribution of the characteristics BOEs is shown, along with the respective respondent BOE, and its mapping down

Figure 6. Simplex plot based representation of final respondent BOEs, and subsequent mappings, using OBR in configuration of RCaRBS system

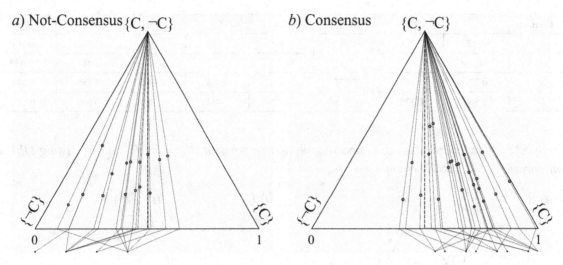

a) Not-Consensus $\{C, \neg C\}$ *b)* Consensus $\{C, \neg C\}$

to the base line of the simplex plot over the domain 0 to 1 (following RCaRBS). Also shown below the simplex plots are the actual levels of strategic consensus associated with each of the two respondents.

The process of positioning the predicted level of strategic consensus of a respondent can be undertaken for all 38 considered respondents, see Figure 6 (respondents partitioned based on having actual levels of strategic consensus less than or greater than 0.5 - in terms of their standardised values).

In Figure 6, the respondent BOEs of the 38 respondents are mapped to the base of the simplex plots, giving their predicted level of strategic consensus, and below them their actual levels of strategic consensus. Inspection of the two simplex plots shows the general trend of the predicted levels of strategic consensus are to the left and right in Figures *6a* and *6b* for respondents with actual levels of strategic consensus less than or greater than 0.5.

Consideration of the contribution of the individual characteristics can be graphically gauged

from combining stages *a* and *b* in Figure 1, for the individual characteristics C1, ..., C8, see Figure 7.

The graphs in Figure 7 are similar to those presented in Figure 4 (part of the CaRBS analysis). These graphs, in terms of direction of contribution, follow the signs of the k_i values in Table 6. In the case of characteristic C2 (Social services dummy variable), the k_i values found in the CaRBS (−3.000) and RCaRBS (2.238) analyses are of different sign. However, in the case of the RCaRBS analysis, the low A_i value means particular predominance of ignorance across its domain of evidence. Despite this minor inconsistency, the findings for the perceived organizational characteristics are broadly the same as those presented for the CaRBS analysis,

FUTURE TRENDS

The future trends associated with inference from the work in this chapter are twofold. Firstly there is the potential for the continued technical development of evidence-based data mining techniques. In particular, the CaRBS and RCaRBS analyses

Figure 7. Contribution graphs for organization characteristic values in terms of their characteristic BOEs, for, C1, ..., C8 (using OBR in configuration of RCaRBS system)

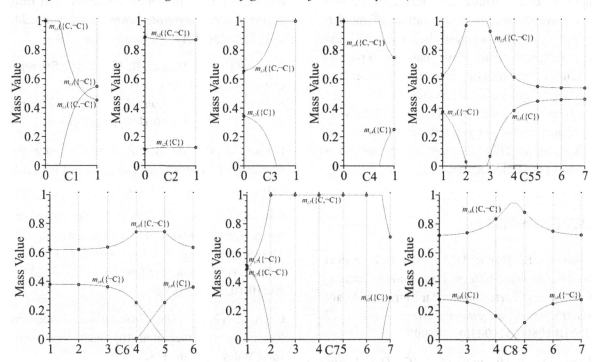

presented here, with their fundamentals based on the Dempster-Shafer theory, furnish a good example of how such novel non-parametric approaches may reveal new insights in a host of areas where data mining is an important consideration.

Secondly, there is scope for greater application of CaRBS and related techniques to other relevant issues in organizational research. To date, studies of organizational behaviour and outcomes have predominantly drawn on parametric techniques such as multiple regressions. Indeed, even relatively established non-parametric techniques, like neural networks, have had only limited impact in this field.

This chapter therefore represents an important response to the growing clamour for the introduction of novel and innovative alternatives to conventional approaches to data mining and analysis within organization and management science.

CONCLUSION

The acquisition of data-based knowledge is essential in organizational research; nowhere more so than in studies of public and governmental organizations. By providing vital information on the interrelationships between key organizational variables, data mining can enable public policy-makers and managers to address the implications of organizing within the complex networked settings in which they increasingly operate. Indeed, given heightened governmental interest shown in strategic planning in the public sector (see Bryson, 2004), the preliminary analysis presented here illustrates how organizational design has important implications for strategic management in public organizations.

However, despite calls for more use of unconventional techniques to explore organizational data across the public and private sectors, as yet, the prevalence of Gaussian regression based forms of analysis, has restricted the impact of data mining approaches within the field of organizational studies. Nevertheless, as the limitations of standard linear regression analysis become ever more apparent, it is highly likely that a more positive attitude towards notion of data mining will emerge amongst organizational researchers.

It is hoped that this chapter offers some evidence on the, as yet, untapped potential for uncertain modelling of organizational behaviour to move the field forward.

REFERENCES

Andrews, R., Boyne, G. A., Law, J., & Walker, R. M. (2009). Strategy Formulation, Strategy Content and Performance: An Empirical Analysis. *Public Management Review*, *11*(1), 1–22. doi:10.1080/14719030802489989

Berry, M. J. A., & Linoff, G. (1997). *Data Mining Techniques for Marketing, Sales, and Customer Support*. New York: Wiley.

Beynon, M. J. (2005a). A Novel Technique of Object Ranking and Classification under Ignorance: An Application to the Corporate Failure Risk Problem. *European Journal of Operational Research*, *167*, 493–517. doi:10.1016/j.ejor.2004.03.016

Beynon, M. J. (2005b). A Novel Approach to the Credit Rating Problem: Object Classification Under Ignorance. *International Journal of Intelligent Systems in Accounting Finance & Management*, *13*, 113–130. doi:10.1002/isaf.260

Bourgeois, L. J. (1980). Performance and Consensus. *Strategic Management Journal*, *1*, 227–248. doi:10.1002/smj.4250010304

Bourgeois, L. J. III. (1985). Strategic goals, perceived uncertainty, and economic performance in volatile environments. *Academy of Management Journal*, *28*(3), 548–573. doi:10.2307/256113

Bowman, C., & Amrosini, V. (1997). Perceptions of strategic priorities, consensus and firm performance. *Journal of Management Studies*, *34*, 241–258. doi:10.1111/1467-6486.00050

Boyne, G. A., & Walker, R. M. (2004). Strategy content and public service organizations. *Journal of Public Administration: Research and Theory*, *14*(2), 231–252. doi:10.1093/jopart/muh015

Bryson, J. M. (2004). *Strategic Planning for Public and Nonprofit Organizations* (3rd ed.). San Francisco: Jossey-Bass.

Canongia Lopes, J. N. (2004). On the classification and representation of ternary phase diagrams: The yin and yang of a T–x approach. *Physical Chemistry Chemical Physics*, *6*, 2314–2319. doi:10.1039/b315799g

Chen, Z. (2001). Data Mining and Uncertain Reasoning: An Integrated Approach. New York: John Wiley & Sons, US.

De Mantores, R. L. (1990). *Approximate Reasoning Models*. Chichester, UK: Ellis Horwood.

Dempster, A. P. (1967). Upper and lower probabilities induced by a multiple valued mapping. *Annals of Mathematical Statistics*, *38*, 325–339. doi:10.1214/aoms/1177698950

Dempster, A. P. (2008). The Dempster-Shafer Calculus for Statisticians. *International Journal of Approximate Reasoning*, *48*, 365–377. doi:10.1016/j.ijar.2007.03.004

Dess, G. G. (1987). Consensus on strategy formulation and organizational performance: competitors in a fragmented industry. *Strategic Management Journal*, *8*(3), 259–277. doi:10.1002/smj.4250080305

Dess, G. G., & Origer, N. K. (1987). Environment, structure, and consensus in strategy formulation: a conceptual integration. *Academy of Management Review*, *12*(2), 313–330. doi:10.2307/258538

DeTienne, K. B., DeTienne, D. H., & Joshi, S. A. (2003). Neural networks as statistical tools for business researchers. *Organizational Research Methods, 6*, 236–265. doi:10.1177/1094428103251907

Dutton, J. E., Fahey, L., & Narayanan, V. K. (1983). Toward understanding strategic issue diagnosis. *Strategic Management Journal, 4*(4), 307–323. doi:10.1002/smj.4250040403

Fan, H.-Y., & Lampinen, J. (2003). A Trigonometric Mutation Operation to Differential Evolution. *Journal of Global Optimization, 27*, 105–129. doi:10.1023/A:1024653025686

Hart, S., & Banbury, C. (1994). How Strategy-making Processes can make a Difference. *Strategic Management Journal, 15*(3), 251–269. doi:10.1002/smj.4250150402

Homburg, C., Krohmer, H., & Workman, J. P. Jr. (1999). Strategic consensus and performance: the role of strategy type and market-related dynamism. *Strategic Management Journal, 20*(4), 339–357. doi:10.1002/(SICI)1097-0266(199904)20:4<339::AID-SMJ29>3.0.CO;2-T

Kellermanns, F. W., Walter, J., Lechner, C., & Floyd, S. W. (2005). The Lack of Consensus about Strategic Consensus: Advancing Theory and Research. *Journal of Management, 31*, 719–737. doi:10.1177/0149206305279114

Kim, D. (1999). Normalization methods for input and output vectors in backpropogation neural networks. *International Journal of Computer Mathematics, 71*(2), 161–171. doi:10.1080/00207169908804800

Meier, K. J., O'Toole, L. J. Jr, Boyne, G. A., & Walker, R. M. (2007). Strategic management and the performance of public organizations: testing venerable ideas against recent theories. *Journal of Public Administration: Research and Theory, 17*(3), 357–377. doi:10.1093/jopart/mul017

Meilich, O. (2006). Bivariate models of fit in contingency theory: Critique and a polynomial regression alternative. *Organizational Research Methods, 9*, 161–193. doi:10.1177/1094428105284915

Meyer, A. D., Tsui, A. S., & Hinings, C. R. (1993). Configurational approaches to organizational analysis. *Academy of Management Journal, 36*(6), 1175–1195. doi:10.2307/256809

Miles, R., & Snow, C. (1978). *Organizational Strategy, Structure and Process.* London: McGraw Hill.

Miller, D. (1986). Configurations of Strategy and Structure: Towards a Synthesis. *Strategic Management Journal, 7*(3), 233–249. doi:10.1002/smj.4250070305

Moore, M. H. (1995). *Creating public value: strategic management in government.* Cambridge, MA: Harvard University Press.

Murphy, C. K. (2000). Combining belief functions when evidence conflicts. *Decision Support Systems, 29*, 1–9. doi:10.1016/S0167-9236(99)00084-6

Priem, R. L. (1990). Top management team group factors, consensus, and firm performance. *Strategic Management Journal, 11*(6), 469–478. doi:10.1002/smj.4250110605

Radhakrishnan, T., & Nandan, U. (2005). Milling force prediction using regression and neural networks. *Journal of Intelligent Manufacturing, 16*, 93–102. doi:10.1007/s10845-005-4826-4

Roesmer, C. (2000). Nonstandard Analysis and Dempster-Shafer Theory. *International Journal of Intelligent Systems, 15*, 117–127. doi:10.1002/(SICI)1098-111X(200002)15:2<117::AID-INT2>3.0.CO;2-2

Safranek, R. J., Gottschlich, S., & Kak, A. C. (1990). Evidence Accumulation Using Binary Frames of Discernment for Verification Vision. *IEEE Transactions on Robotics and Automation, 6*, 405–417. doi:10.1109/70.59366

Schubert, J. (1994). Cluster-based specification techniques in Dempster-Shafer theory for an evidential intelligence analysis of multiple target tracks. Department of Numerical Analysis and Computer Science Royal Institute of technology, S-100 44 Stockholm, Sweden.

Shafer, G., & Srivastava, R. (1990). The Bayesian and belief-function formalisms: A general perspective for auditing. In Shafer, G., & Pearl, J. (Eds.), *Readings in Uncertain Reasoning*. San Mateo, CA: Morgan Kaufman Publishers, Inc.

Shafer, G. A. (1976). *Mathematical theory of Evidence*. Princeton, NJ: Princeton University Press.

Smets, P. (1990). The Combination of Evidence in the Transferable belief Model. *IEEE Transactions on Pattern Analysis and Machine Intelligence, 12*(5), 447–458. doi:10.1109/34.55104

Snow, C. C., & Hrebiniak, L. G. (1980). Strategy, Distinctive Competence, and Organizational Performance. *Administrative Science Quarterly, 25*(2), 317–336. doi:10.2307/2392457

Srivastava, R. P., & Liu, L. (2003). Applications of Belief Functions in Business Decisions: A Review. *Information Systems Frontiers, 5*(4), 359–378. doi:10.1023/B:ISFI.0000005651.93751.4b

Storn, R., & Price, K. (1997). Differential Evolution – A simple and Efficient Heuristic for Global Optimization over Continuous Spaces. *Journal of Global Optimization, 11*, 341–359. doi:10.1023/A:1008202821328

Westphal, C., & Blaxton, T. (1998). *Data Mining Solutions: Methods and Tools for Solving real-World Problems*. New York: Wiley.

Yang, J.-B., Liu, J., Wang, J., Sii, H.-S., & Wong, H.-W. (2006). Belief Rule-Base Inference Methodology Using the Evidential Reasoning Approach—RIMER. *IEEE Transactions on Systems, Man, and Cybernetics. Part A, Systems and Humans, 36*(2), 266–285. doi:10.1109/TSMCA.2005.851270

Zadeh, L. A. (1975). Fuzzy Logic and Approximate Reasoning (In Memory of Grigore Moisel). *Synthese, 30*, 407–428. doi:10.1007/BF00485052

KEY TERMS AND DEFINITIONS

Confidence Factor: A function to transform a value into a standard domain, such as between 0 and 1.

Equivalence Class: Set of objects considered the same subject to an equivalence relation (e.g. those objects classified to x).

Evolutionary Algorithm: An algorithm that incorporates aspects of natural selection or survival of the fittest.

Focal Element: A finite non-empty set of hypotheses.

Mass Values: A positive function of the level of exact belief in the associated proposition (focal element).

Objective Function: A positive function of the difference between predictions and data estimates that are chosen so as to optimize the function or criterion.

Simplex Plot: Equilateral triangle domain representation of triplets of non-negative values which sum to one.

Uncertain Modelling: The attempt to represent uncertainty and reason about it when using uncertain knowledge, imprecise information, etc.

Chapter 15
Data Mining in the Context of Business Network Research

Jukka Aaltonen
University of Lapland, Finland

Annamari Turunen
University of Lapland, Finland

Ilkka Kamaja
University of Lapland, Finland

ABSTRACT

In the field of information technology (IT) enabled business networks and research the traditional data mining approach is theoretically and practically inadequate for knowledge eliction and management requirements in inter-organizational collaborative business environments. The issues are mostly related to fundamentally and philosophically narrow conceptions of the meaning of information, and are grounded to the metatheoretical implications of positivistic, nomothetic and objective view of reality that restricts the feasibility of research oriented application based on them. Here a novel research framework for network-wide knowledge discovery is presented that is based on sociologically anti-positivistic, ideographic and subjective view of society construed from social facts. The theoretical framework is further developed here by synthesizing it with and extracting results from existing research models and artefacts originated in analyzing a variety of business networks (for example, a case study concentrating on modeling the IT enabled service provision of local travel industry value chain). The main contribution here is the explication and elaboration of existing and emerging business network research theories and related stakeholder-level practical considerations focusing on topics such as: multidisciplinary research conceptualizations, information asymmetry reduction by benefiting from contract law oriented functional principles, and network-wide knowledge governance approaches.

DOI: 10.4018/978-1-60566-906-9.ch015

INTRODUCTION

Typically, commercial organizations pursue to find optimal ways to use, manage, administer, and share the critical business information owned by them. In its static form, information (or knowledge) can reside in various internal and external data sources. Traditional *data mining* then consists of techniques that enable the organization to utilize these data repositories (for example databases, data marts, or data warehouses) to support timely access to relevant information (*business intelligence*) and to extract new knowledge for business purposes. However, organizational knowledge also has a tacit and dynamic nature – especially in the context of inter-organizational (customer) relationships – that does not easily comply with the contemporary methods of knowledge discovery (KD). The same applies to the information content that many organizations (specifically SMEs) still have only in the form of unstructured, unorganized, and uncategorized (paper or electronic) business documents.

The intra-organizational and data-centered perspective to business information and data mining emerges mostly from objective and positivistic assumptions of reality. However, considering the nature of inter-organizational communications and information flows, it seems evident that there is a need for a more subjective, relativistic and anti-positivistic view in business and research.

Also, the multidisciplinary character of scientific work that concentrates on the complex phenomena of network-oriented knowledge discovery requires the application of appropriate methodologies and explicit and shared research conceptualizations. In the University of Lapland, a related example is an on-going two-year PROVEM-research project that concentrates on modeling and analyzing the service provision of a local travel industry network, which is examined through three partly overlapping research areas; customer value chains, knowledge management and information modeling, and the legal perspec-

tives of inter-organizational business relationships and agreements.

In addition to the above intrinsic limitation of the contemporary data mining approach, it is not very well applicable to tackling *information asymmetry*, especially in business networks based on customer-centric service provision. In the world of economy, problems arise when one party of a business transaction has more information than the other because this type of a situation has negative implications on business relationships based on trust and power (Aaltonen, 2007; Gratzer & Winiwarter, 2003). To enable the reduction of information asymmetry (Turunen, 2005), the mentioned travel industry network research is in a good position to develop frameworks based on organizational information modeling. These frameworks can be used to expand the traditional data mining paradigm by analyzing the characteristics of inter-organizational information flows and, for example, by specifying the preliminary requirements of the information-intensive governance of business relationships.

In order to address these complex phenomena, this chapter is organized as follows: the first section "Theoretical background" addresses the theoretical aspects of knowledge discovery research in business network context by introducing a novel information technology discipline and its philosophical base grounded on the idea of socially construed reality. The main contribution of this work is then presented in the section "Multilevel model for network-wide knowledge discovery" which first exposes the logical structure of traditional and here proposed novel KD-process by using the construct of sociological paradigms, then in the section "Multidisciplinary concept analysis of the domain area" the key terminology and the conceptual foundations of the main research areas (i.e. business networks, organizational IT and contract law) in the on-going business network project is depicted, and finally these constructs are combined in the section "Preliminary research framework" to an overall multilevel model and a research framework (a prerequisite for a related research program). The more practically oriented discussion about linkage of the developed model to the anti-positivistic characterization of inter-organizational business information, and information asymmetry reduction using functional principles in contract law is the topic in the section "Network-wide knowledge discovery and communicative information", which also contains an analysis of a information technology enabled travel industry network which is used to extract preliminary business requirements and discuss about the feasibility of the proposed model at stakeholder-level. Finally, in the section "Future trends and conclusion", the main themes of this chapter are projected as prospective future knowledge discovery trends and research enablers, and a concluding summary is given.

THEORETICAL BACKGROUND

The theoretical background of this work is based on the Discipline of Information Technology (DIT), a new science concept within information technology. (Kamaja 2009) It is used here to show the nature and main characteristics of the required paradigm shift in research and in business from the traditional organizational data mining to the novel network-wide knowledge discovery. The construction, substance, and theoretical background of DIT have been presented against philosophy of science and conceptual theory (Kamaja 2009), and its frame of reference consists of eight components or levels (Figure 1): (1) *background*, (2) *technological*, (3) *scientific-theoretical*, (4) *philosophical level of science*, (5) *metatheoretical*, (6) *organized activity and management*, (7) *scientific program*, and (8) *theory*.

In what follows, the two important metatheoretical sets of DIT in relation to the content of this research are presented: first, the model of *socially construed reality* (Searle 1995), and second, the utilization of *sociological paradigms* (Burrell

& Morgan 1979) within philosophy of science in conceptual domain area context analysis.

Socially Construed Reality and Social Facts

As stated above, the first metatheoretical set of DIT is the *construction of social reality* (Searle, 1995), which is based on the following three ontological premises: (i) the existence of one world, (ii) the existence of an external world is a prerequisite for our thinking, and (iii) the fact that conscious states are subjective. A fact is a term expressing "the way things are in the world". The core of the construction of social reality is formed by the concepts of fact, social fact, and epistemic community where the structure of perception is based on the *psychology of thought* (Saariluoma, 1990).

Facts depending on the observer are ontologically subjective and facts not depending on the observer are ontologically objective. Ontologically subjective but epistemologically objective facts, referred to as *social facts*, thus become the salient categories. A social fact is a fact containing collective intentionality, that befalls those actors (two or more) who possess a belief, desire, objective, or some other intentional state and who know they share this state. According to collective intentionality, instead of thinking that *I* am striving for something an individual thinks that *we* are striving for something, which creates a *"sense of collectivity."* Consequently, the intentionality possessed by each individual derives from their shared collective intentionality. Social facts thus stem from one's belief that one shares his or her intentionality with someone else; they are essentially facts possessed by an individual as a member of a community. Classical example of these is money, which takes on its meaning only if we all believe in its value. This is basically the nature of all concepts shared by us. Their meaning does not depend on the observer but they are not included in the world itself either; they are ontologically subjective, and at the same time

Figure 1. The components (levels) of DIT

Level	Component	Description
1	Background	Includes the original science concept of information technology (IT) that is based on the frame of reference of the Association for Computer Machinery and the Institute of Electrical and Electronics Engineers (ACM/IEEE) and their concept of computing divided into five computer-related fields of science: Computer Science (CS), Information Systems (IS), Computer Engineering (CE), Software Engineering (SE), and the original area of information technology (IT).
2	Technologcial	The technological substance of DIT is based on the corresponding substance of IT complying with ACM/IEEE.
3	Scientific-theoretical	Includes the creation of a conceptual and theoretical basis for science, the definition of a theory and theoretical meaning, the specification of the requirements of critical and advanced science, and the definition of the characteristics of scientific identity, which requires that its research objects, phenomena, and substance have individual qualities in comparison to other sciences.
4	Philosophical level of science	Presents ontological and epistemological choices and the picture of man. An ontological choice is based on the *three-world ontology* (Popper, 1972): (1) the physical world, (2) the world of mind, and (3) the world of constructions. The structure of perception is based on the psychology of thought, which forms the core of an epistemological choice (Saariluoma, 1990).
5	Metatheoretical	Covers two sets of models: (i) the first set is based on philosophical construction of social reality, social facts, and epistemic societies (Searle, 1995), and (ii) the second set builds on a theory of four sociological paradigms in relation to organizational analysis (Burrel & Morgan, 1979).
6	Organized activity and management	The most important theoretical frame of reference is the multiperspective representation view of organization theory (Hatch & Cunliffe, 2006), that presents three overall conceptions of the (alleged) appearance of the surrounding world: (i) *modern*, (ii) *symbolic* (interpretational), and (iii) *postmodern* perspectives. For each perspective, the theory introduces ontological and epistemological hypotheses, focusing on the organizational viewpoint and organization research.
7	Scientfic program	The core and protective layer of a research program are constructed in which the core contains the fundamental assumptions, theoretical concepts, and theories. The core of DIT consists of a *three-world ontology* (Popper, 1972) and the epistemology consists of the structure of perception based on the psychology of thought and conception of *social facts* (Searle, 1995). It is structurally surrounded by a protective layer that includes the theories and concepts gradually generated by the field of science in question.
8	Theory	The defined theory of DIT will guide DIT-related research where the focus is in information and its significance to the operation of an organization.

these features of our society exceed epistemic subjectivity. (Searle 1995)

Sociological Paradigms and Conceptual Analysis

DIT's second metatheoretical construct consists of conceptual areas and sociological paradigms within philosophy of science. (Burrell & Morgan 1979) This model encompasses (i) four concept areas within philosophy of science (ontology, epistemology, human nature, and methodology) with two opposing concepts forming a pair within each, (ii) two key dimensions (subjectivity – objectivity and regulation – radical change) that form a four-sector model, (iii) a paradigm from the social sciences connected to each sector (i.e. radical humanism, radical structuralism, interpretatism, and functionalism), and (iv) the generally accepted scientific conceptions assigned to each paradigm and agreeing with their requirements.

Based on the above proposed developments in philosophy of science in relation to conceptual theory and supported by the multidisciplinary

Figure 2. The four sociological paradigms (Burrell & Morgan, 1979) used to organize contextual domain areas

	Subjective	Objective
Radical change	**Radical humanism** (A): Nominalism, anti-positivism, ideographic, voluntarism (B.1): Critical theory (B.2): Postmodernism (C): Business ecosystems and commercial markets (in turbulent, external consumer driven competitive environments), SMEs (D): Internet	**Radical structuralism** (A): Realism, positivism, nomothetic, determinism (B.1): Conflict theory (B.2): - (C): - (D): Communities of social media
Regulation	**Interpretatism** (A):Nominalism, anti-positivism, ideographic, voluntarism (B.1): Hermeneutics, phenomenology (B.2): Symbolic interpretation (C): Business networks (supply chains?) (D): Personal computing, semantic webs, etc.	**Functionalism** (A): Realism, positivism, nomothetic, determinism (B.1): Objectivism, integrative theory (B.2): Modernism (C): Big hierarchical and bureaucratic organizations (also the "internal stability features" of private enterprises) (D): Classical information systems, traditional data mining

nature of DIT, the two-dimensional framework of sociological paradigms is employed here as a theoretical construct to organize the following categories of conceptual domain areas: (A) philosophy of science, (B) scientific views, (C) business network research, and (D) organizational IT. On the one hand, the alignment of the individual concepts within these domain areas (Figure 2 below) is based on existing philosophical and sociological theories. On the other, it is based on a preliminary analysis of the research conceptualizations relevant to this chapter.

As they have originally been devised for it, the four sociological paradigms are well suited to position the various orientations and principles within philosophy of science (A) (Burrell & Morgan 1979) in relation to scientific views (B)

(Hatch & Cunliffe, 2006). In philosophy of science, the conceptual areas and opposing pairs are defined as follows (Burrell & Morgan, 1979): (i) *ontology*: nominalism - realism, (ii) *epistemology*: anti-positivism - positivism, (iii) *methodology*: ideographic - nomothetic, and (iv) *human nature*: voluntarism - determinism. In respect to the classical scientific views like critical theory, conflict theory, phenomenology, objectivism, and hermeneutics (B.1), they are usually separated by a degree of commitment to a set of philosophically-oriented principles. An organizational interpretation of the these principles is the above described *multiperspective view* (Hatch & Cunliffe 2006) that consists of three mutually exclusive principles (B.2): postmodernism, modernism and symbolic interpretation that have been mapped respectively to the paradigms of radical humanism, interpretatism and functionalism.

When the same approach is applied to organizing conceptual domain area contexts related to this research, i.e. business network research (C) and organizational information technology (D), the important theoretical relationships of the context areas can be shown. It is possible to carry out a sociological analysis of these domain area-specific conceptualizations, and this possibility has useful methodological implications. The core conceptualizations in business-oriented network research (C) are usually centered on the structural analysis of the topology, organization, and functions of *net-like structures*, which in their most generic form consist of a number of interconnected nodes. In respect to the surroundings (or environments) of the constellations of member organizations and depending on the chosen unit of research analysis, a set of net-like structures can be identified: business ecosystems, industry domain areas, virtual enterprises, collaborative business networks (CBN), industrial business networks, supply chains, large multinational corporations, SMEs, and micro-enterprises. After aligning these to the paradigmatic framework, also the concepts in the domain area of *organizational information technology* (D) can be positioned accordingly. The preliminary domain area analysis conducted as part of this research suggests that this category consists of the following set of relevant concepts: the Internet, communities of social media, personal computing, traditional information systems, and data mining.

In sum, the theoretical benefit of applying the paradigmatic framework to the mapping of several contextual domain areas is that it enables us to show the conceptual interconnectedness of the entities essential to this research. The paradigmatic nature of framework means that concepts, models, and theories in each segment are closely interrelated and thus, in the strictest sense of the theory, even mutually exclusive. The proximity of entities such as data mining, classical information systems (for

example databases), nomothetic methodology, positivism, and large hierarchical companies and the fact that they are all attached to the objective-regulative (i.e. functionalistic) paradigm suggest that the concept of traditional organizational data mining is reflecting only the objective view of society and the positivistic conception of data as well as the cumulative nature of information that is mostly stored in static data sources of large, hierarchically regulated organizations. In order to support knowledge discovery in the contexts of business network research and operations, the improvement of classical data mining methods with some new algorithms is clearly not sufficient. Instead, a more paradigmatic shift from a positivistic and objective view of reality to an anti-positivistic and subjective view of KD in socially construed reality is needed both in research and in business management. This applies particularly to organizations in modern commercial business ecosystems and competitive electronic markets.

MULTILEVEL MODEL AND RESEARCH FRAMEWORK FOR NETWORK-WIDE KNOWLEDGE DISCOVERY

The main objective of this chapter is to develop a theoretically grounded and practically feasible model for network-wide knowledge discovery in real-world business network research contexts The starting point for this is the differentiation of the logical structure of the KD-process into the traditional data mining approach (the positivistic and organizational view) and a progression from socially construed reality to the evolution of epistemic society (the anti-positivistic network oriented view). This analysis is grounded on the previously outlined theoretical background of philosophy of science, the four sociological paradigms and the model of the discipline of information technology (DIT). Then a preliminary conceptual analysis of the phenomenon under

Figure 3. Layered progression of knowledge discovery: positivistic and anti-positivistic paradigms

Logical layers and transitions	Objective view of society (positivistic paradigm)	Subjective view of society (anti-positivistic paradigm)
Layer 0: Networks/communities	-	Evolution of epistemological society by communicative knowledge discovery
Transition 1 -> 0: "Evolutionization"	-	Information asymmetry reduction Functional principles of contract law: reasonableness, good faith and trust
Layer 1: Stakeholder/organization specific	Information pattern presentations: reports and analyzes supporting organizational decision making	Innovations and insights. Critical knowledge assets. Communicative patterns.
Transition 2 -> 1: Functionalization	Traditional data mining	Information intensive governance and network-wide "data mining"
Layer 2: Storage and persistence	Datasources & databases	Object-relational and semantic repositories, ontologies
	RDBMS (ER-paradigm)	OODBs, RDFS- and OWL-repositories
Transition 3 -> 2: Aggregation (information)	Ad-hoc cumulation	Aggregation, interpretation, classification,
		Multidisciplinary Concept Evolution (MCE)
Layer 3: Gathered observations and content corpus representations	Static, numeric and/or symbolic data	Social facts and conceptualizations Dynamic, interpretative and relative information flows.
		Natural language processing, TAT-tools, like ATLAS.ti
Transition 4 -> 3: Observations (socialization?)	-	Observations (based on mental models or schemas), pre-conceptualizations. Sub-conscious cognitive processes
Layer 4: Sources and informants Entities and events	Objective reality based on the world view of realism.	Socially construed reality (Searle, 1995; Popper, 1972), communicative behavior

study is conducted from the relevant research area perspectives, and finally based on these the research framework for network-wide knowledge discovery is presented.

Logical Structure of the Knowledge Discovery Process

By utilizing the sociological framework for organizing the relevant conceptual domain contexts, this section presents the nature and characteristics of a paradigmatic shift from traditional data mining to the requirements and possibilities of network-oriented knowledge discovery. First, both the anti-positivistic and positivistic scenario is presented in detail. The discussion is concluded with a logical structure diagram of the process-oriented progression of KD from the fundamental

level of real-world phenomena to the level of communities and networks (Figure 3).

Positivistic View: Traditional Data Mining

According to positivism, truth is reached through competent methods and reliable measurement, which allows us to test it in the objective world; knowledge is cumulative and allows us to make progress and develop. The nomothetic approach examines the orderliness of phenomena and their causal connections through statistical generalizations. It typically involves the utilization of one theory per case and at least a moderate number of statistical observations. Quite often it entails the testing of theory-based hypotheses that are analyzed statistically using accrued observational material. Traditional data mining is carried out according to the principles of nomothetic methodology. It makes use of statistical calculations to establish dependencies and correlations between variables and to find out the basic distribution of variables.

One typical case of data mining can be found in the area of tourism, where a travel agency systematically gathers customer satisfaction feedback after each trip from all the travelers. The feedback survey is implemented on the Internet using a typical questionnaire form. Most of the gathered data is classified and encoded, for example, the information related to customer satisfaction and the customers' backgrounds. In this case, the data source consists of these numeric representations that can manually be stored in database, and by using traditional data mining (KDD) techniques reports can be generated from these. This body of information represents quantitative information. Among the concepts of philosophy of science, the two dominant pairs in this case are the ones related to epistemology and methodology; thus, the information in this example is epistemologically positive and methodologically nomothetic.

Possibilities of the Anti-Positivistic View: A Case for Network-Wide Data Mining

According to the interpretive scientific view, all knowledge is relative to the person who possesses it, and it can only be understood personally through the one who has been part of it. Truth is constructed socially through the objective knowledge of several interpreters, and therefore it varies with time. The *epistemic community* then, is based on these theories on the construction of social reality and on social facts (Searle, 1995).

The previously presented example of a tourism industry customer satisfaction form can also have text fields for customer opinions, comments, and other informal information. For example, customer feedback could have been gathered under the questionnaire-heading "Other issues related to the trip.", where one customer might have answered: "birds' singing in the morning brought tears in my eyes", while the other response could be: "fresh air gave me a good night's sleep". This kind of content represents anti-positivistic and ideographic information; in terms of scientific classification it represents subjectivity and the symbolic-interpretive view.

One of the salient questions of this work is whether some form of knowledge discovery can be applied to this kind of ideographic and anti-positivistic information. The positive response from the writers of this chapter is based on two epistemological findings: new types of methodological solutions and epistemological objectivity realized through epistemic communities. A methodological solution can be described as *an extended content analysis of qualitative material*. The phases to be implemented in research are: (1) the recognition and definition of key concepts, (2) finding the key concepts from a text and abstracting (interpreting) these text passages, and (3) the aggregation of the abstracted concepts.

Layered Comparison of the Positivistic and Anti-Positivistic Views

As stated above, traditional data mining exhibits the positivistic and objective world view. The novel approach to network-wide knowledge discovery proposed here is based on the anti-positivistic view of socially construed reality. In order to show in detail the differences between these paradigms, a generalized, layered logical structure (including the transitions between them) of the KD-process has been created (Figure 3). This model consists of: (i) five logical representation layers, (ii) four transitions between them producing higher level representations, and (iii) the corresponding positivistic and anti-positivistic substance matter of the knowledge discovery process.

The starting point of the KD (from bottom-up) is the level of sources and informants (Layer 4) that consists of the entities and events of the phenomena under investigation. By making observations and by the process of socialization (Transition 4 -> 3) a higher-level content corpus representation (Layer 3) is achieved. The aggregation (Transition 3 -> 2) of gathered observations enables the persistent storage (Layer 2) of newly generated information. In order to reach the stakeholder- or organization-specific representation level (Layer 1), the persistence-layer substance is functionalized (Transition 2 -> 1). Here, it is important to note that within the positivistic world view this step manifests itself as the traditional data mining process and in the anti-positivistic case it is achieved by following the knowledge discovery methods proposed in this chapter; these methods are based on information-intensive governance and communicative information flow. Finally, the network operations and representation level (Layer 0) can be seen as the result of a semi-autonomous, self-organizing emergence (Transition 1 -> 0) whereby the higher-level organizational structures are formed and through which they evolve.

MULTIDISCIPLINARY CONCEPT ANALYSIS OF THE DOMAIN AREA

The research here focuses on inter-organizational knowledge discovery and the related real-world phenomena that are intrinsically multidisciplinary. There are some scientific views and research approaches in literature that are applicable to research settings where a common set of issues and problems are explored from varying but overlapping perspectives. The scientific challenges of developing, creating, and utilizing novel business models and practices based on network-wide knowledge and enabled by information technology will be confronted by the theoretical backgrounds of philosophy of science and DIT theory presented in the previous section. In this kind of research mutually shared conceptualizations are required on which the higher-level science artifacts (i.e. constructs, models, methods, and implementations) can be based (Aaltonen *et al.*, 2006).

Methodologically the work presented here has been founded on the constructive research approach (CRA) which is a form of action research that uses case-study methods to solve predetermined real-world problems and to generate new scientific knowledge of the area under study (Aaltonen *et al.*, 2006; Kasanen *et al.*, 1993). In the sub-sections below, the results of the multidisciplinary domain analysis supporting the objectives of this work is outlined. The preliminary research conceptualizations are presented in form of key terminology in the following research areas: (i) business networks, (ii) organizational IT, and (iii) contract law. Finally, the content of the shared conceptual domain area of all the individual research fields is specified.

Networks and Business Environments

According to the most generic specification, a *network* is a net that consists of point-like nodes and connections between them. In alignment with the graph theory and depending on how the nodes and links are characterized, a set of layered topologies that exhibit various connectivity structures and patterns (for example social communities and business environments) can be represented and analyzed. Below, an overview is given of nets embedded in various business environments which are a specific case of net-like structures (refer to Figure 4 for details (Aaltonen *et al.*, 2007b; Choi & Stahl, 1997; Håkansson & Johanson, 1992; OASIS, 2006)), followed by a brief discussion on the governance and informa-

Figure 4. Mapping the elements of various net-like structures (Aaltonen et al., 2007b)

Net-like structures	Economic markets (Choi & Stahl, 1997)	Industrial Networks (Håkansson & Johanson, 1992)	Service paradigm (OASIS, 2006)
environment	market	network	context
nodes	participants	actors	services (agents)
resourses	products and services	resources	capabilities
dynamics	transactions / processes	activities	interaction
connectivity	relationships, economic exchange: trust and power relations, information flows	actor bonds resource tiers activity links	composition, choreography, orchestration

tion technology adoption in business networks within the travel industry.

Net-Like Structures

It is useful to employ the *net-like structure* in the identification and specification of the common features of nets. A net is a net-like structure if it consists of: (i) nodes (or actors), (ii) connectivity, meaning the links or relationships, (iii) the environment, which is the logical context or scope of the net in question, (iv) resources (or assets) that can be consumed or transferred between the nodes, and (v) the dynamics, which represents the various interactions and communications between the actors of a net. Even if the context or the level of organizational and structural complexity vary considerably between nets, it is still possible to align them by, for example, comparing the common constitutional elements in each case.

BUSINESS NETWORKS

Networks are a form of governance between the arms-length relationships of markets and the highly integrated organizations of hierarchies. The specialization of nodes and low transaction costs between nodes are the key characteristics of networks. Transactions and relationships are usually coordinated by shared information systems.

Business networks consist of actors, resources, activities and their interconnections. Actors perform interconnected transformation and transfer activities that demand resources. Through network the actors may gain access to resources controlled by other actors. (Håkansson & Johanson, 1992) Activities are connected with flows of information, materials, finance and influence and ultimately they create value for the customers (Parolini, 1999). Business networks that exist mainly for collaboration are called *collaborative business networks (CBN)*, and they aim in bringing together the knowledge, expertise and other resources of the actors (Kotler *et al.*, 1993).

GOVERNANCE OF BUSINESS NETWORKS

The governance of business networks is a compromise between control and emergence: control deteriorates innovation and flexibility and emergence erodes routines and predictability (Choi *et al.*, 2001). Networks are managed and coordinated in terms of knowledge, communication, decision making, price, authority and social relationships (Kohtamäki, 2005; Zettinig, 2003). The fundamental network management functions are: (1) *framing:* forming a vision of value creation and communicating it, (2) *activating:* realizing the structure and pattern of actors, resources and activities to create value, (3) *mobilizing:* building commitment among actors toward mutual value creation, and (4) *synthesizing:* monitoring and measuring value creation and facilitating interaction (Järvensivu & Möller 2008).

DOMAIN SPECIFIC BUSINESS NETWORKS: TOURISM INDUSTRY

Tourism is a network industry par excellence due to its fragmented nature, actor interdependence, collective resources and production (Scott *et al.*, 2008). A traditional tourism value chain consists of four stages: suppliers of basic tourism services, tour operators (wholesale), travel agents (retail) and consumers (tourists). A central problem therein is the matching of demand and supply (the issue of *supply chain management, SCM*), which emphasizes the role of intermediaries.

A tourism network can be defined as a set of formal, co-operative relationships between organizations that is formed to achieve a particular purpose in the tourism business. Tourism production networks consist of producers and users of different services and are coordinated by interaction between actors. These networks rely on the creation, gathering, communication and application of operative type of information,

learning and exchange of knowledge that is guiding day-to-day activities.

Organizational Information Technology

In this section the main conceptual entities relevant to this work that belong to the intersection of information technology and knowledge intensive organizational management and operations are presented. An overview about the hierarchy of the internal conceptual structure of information is given followed by a short description of traditional data mining.

DATA, INFORMATION, AND KNOWLEDGE

The core substance of information technology in general and *information system* sciences in particular is the representation and processing of *information*. Also in modern organizations the utilization and management of various forms of business information are among the critical success factors in competitive IT-enabled trading environments. However, the conception or the understanding of information varies considerably when viewed from the disparate perspectives of business and technology. When applying the results of this research in the contexts of business and science, it is therefore essential to explicate the meaning of information in a mutually agreed way, and optimally set it in a philosophically reasoned and logically sound relationship with *data* and *knowledge*. Thus in short, knowledge is applicable or usable collection of information, which consists of processed or interpreted facts, symbols or marks (i.e. data).

Also, the typical hierarchical relationship between data, information, and knowledge is based on the inherent level of abstraction in each (data at the lowest level and knowledge at the highest). Furthermore, it is based on the idea of containment or the "prerequisite principle," which simply means that information cannot emerge before some data is processed and/or interpreted and that knowledge emerges only if there is information available and if it is applied or used for some particular purpose. In system-analytical thinking, this hierarchical continuum is sometimes extended to entail the notions of *understanding* and *wisdom*, in which case the presupposition is that all five categories exist in and represent the content of the human mind (Ackof 1989).

DATA MINING

Traditional *data mining* (DM) typically occurs in the organizational context where existing structured and static data sources (i.e. databases) function as the source of the actual information and knowledge extraction process. Based on this, data mining is sometimes referred to as *knowledge discovery in databases* (KDD), but there are several other definitions for DM in literature:

- the step in the process of knowledge discovery in databases that inputs predominantly cleaned and transformed data, searches the data using algorithms, and outputs patterns and relationships to the interpretation/evaluation step of the whole knowledge discovery process in databases (Fayyad *et al.*, 1996)
- the science of extracting useful information from large datasets (Hand *et al.*, 2001)
- the process of the exploration and analysis, by automatic and semi-automatic means, of large quantities of data in order to discover meaningful patterns and rules (Berry & Linoff, 1997)

As can be inferred from these descriptions, the requirements of networked business governance and the characteristics and demands of the inter-

organizational operating environments of target organizations are mostly outside the scope of traditional DM. Also, within the field of data mining itself, it is widely accepted that traditional techniques and methods may be inadequate when vast amounts of multi-dimensional data are distributed among heterogeneous data sources and shared by various stakeholders.

Contract Law and Functional Principles

Contract law is defined as a branch of law where the main focus is on a contracting party's free will to commit itself to a binding obligation. A contractual obligation may be fulfilled instantly or during a longer period of time. In latter cases a contract may be defined as a *long-term contract*, which is actually a contract governing continuous, long-lasting, and cooperative contractual relationships. (Nysten-Haarala 1998) In long-lasting relationships contracts are often used for information asymmetry reduction.

CONTRACTUAL PRINCIPLES

Contractual principles derive directly from contract law and are sometimes defined as a cohesive element of contract law. (Pöyhönen, 1988) In order to reduce information asymmetry, contractual relationships build up an internal governing method; they work together to govern a long-term relationship. In this writing, although contract law is not applicable to all kinds of network structures, some of its principles are chosen for describing the governance of networks, enabling knowledge sharing, and for reducing information asymmetry. Here, these principles are called functional principles, the term *functional* coming straight from the governing and activating nature of these principles.

FUNCTIONAL PRINCIPLES

Functional principles constitute the most operative frame of network governance. Here, the functional principles are defined as fairness/equality, good faith/fair dealing and trust/confidentiality. *Fairness/equality* concentrates on balancing a relationship and by these means reducing information asymmetry. *Good faith/fair dealing*, on its part, makes relationships and networks operative and functional together, and *trust/confidentiality* consolidate and improve activity itself.

Shared Conceptual Domain Area

In a multidisciplinary research setting it is typical that some of the key concepts are shared by several individual research areas. Here, the justification for the following preliminary discussion about phenomena such as *information asymmetry, information intensive business governance,* and *network-wide knowledge management* is that they form the central terminology for the ultimate conceptualization and methodological specification of the proposed network-wide knowledge discovery research.

INFORMATION ASYMMETRY

In relation to net-like structures and economic markets, *information asymmetry* refers to a condition in which at least some relevant information is known only to some parties involved. One of the gravest effects of information asymmetry is that it causes markets to become inefficient, since all the market participants do not have access to information they need for their decision making processes. By these means, information asymmetry deals with the study of decisions in transactions where one party has more or better information than the other. This creates an imbalance of power which can sometimes cause the transactions to become distorted. On the other hand, informa-

tion asymmetry may easily be considered the prototype of modern exchange this being carried out in asymmetric informational environment. (Lauriala 2001)

In some exchange trade environments and economic markets information asymmetry may sometimes be desired or even a necessity for creating innovation and growth. (Lamberton 1998) But, asymmetric information changes the overall operational patterns of cooperative relationships in such a way that it becomes impossible to predict the acts of the other party (Virtanen 2001), especially when the parties act only for their own good. It seems quite clear that this does not work for the good of exchange. This implies that increasing mutual communication and thereby decreasing information asymmetry seems to work for the best for the society. (Turunen 2005)

INFORMATION INTENSIVE BUSINESS GOVERNANCE

Referring to the above discussion about the importance of explicating, especially in multidisciplinary research settings, the understanding of the key concepts and their relationships, idea of the proposed *information intensive business governance (IIBG)* is here discussed in order to differentiate it from the more traditional business management conventions.

Business governance has traditionally been divided into the following separate functional management areas: human resources, operations or production, strategic management, marketing, finance and lately also information technology. In modern enterprises operating in complex IT enabled competitive and collaborative network environments, organizational governance is more properly defined in terms of the identified critical business activities (processes) or objects (assets) that are subject to management. The predominant management practice is the *process-based view (PBV)* of business, where the strategic business objectives and visions are to be realized through detailed modeling and engineering, and by the cost-effective performance of the core business processes. In contrast to this, the *resource-based view (RBV)* of a firm (Barney, 1991) focuses the management to the allocation, utilization, and optimal alignment of the demand and supply of critical business resources or assets. While there are many business resource categorization schemes (Aaltonen *et al.*, 2007b), in the resource based strategic management practice the categories used are: financial assets and tangible, intangible and human resources. In this scheme, the intangible resources are of importance because they are information based assets including competencies and reputation (Løwendahl, 1997). Thus, information intensive business governance is an organizational management approach that emphasizes knowledge and information intensive assets as being the core competencies and enablers of successful business.

NETWORK-WIDE KNOWLEDGE MANAGEMENT

As has been stated above, the governance of networks is a complex and controversial issue. However, there seems to be a general agreement that it should be built on trust and norms and that decision rights should be allocated in relation to expertise. But when the dimension of knowledge is added to the subject matter of network-wide governance, many business- and research-oriented issues emerge. In practice, the *inter-organizational knowledge management* here means the utilization of the results of network-wide data mining that should be made available to business stakeholders in some form of a shared knowledge repository. To solve the problems in designing, developing, operating, and managing such a *network-wide knowledge base* in mutual understanding could prove to be very challenging. For example, in supply chain type networks the naturally existing level of knowledge integration is naturally low

because the relationships are instrumental and the communication is directly tied to production issues.

Also, knowledge is often partitioned in relation to expertise and decision rights, but at the same time there is a need for knowledge redundancy in network nodes. (Konsynski & Tiwana, 2004) Widely adopted ICT supports innovative ways to create cooperative alliances. The exchange of information and the ability to interact are key elements in executing business processes in a business network (or a business web). And to succeed in network-wide process- and system-level interoperability, which is a necessity for business webs (Hakolahti & Kokkonen, 2006), inter-organizational agreements are needed to enable the management of supporting collaborative business operations and resource-related knowledge bases.

Network-Wide Knowledge Discovery Research Framework

The main topic here is to advance the model-oriented work conducted so far to a preliminary research framework that provide network-wide support for identifying and representing the existing organizational information contents and inter-organizational information flows. This is done within the field of multidisciplinary business network research from the perspective of data mining in order to enable: (i) network-wide knowledge discovery and management, (ii) information intensive business governance, and (iii) the reduction of information asymmetry. Below, an overview of the preliminary *research framework for network-wide business knowledge discovery and management* is given (Figure 5), where the contents (i.e. the models, constructs, and methods) have been divided into five scientific substance levels (Kamaja, 2009) (from bottom up): (i) philosophy of science and metatheory, (ii) general theories of science, (iii) special theories of science, (iv) the analytical level, and (v) the

Figure 5. The multilevel research framework for network-wide business knowledge discovery

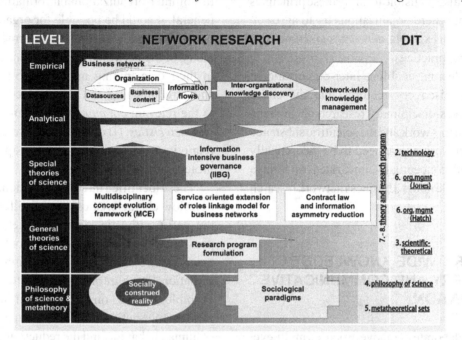

empirical level. The theoretical justification of organizing the elements of the model is based on the DIT, the components of which are here mapped to the relevant levels of the framework.

According to DIT, there are two metatheoretical constructs at the level of philosophy of science and metatheory: *the socially construed reality* (Popper, 1972; Searle, 1995) and the *four sociological paradigms* (Burrell & Morgan 1979). The higher, general and special theories of science can be built on these constructs. One way to achieve this is to *formulate a research program* by using DIT's organization theory constructs, i.e. the Hatch's multi-perspective view. In concrete terms, during the prior and on-going DIT-compliant business network projects at the University of Lapland, the semantic aspects of inter-organizational business communication (for example, interoperability issues), and the challenges in collaborative research have been addressed partly by developing a *multidisciplinary concept evolution (MCE) framework* (Aaltonen et al., 2006; Aaltonen et al., 2007a) that supports

a multi-perspective domain area analysis and the sharing of research conceptualizations. Also, a preliminary *service-oriented extension of the roles linkage model for business networks* has been proposed (Aaltonen, 2007) preparing a way for the service-centered structural analysis of industrial networks. The model aims to make it easier to align the roles that individual enterprises play in business networks with the IT-oriented service paradigm based descriptions of corresponding linkages or business relationship generalizations. In addition, generic business information conceptualization models that rest on the semantic and dynamic extension of resource based view of a firm are useful for an organization in categorizing and classifying knowledge based business resources (Aaltonen et al., 2007b) as a prerequisite for successful information intensive business governance (IIBG). In relation to the characteristics of inter-organizational information flow and *information asymmetry reduction* the functional principles originating from *contract law* can be capitalized in ongoing and future research programs. It is also plausible to apply these principles in situations where organizations try to agree on the terms of, for example, *network-wide knowledge management* practices.

In conclusion, enabling inter-organizational knowledge discovery requires that the entire complex cross-disciplinary research phenomena presented in this work and the scientific substance of the framework above need to be theoretically aligned and conceptually integrated to form a seamless whole under a business network research program.

NETWORK-WIDE KNOWLEDGE DISCOVERY AND COMMUNICATIVE INFORMATION

In order to elaborate the above proposed multilevel knowledge discovery research model and framework, some practical requirements, enablers, and implications are discussed in more detail in this section that is organized to sub-sections as follows: (i) specification of the inter-organizational information flows in respect to the anti-positivistic view of society, (ii) discussion about information asymmetry reduction through contract law-oriented functional principles, and (iii) presentation of the case study results of an existing tourism network where the main information and knowledge transfer between the key actors were identified.

Anti-Positivistic Characterization of Inter-Organizational Business Information

Decreasing information asymmetry needs to be founded on open access to information or on increased exchange of information. Thus information itself and its communication need to be based on some common rules or basic principles of circulating information and getting access to it. Such information intensive governance of business relationships must observe the main characteris-

tics of inter-organizational information flows. In general, it could be possible for organizations to pursue to reduce the overall information asymmetry of the networks they are members of, also in their data mining initiatives, by identifying and strengthening the enablers corresponding to the relevant *communicative information flow characteristics*: (i) dynamics, (ii) semantics, (iii) relativity, (iv) usability, and (v) openness and protectability (Figure 6).

These identified inter-organizational information flow characteristics are a manifestation of a the anti-positivistic view of society presented previously. In business network context, the dynamic nature of information (i.e. information as a relationship) (Czerniawska & Potter, 1998), for example, is based on the view that inter-organizational transactions reflect the transient patterns of human behavior, and the reduction of information asymmetry could in this case be achieved by increasing the accessibility to and availability of information. The networked organizations could also benefit from recognizing and reacting to the other information flow aspects in their business relationships. In line with past and ongoing multidisciplinary research done at the University of Lapland, these notions and insights are elaborated below. The main contributions here originate from the domain areas of contract law, and analysis of digitally enabled business relationships and networks in the field of tourism.

Information Asymmetry Reduction by Contract Law-Based Functional Principles

In respect to the principles of contract law and in order to reduce information asymmetry, information intensive governance can be based on the following functional principles: fairness/equality (reasonableness), good faith/fair dealing, and trust/confidentiality. Choosing and using these principles taken from contract law is justified by the cooperative nature of networks and their

Figure 6. Inter-organizational information flow characteristics and asymmetry reduction enablers

Characteristic	Description	Information asymmetry reduction (and network-wide knowledge discovery) enablers
dynamic nature (information as a relationship (Czerniawska & Potter, 1998)	Inter-organizational business transactions (transfer activities) reflect the transient and variable patterns of human behavior.	Increase accessibility and availability of information
interpretation and semantics	To share information it is first conceived and semantically "annotated" by the participants.	Explicate the meaning; -> requires the construction of common and shared conceptualizations, ontology engineering (Aaltonen *et al.*, 2007a)
relativity	The stakeholders asses the information according to varying value functions (Shapiro & Varian, 1999)	Explicate the value functions -> requires semi-formal value creation models
usability	Communicating information makes it usable for a wider range of actors and functions.	Makes it possible to target the information more precisely -> customer intensive network analysis methodology
openness & legal protectability	The transparency (but also the vulnerability) of information increases in communicative actions.	Implement property rights management, privacy and information security guidelines and policies -> inter-organizational information security model (Aaltonen *et al.*, 2008)

relationships. Mainly the same principal basis that makes a network functional operates on the background of contract law as well. These very three principles are chosen because of their dynamic nature, their strong emphasis on reciprocity and mutuality, and their intrinsic relevance to the proposed anti-positivistic network-wide KD-process.

Fairness/Equality as Interpretation and Relativity

Information is an activity and it is experienced rather than possessed. (Shapiro & Varian, 1999) In the business network environment, information is based on inter-organizational business transactions where human behavior and communication constitute the core. This view makes information relative. As information seems to be based on fluent communication, it seems plausible to build instruments enabling the reduction of information asymmetry based on the functional nature of information.

On the other hand, communicative actions increase the transparency of information and bring some openness to information flows. Information often builds up the basis of network relationships, which are generally collaborative and more or less based on information. Openness is a content-related element and it is supported and increased by pursuing fairness and equality in collaboration. (Saunders *et al.*, 2004) At the same time, and as a result of fairness, openness works for decreased information asymmetry.

The concept of fairness is best known from Nordic contract law, where the focus is usually placed on a real mutual balance between parties. And vice versa; the very aim of fairness is to decrease the unbalance and asymmetry caused by the economic or informational inequality of the parties. One of the prerequisites of fairness is that the contracting parties openly disclose unusual issues known to them. (Atiyah, 1979) In this way, every actor of the network gets the same information. By these means, interpreting information while making it relative serves for enabling fair and equal access to it. Thus information, at its content level, becomes more accessible to all stakeholders.

As a single instrument for information asymmetry reduction fairness/equality is relatively weak, as it is mainly fixed to content-related issues. It may be improved and strengthened through some more operative principles, like good faith/fair dealing, which works for openness as well, but in a more functional manner. As these principles operate side by side they are closely linked to each other. This linkage emphasizes and ensures that the collaborating parties observe each other's advantages as far as it is reasonable.

Good Faith/Fair Dealing Constituting Information Usability

Business networking is generally based on the common goal setting of partners. The goal is often based on information, and the purpose of the network is to create added value or synergy. (Balloch & Taylor, 2001) On these grounds, networking is defined as a functional entity, and this entity requires coordinating the roles of the stakeholders in order to enable knowledge sharing. Good faith/fair dealing works for ensuring a common set of goals, and it operates for increasing the communication among the networking parties. By these means good faith/fair dealing on its part reduces information asymmetry.

As a general principle, good faith/fair dealing is in a close relation to contract law, in this case with a European one, and it thereby constitutes a mirror through which the content of the principle may be examined. The Commission of European Contract Law has laid down the principles of European contract law (Commission of European Contract Law, 1999), including good faith, fair dealing, and cooperation. In this document its is stated (Article 1:201) that each party must act in accordance with good faith and fair dealing, an obligation the parties are not allowed to exclude or limit. In this way good faith/fair dealing sup-

ports network activities and makes them more transparent.

Functionality in network relationships is based especially on the above principle and it enables the communication of information, but it is communication that makes information usable for a larger group of stakeholders. For example, in a long-term contract good faith/fair dealing requires that the parties observe not only their own interests, but also the interests of the other contracting party. (Annola 2003) Often this is the most significant issue when building up a long-term relationship or when operating in one; cooperation may not even be started without a mutual core of interest.

In general, good faith/fair dealing is bound closely to fairness/equality, and both are founded on the enabling and ensuring of communication. Fairness/equality supports relative and interpretative content for all parties, but good faith/fair dealing principally concentrates on communication. These principles even seem to suggest that communication needs to be carried out in such a way that all the stakeholders are treated on a completely similar basis. In this way they operate together and support each other through a functional linkage. This complex is functionalized further by trust.

Trust/Confidentiality Increasing Accessibility

Information asymmetry is often reduced by granting access to information and increasing its availability. Both fairness (by explicating the meaning and value of information) and good faith/fair dealing (by increasing its usability) improve access to information. Granting access to information is, again, based on communication that is best described as a part of information, when information is seen as an activity rather than a possessable object. (Shapiro & Varian 1999) Because of this it is less like an inflexible object to be implemented in unchangeable conditions. This makes information operate like a relationship that does not exist in isolation but is rather linked to its more fundamental meaning. In terms of its very essence, *information is communicative* and thereby a dynamic asset.

Successfulness of the communication by which the access to these assets is provided is mainly based on the capability of the parties to trust each other; all the advantages reached by communication are derived from the trust/confidentiality of the relationship, which is seen as a continuous process that includes obtaining and experiencing new knowledge about the relationship, sharing information with the networking partners, and being habituated to trust-based acts.

As mutual trust between parties is required to create a solid base for commitments needed for cooperation, the reciprocity thus constitutes the essence of trust (Atiyah, 1981) and it operates for strengthening the relationships of parties. Each level of trust has a corresponding level of information sharing and in communicating information trust is strengthened accordingly. The more partners trust each other, the more they are expected to share information. (Saunders *et al.*, 2004)

KNOWLEDGE DISCOVERY REQUIREMENTS IN IT-BASED TOURISM INDUSTRY NETWORKS

As indicated previously in the domain area analysis of the travel business networks the intermediaries, like an incoming tour operator (ITO), are the key actors in the tourism industry. Therefore, an existing ITO was selected as the focal company of the case study, where a specific travel industry network in Lapland area is described in terms of its main actor roles, activities and information flows (Figure 7), and as part of this research is linked to the anti-positivistic information characteristics and related knowledge discovery requirements.

An ITO connects the networks of customers and suppliers. Its main function is to match the demand for and supply of tourism services and packaged tours. These intermediaries operate in some geographical destination and they compete for customers and tourism-related resources provided by different suppliers. The key resources for a packaged tour are hospitality services (accommodation and food), arranged activities for travelers, and transportation services to take groups of travelers from their accommodations to activities and attractions. The customers of incoming tour operators are often outgoing tour operators residing in the departure areas of travelers. They market and sell packaged tours to end customers and are responsible for transporting them to the destination area. These kind of information technology-oriented tourism business networks can be evaluated by analyzing digital enablers and service supply network activities, the activities of which consist of several types (Rai *et al.*, 2005): (i) *service design*, (ii) *sourcing*, (iii) *logistics*, (iv) *production*, and (v) *asset management*.

The essential analytical question here is, how are the main service supply network activities within travel industry (i.e. the service design and realization, and asset management) supported by inter-organizational knowledge discovery in respect to the relevant generic anti-positivistic information flow characteristics. To answer this, a set of inter-organizational *information flow content types* that relate to each group of activities in the network under study can be identified: (i) service specifications, (ii) demand and sales information, (iii) consumer information, (iv) service realization, and (v) feedback information. For these, it is possible to define the preliminary KD requirements that take into consideration the generic information flow characteristics. For example, during the service design activities the business innovations are either transformed to concrete *service specifications,* or existing services are adjusted in response to changing environments. These activities would benefit from information about the customer and partner feedback for new products or from support to the identification of important service components. Also, in a more

Figure 7. Actors, activities and information flows in the tour operating network

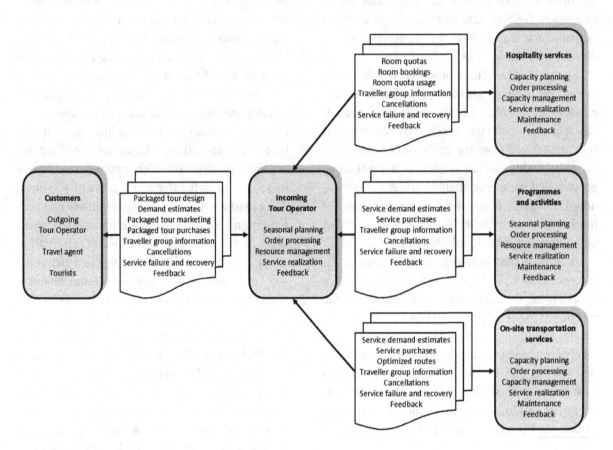

production oriented view, the overall network-wide performance (service realization activities) could be enhanced if knowledge about the business rules for service execution optimization and recovery tactics were available. For organizations to succeed in capitalizing on these types of network-wide knowledge discovery or asset management services they would additionally have to respond to a number of specific issues and requirements related to the generic information flow characteristics:

- **dynamics** - How is the service consumed and what resources are tied to it?
- **semantics** - Requires that commonly understood and compatible service specifications are shared by the consumers, intermediaries and suppliers.

- **relativity** - Different value in service design for consumers and intermediaries should be reflected in the service specifications.
- **usability** - Taking into consideration the different information needs for consumers and intermediaries, and the ability to combine and compare service specifications increases their usability.
- **openness** - Openness and distribution of service information should be based on information needs that is regulated and sanctioned by, for example, immaterial rights, privacy, security policies based on network-wide information security models (Aaltonen *et al.*, 2008), and non-disclosure agreements.

To provide yet another perspective to this discussion, the main features and responsibilities of a feasible KD services for the travel industry business networks can be organized in relation to the above mentioned domain specific information flow content types:

- **service specification** - The essential information contents and service components for consumers and intermediaries.
- **demand and sales information** - Demand patterns for different services
- **consumer information** - Combined service consumption patterns and service component significance for whole tourism experience.
- **service realization** - The critical service flow incidents.
- **feedback information** - Differences of tourism experience among consumer groups

In sum, knowledge discovery in the business network environment should support value creation in terms of efficiency, innovation, customer lock-in, and resource availability. These activities should also enable the digitalization of supply network operations in terms of visibility, process integration, measurement, and information sharing. In the latter two cases, the benefits of network-wide KD would be especially high.

FUTURE TRENDS

The main contribution of this chapter is the theoretical analysis of the proposed paradigmatic change to an anti-positivistic research approach in order to support business network-wide knowledge discovery. In this section, the focus is more on the practical future considerations of intra- and inter-organizational data mining. In what follows, the phenomena under study in this work are first reviewed by categorizing the main insights,

comments and prospective business benefits and outcomes to a representative set of trends to which the theoretical and practical research should respond. The result of this is a summary and the identification of the key benefits, overall feasibility and the main issues of developing, using and adopting the proposed network-wide knowledge discovery approach in research and in operations at the stakeholder-level.

Feasibility of Network-Wide Data Mining Approach at Stakeholder Level

Many issues remain unresolved at the business network participant level in relation to information technology adoption in general and it has a severe impact on the feasibility of the organizational data mining. In tourism networks, as in many other similar networked industries with complex interconnected value chain topologies, information systems, applications and databases enable the network-wide creation, sharing and transfer of knowledge. But, in many cases, the coordination of business activities and the sharing of knowledge are hindered by a lack of shared information systems, a lack of legacy/proprietary systems integration, and an unwillingness to implement or use these systems. Also, the practical business benefits of such systems are somewhat uncharted, but they seem to involve a reduction of manual information processing, higher quality of service execution, and improved business planning and decision making. Additionally, important tourism systems (dynamic packaging and journey management) are not being implemented due to inadequate information infrastructures and the high cost of systems integration (Hakolahti & Kokkonen 2006). However, actors in tourism business recognize the need for a cooperative approach to protect against vertical integration led by large international tourism operators. Yet they also recognize the existing culture of independence and competition. (Saloheimo *et al.*, 2007) Also, advances in IT have made customers (i.e. tourists) more experienced and demanding. (Guzman *et al.*, 2008) Based on this it follows:

- *(future trend)* increasing overall organizational IT adoption has a direct positive impact on conventional data mining feasibility and will indirectly lower the barrier for novel network-wide KD approaches.
- *(research enabler)* appropriate, cross-disciplinary, and participatory research methodologies (e.g. action research) should be designed and applied, in which the stakeholder requirements and expectations must carefully be collected and observed.

Knowledge-Centered Business Network Management

The challenges in the field of inter-organizational business governance stem basically from the fact that the typical operational connectivity properties between networked organizations do not easily support and allow for mutual strategic decision making which has a negative impact on the collaborative management of knowledge assets and corresponding information flows. Also, the existing asymmetric trust and power relationships and the competitive nature of modern commercial ecosystems usually prevent the sharing and communication of critical business knowledge. Yet, the existence of some form of knowledge-centered network governance is crucial for the emergence and optimal utilization of the results of knowledge discovery method proposed here. Additionally, there clearly is a need for neutral and trustworthy network actor who specializes on data, information and knowledge gathering, mining and dissemination for the whole network. Based on the findings in this work and especially on the discussion about contractual principles and information asymmetry reduction, it is possible to suggest that:

- *(future trend)* the assimilation of contract law based functional principles and opting long-term cooperative business agreements over transaction cost reduction oriented short-term contracts encourages existing business networks to turn into net-like structures that exhibit and support the characteristics and features of collaborative knowledge based business networks in which the products of network-wide data mining (i.e. business knowledge repositories) can more easily be capitalized by the participants.
- *(research enabler)* in research projects that pursue to analyze and resolve the issues of network governance, it seems evident that these phenomena should be triangulated from multifaceted, cross-disciplinary research angles; particularly combining business network theories with IT-enabled knowledge representation and contract law-oriented functional principles open up promising research prospects.

Information-Oriented Network Analysis and Modeling

Theoretically, this work has engrossed in the philosophical and meta-theoretical foundations of a required paradigm change from positivistic view of reality to the anti-positivistic world view. The essence of the proposed novel approaches, models and methodologies is in the conception of information. It is important to realize that overlooking the opted information and knowledge associated research orientations may hinder research that is directed to information-centered real-world phenomena. Most notably this is evident when the scientific foundations and views are not chosen appropriately but instead the research unconsciously remains constricted, for example, to a prevailing and traditional paradigmatic approach. The negative implications of this can be noticed by comparing the fundamentally different conceptions of *gathered observations* (Layer 3 in Figure 3) under the anti-positivistic world view (social facts) and the positivistic world view (static data). On the positive side of things, a conscious and explicit commitment to developing and designing anti-positivistic research methods will widen the prospects of future scientific work by promoting philosophically and semantically grounded network structure models and behavior models. The information related network research trends and enablers can be thus summarized:

- **(future trend)** the ongoing and escalating sociological and technological paradigmatic change from positivistic view of reality to anti-positivistic view of society has a major theoretical and practical impact on scientific work and information intensive business network research in particular.
- **(research enabler)** as the information and its significance to the operation of a business network organization is in core of DIT theory, the future themes in research should include topics such as information handling, information processes, the role of man in information processes, information quality and detailed analysis of information flow characteristics.

CONCLUSION

The main proposition of this research is that the traditional conception and implementation of organizational data mining fails to address the important needs and requirements of knowledge discovery in modern business organizations operating in highly heterogeneous and inter-connected and networked service provision environments. The philosophically justified sociological paradigm change influences to the theoretical and practical research work that focuses on information intensive collaborative environments and knowledge eliction, and on representation and

discovery initiatives. The multidisciplinary nature of the phenomenon in question draws attention to research area conceptualizations and the sharing of them. All of these theoretical aspects have been discussed in this work that ultimately proposes an anti-positivistic multilevel research model and framework to address these issues in ongoing and future academic work.

One of the specific issues here is the observed strong information asymmetry between many small and medium size business organizations (especially in travel industry). To resolve this, novel conceptual and practical approaches and methods can be developed during the on-going and future research by focusing on the characteristics of inter-organizational information flows and on the requirements of network-wide data mining approaches. In this regard, the aim is to fully enable organizations to utilize content that manifests itself both in the existing internal and external static data sources, and in dynamic and relative knowledge based and information-intensive communications and transactions.

To summarize, the main observation thus is, that in order to enable the provision of research oriented solutions to the phenomena of KD in business networks, the existing approaches and orientations should be extended and elaborated by concentrating on the information and knowledge modeling dimension of business network operations and relationships. This means that successful theoretical and practical results in the future network-wide knowledge discovery research can be expected when the focus is directed to issues in the overall network-wide information intensive business governance, especially when the examination is based and designed in alignment with the meta-theoretical models of discipline of information technology (DIT), functional principles of contract law, and on the anti-positivistic, ideographic and subjective view of social reality construed from social facts.

REFERENCES

Aaltonen, J. (2007). Service oriented extension of roles-linkage model for travel business networks. In Saloheimo, M. (Ed.), *Operative Network Integration: working papers from research project, University of Lapland, Department of Research Methodology Reports, Essays and Working Papers 10* (pp. 166–181). Rovaniemi, Finland: University of Lapland Press.

Aaltonen, J., Krone, O., & Mustonen, P. (2008). Towards Information Security Ontology in Business Networka. In Y. Kiyoki & T. Tokuda (Eds.), *Proceedings of the 18th European-Japanese Conference on Information Modeling and Knowledge Bases (EJC 2008),* (pp. 373-379). Kanagawa, Japan: EJC 2008 Program Committee.

Aaltonen, J., Rinne, J., & Tuikkala, I. (2006). A Multidisciplinary Framework for Concept Evolution: A Research Tool for Business Models. In Maula, M., Hannula, M., Seppä, M., & Tommila, J. (Eds.), *ICEB + eBRF 2006 Frontiers of e-Business Research 2006* (pp. 526–532). Tampere, Finland: Tampere University of Technology and University of Tampere.

Aaltonen, J., Tuikkala, I., & Saloheimo, M. (2007a). Concept Modeling in Multidisciplinary Research Environment. In H. Jaakkola, Y. Kiyoki & T. Tokuda (Eds.), *Proceedings of the 17th European-Japanese Conference on Information Modeling and Knowledge Bases (EJC 2007)* (pp. 143-160). Pori, Finland: Tampere University of Technology.

Aaltonen, J., Tuikkala, I., & Saloheimo, M. (2007b). Towards Semantic Resource Classification in Organizational Environment. In L. Uden, E. Damiani & G. Passiante (Eds.), *Proceedings of the 2nd International Conference on Knowledge Management in Organization (KMO): New trends in Knowledge management* (pp. 183-187). Lecce, Italy: Knowledge Management in Organizations 2007.

Ackof, R. L. (1989). From Data to Wisdom. *Journal of Applies Systems Analysis, 16,* 3–9.

Annola, V. (2003). Sopimuksen dynaamisuus. Talousoikeudellinen rakennetutkimus sopimuksen täydentymisestä ja täydentymisen ohjaamisesta. Turku, Finland: Turun yliopisto.

Atiyah, P. S. (1979). *The Rise and Fall of Freedom of Contract*. Oxford, UK: Clarendon Press.

Atiyah, P. S. (1981). *Promises, Morals and Law*. Oxford, UK: Clarendon Press.

Balloch, S., & Taylor, M. (2001). Partnership working: Introduction. In Balloch, S., & Taylor, M. (Eds.), *Partnership working: Policy and practice* (pp. 1–14). Bristol, UK: The Policy Press.

Barney, J. (1991). Firm resources and sustained competitive advantage. *Journal of Management, 17,* 99–120. doi:10.1177/014920639101700108

Berry, J. A., & Linoff, G. (1997). *Data mining Techniques For Marketing, Sales and Customer Support*. New York: John Wiley & Sons Inc.

Burrell, G., & Morgan, G. (1979). *Sociological Paradigms and Organizational Analysis*. London: Heinemann.

Choi, S., & Stahl, D. (1997). *The Economics of Electronic Commerce*. Indiana: Macmillan Technical Publishing.

Choi, T., Dooley, K., & Rungtusanahan, M. (2001). Supply networks and complex adaptive systems. *Journal of Operations Management, 19*(3), 351–366. doi:10.1016/S0272-6963(00)00068-1

Commission of European Contract Law. (1999). *The Principles of European Contract Law.* Retrieved 17.10.2008 from <http://frontpage.cbs. dk/law/commission_on_european_contract_law/ PECL%20engelsk/engelsk_partI_og_II.htm>

Czerniawska, F., & Potter, G. (1998). *Business in a Virtual World. Exploiting Information for Competitive Advantage.* Houndmills, UK: Palgrave MacMillan.

Fayyad, U., Piatetsky-Shapiro, G., & Smyth, P. (1996). From Data Mining to Knowledge Discovery: An Overview. In Fayyad, U. M., Piatetsky-Shapiro, G., Smyth, P., & Uthurusamy, R. (Eds.), *Advances in Knowledge Discovery and Data Mining* (pp. 1–34). Menlo Park, CA: AAAI Press/The MIT Press.

Gratzer, M., & Winiwarter, W. (2003). The role of the internet in the SME hotel sector in Austria. In C. Chung, C. Kim, W. Kim, T. W. Ling & K. H. Song (Eds.), *Human Society @ Internet Conference 2003*, (pp. 85-95). Seoul, South Korea: Springer-Verlag.

Guzman, J., Moreno, P., & Tejada, P. (2008). The tourism SMEs in the global value chains - the case of andalusia. *Service Business, 2*, 187–202. doi:10.1007/s11628-008-0034-6

Håkansson, H., & Johanson, J. (1992). A model of industrial networks. Indiustrial Networks. A New View of Reality, 1, (pp. 28-34).

Hakolahti, T., & Kokkonen, P. (2006). Business webs in the tourism industry. In Hitz, M., Sigala, M., & Murphy, J. (Eds.), *Information and communication technologies in tourism* (pp. 453–462). Vienna, Austria: Springer. doi:10.1007/3-211-32710-X_58

Hand, D., Mannila, P., & Smyth, P. (2001). *Principles of Data Mining.* Cambridge, MA: MIT Press.

Hatch, M. J., & Cunliffe, A. L. (2006). *Organization Theory modern, Symbolic and Postmodern Perspectives.* Oxford, UK: University Press.

Järvensivu, T., & Möller, K. (2008). *Metatheory of network management - a contingency perspective.* Upsala, Sweden: Helsinki Scool of Economics, Working papers.

Kamaja, I. (2009). DIT – IT:n uusi tiedekäsitys. DIT:n peruspiirteet ja ominaisuudet. Rovaniemi, Finland: Lapin yliopisto, Menetelmätieteiden laitos.

Kasanen, E., Lukka, K., & Siitonen, A. (1993). Constructive approach in management accounting. *Journal of Management Accounting Research, 5*, 243–264.

Kohtamäki, M. (2005). *Strategisen verkoston ohjaus* [Governance of Strategic Network]. Vaasa, Finland: University of Vaasa.

Konsynski, B., & Tiwana, A. (2004). The improvisation-efficiency paradox in inter-firm electronic networks. *Journal of Information Technology, 19*, 234–243. doi:10.1057/palgrave.jit.2000029

Kotler, P., Haider, D., & Rein, I. (1993). *Marketing places.* New York: The Free Press.

Lamberton, D. M. (1998). Information Economics Research: Points of Departure. *Information Economics and Policy, 10*, 325–330. doi:10.1016/S0167-6245(98)00002-X

Lauriala, J. (2001). *Kontrolli, riski ja informaatio: tutkimus kasvuyrityksen rahoittamiseen ja transaktioihin liittyvistä juridisista ja liiketoimintariskeistä sekä niiden hallitsemisesta velvoite- ja yhtiöoikeudellisin keinoin modernin varallisuusoikeuden ympäristössä.* Saarijärvi, Finland: Kauppakaari.

Løwendahl, B. (1997). Strategic Management of Professional Service Firms. Copenhagen: Handelshøjskolens forlag.

Nysten-Haarala, S. (1998). *The Long-Term Contract. Contract Law and Contracting.* Jyväskylä, Finland: Gummerus Kirjapaino Oy.

OASIS (2006). *Reference Model for Service Oriented Architecture.* (SOA Reference Model Technical Committee). 01.08.2006: OASIS

Parolini, C. (1999). *The value net: A tool for competitive strategy*. New York: Wiley.

Popper, K. R. (1972). *Objective Knowledge. An Evolutionary Approach*. Oxford, UK: Clarendon Press.

Pöyhönen, J. (1988). *Sopimusoikeuden järjestelmä ja sopimusten sovittelu*. Vammala, Finland: Vammalan Kirjapaino Oy.

Rai, A., Wareham, J., & Sambamurthy, V. (2005). Designing intelligent service supply networks. In Vervest, P., Preiss, K., van Heck, E., & Pau, L. (Eds.), *Smart busness networks* (pp. 239–254). Berlin: Springer. doi:10.1007/3-540-26694-1_17

Saariluoma, P. (1990). *Taitavan Ajattelun Psykologia* [Psychology of skilled thinking]. Helsinki, Finland: Otava.

Saloheimo, M., Soukka, A., Tuikkala, I., & Aaltonen, J. (2007). Towards ICT-enabled SME supply networks within the tourism industry in Lapland. In Kankaanpää, P., Ovaskainen, S., Pekkala, L., & Tennberg, M. (Eds.), *Knowledge and power in the arctic* (pp. 134–139). Rovaniemi, Finland: University of Lapland.

Saunders, C., Wu, Y., Li, Y., & Weisfeld, S. (2004). Interorganizational Trust in B2B Relationships. In M. Janssen, H. G. Sol & R. W. Wagenaar (Eds.), *Proceedings of the 6th International Conference on Electronic Commerce,* (pp. 272-279) (ICEC 2004). New York: ACM.

Scott, N., Baggio, R., & Cooper, C. (2008). The network concept and tourism. In Scott, N., Baggio, R., & Cooper, C. (Eds.), *Network analysis and tourism* (pp. 15–26). Clevedon, UK: Channel View.

Searle, J. R. (1995). *The Construction of Social Reality*. New York: The Free Press.

Shapiro, C., & Varian, H. R. (1999). *Information Rules. A Strategic Guide to the Network Economy*. Boston: Harward Business School Press.

Turunen, A. (2005). *Innovations as Communication Processes. A Legal Architecture for Governing Ideas in Business*. Saarijärvi, Finland: Lapland University Press.

Virtanen, P. (2001). Määräävän markkina-aseman kontrollointi. Oikeus ja taloustieteellinen vertaileva tutkimus Saksan, Suomen ja EU:n kilpailuoikeudesta. Helsinki, Finland: Suomalainen lakimiesyhdistys.

Zettinig, P. (2003). *Invisible Organisations: Inter-firm Organisational Formation and Form*. Turku, Finland: Turku School of Economics and Business Administration.

KEY TERMS AND DEFINITIONS

Network-Wide Knowledge Discovery: In contrast to intra-organizational and database centered traditional data mining the network-wide knowledge discovery is based on sociologically anti-positivistic, ideographic and subjective view of society construed from social facts in contexts where inter-organizational communication and information flows are the main source of knowledge acquisition and analysis.

Socially Construed Reality: A philosophical view as the construction of social reality is formed by the concepts of facts, social facts and epistemic community where the structure of perception is based on the *psychology of thought*.

Net-Like Structure: A net is a *net-like structure* if and only if it consists of: (i) nodes (or actors), (ii) connectivity features (links or relationships), (iii) the environment (the logical context or scope), (iv) resources (or assets) that can be consumed or transferred between the nodes, and (v) the dynamics, which represents the various interactions and communications between the actors of a net.

Functional Principles: Contractual principles (fairness/equality, faith/fair dealing, trust/confidentiality) derived from contract law that have an operative and activating nature in supporting network governance, knowledge sharing and information asymmetry reduction.

Information Asymmetry: Refers to a condition in which at least some relevant information is (better) known only to some parties (of a net-like structure) and/or there exists an information related power balance having typically negative impact to business transactions.

Information Intensive Business Governance (IIBG): Is an organizational management approach like resource based view (RBV) and process based view (PBV) that emphasizes knowledge and information intensive assets (i.e. knowledge based view, KBV) as being the core competencies and enablers of successful business.

Tourism Value Chain: A supply chain or network in tourist industry, which typically consists of suppliers of basic tourism services, tour operators (wholesale), travel agents (retail) and customers (tourists).

Multidisciplinary Concept Modeling: The creation of multiperspective domain area analyses in form of semi-formal concept specifications that enable the sharing of research conceptualizations and provide support to explicating the semantics of the key domain entities and their relationships.

Chapter 16
Clinical Data Mining in the Age of Evidence–Based Practice:
Recent Exemplars and Future Challenges

Irwin Epstein
City University of New York, USA

Lynette Joubert
University of Melbourne, Australia

ABSTRACT

Clinical Data Mining (CDM) is a paradigm of practice-based research that engages practitioners in analyzing and evaluating routinely recorded material to explore, evaluate and reflect on their practice. The rationale for, and benefits of this research methodology are discussed with multiple exemplars from health and human service settings. While CDM was conceived as a quantitative methodology evaluating the process, intervention and outcomes of practice, it can support qualitative studies encouraging reflectiveness. CDM was originally employed as a practice based research (PBR) consultation strategy with practitioners in clinical settings, but the methodology has been increasingly used by doctoral students as a dissertation research strategy either by itself or in combination with other research methods. CDM has gained international recognition by both social workers and allied health professionals. The authors present CDM as a knowledge-generating paradigm contributing to "evidence-informed" practice rather than "evidence based practice."

INTRODUCTION

In the course of their work, social workers and other allied health professionals routinely generate and record massive amounts of qualitative and quantitative information concerning patient needs, services provided and outcomes achieved. However, other than for accountability purposes, this information

DOI: 10.4018/978-1-60566-906-9.ch016

is rarely retrieved, converted into data-bases and systematically analyzed by those practitioners who have generated it. At the same time, these professionals are under increasing pressure to integrate research into their practice and to employ research-based interventions.

Within social work in the United States and to a lesser extent elsewhere, Evidence-based Practice (EBP) is the prevailing paradigm of practice-research integration (Gambrill, 2006; Gibbs &

Gambrill, 2002) whereby practitioners are encouraged to conduct exhaustive and critical reviews of research literature in quest of interventions that are "proven" to be effective based on the accumulated evidence of randomized clinical trials (RCT's) and meta-analyses of these studies. Alternatively, EBP proponents advocate providing practitioners with "manualized" guides to practice, based on the results of systematic reviews and meta-analyses conducted by academics. Clearly, this idealized model of practice-research integration is fashioned according to western medical practice and drug studies.

Unfortunately however, there are many reasons why this approach to social work knowledge generation and practice integration is problematic. One major reason is that RCT's are not especially suitable for studying social work interventions (Epstein, 2001). Another is that EBP advocates conceptualize practitioners as mere consumers of knowledge, disparaging their accumulated "practice wisdom" as "non-scientific" at best and "quackery" at worst. In so doing, they minimize the potential of practitioners as knowledge producers and further alienate them from the value of research.

This chapter describes an alternative paradigm of practice-knowledge generation that engages practitioners in evaluating and reflecting on their own practice by systematically collecting, analyzing and interpreting client and patient information that practitioners themselves have created. We call this analysis of routinely available information "Clinical Data-Mining" (CDM) (Epstein, 2001). Although CDM was "invented" in the context of American social work practice, it has been effectively disseminated by the authors and applied by social work practitioners in Australia, Hong Kong, Israel, Singapore and Sweden. In addition, the method has been productively employed by allied health professionals other than social workers (e.g., music therapists, occupational therapists, physiotherapists, psychologists, podiatrists, speech pathologists, etc.) as well as by multi-disciplinary

teams of health professionals. Finally, in a few social work doctoral programs, CDM has been accepted as a legitimate research methodology for PhD dissertation research either in combination with other more established research approaches or in its own right.

Thus, in a decade's teaching, training and consultation experience of the authors—together and separately—CDM has proven to be an especially congenial strategy for engaging practitioners in research, for testing research-based knowledge as well as practice wisdom, and for producing practice-relevant knowledge for social work and allied health professions.

The purpose of this paper is to:

- To distinguish between EBP as a Research-Based Practice (RBP) strategy and Practice-Based Research (PBR)
- To define CDM and identify it as one of a number possible PBR strategies
- To distinguish CDM from conventional data-mining, from Secondary Analysis (SA) and from Chart Reviews
- To present and illustrate a typology of CDM approaches
- Describe the basic steps in the CDM process and the methodological variations that are possible offering exemplars of each
- Discuss CDM's strengths as well as its limitations
- Discuss future potential of CDM

BACKGROUND

Although the social work research potential of available information as well as its limitations were clearly articulated decades ago by Shyne (1960), academic researchers largely ignore her prescient writing on the subject. Emphasizing the inadequacies of available agency-based data (e.g., missing information, problems of validity and reliability, etc.) researchers such as Reamer (1996) and Kagle (1998) briefly consider the possibilities and quickly dismiss them. Instead, they as well as their academic colleagues privilege research based on original data collected by researchers, for research purposes, Certainly among academic researchers associated with the EBP project, RCT's employing standardized quantitative measures are viewed as the "gold-standard" to which all social work researchers should aspire (Ell, 1996).

Four decades after the publication of Shyne's paper, in a paper subtitled "Mining for Silver While Dreaming of Gold" Epstein (2001) resurrected her method and working as a research consultant in social work agencies, placed it in the hands of practitioner-researchers. In that paper, Epstein introduced and illustrated CDM as a Practice-based Research (PBR) strategy that practitioners could employ to evaluate and reflect upon their own practice using the information they already had routinely available to them for practice purposes. In this paper, the epistemological assumptions contained within PBR were distinguished from those within Research-based Practice (RBP). The latter are consistent with current thinking in the EBP movement which privileges RCT's with original data-collection based on standardized quantitative methods and summative evaluations.

The implication of the subtitle was that by contrast with RBP strategies, those which fall into the category of PBR might be considered imperfect from the standpoint of the reliability, validity and completeness of the data but they might still employ "gold-standard" logic in generating practice-relevant and highly useful descriptive and quasi-experimental studies. CDM is one such strategy which makes use of available clinical information even if it is less than ideal from a research perspective. And, it has distinct advantages—not the least of which is that it can be implemented unobtrusively in clinical research studies by practitioners with no additional burden on consumers.

A great deal has changed since Shyne's day which makes the analysis of available information

by practitioners much more feasible. Most significant are the following changes in information technology: (1) affordable personal computers with enormous memory storage and rapid information processing capacities; (2) widespread computer literacy among non-researchers as well as researchers; (3) the introduction of "off the shelf" computerized management and clinical information systems in social work and other public and private service agencies; (4) easy to use "point and click" data-analytic software; and (5) search engines that make prior research readily accessible to practitioners as well as to researchers.

What hasn't changed is the fact that for external accountability and internal supervisory purposes, social workers and other health professionals are still obliged to maintain quantitative and well as qualitative records of their clients' demographic characteristics, diagnostic information, service needs and requests, interventions received, short and long-term outcomes achieved and satisfaction with service. Taken together, these two sets of factors significantly increase the potential for the research uses of available information by practitioners.

With this combination of profound technological change and continuing production of information in mind, CDM may be currently defined as *a practice-based research strategy by which practitioner-researchers systematically retrieve, codify, analyze and interpret available qualitative and/or quantitative information concerning client characteristics and needs, services and interventions received and outcomes achieved derived from their own records for the purpose of reflecting upon the practice and policy implications of their findings*. This definition incorporates the latest developments in its application since it was identified as a distinct social work research method (Epstein, 2010).

Thus for example, while CDM was originally conceived as a purely *quantitative* approach, under special circumstances it can support *qualitative* studies. Similarly, while CDM was originally conceived as a *retrospective* research approach, Joubert (2006) has introduced the concept of *prospective* CDM. Additionally, while CDM was originally employed as PBR consultation strategy with practitioners in clinical settings, it has been increasingly used by doctoral students as a dissertation research strategy either by itself or in combination with other research methods. Finally, while CDM was originally thought of as an exclusively social work research method, its use has been extended by Joubert and Epstein (2005) to multi-disciplinary and allied health practice research. Although CDM relies on available data, it differs from secondary analysis in that the information it employs was not originally collected for research purposes. Instead, its unique contribution is to maximize the research potential of information that would otherwise contribute little to knowledge generation via professionals who are not routinely viewed as contributors to the professional knowledge base. Perhaps more important is the way the process of conducting CDM studies offers practitioners an opportunity for "evidence-informed" reflection on who they are serving, what interventions they are providing and what outcomes they are achieving. (Figure 1)

How is CDM Different from Conventional Data-Mining, Secondary Analysis and Chart Reviews?

Although CDM, conventional business uses of data-mining and Secondary Analysis all rely on available information, CDM (as it has been employed) is different in various ways. Separate from the use of it to answer social work and allied health practice-research questions, CDM differs from conventional data-mining approaches in that it makes use of far less sophisticated statistical techniques. In fact, even the use of decision trees, regression and cluster analyses which are the mainstays of conventional data-mining in industry (Rexer, 2008) are rarely used in CDM. Instead,

practitioner-initiated and executed CDM studies rely heavily on univariate and bi-variate analyses in descriptive and quasi-experimental studies. When more sophisticated multi-variate analyses are employed they are most likely to be carried out by more methodologically sophisticated doctoral students in their dissertation research studies.

And while SA is occasionally employed by academic social work researchers as well as doctoral students—particularly those engaged in policy-oriented research—it makes use of available information and existing data-bases that were generated for research purposes to begin with. By contrast, CDM involves the conversion to research purposes of clinically-relevant information that was not generated with research in mind. Therein lies CDM's greatest strength and greatest weakness. Thus, it salvages and exploits informational resources that would otherwise go to waste. At the same time—and here it resembles conventional data-mining—CDM researchers and research consultants must be prepared to struggle with issues of missing data, extreme outliers, the absence of key variables and limited theoretical underpinning.

Despite these acknowledged limitations, over a decade's experience of CDM consultation suggests that it is an extremely effective way to engage social work and other human service practitioners in research on their own practice. In addition, it generates findings as well as theoretical insights that can be shared with other professionals through publications and conference presentations. In social work, this is particularly noteworthy because practitioners are notoriously "reluctant" to read and/or conduct research studies (Epstein, 1987). The exemplars described in this paper are presented as "evidence" in support of the opposing proposition.

In many respects, CDM is an extension of what have traditionally been called "Chart Reviews" whereby practitioners review their own records for the purpose of aggregating particular information about those they are serving. Often this involves

Figure 1. The process of generating practice-based evidence through clinical data mining (Macdonald, Carroll, Albiston and Epstein 2006)

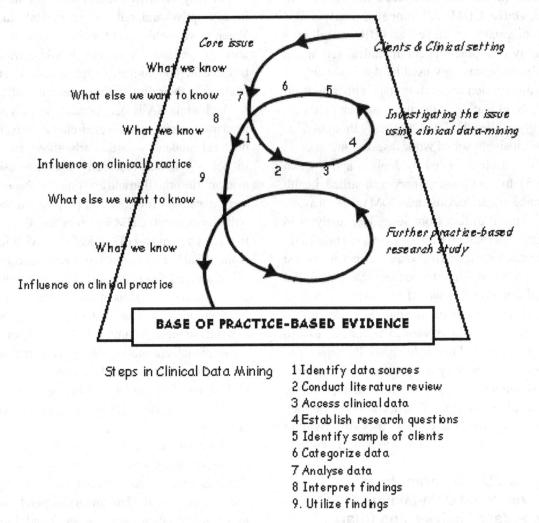

Steps in Clinical Data Mining

1 Identify data sources
2 Conduct literature review
3 Access clinical data
4 Establish research questions
5 Identify sample of clients
6 Categorize data
7 Analyse data
8 Interpret findings
9. Utilize findings

hand percentaging of information about certain categories of service recipients for accountability purposes or to identify unmet needs. What makes CDM different is its broader scope, its use of computerization and data-analytic software and its systematic reflection on practice and programmatic implications of findings. Rather than seeing them as distinct or dichotomous categories, perhaps it is more appropriate to think of simple Chart Reviews and complex CDM studies as representing opposite ends of a continuum reflecting the research use of available clinical information.

PURPOSES OF CDM IN SOCIAL WORK AND ALLIED HEALTH

Although data-mining in other fields is geared to building statistical models that predict and validate decision-making of one kind or another, CDM as the present authors have defined it serves many different purposes within social work and other allied health professions. These are as follows:

- To describe consumer characteristics and needs, services received and outcomes achieved

- To assess the "fidelity" of implementation of intervention models and to evaluate the relationship between interventions for various groups of consumers
- To articulate, refine and enhance "practice wisdom" regarding various forms of intervention
- To identify "best practices" based on available empirical information
- To encourage practitioner "reflectiveness" about what they are doing, with whom and with what effect?
- And ultimately, to promote an Evidence-Informed Practice (McNeill, 2006, Epstein, in press) that is more inclusive than models of EBP that rely entirely on original, non-clinical data-collection

THE ADVANTAGES OF USING CDM AS A RESEARCH METHODOLOGY

While it is clear that in every helping profession, there is a robust academic research enterprise, this program of study tends to emphasize studies based on original data, collected prospectively with standardized research instruments, preferably in an experimental context. Elsewhere, Epstein (2001) has referred to this as "Research-based Practice" (RBP) a term which encompasses but is not limited to the currently dominant EBP model of practice-research integration. The academic emphasis has the dual negative consequence of failing to exploit vast bodies of potentially valuable information and furthering the research/practice antagonism by imposing research-generated burdens on both practitioners and service recipients in clinical settings (Epstein, in press). By contrast, legitimating CDM as a practice-research methodology opens the door to the following:

- The non-intrusive research utilization of enormous quantities of qualitative

and quantitative consumer and program information
- Relatively inexpensive access to large sample sizes and efficient sampling possibilities
- Ease of de-identifying data
- Efficient data-gathering and low levels of study attrition

With the advent of electronic record keeping in some organizations and the introduction of standardized assessment tools into clinical information systems, the potential for CDM is even greater.

THE DISADVANTAGES OF CDM AS A RESEARCH METHODOLOGY

It would be misleading to suggest that CDM doesn't have its downsides and detractors. Wherever and whenever researchers are limited to available information (Shyne, 1960) they inevitably struggle with a host of limitations. Thus, CDM tends to be:

- Labor intensive and dirty—especially when working with non-computerized records
- Plagued by missing data, relatively crude indicators and/or the absence of any information about key study variables
- Limited in terms of capacity to empirically test the validity and reliability of measures
- Vulnerable to methodological as well as organizational problems associated with linking multiple data-sets and dealing with contradictory and ambiguous information.
- Less likely to receive large research grants
- Less likely to be published in journals devoted to EBP "evidence" hierarchy

Despite de-indentification of data, a few academic colleagues have questioned the ethics of conducting retrospective research for a purpose for which consumers have not granted specific consent. Other criticisms have been more epistemologically-based. Hence negative labels such a "cherry-picking", "fishing expedition" or "hunting trip" have been informally leveled at CDM studies implying that they were insufficiently scientific, a theoretical, not driven by hypotheses and not open to refutation.

Leaving the thorny question of what is science aside, while it is true that many CDM studies are exploratory and do not test explicit hypotheses, they implicitly test practice and program theories. Moreover, we would contend that they are as open to discovery (both positive and negative) as any other form of research and this observation has been supported by virtually every CDM study with which the authors have been involved.

BASIC ELEMENTS OF CDM

Essentially, CDM is an inductive approach to research which as a PBR strategy is intended to inform practice decision-making. Hence its inspiration is often a practice-related question concerning consumer needs and/or service outcomes. While the majority of CDM studies involve the use of quantitative data directly (e.g. demographic data) or the conversion of qualitative information into quantitative data (e.g. narrative accounts of patient improvements in mental health) for subsequent analysis, under the right conditions CDM can support qualitative analysis. In other words, qualitative information analyzed as qualitative data (Cordero 2000, Jones 2006, O'Callaghan 2001).

Initially, CDM was conceived by Epstein (2001) as an entirely *retrospective* approach to research but Joubert (2006) has since explored the possibilities of *prospective* CDM which will be described in a subsequent section of this paper. Whether prospective or retrospective, CDM is at best, quasi-experimental and correlational,

relying on the logic of RCT's but avoiding the less desirable aspects of implementing RCT's in human service settings. Nonetheless, our experience with CDM consultation in agency settings suggests that even purely descriptive CDM studies can offer valuable insights about client or patient needs, service delivery and outcomes achieved.

Finally, employing Scriven's distinction (1995) CDM studies are intended to provide *formative* knowledge that will aid in intervention targeting and refinement or program development, the more methodologically sophisticated CDM studies can come fairly close to approximating *summative* findings with sufficient external validity to cautiously support for external generalization. Certainly, by now CDM studies in social work and allied health have garnered sufficient legitimacy to be published in all but the most scientifically "orthodox", peer-reviewed journals.

THE PROCESS OF CDM IN RESEARCH

Most CDM studies conducted in practice settings begin with an expressed desire to do some form of unspecified evaluative research. As practice-research consultants, it is important to help practitioners specify their interest by arriving at a *somewhat* clearer notion of what it is they want to know? Once this established, we follow some fairly predictable steps which underscore the utility and appropriateness of the "mining" metaphor. And while it is important to be somewhat clear about the purpose of the initial data-mining, flexibility is important in order to be open to unanticipated discoveries. On some occasions, these have been quite striking but it is safe to say that every CDM study we have ever conducted with our practitioner colleagues have yielded surprises of one degree or another. The reason for that we suspect is that no matter how perceptive we are as practitioners and/or observers we cannot compete with the analytic capacity of computers to sift through large amounts of data.

Once the general parameters of the inquiry are established, the following steps the CDM researcher should:

- *Prospect* all potential sources of information
- *Assess core samples* for available variables, quality and completeness of information, accessibility, connectivity of information systems, etc.
- *Inventory samples* for potential independent, dependent, explanatory and mediating variables
- *Consult* research literature for *prior claims* as well as *theories, methods of extraction* and *analysis*
- Create original or adapt available *retrieval tools*
- Devise a *sampling strategy*
- Begin *small-scale mining* and devise methods for testing and improving reliability and validity of data that is unearthed
- Once reliability and validity of mining procedures is established, begin *large-scale mining* in accordance with the original sampling plan
- *Analyze* the *findings* using simple or complex techniques depending on the quality of information, the objectives sought and the research resources available
- *Utilize* the *findings* within and outside the practice context

These steps are described in great detail in Epstein's "handbook" devoted entirely to CDM. And while the steps in the process broadly approximate what any applied researcher would do, it is important to underscore the "openness" of this process to unanticipated findings precisely because it begins with what information is available rather than with a literature review, a theory

and sets of specific hypotheses for testing. Hence it is more "exploratory" than conventional research approaches. This unconventionality may be seen as both its greatest strength and its greatest weakness. For engaging practitioners who are either fearful of research or put off by it, CDM is remarkably user-friendly. For academic researchers on the other hand, who have a *stake* in more pristine and less messy forms of knowledge development, CDM is exceedingly uncomfortable.

Finally, while the "mining" metaphor remains remarkably apposite through the various steps of the CDM process, one way that it isn't involves the "raw materials" that are "mined". Unlike mining for precious gems or metals, CDM uncovers and refines sensitive information about vulnerable human beings. Consequently, at some stage in the process, oversight and approval by some external ethics or human subjects committee needs to be secured so that individuals and groups whose information has been analyzed and disseminated are adequately protected in terms of anonymity, confidentiality, etc.

In practice, this approval may be sought relatively early or late in the process, depending on how routinely accessible the information is to those who are doing the data-mining. Certainly, committee approval must be attained prior to external publication or presentation of findings. De-identification techniques and aggregation of findings are helpful here and all the studies the authors have been associated with have achieved approval. Moreover, we as research consultants and teachers and our practitioner-researcher colleagues as well as doctoral students have been personally comfortable that the rights of those whose available information is utilized have not been abrogated. Nonetheless, it is important to note that some academic researchers have objected to CDM studies because they do not routinely involve consenting research subjects for that particular use of their information.

EXAMPLES OF DIFFERENT TYPES OF CDM STUDIES

As research consultants to health, mental health and child welfare agencies and as social work educators, our "hands-on" experience with CDM falls into two broad categories—practitioner-initiated CDM studies and student-initiated CDM studies. The former are generally conducted by social work or multi-disciplinary teams of social workers and members of the allied health professions (Joubert & Epstein 2006). Student CDM Master's and Ph.D. studies are necessarily individually conducted and authored. Predictably CDM doctoral dissertations tend to be the most methodologically sophisticated with regard to data-analytic strategies employed as well as the mixing of CDM with other research methods and/or the use of available as well as original data. On the other hand, practitioner-initiated studies are likely to have more of an organizational impact in the settings in which they were conducted. Both types of studies have resulted in the publications and conference presentations, often by individuals who have never published or presented before. Likewise, CDM PhD's have been a bridge for several practitioners to become social work academics, bringing their clinical expertise and newly acquired research skills to professional education. As such, CDM is beginning to play a human resource development role.

Irrespective of whether the CDM is conducted in a service agency or educational context, we find it most useful for heuristic purposes to present CDM studies in three broad categories—1) needs studies; 2) monitoring studies; and 3) outcome studies Naturally, in their implementation, CDM studies may overlap these categories—especially so because of the importance of exploiting the research potential of all available information. In CDM studies where we are considering all available information as potential data sources, needs, services and outcomes may be reflected.

As indicated earlier, CDM efforts may yield relatively simple descriptive studies using uni-variate statistics or straight forward qualitative description. Or they may employ bi-variate and multi-variate data analyses or complex designs approximating RCT studies (Sainz & Epstein, 2001). Similarly, qualitative CDM may be approached through a complex "constructivist" lens yielding results approximating phenomenological studies (O'Callaghan, 2006). In the exemplars cited below, the potential uses of CDM needs, monitoring and outcome explorations is only suggested.

Need Studies

CDM need studies tend to describe the demographic and psycho-social characteristics of clients, patients and/or service recipients in order to make inferences about unmet needs that existing consumers may bring to the organization.

Perhaps the simplest quantitative exemplar of such a study was conducted by Nilsson (2001) who collected information from the charts of 18 "frequent flyers" in a pediatric diabetes program in an Australian children's hospital. The foregoing label was applied by staff to children who were frequently readmitted to hospital and whose families failed to comply with medical recommendations. Nilsson was able to identify unmet psycho-social needs that these families displayed which were extremely helpful in targeting future prevention and treatment efforts.

A mixed-method CDM needs study was conducted by MacDonald et al. (2006) of the purely social needs of young adults who had experienced their first episode of schizophrenia. Extracting and analyzing (both quantitatively and qualitatively) intake information taken from a self-administered questionnaire given to applicants for clinical services targeted to young adult schizophrenics, they were able to identify the particular kinds of social support these young persons wanted from family and friends.

A larger and more complex CDM needs study involved the purely quantitative analysis of intake information collected in 2 medical clinics in New York, designed to identify women at risk of intimate partner violence. By retrieving ignored questionnaires, converting the information collected to an SPSS data-base, aggregating and correlating the data, Ross, Walther and Epstein (2004) were able to empirically demonstrate the links between witnessing prior violence in one's family of origin, fear of intimate partner violence and mother's concerns about their own potential for abusive behavior toward their children.

Certainly the most ambitious practitioner-initiated, CDM needs study was conducted under the auspices of the Adolescent Health Center at Mount Sinai Hospital in New York City. This project involved several teams of social workers, a psychiatrist, health and occupational counselors, etc. Applicants routinely completed a self-administered questionnaire named "Adquest" that queried them about school, work, family, friends, drugs and alcohol, sex and sexual orientation, experience of racism, etc. Although the staff routinely referred to the questionnaires as "the data-base" they remained untouched and unanalyzed in a file drawer once the intake interview was completed.

While the prior study was clearly the most ambitious CDM needs study, perhaps the most methodologically sophisticated is a PhD dissertation currently close to completion at Hunter College School of Social Work where the first author teaches. Louis Rodriguez is studying men who are "long-term stayers" in homeless shelters that are intended to move them into permanent housing in New York City. Using survival analysis and Cox regression analysis, Rodriguez is seeking to derive and validate an empirically-based predictive model of length of stay with the intention of informing homeless shelter policy and services.

Goldstein (2007) considered a similar length of stay for homeless women in New York City shelters. Although Goldstein initially employed CDM of *available* information on the women and their families supplied by the Department of Homeless services for her dissertation, she did so

in combination with *original* qualitative information gathered in interviews that she conducted.

Monitoring Studies

CDM monitoring studies focus on who is being served for what problems and clinical and program intervention patterns. As such they may be purely descriptive using univariate statistics or qualitative description to render the reality of practice in the agency. Additionally, they may focus on the *quality* of practice by comparing empirical patterns of service provision with accountability requirements from funding sources, notions of "best practice", and/or the "fidelity" with which program models or theories are actually implemented. Here, bi-variate statistics and correlations are employed. Finally, in principle monitoring uses of CDM might involve multi-variate analyses of institutional racism, sexism or other forms of discrimination based on relationships between service provision and demographics, controlling for problem presentation, diagnosis, etc.

The following are some practitioner-initiated and PhD dissertation exemplars of CDM monitoring studies:

- Working as a CDM research consultant with various levels and kinds of practitioners at different health settings in Australia, Joubert has facilitated numerous social work, allied health and multi-disciplinary practice-based research projects. At St. Vincent's Hospital in Melbourne, working with a team of administrators in allied health, social work, occupational therapy and physiotherapy, Joubert and her practitioner colleagues conducted a CDM monitoring study of Emergency Department admissions and discharges the health issues surrounding these (Posenelli, Joubert, Power, Vale, Lewis & Elliot, 2005). In addition to the study findings, their published paper described the ways in which the

CDM process fostered managerial collaboration in future service planning.

- In New York City, Dobrof and her colleagues (Dobrof, Doinko, Lichiger, Uribarri & Epstein 2000) conducted a study of social work services provided to End-Stage Renal Disease (ESRD) patients receiving dialysis treatment at Mt. Sinai Hospital. They were able to both describe the problems of Israeli ESRD dialysis patients but by comparing findings with Dobrof et al.'s study reflect upon differences between the Israeli and American patient populations and the implementation of dialysis services in these two countries. In the comparisons, previously unanticipated differences were surfaced and discussed (Auslander, 2001).

- A CDM doctoral dissertation conducted by Hanssen focused in part on the issue of the "fidelity" of services provided in a single, highly regarded Intensive Family Preservation (IFP) agency in the United States. As a consequence, the two papers published from this quantitative CDM dissertation study in the *Journal of Family Preservation* can be seen as a CDM monitoring (Hanssen & Epstein 2006) and a CDM outcome study (Hanssen & Epstein, 2007). Further exemplars of CDM outcome studies are presented below.

CDM Outcomes Studies

A final set of CDM studies are those that consider the outcomes associated with social work interventions. These studies cannot match RCT's for their capacity to demonstrate causality. At best, they are only approximations to experiments. Or, they may be qualitative accounts "best practices" associated with desirable outcomes. However, though they are not nearly as highly valued as RCT's by those identified with the EBP movement, they do enjoy several advantages over prospective controlled experiments. First, the fact that they are retrospective insures that they are unintrusive and do not require any change in "natural" modes of intervention in order to learn from them. Second, they do not require artificially constructed control groups and the necessary withholding of service to derive useful results. Third, they do not burden service recipients with the completion of standardized research instruments for purely research purposes. Finally, they do not rely on random assignments of clients, patients or service recipients to various interventions or to none at all. For this reason, CDM outcome studies have been comfortably adopted by teams of clinicians working *in situ* as well as by individual clinicians seeking their PhD's.

In fact, for the first author of this paper, the first published CDM outcome study conducted by practitioners has served as a prototype for all subsequent quantitative CDM studies of this kind (Epstein, Zilberfein & Snyder 1997). Thus, the Mount Sinai Hospital liver transplant study involved and extensive, retrospective chart review by a team of social workers and a psychiatrist whose organizational assignment was to assess the psycho-social suitability of candidates for transplant and to provide on-going social work services to those who received transplants (Zilberfein, Hutson, Snyder & Epstein 2001).

Their study could not "prove" the proposition that social work services increased survival rates. As anticipated, Zilberfein and her fellow data-miners found that demographic factors such as race and ethnicity were not associated with survival rates. However, to their surprise they discovered that patients with a documented history of substance abuse fared just as well as those who had no such history. Intrigued by their unanticipated finding, Zilberfein and her colleagues went on to demonstrate that those patients whose records revealed a history of substance abuse but a failure to "link their liver disease to the substances they ingest" had significantly lower survival rates than those who acknowledged this connection (Zilberfein, Hutson, Snyder & Epstein 2001, 102).

A doctoral dissertation conducted by Chan in a palliative care unit for dying cancer patients in Hong Kong employed many of the same steps and techniques first developed in the liver transplant study (Chan 2007). However, rather than focusing on survival, Chan was interested in the psycho-social correlates of patients' having a "good death" and the contribution that being in the palliative care unit made to this outcome. He was able to demonstrate significant T1/T2 improvements on several dimensions and to identify what he refers to as a "paradox of helping". Chan suggests that this interpersonal dynamic is culturally based but there is reason to think that it is universally applicable and clinically relevant.

Working in the context of child welfare in New York City, Cordero pioneered a qualitative CDM outcome study for her doctoral dissertation. More specifically, her focus was on the reunification of foster children with their biological families (Cordero 2000). Working with scrupulously detailed social work records in a highly-regarded private foster-care agency, Cordero studied only successful reunification cases. Although her sample was relatively small (N=18), these represented the entire successful output of the agency for the year which served as her "window" into successful practice. Nonetheless, she was able to employ a typology based on the court-assigned reason official reason for foster placement—i.e., parental neglect, substance abuse or domestic violence and whether they were in kinship or non-kinship foster care.

Employing this typology, she extracted qualitative case information following a three-stage "model" of intervention that included initial assessment, maintenance of a positive foster-care environment and transition back to the biological family. Lessons learned from this study were communicated to the field via presentations and training conducted by Cordero at the agency from which she acquired the data and through publication (Cordero 2004, Cordero & Epstein 2005).

In addition, her work served as the prototype for subsequent qualitative CDM studies.

In another qualitative CDM doctoral dissertation conducted in Australia, O'Callaghan—a social worker and a music therapist—data-mines her own personal practice journals to reflect upon how music therapy with dying cancer patients helps and does not. Employing a "self-dialogic" model of enquiry, qualitative journal entries on over 200 patients and over 350 therapy sessions and Atlas/ti software, O'Callaghan describes and illustrates the cognitive, emotional, spiritual and physical changes that are reported by patients and observed by her during and after music therapy interventions. (O'Callaghan 2005, 223).

Another advantage of CDM versus RCT is demonstrated in the outcomes evaluation portion Hanssen's quantitative CDM study of Intensive Family Preservation referred to earlier. In her ex-post facto application of experimental logic to available data, Hanssen was able to identify demographic and clinical variations that appeared to mediate or intensify the effectiveness of the intervention. Although these wait further testing as hypotheses for future studies, they would not have arisen in an RCT where the guiding assumption is *ceteris paribus,* i.e., all other things being equal.

A final exemplar of a CDM outcome study involves a doubly mixed-method study. Thus, Mirabito's doctoral dissertation (Mirabito 2000) involved both available and original data-collection and quantitative as well as qualitative analysis. Conducted at Mount Sinai Hospital's Adolescent Health Center (AHC) in which the CDM need studies described earlier (Peake, Epstein & Medeiros 2004) was conducted. Based upon original interviews and the qualitative data they generated, Mirabito constructed a practitioner-based theory that "unacknowledged" terminations or "drop-out" without any accompanying clinical process occurred frequently with those adolescents who were most resistant to treatment and with whom treatment was least effective. This theory was logical, persuasive and consistent with her expectations.

The quantitative CDM portion of her study allowed Mirabito to test this theory with available quantitative retrospective data extracted from the case records of 100 systematically sampled, closed cases selected from the prior year. Most intriguing to Mirabito were those young persons who did extremely well in treatment had very positive relationships with their therapists but ended it with no acknowledgement. Thus, Mirabito's mixed methodology represents a highly creative approach to practice-theory development and testing. Her findings suggested a more flexible treatment termination policy in the agency and a more sensitive and differentiated approach to young persons with various clinical profiles.

Joubert (2006) applied CDM prospectively in a practice based evaluation conducted by a multi-disciplinary care coordination team in the emergency department at Sunshine Hospital, in the western suburbs of Melbourne, Australia. Using a prospective data mining methodology, the team had the opportunity to analyze and evaluate outcomes relating to patients' representation rates in emergency, the number of admissions to hospital and the length of stay in hospital. The evaluation process utilized existing assessment tools for data collection in an attempt to meet the needs of a busy team who were implementing the evaluation as part of their practice. The design was prospective and quasi-experimental with the team collecting data over a period of a month and used CDM in analyzing an existing hospital database to create a comparison group.. The outcomes of the study impacted on practice, and demonstrated the importance of acknowledging transdisciplinary profession specific skills by means of pathway protocols for referral between team members.

Joubert (2006) used retrospective and prospective CDM to explore the relationships between the process of assessment and discharge planning in a multidisciplinary team at St Vincent's health service. The team explored the role of family and informal support systems in strengthening the older person's quality of life and capacity for independent living. Both quantitative and qualitative data from 50 patients recruited into study were collected using routine assessment forms. In phase 1, quantitative data was collected through the hospital's patient administrative system and medical record audit using retrospective data mining. In phase 2, the allied health team used their post-discharge semi-structured interview schedule in a telephone interview with elderly patients and their careers. The interview schedule was refined as a result of this analysis to include more items exploring family resilience and informal social networks as routine practice in the geriatric assessment units in the health service.

Although the exemplars cited above all involve studies of social work interventions or related interventions to one degree another, some recent CDM doctoral dissertations illustrate how the "mining" of available information can be used to reflect on broader social work issues at higher levels of abstraction. Although some might define these studies as "non-clinical" their methodological inspiration and inherent logic was based upon prior CDM studies.

Thus for example, in what is essentially and N=1 study of a single, community mental health organization, Schwartz (2006) used available, quantitative clinical and management data to reflect on the impact that privatization had on the agency. More specifically, she demonstrated that in this agency privatization did not have the negative organizational impact that the social work literature on privatization would suggest.

The most recently completed data-mining dissertation with which the first author of this chapter was associated is a national study conducted by Williams-Gray of over 100 organizations that have gone through an accrediting process. Viewing the accreditation process as analogous to an "intervention" Williams-Gray was interested in determining whether and how the accreditation process contributed to organizational capacity-building. Her findings demonstrated that within narrow limits—i.e., the development of capacity to collect and manage computerized information—it did.

Moving from Schwartz's N=1 study to William's Gray N=256 study to a CDM study of many thousands, Saracosti (2007) employed a CDM strategy to study the effectiveness of the first year's implementation of a very broadly focused anti-poverty initiative sponsored by the Chilean government and targeted to the entire nation. In her doctoral dissertation, Saracosti used available but previously unanalyzed quantitative data to test the broad theory of social capital formation that served as an underpinning of this national, anti-poverty program.

THE FUTURE OF CDM IN SOCIAL WORK AND ALLIED HEALTH STUDIES

The exemplars cited above provide a picture of the potential of CDM as a knowledge-generating strategy in social work and other helping professions where RCT's present serious ethical and professional limitations. Accordingly, our experience in providing CDM consultation to practitioners who were indifferent to or hostile to research indicates that CDM is not only compatible with their practice norms and values but contributory to their practice reflection and to their appreciation of the value of empirical testing. In addition, it encourages them to research and understand research literature in contexts in which they are conducting their own CDM research studies.

Additionally, doctoral students—particularly those who are concurrently practitioners or identified with practice—find CDM an intriguing and attractive methodology that allows them to efficiently use available agency data rather than dealing with the problems of collecting original data or introducing intrusive experimental designs in natural settings. Finally, the recent introduction

of Propensity Score Matching (citations) to social work research brings with it the potential for use in CDM studies with large quantitative data-bases. With this refined statistical tool, CDM studies can come closer to approximating RCT's in a way that Sainz & Epstein (2001) crudely adumbrated in the first collection of CDM studies.

Unfortunately however many academic researchers and research journals—particularly in the United States where EBP is currently dominant—are resistant to CDM as a practice-research strategy. This resistance represents a real paradigm conflict that has unfortunate consequences for the continued development and dissemination of the approach. Thus for example, for three consecutive years several submissions for conference presentations based on CDM dissertations and on CDM as a dissertation "model" have been rejected by the main social work research conference in the United States. Likewise, the journal connected to this conference robustly rejected submissions based on one of the CDM dissertations cited above on methodological grounds and because there had been several prior RCT's conducted in this area. Notwithstanding these prior research efforts, submission of the same papers to a journal identified with the particular intervention model that the CDM study explored received immediate and enthusiastic acceptance.

Despite the resistance there are reasons to be positive about the future of CDM. The authors are aware of practitioner-initiated and academically-supported CDM projects currently underway or recently completed in Australia, Hong Kong, Ireland, Israel, New Zealand, Singapore, Sweden and the United States. More CDM doctoral dissertations are underway. Another collection of CDM studies in allied health is in the planning stage in Australia. And in addition to this chapter, the first author is currently under contract with a major publisher to write a CDM "handbook" for a series devoted to otherwise "established" social work research methodologies. Publication of the CDM handbook and the current chapter should contribute to legitimating CDM in the United States and on the world stage.

Another way to approach this paradigmatic opposition is to view CDM/RCT or the RBP/PBR distinction as false dichotomies. Thus Epstein (2009) has argued that viewing them in conflicting terms has negative consequences for practice-research integration. Instead, borrowing a concept introduced by McNeill (2006), he advocates a methodologically pluralist model of "evidence-informed practice" which, rather than placing different methodologies on a hierarchy, accepts the contributions and limitations of every knowledge-generating strategy and epistemological paradigm.

CONCLUSION

Clinical Data Mining (CDM) is a practice-based research (PBR) methodology, different from conventional data-mining, Secondary Analysis (SA) and Chart Reviews. While CDM studies are intended to provide *formative* knowledge that will aid in intervention targeting and refinement or program development, the more methodologically sophisticated CDM studies can come fairly close to approximating *summative* findings with sufficient external validity to cautiously support for external generalization. Although regarded as less than ideal from an empirical research perspective, CDM can be implemented unobtrusively in clinical research studies by practitioners, with no additional burden on consumers. Originally conceived as retrospective analysis, studies using a prospective CDM methodology are offering the opportunity to monitor careful data collection while still focused on routinely available information. CDM is rapidly gaining international recognition as a PBR methodology by social workers and allied health professionals as well as being used increasingly in doctoral dissertations. The authors demonstrate the considerable contribution made by CDM as a practice based

research methodology within a methodologically pluralist model of 'evidence–informed practice".

REFERENCES

Auslander, G., Dobrof, J., & Epstein, I. (2001). Comparing social work's role in renal dialysis in Israel and the United States: The practice-based research potential of available clinical information. *Social Work in Health Care, 33*(3/4), 129–152.

Blumenfield, S., & Epstein, I. (2001). Introduction: Promoting and maintaining a reflective professional staff in a hospital-based social work department. *Social Work in Health Care, 33*(3/4), 1–14.

Bush, I., Epstein, I., & Saines, A. (1997). Social work utilization of social sciences literature: A content analysis of practice journal citations. *Social Work Research, 21*, 45–56.

Chan, W. (2007). *A clinical data-mining study of the psycho-social status of Chinese cancer patients in palliative care.* Doctoral dissertation, University of Hong Kong, Hong Kong.

Chan, W., Epstein, I., & Chen, C. (2008). (submitted to). Family predictors of psychosocial outcomes among Hong Kong Chinese cancer patients in palliative care: living and dying with the "support paradox". [Palliative Medicine.]. *Paper*.

Chow, A. (2005). *The bereavement experience of Chinese persons in Hong Kong.* Doctoral dissertation, University of Hong Kong, Hong Kong.

Ciro, D., & Nembhard, M. (2005). Collaborative data-mining in an adolescent mental health service: Clinicians speak of their experience. In K. Peake, I. Epstein & D. Medeiros, (Eds.), Clinical and research uses of an adolescent intake questionnaire: What kids need to talk about (pp. 305-318). Binghampton, NY: Haworth Press.

Cloward, R., & Epstein, I. (1965). Private social welfare's disengagement from the poor: The case of family adjustment agencies. In *Proceedings of the annual social work day conference*. University of Buffalo. Reprinted in Brager, G., & Purcell, P. (Eds.), (1967). *Community action against poverty*. New Haven, CT: College & University Press (pp. 40-63).

Collins, M., Schwartz, I., & Epstein, I. (2001). Risk factors for adult imprisonment in a sample of youth released from residential child care. *Children and Youth Services Review, 23*, 203–226. doi:10.1016/S0190-7409(01)00133-5

Cordero, A. (2000). *When reunification works: A family strengths perspective*. Doctoral dissertation, Graduate Faculty in Social Welfare, The City University of New York, New York.

Cordero, A. (2004). When family reunification works: Data-mining foster care records. *Families in Society, 85*(4), 571–580.

Cordero, A., & Epstein, I. (2005). Refining the practice of reunification: "Mining" successful foster care case records of substance abusing families. In Mallon, G. P., & Hess, P. M. (Eds.), *Child Welfare for the Twenty-First Century: A Handbook of Practices, Policies and Programs*. New York: Columbia University Press.

Dobrof, J., Dolinko, A., Lichtiger, E., Uribarri, J., & Epstein, I. (2000). The complexity of social work practice with dialysis patients: Risk and resiliency factors, interventions and health-related outcomes. *Journal of Nephrology Social Work, 20*, 21–36.

Dobrof, J., Dolinko, A., Lichtiger, E., Uribarri, J., & Epstein, I. (2001). Dialysis patient characteristics and outcomes: The complexity of social work practice with end stage renal disease. *Social Work in Health Care, 33*(3/4), 105–128.

Dobrof, J., Ebenstein, H., Dodd, S., & Epstein, I. (2006). Caregivers and professional partnership caregiver resource center: Assessing a hospital support program for family caregivers. *Journal of Palliative Medicine, 9*(1), 196–205. doi:10.1089/jpm.2006.9.196

Epstein, I. (1987). Pedagogy of the perturbed: Teaching research to the reluctant. *Journal of Teaching in Social Work, 1*, 71–89. doi:10.1300/J067v01n01_06

Epstein, I. (1992). Changing models of practice in research utilization. In Grasso, A. J., & Epstein, I. (Eds.), *Research utilization in the social services: Innovations for practice and administration* (pp. 7–10). Binghampton, NY: Haworth.

Epstein, I. (1995). Promoting reflective social work practice: Research strategies and consulting principles. In Hess, P., & Mullens, E. (Eds.), *Practitioner-researcher partnerships: Building knowledge from, in and for practice* (pp. 83–102). Washington, DC: NASW Press.

Epstein, I. (1996). In quest of a research-based model for clinical practice: Or, why can't a social worker be more like a researcher? *Social Work Research, 20*, 97–100.

Epstein, I. (2001). Using available clinical information in practice-based research: Mining for silver while dreaming of gold. In I. Epstein & S. Blumenfield (eds.), Clinical data-mining in practice-based research: Social work in hospital settings (pp. 15-32). Binghamton, NY: Haworth Press.

Epstein, I. (2005). Following in the footnotes of giants: Citation analysis and its discontents. *Social Work in Health Care, 41*(3/4), 93–101. doi:10.1300/J010v41n03_04

Epstein, I. (2007). From evaluation methodologist to clinical data-miner: Finding treasure through practice-based research. In Rehr, H., & Rosenberg, G. (Eds.), *The Social Work – Medicine Relationship: 100 Years at Mount Sinai* (pp. 107–111). Binghamton, NY: Haworth Press.

Epstein, I. (2008). *Clinical Data-Mining: Integrating Practice and Research.* Oxford, UK: Oxford University Press.

Epstein, I. (2009). Promoting harmony where there is commonly conflict: Evidence-informed practice as an integrative strategy. *Social Work in Health Care, 48*(3), 216–231. doi:10.1080/00981380802589845

Epstein, I. (2010). *Clinical data-mining: Integrating practice and research.* New York, N.Y.: Oxford University Press.

Epstein, I., & Grasso, A. J. (1990). Using agency-based available information to further practice innovation. In Weissman, H. (Ed.), *Serious play: Creativity and innovation in social work.* New York: NASW Press.

Epstein, I., Grellong, B., & Kohn, A. (1992). Models of university-agency collaboration in research. *Research on Social Work Practice, 2,* 350–357.

Epstein, I., & Hench, C. (1979). Behavior modification in the classroom: Education or social control? *Journal of Sociology and Social Welfare,* (September): 223–229.

Epstein, I., & Tripodi, T. (1978). *Research techniques for program planning, monitoring and evaluation.* New York: Columbia University Press.

Epstein, I., Zilberfein, F., & Snyder, S. (1997). Using available information in practice-based outcomes research: A case study of psycho-social risk factors and liver transplant outcomes. In E.J. Mullen, & J.L. Magnabosco, (eds.), Outcomes measurement in the human services: Cross-cutting issues and methods (pp. 224-233). New York: NASW Press.

Freedman, C., Joubert, L., & Russell, N. (2005). Practitioner evaluation of a brief intervention approach in emergency services: The Sunshine Hospital Quick Response Team. *Social Work Research and Evaluation, 6*(2), 207–216.

Gambrill, E. (2006). Evidence-based practice and policy: Choices ahead. *Research on Social Work Practice, 16*(3), 338–357. doi:10.1177/1049731505284205

Gibbs, L., & Gambrill, E. (2002). Evidence-based practice: Counter arguments and objections. *Research on Social Work Practice, 12,* 452–476. doi:10.1177/1049731502012003007

Goldstein, A. (2007). *"A place of my own" Homeless families in the New York City shelter system: The long-term stayers.* Doctoral dissertation, Graduate Faculty in Social Welfare, The City University of New York, New York.

Grasso, A. J., & Epstein, I. (Eds.). (1992). *Research utilization in the social services: Innovations for practice and administration.* Binghampton, NY: Haworth Press.

Grasso, A. J., & Epstein, I. (Eds.). (1993). *Information systems in child, youth and family agencies: Planning, implementation and service enhancement.* Binghampton, NY: Haworth Press.

Hanssen, D. (2003). *Looking inside the black box of intensive family preservation services.* Doctoral dissertation, Graduate faculty in Social Welfare, The City University of New York, New York.

Hanssen, D., & Epstein, I. (2006). A "black box" study of intensive family preservation services: Utilization of clinical data-mining. *Family Preservation, 9,* 7–22.

Hanssen, D., & Epstein, I. (2007). Learning what works: Demonstrating practice effectiveness with children and families through retrospective investigation. *Family Preservation, 10,* 24–41.

Hughes, D., Elkin, C., & Epstein, I. (2004). Long-term Counseling: A feasibility study. of extended follow-up services with high-risk EAP clients. *Journal of Workplace Behavioral Health, 22*(2/3), 27–41.

Hughes, D. C., Leung, P., & Naus, M. J. (2008). Using a single-system analysis to assess the effectiveness of an exercise intervention on quality of life for Hispanic breast cancer survivors: A pilot study. *Social Work in Health Care, 47*(1), 73–91. doi:10.1080/00981380801970871

Hutson, C., & Lichtiger, E. (2001). Mining clinical information in the utilization of social services: Practitioners inform themselves. *Social Work in Health Care, 33*(3/4), 153–162.

Jones, S., Statham, H., & Solomou, W. (2006). When expectant mothers know their baby has a fetal abnormality: Exploring a crisis of motherhood through qualitative data-mining. *Journal of Social Work Research and Evaluation, 6*(2), 195–206.

Joubert, L. (2006). Academic-practice partnerships in practice research: A cultural shift for health social workers. *Social Work in Health Care, 43*(2/3), 151–161. doi:10.1300/J010v43n02_10

Joubert, L., & Epstein, I. (Eds.). (2005). Special Issue. Multi-disciplinary data-mining in allied health practice: Another perspective on Australian research and evaluation [Special Issue]. *Journal of Social Work Research and Evaluation, 6*(2).

Joubert, L., & Power, R. (2006). Using data-mining to explore the outcomes of an integrated care program: Looking for meaning behing key outcome indicators. *Social Work Research and Evaluation, 6*(2), 185–194.

Kabillo, R. (2005). *Family functioning and adolescent psychopathology: A comparison of content and process scoring indices on the McMaster Family Assessment Device in terms of association with adolescent clinical indicators of depression, self-esteem and behavior.* Doctoral dissertation, School of Psychological Science, Faculty of Science, Technology and Engineering, La Trobe University, Bundoora, Victoria, Australia.

Kapp, S., Schwartz, I., & Epstein, I. (1994). Adult imprisonment of males released from residential childcare: A longitudinal study. *Residential Treatment for Children & Youth, 12*, 19–36. doi:10.1300/J007v12n02_03

Kochkine, V. (2006). *Depressive symptoms and academic achievement in immigrant and American-born adolescents of diverse ethno-cultural backgrounds: A cultural data-mining exploration.* Doctoral dissertation, Graduate faculty in Social Welfare, The City University of New York, New York.

Kogan, G. (in progress). *A conceptual and empirical data-mining study of bullying and social power.* Doctoral dissertation, Graduate faculty in Social Welfare, The City University of New York, New York.

Lo, H. (in process). *A clinical data-mining study of symptom presentation of depression, anxiety and Cognitive Behavioral Therapy outcomes in a community–based mental health program.* Doctoral dissertation, University of Hong Kong.

Macdonald, E. M., Carroll, A., Albiston, D., & Epstein, I. (2006). Social relationships in early psychosis: Clinical data-mining for practice-based evidence. *Journal of Social Work Research and Evaluation, 6*(2), 155–166.

Markoff, J. (2006). Taking spying to higher level, Agencies look for more ways to mine data. *New York Times,* February 25th. Technology, 1-4.

Mason, J., Edlow, M., Lear, M., Scopetta, S., Walther, V., Epstein, I., & Guaccero, S. (2001). Screening for psycho-social risk in an urban prenatal clinic population: A retrospective, practice-based research study. *Social Work in Health Care, 33*(3/4), 33–52.

McCracken, S., & Marsh, J. C. (2008). Practitioner expertise in evidence- based practice decision-making. *Research on Social Work Practice, 18*(4), 301–310. doi:10.1177/1049731507308143

Mirabito, D. (2000). *Keeping the door open or keeping the door shut: How and why adolescents terminate from mental health treatment?* Doctoral dissertation, Graduate faculty in Social Welfare, The City University of New York, New York.

Mirabito, D. (2001). Mining treatment termination data in an adolescent mental health service: A quantitative study. *Social Work in Health Care, 33*(3/4), 71–90.

Mullen, E. J., & Bacon, W. (2004). A survey of practitioner adoption and implementation of practice guidelines and evidenced-based treatments. In Roberts, A. R., & Yeager, K. (Eds.), *Evidence-based practice manual: Research and outcome measures in health and human services* (pp. 193–199). New York: Oxford University Press.

Nilsson, D. (2001). Psycho-social problems faced by "frequent flyers" in a pediatric diabetes unit. *Social Work in Health Care, 33*(3/4), 53–70.

O'Callaghan, C. (2001). *Music therapy's relevance in a cancer hospital researched through a constructionist's lens*. Doctoral dissertation, University of Melbourne, Melbourne.

O'Callaghan, C. (2005). Qualitative data-mining through reflexive journal analysis: Implications for music therapy practice development. *Journal of Social Work Research and Evaluation, 6*(2), 217–229.

O'Callaghan, C. (2008). Lullament: Lullaby and lament-therapeutic qualitaties actualized through music therapy. *American Journal of Hospice and Palliative Medicine, 25*(2), 93–99. doi:10.1177/1049909107310139

Osmond, J., & O'Connor, I. (2004). Formalizing the unformalized: Practitioners' communication of knowledge in practice. *British Journal of Social Work, 34*(5), 677–692. doi:10.1093/bjsw/bch084

Payton, G. (1970). Webster's Dictionary of Proper Names. Springfield, MA: G & C Merriam, C O.

Peake, K., Epstein, I., & Medeiros, D. (Eds.). (2005). *Clinical and research uses of an adolescent intake questionnaire: What kids need to talk about*. Binghampton, NY: Haworth Press.

Peake, K., Mirabito, D., Epstein, I., & Giannone, V. (2005). Creating and sustaining a practice-based research group in an urban adolescent mental health program. *Social Work in Mental Health, 3*(1/2), 39–54. doi:10.1300/J200v03n01_03

Posenelli, S., Joubert, L., Power, R., Vale, S., Lewis, A., & Elliot, R. (2005). Managerial collaboration through allied health data-mining: The St. Vincent's Health experience. *Journal of Social Work Research and Evaluation, 6*(2), 167–176.

Pottick, K., Bilder, S., Vander Stoep, A., Warner, L., & Alvarez, M. (2007). US Patterns of mental health service utilization for transition-age youth and young adults. *The Journal of Behavioral Health Services & Research*, 1–16.

Proctor, E., & Rosen, A. (2008). From knowledge production to implementation: Research challenges and imperatives. *Research on Social Work Practice, 18*(4), 285–291. doi:10.1177/1049731507302263

Reeser, L., & Epstein, I. (1990). *Professionalization and activism in social work: The 60's, the 80's and the future*. New York: Columbia University Press.

Rexer, K., Gearan, P., & Allen, H.N. (2007). Surveying the field: Current data mining applications, analytic tools, and practical challenges. *Data Mining Survey Summary Report*, 1-7.

Rodriguez, L. (2008). *Exploring pathways to independence: A data-mining study to research predictors of long-term stay among homeless men in the New York City family shelter system*. Doctoral dissertation, Graduate faculty in Social Welfare, The City University of New York, New York.

Ross, J., Walther, V., & Epstein, I. (2004). Screening risks for intimate partner violence in primary care settings: Implications for future abuse. *Social Work in Health Care*, *38*(4), 1–24. doi:10.1300/J010v38n04_01

Sainz, A., & Epstein, I. (2001). Creating experimental analogs with available clinical information: Credible alternatives to 'gold standard' experiments? *Social Work in Health Care*, *33*(3/4), 163–184.

Sales, E., Lichtenwalter, S., & Fevola, A. (2006). Secondary analysis in social work research education: Past, present and future promise. *Journal of Social Work Education*, *42*(3), 543–558. doi:10.5175/JSWE.2006.200404136

Saracostti, M. (2008). *Social networking as a strategy to overcome poverty in Chile: A data-mining evaluation of the Chile Solidario System*. Doctoral dissertation, Graduate faculty in Social Welfare, The City University of New York, New York.

Schwartz, D., Kaufman, A. B., & Schwartz, I. M. (2004). Computational intelligence techniques for risk assessment and decision support. *Children and Youth Services Review*, *26*(11), 1081–1095. doi:10.1016/j.childyouth.2004.08.007

Schwartz, E. (2007). *Effective privatization of a community mental health agency: Assessing and developing an agency's readiness to change*. Doctoral dissertation, Graduate faculty in Social Welfare, The City University of New York, New York.

Scriven, M. (1995). The logic of evaluation and evaluation practice. In Fournier, (Ed.), Reasoning in evaluation: Inferential links and leaps (New Directions for Program Evaluation, No. 68, pp. 49-70). San Francisco. Jossey-Bass.

Shaw, I. (2005). Practitioner research: Evidence or critique? *British Journal of Social Work*, *35*(8), 1231–1248. doi:10.1093/bjsw/bch223

Shyne, A. B. (1960). Use of available material. In N.A. Polansky (ed.), Social work research (pp. 106-124). Chicago: University of Chicago Press.

Tripodi, T., & Epstein, I. (1978). Incorporating knowledge of research methodology into social work practice. *Journal of Social Service Research*, *2*, 65–78. doi:10.1300/J079v02n01_06

Tripodi, T., & Epstein, I. (1980). *Research techniques for clinical social workers*. New York: Columbia University.

Tripodi, T., Epstein, I., & MacMurray, C. (1970). Dilemmas of evaluation. *The American Journal of Orthopsychiatry*, *40*, 850–857.

Tripodi, T., Fellin, P., & Epstein, I. (1978). *Differential social program evaluation*. Itasca, IL: F.E. Peacock.

Vonk, E., Tripodi, T., & Epstein, I. (2006). *Research techniques for clinical social workers* (2nd ed.). New York: Columbia University Press.

Wai, F. (2007). *Data-mining as a methodology for explaining written narratives: An application on understanding the breast cancer experience among Hong Kong Chinese women*. Doctoral dissertation, University of Hong Kong.

Williams-Gray, B. (in progress). *Accreditation as an intervention and a means for expanding organizational capacity: A data-mining study.* Doctoral dissertation, Graduate faculty in Social Welfare, The City University of New York, New York.

Zilberfein, F., Hutson, C., Snyder, S., & Epstein, I. (2001). Social work practice with pre- and post-liver transplant patients: A retrospective self-study. *Social Work in Health Care, 33*(3/4), 91–104.

KEY TERMS AND DEFINITIONS

Research-Based Practice (RBP): The use of research-based concepts, theories, designs and data-gathering instruments to structure practice so that hypotheses concerning cause-effect relationships may be rigorously tested.

Practice-Based Research: The use of research-inspired principles, designs and information gathering techniques within existing forms of practice to answer questions that emerge from practice in ways that inform practice.

Clinical Data Mining: Practice-based research methodology that engages practitioners in analyzing and evaluating routinely recorded material to explore, evaluate and reflect on their practice.

Formative Knowledge: Collecting data for a specific period of time to improve implementation, to solve unanticipated problems and to record whether participants are progressing towards desired outcomes.

Summative Findings: Data that enables a judgement to be made about a program's worth.

Reflective Practice: Involves thoughtfully considering one's own experiences in applying knowledge to practice while being coached by professionals in the discipline. It has been described as an unstructured self regulated approach directing understanding and learning.

Chapter 17
Data Mining and the Project Management Environment

Emanuel Camilleri
Ministry of Finance, Economy and Investment, Malta

ABSTRACT

The chapter illustrates how data mining and knowledge management concepts may be applied in a project oriented environment for both the private and public sectors. It identifies the project environment success roadmap that consists of four levels leading to project corporate success. Processes that control the dataflow for generating the projects data warehouse are identified and the projects data warehouse contents are defined. The rest of the chapter shows how data mining may be utilised at each project success level to increase the chances of delivering profitable projects that will have the intended impact on the corporate business strategy. The general conclusion is that there is a need to structure and prioritise information for specific end-user problems and to address a number of organizational issues that may facilitate the application of data mining and knowledge management in a project oriented environment. Finally, the chapter concludes by identifying the issues that need to be addressed by private and public sector organizations so that data mining may be utilised successfully in their decision making process.

INTRODUCTION

According to Bala (2008), data mining deals with the principle of extracting knowledge from large volume of data and picking out relevant information that finds application in various business decision-making processes. By its very nature the project oriented environment deals extensively with data, information and knowledge for a wide spectrum of decision-making scenarios. This direct and robust linkage of data mining with a project oriented environment will be illustrated throughout this chapter by demonstrating how data mining may be applied to resolve issues raging from assessing whether a proposed project is aligned with the strategic direction of an entity to the delivery of the project outputs and outcomes.

DOI: 10.4018/978-1-60566-906-9.ch017

Two critical points must be emphasized. Firstly, no matter what your profession is, whether it is marketing, engineering, manufacturing or ICT development and whether you work for the private or public sector, you will at one time or another be involved in undertaking projects. Secondly, to keep clients satisfied, private and public sector organizations are continually faced with the development of products, services, and processes with very short *time-to-market* windows combined with the need for cross-functional expertise. In this scenario, the application of data mining in a project oriented environment becomes a very important and powerful tool for those organizations that understand its use and have the competencies to apply it.

A project management environment provides many challenges. As a project moves through its life cycle the issues involved become numerous. Some of these issues include managing the project portfolio; having a mechanism in place to capture and share project lessons learnt; maintaining the critical project data flow processes; defining project scope; preparing project bids; planning and controlling projects; and assessing project risk. Hence, the road leading to success in a project oriented environment is a long and difficult one. Many of the concerns related to the issues highlighted above may be mitigated through the application of data mining tools by the thorough sifting and analysis of data related to projects previously undertaken.

Private and public sector organizations that are involved in delivering projects normally possess a tremendous amount of data related to past and current projects. This voluminous historical projects data is often by itself of low value. However its hidden potential needs to be exploited for various purposes within the project life cycle to ensure the achievement of the business objectives and more specifically corporate success. Executive management must seek ways to exploit data to add value to processes and create a new reality in terms of establishing innovative practices by capturing intelligence and knowledge across the organization. Hence, the project oriented environment with its extensive data generating capability and capacity has a direct potential link with data mining application concepts for private and public sector organizations.

Data mining techniques have been successfully applied to various private sector industries in marketing, financial services, and health care. Governments are using data mining for improving service delivery, analyzing scientific information, managing human resources, detecting fraud, and detecting criminal and terrorist activities. However, literature is scarce regarding the application of data mining to a project oriented environment. Generally, the purpose of this chapter is to show how data mining concepts may be applied in a project oriented environment. It will examine the so called project success framework and show how data mining may be utilised at particular stages to increase the chances of delivering successful projects that will have the intended impact on the corporate business strategies of private and public sector organizations.

DATA MINING AND THE PROJECT MANAGEMENT ENVIRONMENT CONTEXT

Cooke-Davies (2002) argue that the ultimate aim of an organization should be to introduce practices and measures that allow the enterprise to resource fully a portfolio of projects that is rationally and dynamically matched to the organization's business objectives and corporate strategy. These practices and measures cover a spectrum of tasks, such as transforming data to information and information to knowledge thus optimizing the information value chain of an organization and therefore its ability to bring projects to a successful conclusion. Sutton (2005) identifies four distinct levels of project success, with each level having its own discipline, tools and techniques. Thus, excellence

Figure 1. Project success road map - Sutton's project success framework

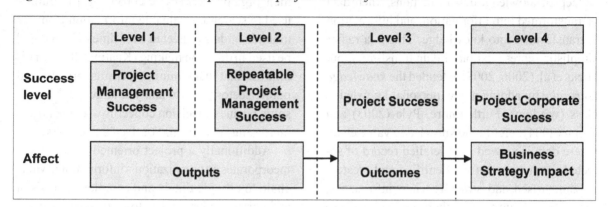

at each level is viewed as being critical for absolute project success. The project success framework put forward by Sutton (2005) shown at Figure 1 takes a holistic corporate approach by linking project delivery to corporate strategy. It provides a road map which leads to an organization being successful in a project oriented environment. The objective is to apply data mining techniques as one travels along the project success road map.

It is important to note that there is a definite tangible distinction and focus between the four success levels proposed by Sutton (2005). Project management success refers to whether a specific project has produced the desired output (project deliverables) while project success refers to whether a specific project has produced the desired outcomes (project objectives). Hence, project output and outcomes are viewed as being separate. Repeatable project management success refers to the organization's ability to consistently execute projects that have produced the desired output.

Furthermore, a project corporate success refers to whether the outcomes produced have the intended impact on the business strategy of the organization. Sutton (2005) insists that project failure may occur at any one of the four levels. Therefore, managers are to understand where and how they are failing and then target the measures that produce the greatest likelihood of success. The application of data mining techniques is viewed as providing an opportunity for management to produce the best likelihood of success at each of the four project success levels. Therefore, the objective is to identify how data mining may be applied at each project success level to facilitate corporate success.

In addition, an organization's value chain becomes an important notion when examining the application of data mining to the project oriented environment. One should note that when referring to an organization's value chain we are in reality referring to two separate concurrent but complementary value chains. One portrays the physical value chain and the other depicts the informational value chain. Hence, the physical value chain is the transformation of tangible resources, such as materials and labour, to a finished product or service; while, the informational value chain consists of the data necessary to transform tangible resources to a finished product or service. Both value chains are necessary, each supporting the other, and ultimately they shape the basis of the organization's business survival.

Admittedly in the knowledge management literature there is a major difficulty in the use of consistent vocabulary (Hicks et al., 2006). The informational value chain in this context was viewed to be similar to the *knowledge hierarchy* as defined by Nissen (2000). This researcher viewed the *knowledge hierarchy* as the traditional concept of knowledge transformations, where data is transformed into information, and information is transformed into knowledge. This is a rather simplistic representation of data transformation. Hicks et al. (2006, 2007) extended the *knowledge hierarchy* by adding a new personal knowledge class (wisdom). Furthermore, Pyle (2003) and Wong (2004) refer to the knowledge value chain where data is viewed as a detailed record of selected events that is first identified and created, is summarised and structured into information for a specific purpose, is then transformed into knowledge from information by a structured framework. Reference to the informational value chain in this text should be viewed as incorporating the notions presented by these researchers. Data mining or knowledge discovery refers to the process of finding interesting information in large repositories of data (Ayre, 2006). Therefore, the informational value chain is viewed as fundamental to the application of data mining in private and public sector entities.

Moreover, data mining is the process of analysing data from different perspectives and summarising it into useful information; information that can be used to increase revenue, cut costs, or both (Palace, 1996). Hence, the focus of data mining in the project oriented environment context is the exploitation and application of the organization's vast repository of projects data to the projects that are in the pipeline or are being implemented. The aim is to ensure the maximum return on project completion with the consequence that the undertaken projects will have the intended impact on the private and public sector organizations' business strategy.

APPLICATION OF DATA MINING: THE PROJECT MANAGEMENT ENVIRONMENT

Managers are not interested in what data mining is, rather, they want to know what it will do for their organization (Pyle, 2003). Data mining is used to search for valuable information from the mounds of data collected over time, which could be used in decision making (Keating, 2008). This implies that data mining permits private and public sector users to analyze large databases to solve business decision concerns with the aim of increasing revenue and/or decreasing costs.

Additionally a project oriented environment incorporates an organization's informational value chain to provide timely and complex analysis of an integrated view of data to strengthen the organization's competitive position. This section will address two essential aspects. The first aspect is related to the contents of the data warehouse and the organizational processes that contribute to populate it. The second aspect is the application of data mining methods as a project travels along the four project success levels.

THE HEART OF THE MATTER: PROCESSES AND THE PROJECTS DATA WAREHOUSE

Management have six types of resources at their disposal to carry out the projects under their responsibility. These are money, people, materials, equipment, energy and data. The focus of this section is data and the processes needed to support the data flow. Datta (2008) makes reference to the basic elements of data mining, two of which are; (a) extracting, transforming, and loading transaction data onto the data warehouse system; and (b) storing and managing the data in a multidimensional database system. However, for these elements to occur management must have the proper processes in place. These processes permit the communication and dissemination of information and knowledge to the relevant people thus achieving the three remaining data mining elements, namely, data access by relevant professionals; analysis of data by suitable application software; and presenting results in a meaningful format to various organizational users.

In an environment where projects are conducted by individuals in isolation, the processes will most likely be undemanding and involve only a few persons. However, in project oriented organizational environments the processes that determine the information flow can be quite intricate. Figure 2 provides a concise view of the complexity of the functions and processes that control project information flow in a private or public sector project oriented environment. Each functional area may generate a combination of data, information and knowledge that are required to be stored in a projects data warehouse for retrieval, analysis and compilation of meaningful reports to resolve complex problems. Figure 2 shows the strong integration of the various functional areas that contribute to the physical and informational value chains. The informational value chain consists of data from external and internal sources that combine to provide a holistic and complete picture of the organizational project oriented environment at any one point in time.

Figure 3 illustrates that ICT plays a crucial role in bringing together the processes and data to populate the projects data warehouse that may be mined to determine operational patterns and resolve specific concerns for private and public sector organizations. Figure 3 demonstrates a number of fundamental features. Firstly, input data may consist of raw data that act as the input transactions for Management Information Systems (MIS) which generate the transactional databases or/and may consist of documented project experiences, such as, business strategies; contracts and projects scopes; various concerns and solutions; and various conflicts and conflict resolution that are entered directly into the projects data warehouse without an MIS filtering.

Secondly, MIS provides information for the projects data warehouse and may also utilise its transactional databases as an input source for Decision Support Systems (DSS) and Executive Information Systems (EIS). Thirdly, DSS and EIS may after executing the relevant business models provide information and knowledge to the projects data warehouse. Finally, the projects data warehouse will consist of data, information, and knowledge that will be used by data mining methods for the resolution of a wide spectrum of project related concerns. The long term objectives are to reconcile the varying views of data; provide a consolidated view of enterprise data; create a central point for accessing and sharing analytical data; and develop an enterprise approach to business intelligence and reporting.

This concept is inline with the five tier knowledge management hierarchy of Hicks et al., (2007), where the data warehouse is populated from various sources, including individual experience; databases; learning systems; DSS and EIS; knowledge pooling; best practices; expert systems and corporate strategy. It is important to note that the processes needed to support the data flow and the respective critical data sets that are generated by them are essential to the four project success levels. Finally, the concept is applicable to both the private and public sectors, irrespective of the industry or government department they represent.

THE ROAD TO SUCCESS: PROJECT MANAGEMENT SUCCESS (OUTPUTS)

Sutton's (2005) project success Levels 1 and 2 refer to the project management function. Success Level 1 refers to the successful completion of an individual project. However, Success Level 2 refers to repeatable project management success, that is, the organization's ability to consistently execute projects that have produced the desired deliverables. The emphasis of Success Level 1 is related to the tasks that achieve project scope; project planning and control; and project risk

Figure 2. Processes controlling project information flow and data warehouse contents

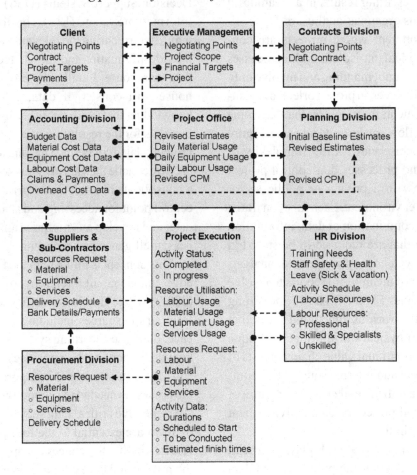

management. While the focus of Success Level 2 is having a definite project management standard and ensuring its compliance throughout the organization. Both success levels are related to project planning, control and execution. The literature revealed a number of potential areas where data mining applications may be applied to project management success. These potential data mining application areas are discussed below.

Project Proposal Preparation and Project Scope

Project proposal and project scope are interconnected. A project proposal is an initial definition of the project outputs and outcomes, and precedes

the project scope. Project scope defines in detail what needs to be done and what is excluded from the project. A project scope is only undertaken when a project proposal has been accepted by the client and is usually an annex of a formal legal contract between the client and the organization executing the project.

If a project proposal is issued as part of a competitive tender process then timeliness, quality and accuracy of the bid preparation become critical. However, at the project scope stage quality and accuracy become the most important elements. It should be emphasised that the project proposal and project scope establish the overall project time and cost parameters, and normally also define the payment terms and payment schedule.

Figure 3. Project data warehouse & data mining

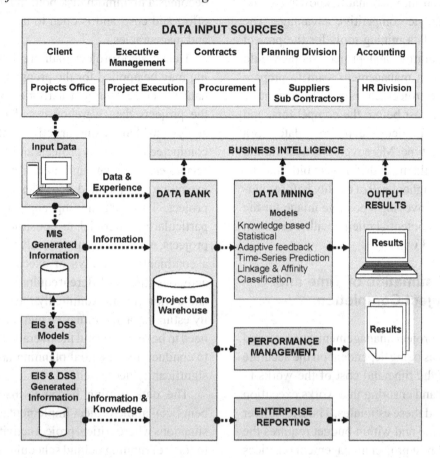

Therefore, an organization must overcome three major hurdles: to outclass its competitors by promptly providing a precise and accurate project bid; to be awarded the project; and to execute the project within the defined project scope and the established contractual parameters to achieve its estimated profit margin.

Nemati and Barko (2002) argue that we are living in an age where information is quickly becoming the differentiator between industry leading firms and second rate organizations. The application of data mining at this level would focus on the analysis of the projects data warehouse to find similar project requirements configuration for projects that have already been undertaken by the organization. This may be achieved through text mining and rules generation using classification

and association of the projects data warehouse (previous project scopes and contracts). A software tool may be used to automatically summarise text data and extract valuable rules that may be further transformed into a semantic network which may provide a concise and accurate summary of the analysed text. Nayak and Qiu (2004) have successfully applied this data mining technique to analyse software problem reports in pure text for the accurate prediction of time and cost in fixing software problems at a global telecommunication company.

This data mining application goes beyond the concept of exploring patterns and relationships within the projects data warehouse to discover hidden knowledge; it would aim at enhancing the decision-making process by transforming data and information into actionable knowledge and gaining a strategic competitive advantage. The application of data mining tools for the project proposal preparation and project scope would allow the project management team to prepare project bids and project scopes quickly, accurately and at a lower cost before the competitors, and to be aware of particular concerns related to a specific project type. Moreover, this data mining application would mean that project bids may be submitted to a higher level of quality before competitors, thus conveying a positive image for the organization to potential clients with a resultant increase in good will.

Accurate Estimation of Time and Cost to Project Completion

Traditionally project management success and failure is seen as being dependent on the accurate estimation of the time and cost of the works to be completed and ensuring that works execution does not exceed these estimates. Thus, to deliver a project on time and within budget requires the application of best project management practices and tight control of the projects undertaken.

An essential step within the project planning stage is the accurate preparation of activity utility data. The preparation of activity utility data is concerned with estimating the duration and cost that each activity within a project will take to be completed. Furthermore, an individual activity may be conducted by alternative methods using different types and combination of resources. Hence, the duration and cost activity estimate will need to be established for each alternative method. These calculations become important during project execution particularly when a project slips behind schedule and certain critical activities need to be expedited. However, a large and complex project may consist of hundreds of activities, with many activities having different execution methods. Therefore, the preparation of activity utility data for a particular project

becomes a mammoth task both in terms of work effort and cost; and is open to the risk of errors and inaccuracies.

Hence, at the project planning stage, data mining may be applied for the preparation of utility data for current project activities by analysing the projects data warehouse and using cluster analysis to identify similar activities that had been conducted in previous projects and extracting the related estimate data and alternative methods of executing the planned activities of the current project. This data mining application may be particularly beneficial to construction industry projects, where the resultant analysis may provide a combination of ways of executing particular activities utilising different equipment, crew sizes, and working hours. Admittedly, the resultant activity estimates and alternative methods would still need to be reviewed but the overall effort and cost to conduct this essential planning task would be significantly decreased.

The data mining becomes also extremely beneficial at the project implementation stage in situations where critical project activities are close to (or are) running behind schedule or when non-critical activities are approaching being critical. In this situation data mining may be utilised to analyse similar activities from the projects data warehouse of current and previous projects, and suggest alternate methods to carry out the specific activity to recover lost time at an optimal cost. The overall objective in the application of data mining at this level is to ensure that the optimum economic project solution is being implemented with a change in project circumstances.

The application of data mining methods for the project planning and control stage embraces a number of different approaches. Iranmanesh and Mokhtari (2008) contend that traditional methods to deal with the complex task of controlling and modifying the baseline project schedule during project execution to measure and communicate the real physical progress of a project are not adequate, since these methods often fail to predict the total duration of a project to completion. These researchers have applied the decision tree, neural network and association rule data mining tools to predict the total project duration in terms of Time Estimate at Completion. To calculate the Time Estimate at Completion, the Iranmanesh and Mokhtari (2008) model applies six input parameters, namely, actual cost of work performed; budget cost of work performed; budget cost of work scheduled; actual duration; earned duration; and planned duration.

The three data mining methods provided consistent results in that the neural network showed that the cost performance index (budget cost of work performed divided by actual cost of work performed) had the largest weighting among all indexes to predict project completion time; whilst the decision tree and the association rule methods predicted consistent Time Estimate at Completion results. The objective of the study was to enable the applied data mining tools to accurately forecast the project completion time during the project execution stage so that the project team may assess and monitor project risk by measuring project progress in time and monetary terms and take proactive preventative actions to mitigate any adverse conditions.

Occupational Health and Safety

Many projects involving the output of physical items, such as in the engineering and construction environments, regularly encounter occupational health and safety issues. The consequences of accidents during project execution may turn out to be very harmful both in terms of human causalities and project cost escalation. For example, the West Gate Bridge in Melbourne, Australia collapsed during construction in 1978. Approximately 2000 tonnes of steel and concrete came crashing down taking the lives of thirty-five workers with many others injured. The report from the Royal Commission (VPRS 2591/P0, unit 14) stated: "*Error begat error ... and the events which led to the*

disaster moved with the inevitability of a Greek Tragedy." The project was finally completed after ten years at a cost of A$202 million. While project cost escalation issues may somehow be resolved in the long-term, human lives are irreplaceable.

A data mining method that may be applied to reduce such tragic incidents would be very cost effective in terms of human causalities and project expenditure. NASA Engineering and Safety Centre (NESC) was established to improve safety through engineering excellence within NASA programs and projects (Parsons, 2007). One of NESC's objectives is to find methods that enable it to become proactive in identifying areas that may be precursors to future problems. Parsons (2007) argues that problems are better prevented than solved. Hence, the goal is to find a method to uncover adverse patterns. Parsons (2007) contends that NASA's research findings indicate that clustering techniques in their particular environment are a key component.

However, cautions show that there is a disparity between the generation of data and the true interpretation (or understanding) of the meaning within the data. The findings suggest that when data is dynamic, voluminous, noisy, and incomplete then learning algorithms are the most ineffective and discovery algorithms such as clustering are optimal. Furthermore, when the data mining objective is exploration, clustering should be used as the optimal unsupervised learning technique (Parsons, 2007).

Hence, in a project oriented environment, data mining tools such as, learning and discovery algorithms may be used to determine which project activities, skills or/and resources may be more prone to occupational health and safety issues so that appropriate steps are taken to mitigate or prevent adverse occurrences. Furthermore, decision trees and association rules may be used to detect anomalies in the way project activities are being carried out in relation to past projects and current regulatory standards (e.g. engineering, construction, and occupational health and safety standards). The data mining methods applicable will depend on the organizational environment in terms of the data, information and knowledge characteristics, such as quality, volume, integrity and completeness.

Preventative Maintenance of Plant and Equipment

Many project oriented organizations, particularly those involving engineering and construction, increasingly rely on profits generated from the high utilisation of plant and equipment. The unscheduled disruption in the use of plant and equipment during project execution not only incurs direct costs of labour, replacement parts and consumables, but also the consequential costs of delays to contract, possible loss of client goodwill and ultimately, loss of profit. The findings of a study conducted by Barber et al. (2000) regarding the cost of quality failures in two major road projects suggest that the cost of failures may be a significant percentage of total costs, and that conventional means of identifying them may not be reliable. Moreover, these types of costs will not be easy to eradicate without widespread changes in attitudes and norms of behaviour within the industry and improved managerial co-ordination of activities throughout the supply chain.

Srinivas and Harding (2008) propose a data mining integrated architecture model that provides a mechanism for continuous learning and may be applied to resolve concerns regarding process planning and scheduling, including extracting knowledge to establish rules for identifying maintenance interventions. Wang (2007) illustrates the use of data mining to solve a scheduled maintenance problem in a manufacturing shop which may also be applicable to a project environment. Wang's data mining application has two objectives: classification - to determine what subsystems or components are most responsible for downtime, the "root cause"; and prediction - to forecast when preventative maintenance would be

most effective in reducing failures. Finally, the generated information may be used to establish maintenance policy guidelines, such as planned plant and equipment maintenance schedule. In this example classification and prediction were achieved by utilising decision trees.

Wang (2007) applied the decision tree approach to classify machine health, with equipment availability being the target dependent variable. The developed model determined the most sensible plant and equipment that are most responsible to the low equipment availability. Therefore, the aim was to detect the plant and equipment with a low availability index thus focusing on specific apparatus (or group of apparatus) in order to make the maintenance effort more effective thus saving time and cost. The generated nodes on the decision tree consisted of the different plant and equipment that are classified by the evaluation of the equipment availability value. Hence, those responsible for maintenance are able to examine specific plant and equipment responsible for the low availability in this part of the classification and take the necessary action. Furthermore, the model is able to provide accurate knowledge about the specific component that is the "root cause" of failure within the indicated plant and equipment.

Project Risk Management

According to Hubbard (2009, p46.) risk management is the identification, assessment, and prioritization of risks followed by coordinated and economical application of resources to minimize, monitor, and control the probability and/or impact of unfortunate events. There are many causes of negative risks in project execution, including delays in the delivery of adequate supplies; inadequate quality levels of procured items; high turnover of project team members; and a host of other potential adverse elements. These risk sources can be damaging to a project, such as having delays in project delivery dates and budget overruns. The consequences of these risk occurrences include financial loss; demoralisation of project team members; and harming the reputation of the project manager. Project risk management endeavours to foresee and deal with uncertainties that jeopardise the objectives, and the time and cost schedules of a project.

The basis for the project risk management process is information and knowledge. Earl (2001) argues that knowledge is a critical organizational resource and mentions examples from industry about how various organizations build and utilise their knowledge base. For example, he refers to BP Amoco's philosophy of productivity through knowledge reuse and accelerated learning which is articulated by their expression: *"Every time we drill another well, we do the next one better."* Earl (2001) illustrates how a typical productivity-through-knowledge project at BP follows a number of stages, including: documenting the current work process; gathering, summarising and codifying knowledge and expertise on critical tasks; and conducting post project reviews to assess initial goals, examine what actually happened, and assess the variance between outcome and intent. Hence, both the positive and negative aspects of executed projects are documented for future utilisation.

The above process ensures that new learning and experience is added and validated by the project team and expert facilitators. This way a projects data warehouse is maintained with knowledge and expertise that has the potential, if suitably applied, to identify and quantify risk so that an appropriate risk response may be undertaken by the project manager.

Datta (2008) identifies risk analysis as a key data mining application area where hidden rules may not be obvious to the decision maker. Data mining is extremely useful in facilitating project risk management. For instance, risk identification basically addresses the question: What might go wrong? The aim of this process is to identify and specifically name the project risks and their characteristics. Data mining can be applied through the analysis of the projects data warehouse, seeking learning classification and association rules to determine the attributes of the potential identified risks. The analysis would closely examine the current project plan for areas of uncertainty when compared to projects that have already been implemented. Hence, the objective of the analysis would be to examine the project plans to search for issues that could cause the project to be behind schedule. The outcome of the analysis would be a full risk inventory that would categorise risk under a number of major headings consisting of two components, namely, the likely cause of the specific condition, for example, a sub-contractor not meeting the delivery schedule; and the general impact of the risk on the project, for example, milestones will not be achieved and/or the budget will be exceeded.

When the risk identification process is completed, the project manager will closely interpret the analysis containing the resultant risk inventory and decide on a risk by risk basis which project risks are to be further investigated through risk quantification. The risk quantification process would result in a prioritised list of project risk elements that will need a response from the project manager to take advantage of the risk if it has a positive trait or to take action to mitigate any adverse circumstances should the risk have a negative attribute. Turner and Zizzamia (2008) apply a similar approach using a data mining predictive modelling for an insurance claims management scenario. They maintain that predictive modelling provides a better understanding of a claim, allowing it to identify and prioritise an appropriate and immediate response. Their predictive model has the potential to analyse hundreds of risk attributes based on the available data to produce a numerical score (and rational) indicating exposure level and complexity. Turner and Zizzamia (2008) argue that by using the predictive model to explore and pinpoint exposure, risk managers can optimise resource deployment and minimise the process duration.

In a project management scenario, decision tree analysis provides a way of presenting a balanced view of the risks and pay-outs associated with each possible alternative strategy. This type of application has the objective of answering the following questions: What is the probability of meeting the project scope, taking into account all known and quantified risks? By how much will the project be delayed? What level of contingency does the organization need to allocate in terms of time and cost to meet the desired level of certainty taking into consideration the predicted project delay? Where in the project are the most risks, taking into consideration the project network and all the identified and quantified risks?

Using decision tree analysis as a data mining tool is valuable because it visibly defines the decision to be resolved by showing all options and associated cost calculations; permits management to fully assess all the likely consequences of a decision; provides a feasible framework for calculating the outcome values and respective probabilities of achieving them; and help management to evaluate the available information to arrive at the best decisions by selecting the better alternative. Statistical methods can also be used to assess the impact of all identified and quantified risks. The outcome of the statistical analysis is a probability distribution of the project's cost and completion date based on project risks to predict schedule risk. Schedule risk is the probability that a project will go beyond its calculated time schedule and cost.

The data mining application may also provide the possible risk response based upon the project risk identification and quantification, thus itemising the options available and defining the appropriate actions to enhance the opportunities and minimise the threats. The aim of the project manager at this stage would be to closely examine the data mining results and select the best approach to address each risk that merit attention and propose particular actions for implementing the selected risk policy. Furthermore, the project

risk data mining application should be viewed as being a continuous process that will regularly monitor and control risk during the entire project implementation life cycle. The continuous monitoring and control of risks will identify any change in the risk status or if a particular risk has developed into an issue. The inventory of project risk is not static and constantly changes as the project is being implemented, thus new risks evolve and other risks disappear. Hence, the data mining risk reviews allow the project manager to reassess and modify the risk ratings and prioritisation throughout the project lifecycle until its successful completion.

Repeatable Project Management Success

As stated previously repeatable project management success is the organization's ability to consistently execute projects that have produced the desired output. The emphasis here is on "consistency" in implementing projects successfully. Consistency in a project management context is normally achieved by having and adhering to a uniform project management standard throughout the organization. Therefore, the objective is to ensure that the stages and steps in the project implementation life cycle do not deviate from the project management standard by detecting anomalies in the way the project is being implemented. This is particularly applicable to projects that have a specific implementation framework, for instance, computer application software development and conducting research and development projects.

According to Eberle and Holder (2007) detecting anomalies in various data sets is an important endeavour in data mining, particularly for handling data that cannot be easily analyzed. Anomaly detection in data mining is related to the discovery of events that generally do not conform to expected normal behaviour. Such events are often referred to as anomalies, outliers, exceptions, deviations, and other similar designations depending on the application domain. Although deviations may be infrequent events, their occurrence may have serious consequences and therefore their detection becomes extremely important. Most anomaly detection methods use a supervised approach that requires some sort of baseline of information from which comparisons or training can be performed (Eberle & Holder 2007). There are generally two steps in anomaly detection schemes:

- Building a profile of the "normal" behaviour. These profiles may be patterns or summary statistics of the overall population.
- Using the "normal" profile to detect anomalies. Anomalies being observations whose characteristics differ significantly from the normal profile.

In a project management standard compliance application, anomaly detection can be based on supervised learning whose goal is to develop a group of decision rules that can be used to determine a known outcome. For instance, the project management standard would form the basis of the data mining learning model, defining classes and providing positive and negative examples of objects belonging to the classes. Supervised learning algorithms can be utilised to construct decision trees or rule sets that work by repeatedly subdividing the data into groups based on identified predictor variables which are related to the selected group membership. The supervised learning algorithms, such as classification, create a series of decision rules that can be used to separate data into specific determined groups.

Typically, the major difficulty in detecting anomalies in a data mining context is to know what is "normal". For instance, Eberle and Holder (2007) assume that an anomaly is not random and that an anomaly should only be a minor deviation from the normal pattern. They argue that anyone who is attempting to hide devious activities would not want to be caught, and therefore, they would want their activities to look as real as possible.

This does not appear to be a concern in a project management standard compliance application, since the "normal" is established by the project management standard being used. Another concern is having noisy data that may hamper efforts to detect deviations. However, the type of data being generated in a project oriented environment will be mostly filtered and therefore clean, hence noisy data should not present an obstacle for this type of application.

Furthermore, the project management standard may be codified or labelled through a standard work breakdown structure (WBS) framework that would be mirrored by the WBS milestones for the projects being implemented. Hence, the detection of any deviation from the project management standard by a specific project is a practical application that may be easily achieved by the above data mining method. This would ensure that projects are implemented to the desired quality at a cost effective level; and that the organization's ability to consistently execute projects that have produced the desired output is realised, thus achieving the primary objective of repeatable project management success.

THE ROAD TO SUCCESS: PROJECT SUCCESS (OUTCOMES)

This is Sutton's (2005) project success Level 3. Project management is often viewed as the application of knowledge, competencies, methods, and tools to achieve the defined project tasks in order to satisfy stakeholder requirements and expectations from a project. This view takes into consideration two aspects, namely, project outputs, that is, the actual deliverables; and project outcomes that is, the project purpose and objectives. The previous section addressed how data mining tools may aid in attaining the project outputs; this section will focus on how data mining may aid in achieving the project outcomes.

Active Project Stakeholders and the Perception of Project Success

An essential factor to a project's level of success will depend on the perceptions of different stakeholders that have an interest in the project. Therefore, a critical consideration is whether or not the project achieves its purpose and objectives, that is, does the project do what it is supposed to do? The answer to this question is very subjective because it depends on the eyes of the beholder, namely the different stakeholders' perceptions. For example, in a building construction project, the outcomes are closely related to the users of the building. Is the building functional for the purpose it was built? Does it accommodate different individuals' general needs? For instance, does the building design cater for individuals with special needs? Hence, project outcomes are more difficult to achieve because they take into consideration the operational aspects of the deliverables after the project has been implemented.

The difficulty with achieving project success as distinct from project management success is the variety of the stakeholders that need to be satisfied. These stakeholders may include consumer groups, environmentalists, local communities, general public, mass media, shareholders, creditors and many others depending on the nature of the project. Hence, each industry type may have different active stakeholders. However, it should be noted that individual entities normally conduct projects that are specific to their industry. Therefore, these individual entities are in a position to identify and know their influential and active stakeholders.

According to Rennolls and Shawabkeh, (2008) knowledge of various forms is recognized as a crucial business asset, to be utilized for the development of new products and services, and hopefully leading to competitive advantage. They argue that knowledge management has been high on corporate agendas, with the main concerns (apart from IT infrastructure) being people and culture, and communication and collaboration.

Hence, gaining knowledge of the stakeholders' needs, characteristics, and attitudes are achievable and are fundamental in influencing their perceptions. This may be translated into the application of data mining methods to establish a mechanism for building a knowledge warehouse and developing a learning organization, and utilising it for the purpose of facilitating the achievement of the project outcomes. This process may consist of capturing, storing, analysing and sharing project lessons learnt about past project outcomes and profiling stakeholders' needs, attitudes and characteristics.

Building a Knowledge Warehouse and Developing a Learning Organization

The generation of a knowledge warehouse and the development of a learning organization require continuous attention and effort. The major reasons for this are: (a) knowledge may be obtained from both the organization's internal and external environments, therefore knowledge is infinite; and (b) knowledge must be relevant to the organization's needs, however deciding what is relevant may not be a straight forward matter. Hence, perfection is not entirely possible. Having said this however, even the imperfect achievement of a knowledge warehouse and the creation of a learning organization will have a tremendous positive effect on the project success performance rating. Currently, the maturation of data mining supporting processes which would take into account human and organizational aspects is still living its childhood (Pechenizkiy et al., 2008).

There are a number of activities that may help an organization to build and retain knowledge and thus develop a learning organization. For example, knowledge about project outcomes may be possible by collecting and storing remarks (and their source) appearing in the mass media, such as the press, internet, virtual media, and televised and broadcast media about projects that are relevant to the particular industry in which the organization is involved with. These projects may include project proposals or projects being undertaken within a similar cultural and operational environment, and not necessarily conducted by the organization itself.

Academic literature suggests that a learning organization knows how to retain knowledge, appreciates the value of sharing collective knowledge, and grows more knowledgeable with each activity it performs (Day and Rogers, 2006). The aim is to build a knowledge warehouse about the outcomes of projects, and the identification and profiling of influential stakeholders. The knowledge source in this case will be mainly external and could come from anywhere and at any time. The type of knowledge to be collected will vary but the content of critical reviews and their source are obviously most relevant. This will enable the organization to gain knowledge about what society thinks about specific projects (likely outcomes) and identify the influential stakeholders. However, in generating a knowledge warehouse it is important to examine ethical considerations, particularly data protection legislation in relation to the creation of stakeholder profiles. It is emphasised that reference about influential stakeholders should not be viewed as individuals but as generic designations.

Another means of collecting knowledge is through the maintenance of an electronic journal, documenting specific unique experiences during project implementation. This knowledge will be mainly from internal sources, however, external information sources are also possible, particularly from contractors and sub-contractors that are involved in the project. This knowledge source will involve projects specifically undertaken by the organization. Special focus should be given to factors related to satisfying project outcomes and specifically to remarks and other feedback from clients, potential end users of the project deliverables and society in general.

Finally, the creation of a learning organization is facilitated by conducting a post project imple-

mentation review, specifically when the project outputs have shifted to the operation stage, where project outcomes are brought to fruition. The post project implementation review evaluates the project at completion to assess what went right and wrong with the project so that experience gained from a project is not lost. The organization should have the proper mechanisms for capturing lessons learnt through the documentation of the good and bad things in the management of the project and capture all comments and recommendations for improvements. Day and Rogers (2006) suggest that project reviews should occur after major events and milestones because data collected close to the event eliminates the bias of hindsight. Such a process facilitates a commitment to long-term relationships amongst the project teams and stakeholders with the primary objective of having continuous improvement through learning from project experience.

This data mining mechanism ensures that knowledge gained by individuals is retained for the benefit of the organization. A lack of such mechanism will mean that knowledge is likely to be lost, especially if the individual ceases membership to the organization. When employees leave an organization, they carry with them invaluable tacit knowledge which is often the source of competitive advantage for the business (Nagadevara et al., 2008). Knowledge lost to the organization is likely to be knowledge gained by a competitor. Therefore, data mining in a project management environment has the potential of allowing the storage, retrieving and analysing of project experience and knowledge that is shared throughout the organization for the achievement of the defined project outcomes and not hoarded by any particular individual.

Utilisation of the Knowledge Warehouse

The terminology of machine learning and data mining methods does not always allow a simple match between practical problems and methods; while some problems look similar from the user's point of view, but require different methods to be solved, some others look very different, yet they can be solved by applying the same methods and tools (Van Someren and Urbancic, 2006). Applying the appropriate data mining tools for problem solving in practice depends on experience and an innovative approach in the way a knowledge warehouse is utilised.

The focus in the utilisation of the knowledge warehouse to achieve project success is to share project lessons learnt about the outcomes from previous projects and stakeholder profiling. The aim is to predict stakeholder reactions to a project, taking a proactive approach to mitigate any adverse stakeholder reactions to the project, thus influencing the eventual project outcomes. According to Datta (2008), data mining can facilitate in identifying and exploring patterns of information from massive client focused databases and can help to select, explore and model large amount of data to discover previously unknown patterns, for the advantage of business. This application would be similar to a marketing environment related to launching a new product or service, where predicted reactions to the project by different stakeholders are viewed as the likely project outcomes, and the stakeholders are associated to different types of clients, with each stakeholder type having different requirements, attitudes and attributes.

The objective of this data mining application would be to identify the various stakeholders that are likely to have an interest in a proposed project; to identify the likely attitude to a proposed project by the identified stakeholders; to ascertain the characteristics of each stakeholder type; to itemise decisions taken in prior projects and their respective impact on stakeholder attitudes and project outcomes; and to provide suggestions that are likely to have a positive impact in changing stakeholder attitudes and therefore are likely to influence project outcomes. Stakeholder segmen-

tation analysis would be an appropriate method in this situation.

The stakeholder segmentation analysis would aim at identifying groups of stakeholders that have common attributes and that have an interest in a proposed project. The stakeholder attributes are likely to represent attitudes and resultant behaviours. This stakeholder segmentation analysis may be based on supervised learning algorithms that take the form of a hierarchical decision tree structure such that small segments form larger stakeholder segments, with each small segment representing a stakeholder type. Furthermore, using the knowledge about the attributes of each stakeholder type and the decisions taken in former projects and their respective impact on stakeholder attitudes and project outcomes, this data mining application may create a series of decision rules that may be used to generate ideas that are likely to positively change stakeholder attitudes to the proposed project for each stakeholder segment with the aim of favourably impacting the outcomes of the proposed project.

FINAL DESTINATION: PROJECT CORPORATE SUCCESS

Project corporate success is Sutton's (2005) project success level 4. The consequence of business endeavours that do not support the business strategy is the misuse and under utilisation of corporate resources. Hence, it is essential that projects are aligned with the organization's strategic direction and that their completion results in a positive impact on the organization's business objectives (Cleland and Ireland, 2006). Applying data mining methods in a project oriented environment can facilitate corporate success. In a practical sense, this means using data mining techniques to sustain organizational initiatives by having a proper project selection processes and best practice in project portfolio management.

Proper Project Selection: Strategic Fit of Projects

According to Cleland and Ireland, (2006) projects are essential to the survival and growth of organizations. They argue that failure in the management of projects in an organization will impair the ability of the organization to accomplish its mission in an effective and efficient manner. Data mining may be used to determine if a project proposal is aligned with the corporate business strategy before a decision is made about whether to pursue it. Similar to the other data mining examples, this application is based on having and utilising the relevant information stored in the projects data warehouse (refer to Figure 3). A combination of decision tree learning and statistical methods may be used to construct a predictive model. The aim of this application is to conduct an analysis of the project proposal and the relevant information items held in the projects data warehouse to determine a strategic fit index for particular project proposals. The strategic fit index would be based on assessing the following:

a.   The extent to which a proposed project fits within the organization's activity boundary.
b.   Human and financial resource implications of the proposed project to ensure that it does not expose the organization to the risk of economic non-sustainability.
c.   Stakeholder values and expectations related to the proposed project to ensure that unrealistic project execution time frames that often lead to ineffective outcomes, do not occur.
d.   Long-term influence of the proposed project on the organization to ensure that undertaking a major project does not restrict the organization from conducting other concurrent projects and hence adversely impact the organization's potential for future growth.

This data mining application will evaluate the strategic fit of a proposed project and will also rank proposals in order of priority, since a high strategic fit index means a higher project ranking.

Project Portfolio Management: Project Partnerships and Analysis of Project Bids

Undertaking a major project can be viewed as a partnership between the project owner (client), the organization executing the project, and suppliers. The failure of one partner could be detrimental to the project and is likely to result in a financial loss to some or all of the partners. The extent of harm to the project will depend on the failing partner. For example, if the client fails, the project will likely be abandoned. However, if a supplier fails, the project will probably experience a delay with a resultant financial loss, but the project as a whole will likely survive. Project portfolio management in this text will take the view of the organization executing the project and consider a data mining application for determining the financial reliability of the client and contractors in the supply chain.

Van Someren and Urbancic (2006) cite an example that uses data mining for predicting financial risk in the banking industry by evaluating credit worthiness to forecast the financial state of a person, company or other entity by exploring the characteristics of their current financial state and economic conditions. This example is based on a Bayesian model using information about similar clients and contractors whose status is known to establish a comparable appraisal baseline. The input to the model is a mixture of numerical and nominal data that is normally available in financial statements. Furthermore, Hensher and Jones (2007) using published financial data apply a mixed logit model (or random parameter logit) to predict corporate bankruptcy. They argue that the development of more powerful and accurate forecasting methodologies to predict corporate bankruptcy is of importance to a range of user groups, including shareholders, creditors, employees, suppliers, ratings agencies, auditors and corporate managers.

A similar approach may be used to assess the financial reliability of the project partners, in this case, the client and contractors in the supply chain. However, it should be noted that the generated knowledge from the prediction model will need to be presented in a manner that is easily understood by the decision makers. There is no doubt that these data mining applications will enable the organization to understand and assess the financial reliability of potential partners and enable private and public sector organizations to choose their partners carefully and thus avoid partial or project failure.

FUTURE TRENDS

The applications described above are based on the ability to have a well synchronised team utilising the extensive knowledge that an enterprise possesses. To engage in innovative project management practices such as, supply chain management and the sharing of information and knowledge across the entire organization requires the acceptance of a collaborative spirit. Computer-supported cooperative work (CSCW) systems are computer-based tools that support collaborative activities that meet the requirements of normal collaborative efforts among people (Zhu, 2006).

Future research should attempt to link data mining tools to CSCW. The future widespread use of data mining lays in the ability and capacity of an organization to implement an enterprise knowledge framework that permits individuals to collaborate in the gathering, storing, analysing and sharing of data, information and knowledge across the organizational boundaries, be they private or public entities. An enterprise approach to knowledge management will increase an organization's capacity to apply data mining tools for

strengthening its competitive position and thus ensure corporate success.

CONCLUSION

This chapter has examined data mining and the project management environment. It has shown a number of applications where data mining and knowledge learning may be used at various stages in the project management lifecycle with the ultimate goal being to achieve corporate success in private and public sectors. Data collected on its own is not of much use and has to be converted into information and knowledge so that it can be used (Datta, 2008). Data mining is an analytical process specifically designed to explore the considerable magnitude of data from different perspectives in search of consistent patterns and relationships between variables and summarising the findings into useful information and knowledge that can help an entity to increase its revenue and/or decrease its costs.

In the context of enterprise resource planning, data mining involves the search for patterns from statistical and logical analysis of large transaction data sets that can help in decision-making (Monk & Wagner, 2005). A proper project management environment integrates an organization's information value chain with its decision making process to increase its ability for making effective decisions in the implementation of projects.

On the other hand, there is a growing gap between more powerful storage and retrieval systems and the users' ability to effectively analyse and act on the information they contain. Both relational and on-line analytic processing (OLAP) technologies have immense potential for navigating voluminous data warehouses. However there is a need to structure and prioritise information for specific end-user problems and to address a number of organizational issues that may facilitate the application of data mining and knowledge management in a project oriented environment. Some of the major organizational issues that are applicable to both the private and public sectors include:

a. Ensuring that data mining applications focus and support the strategic direction of the organization to gain a competitive advantage and satisfy clients' satisfaction;

b. Recognising that data, information and knowledge are a corporate asset that should be proactively managed like every other major asset;

c. Respecting ethical values by ensuring that individuals are not the end target of profiling exercises since this may be in conflict with data protection legislation;

d. Ensuring the support of executive management for sharing data, information and knowledge across the organizational boundaries;

e. Recognising that data mining applications do not follow the conventional data processing way of thinking but require an innovative and creative mindset;

f. Recognising that information and particularly knowledge are dynamic and therefore must be constantly rejuvenated through continuous regeneration;

g. Recognising that the contents of a data warehouse depends on well defined data flow procedures and processes;

h. Ensuring that appropriate security measures and procedures are in place to protect the data warehouse from unauthorised access and/or deliberate and non-deliberate destruction;

i. Ensuring that an appropriate organization structure is in place for knowledge management and its associated data mining functions.

j. Selecting suitable analytical software tools that are compatible with the existing ICT infrastructure and the projects' data warehouse.

Finally, it is essential to have a senior management executive who will act as the organization's data mining champion to guarantee the long-term sustainability of the data mining investment. These measures will ensure that using data mining in a project oriented environment will help an entity to achieve corporate success at unprecedented levels.

REFERENCES

Ayre, L. B. (2006). *Data Mining For Information Professionals.* Retrieved May 6, 2008, from http://techessence.info/files/Ayre_DataMiningForInformationProfessionals_June2006.pdf.

Bala, P. K. (2008). A technique for mining generalized quantitative associated rules for retail inventory management. *International Journal of Business Strategy, 8*(2), 114–127.

Barber, P., Graves, A., Hall, M., Sheath, D., & Tomkins, C. (2000). Quality failure costs in civil engineering projects. *International Journal of Quality & Reliability Management, 17*(4/5), 479–492. doi:10.1108/02656710010298544

Cleland, D. I and Ireland, L. R. (2006). Project management: strategic design and implementation, (5th Ed.). Clarksville, TN: McGraw-Hill.

Cooke-Davies, T. (2002). The "real" success factors on projects. *International Journal of Project Management, 20,* 185–190. doi:10.1016/S0263-7863(01)00067-9

Datta, R. P. (2008). Data Mining Applications and Infrastructural Issues: An Indian Perspective. *ICFAI Journal of Infrastructure, 6*(3), 42–50.

Day, R., & Rogers, E. (2006). Enhancing NASA's Performance as a Learning Organization. *NASA Ask Magazine, 22,* 36–39.

Earl, M. (2001). Knowledge Management Strategies: Toward a Taxonomy. *Journal of Management Inquiry, 18*(1), 215–233.

Hensher, D. A., & Jones, S. (2007). Forecasting Corporate Bankruptcy: Optimizing the Performance of the Mixed Logit Model. *Abacus, 43*(3), 241–264. doi:10.1111/j.1467-6281.2007.00228.x

Hicks, R. C., Dattero, R., & Galup, S. D. (2006). The five-tier knowledge management hierarchy. *Journal of Knowledge Management, 10*(1), 19–31. doi:10.1108/13673270610650076

Hicks, R. C., Galup, S. D., & Dattero, R. (2007). The Transformations In The Five Tier Knowledge Management Transformation Matrix. *Journal of Knowledge Management, 8*, 1.

Hubbard, D. (2009). *The Failure of Risk Management: Why It's Broken and How to Fix It.* Hoboken, New Jersey: John Wiley & Sons.

Iranmanesh, S. H., & Mokhtari, Z. (2008, August). Application of Data Mining Tools to Predicate Completion Time of a Project. In Proceedings of World Academy of Science (Vol. 32, pp. 234–239). Engineering and Technology.

Keating, B. (2008). Data Mining: What is it and how is it used? *The Journal of Business Forecasting, Fall*, 33-35.

Monk, E., & Wagner, B. (2005). *Concepts in Enterprise Resource Planning* (2nd ed.). Boston: Thomson Course Technology.

Nagadevara, V., Srinivasan, V., & Valk, R. (2008). Establishing a link between employee turnover and withdrawal behaviours: Application of data mining techniques. *Research and Practice in Human Resource Management, 16*(2), 81–99.

Nayak, R., & Qiu, T. (2004). Data Mining Application in a Software Project Management Process. In *proceedings of Australian Data Mining Conference*, Cairns, Australia.

Nemati, H. R., & Barko, C. D. (2002). Enhancing Enterprise Decisions Through Organizational Data Mining. *Journal of Computer Information Systems*, (Summer): 21–28.

Nissen, M. E. (2000). An extended model of knowledge-flow dynamics. *Communications of the Association for Information Systems, 8*, 251–266.

Palace, B. (1996). Data Mining: What is Data Mining? *Anderson Graduate School of Management at UCLA*. Retrieved November 20, 2008, from http://www.anderson.ucla.edu/faculty/jason.frand/teacher/technologies/palace/datamining.htm

Parsons, V. S. (2007). Searching for "Unknown Unknowns.". *Engineering Management Journal, 19*(1), 43–46.

Pechenizkiya, M., Puuronenb, S., & Tsymbalc, A. (2008). Towards more relevance-oriented data mining research. *Intelligent Data Analysis, 12*, 237–249.

Pyle, D. (2003). Making the Case. *IBM Database Magazine, 8*(4). Retrieved November 20, 2008, from http://www.ibmdatabasemag.com/showArticle.jhtml?articleID=15300105

Rennolls, K and AL-Shawabkeh, A. (2008). Formal structures for data mining, knowledge discovery and communication in a knowledge management environment. *Intelligent Data Analysis, 12*, 147–163.

Srinivas and Harding. J. A. (2008). A data mining integrated architecture for shop floor control. In Proc. IMechE Part B: J. Engineering Manufacture, 222, 605-624.

Sutton, B. (2005). *Why Projects Fail – Mastering the Monster (Part 2), Examining the underlying reasons for project failure, and how to use that knowledge to get your projects back on track.* ArchItect, Bearpark Publishing Ltd. Retrieved November 19, 2008, from http://www.itarchitect.co.uk/articles/display.asp?id=224

Turner, K., & Zizzamia, F. (2008). Predicting Better Claims Management. *Risk Management*, *55*(7), 52–55.

Van Someren, M., & Urbancic, T. (2006). Applications of machine learning: matching problems to tasks and methods. *The Knowledge Engineering Review*, *20*(4), 363–402. doi:10.1017/S0269888906000762

Vanhoof, K., Bloemer, J., & Pauwels, K. (1997). A case of loyalty and satisfaction research. In M. Van Someren, & G. Widmer (Eds.). *Proceedings 9th European Conference on Machine Learning, Prague, Czech Republic (ECML)* (pp. 290-297). Berlin: Springer.

Wang, K. (2007). Applying data mining to manufacturing: the nature and implications. *Journal of Intelligent Manufacturing*, *18*, 487–495. doi:10.1007/s10845-007-0053-5

Zhu, H. (2006). Role mechanisms in collaborative systems. *International Journal of Production Research*, *44*(1), 181–193. doi:10.1080/00207540500247495

KEY TERMS AND DEFINITIONS

Data Mining or Knowledge Discovery: The process of analyzing data from different perspectives and summarizing it into useful information.

Data Warehouse: A repository of an entity's electronically stored data designed to facilitate the transformation and loading of data for retrieval, analysis, and decision making purposes.

Informational Value Chain: The data necessary to transform tangible resources to a finished product or service.

Physical Value Chain: The transformation of tangible resources, such as materials and labor, to a finished product or service.

Project: A finite (temporary) piece of work that has a beginning and an end.

Project Corporate Success: Whether the project outcomes produced have the intended impact on the business strategy of the organization.

Project Management: The application of knowledge, competencies, methods, and tools to achieve the defined project tasks in order to satisfy stakeholder requirements and expectations from a project.

Project Management Success: Whether a particular project has produced the desired project deliverables (outputs).

Project Success: Whether a particular project has produced the desired project objectives (outcomes).

Repeatable Project Management Success: The organization's ability to consistently execute projects that have produced the desired outputs.

Chapter 18
User Approach to Knowledge Discovery in Networked Environment

Rauno Kuusisto
Finnish Defence Force Technical Centre, Finland

ABSTRACT

Collaboration and networking demands are increasing and lots of organizational communicative activities have moved into technical networks. Need to understand not only how to refine right information contents out of the available data mass but also what type of information is important in various information using situations has increased. This chapter delves into the problem area of finding ways to support users to find relevant, specific types of information that is related to various phases of operating in network. Establishing a network, planning operations and managing operations differ from each others what comes into information requirements. It will be shown via four generalized cases that information requirements vary depending on what phase of networking activity the organization is. Via those cases that are based on sufficiently broad empirical material it will be cleared that knowledge requirements differ from situation to another. This leads to a conclusion that flexible data mining and knowledge discovery systems shall be constructed.

INTRODUCTION

The increasing amount of various available data and information has been a powerful engine for the research of data mining and knowledge discovery. Methodology and procedure discovery and development to sort out relevant and reliable information out of vast masses of ever evolving and increasing

data space have been successfully developed. In addition, a great amount of solutions that help to discover relevant key words or key expressions exist. However those solutions are mainly targeted to marketing development purposes, not for networking purposes. For networking purposes lots of social media tools and other more sophisticated collaboration solutions exist, but they do not answer the challenge of finding comprehensively right type of information. They rather support people to find

DOI: 10.4018/978-1-60566-906-9.ch018

other people who are interested in same kinds of areas and items leaving information discovery on the responsibility of the users. So, the question "How to do it?" is frequently expressed and answered in case of knowledge discovery. A less studied area is what kind or type of information shall be discovered for certain information using situations. This kind of situations exist e.g. in networked business environment and inter-authority collaboration situations. The question "What to do?" that is relevant in this kind of situations is expressed more seldom under the topic of knowledge discovery.

The purpose of this chapter is to introduce a less frequently expressed perspective to knowledge discovery. This chapter describes an example of high-level ontology to solve challenges faced when developing algorithms for networking in emergent and evolving communication environment. Algorithms are not introduced. The focal point is to introduce the difference of information requirements between various phases in collaboration situations. Via those differences it will be demonstrated that knowledge discovery requirements vary also from situation to another. Information is dealt not with content but with framework level. This allows finding general phenomena of inter-working situations thus making possible to solve general knowledge discovery algorithms in complex collaboration environment. Empirical material is collected in the context of authority cooperation.

The working environment of organizations has changed due the extensive use of information technology. Organizations are more or less interrelated to each others and lots of activities are executed using technical tools and networks. Relationships are changing more or less frequently making working environment challenging. New relationships are constructed while others are in execution phase containing planning and decision-making. Those phases differ from each others thus requiring different type of information exchanged. Organizations are interdependent with

each others with certain cross-organizational and non-organization specific processes. They have common interests concerning certain objectives in certain situations. Information technology glues organizations together in two ways. It enables collaboration and the use of non-organizational specific services, and it enables somewhat free information publishing and gathering. The organization independent information domain makes inter-organizational relationships complex and emergent by nature. This emergence cannot be controlled, but the content of mutually available information can be structurized to some degree by using processual and technological tools. Knowledge discovery is about combining information to find hidden knowledge. This chapter describes what type of knowledge shall be discovered when acting in evolving cooperation environment. Knowledge discovery can be seen as a tool to enable more sophisticated way for organizations to optimize their efforts to gain their goals on adequate networking level.

Cross-organizational collaboration situations in inter-authority context are analyzed to increase understanding about the activity environment, where knowledge discovery needs may occur. It will be shown that information needs will vary depending on the phase of activity of an actor. The main research question is: "What type of information shall be discovered to serve actors' needs during different phases of its activity?" This question is dealt with examples based on empirical findings of several collaboration situations of inter-working authorities. The analysis of these cases is based on multi-theoretical model of human information handling.

Information domain can be divided in two main areas. First one is the contents of the information. Content is typically defined by requirements of doing something. Content is related to subject of particular interest. The other main area is the information framework. This can be referred as the universal level of the information domain. This universal level describes the information phenomena of the situation under concern. It defines general information exchange features of getting together and dealing with challenges no matter what they are. This universal framework can be illustrated, like it is done in this study, with a human oriented information categorization model. The model acts as a frame of reference to typify information requirements in different phases of networking activity. The model is an approach to the ontology of human information handling in a context of a complex adaptive social system (Holland 1996). Theoretical basis for modeling this human information exchange is based on philosophy of communication and cognition, theory of knowledge management, sociology, and decision-support systems.

Approach to information is framework and universally oriented pursuing to increase understanding about information exchange situations offering user focused approach to develop dynamic knowledge discovery solutions. The scientific approach is hermeneutical supported by validating empirical results. The research approach is cross-disciplinary. The ultimate goal of this paper is to open novel viewpoints to extract useful knowledge from available data. Basic hypothesis is: "Understanding the varying nature of information requirements of a networking organization at information framework level offers enhanced departure point to develop more user supportive knowledge discovery solutions."

THEORETICAL BACKGROUND AND METHODOLOGY

Complex Adaptive Systems

The problem area is approached using complex adaptive systems (CAS) theory as a comprehensive frame of reference (Holland 1995, Kauffman 1995, Ball 2004). The change of working environment phenomena is demonstrated via CAS-base hypotheses of traditional and networked acting

circumstances. The viewpoint is information that is required to successful networking.

The theory of complex adaptive systems (CAS) by (Holland 1995) aims at to explain the chaotic nature of multi-actor interactive system on the viewpoint of one actor. The CAS theory seeks understanding of the adaptive behavior of an entity in its acting environment by categorizing its basic features. CAS theory divides these basic elements in four properties and three mechanisms. Properties are aggregation, nonlinearity, flows and diversity. Mechanisms are tagging, internal models and building blocks.

- Aggregation is a property of an entity. It defines that an entity seeks to categorize same kind of things in same kinds of classes. All new perceptions are then situated into these classes to ease to understand the outer world. On the other hand, aggregation aims to explain, what a complex adaptive system does as a whole. It seeks to gain understanding about the behavioral phenomena of entities defined by certain plethora of classes.

- Tagging is a mechanism that gives a descriptive symbol for an aggregate. Tag is a name or symbol to gather correspondence entities together.

- Flow is property that tells what transfers between nodes. Nodes act like processors that refine or redirect flows. Nodes, connectors and flows vary over time. Flow has two properties. The first one is called multiplier effect. It means that additional resource injected into a system produces a chain of changes via affecting the internal behavior or redirecting properties of nodes. The second property is a feedback process, where output of a process has effects on the input stage of the process. In CAS environment several such feedback processes and interacting relationships are taking place simultaneously, because nodes are connected together via evolving connector network.

- Building blocks form the mechanism that enables to construct models in a simple way. Each block is tagged aggregation. Second level aggregations and models can be formulated by combining certain simple enough building blocks. Blocks are combined together in space in a certain order to form such models that can be tagged to be meaningful for the node.

- Nonlinearity is property that expresses that the outcome of the whole is not the sum of its parts. The outcome of multi-actor inter-action situation cannot be deterministically counted by knowing the features of all entities.

- Diversity is property that tells that wholeness contains certain amount certain kinds of nodes that have suitable role in that wholeness. If a specific node is removed it will be replaced during time with another similar kind of nodes or its roles are transferred to other nodes.

- Internal modeling (or schema) is mechanism that causes certain behavior of an entity, when certain stimulus occurs. (Holland 1995, 10-40)

The world can be considered as a complex system of complex systems. It is neither random nor accidental. It is a collection of systems' elements with certain kinds of universal features and the continuum of their interrelations. This makes the world act in a non-deterministic way. This apparently fuzzy behavior becomes understandable if we perceive the system at the right structural level. (see Ball 2004; Kauffmann 1995).

This study focuses on the property called "aggregation" supported by "tagging", "flow" and "building blocks". It will be shown that shifting from content based knowledge discovery thinking towards situation based thinking will give a novel

opportunity to construct such knowledge discovery practices that will support networked people to gather and release relevant information on the viewpoint of the situation they are dealing with.

So, let's generate hypotheses concerning aggregation both in content based approach and framework based approach. First, content based aggregation added with network features (motivation of networking, information flow characteristics and building blocks):

- People like to categorize the exchanged information. Typically information is defined by subject of interest thus being categorized by content. The behavior of the wholeness is judged on behalf of aggregation of those content based information categorization models.

- Social communication networks are defined by subject of interest. The name – tag – of interest guides people to form networks with such people, who express same kind of tags.

- Information flow between various interactive entities is controlled by content and amount. Second order effects are typically not taken account.

- Because of the content based strategy orienting towards interaction the building blocks of creating common models for releasing and receiving relevant information may be different amongst different communicative actors during networking situations. This makes communication challenging, while different actors are speaking on different context.

And secondly, framework based hypothesis:

- Aggregation shall be done on the basis of networking context and situations requirements instead of communicated information content. Second order aggregation describes in that case the nature of networking instead of the meaning of each collaborative party.

- Tagging is formed in addition to defined content also around the phase of networking activity. Tagging supports context and situation based aggregation.
- Information flows are controlled by the demands of networking context and situation instead of one or several parties' agreements of releasable information. Each networking party releases such information that is relevant for tagged networking aggregation.
- Building blocks are situations instead of organizations or other actors. The outcome of the comprehensive context will be constructed as a system of situations rather than system of actors.

High-Level Information Exchange Ontology

Actors´ interests to information can be categorized in several ways, e.g. on time axis, based on information content, based on the role of a particular actor or based on the phase of activity. Information interests differ from one situation to another and also from one actor to another. All these interest viewpoints exist during the situation where actors are involved. A unified and abstract enough structure of describing information shall be needed to get an idea, what type of information various networking situations may require and further on to structurize various knowledge discovery situations in an equal way.

Pardo et. al (2004) take a holistic view to this area and approach challenges via components of social processes, resources and technical and social artifacts in the contexts of technology, business processes, inter-organizational structures and policies in social environment. They construct a four layered model defined by context. Every layer contains similar integration components

producing a system with integrating processes in the focus. However this model does not take account the general level ontology of the exchanged information. Wang & Wei (2007) take value chain and process approach to the issue. Neither have they provided an approach to the exchanged information itself concentrating to the ways to collaborate.

However, the approach here will be the information itself despite the processes viewpoint is important. For that reason, a high-level abstraction of human information exchange ontology is shortly introduced here. This ontological model has been developed, iterated and applied frequently during last few years (2004–2008). The model is based on communication philosophy (Habermas 1984, 1989), sociology (Parsons 1951; Luhmann 1999), cognition philosophy (Bergson 1983; Damasio 1999; Merleau-Ponty 1968), organizational culture (Schein 1992; Hofstede 1984), knowledge management (Polanyi 1966; Maier 2002; Nonaka & Takeutchi 1995) and decision support systems (Turban et.al 2005; Marakas 2003). Various development variants of the model have been published frequently (e.g. Kuusisto 2006, 2007 and 2008;2008 Kuusisto et.al 2007; Kuusisto & Kuusisto 2008). The up-to-date version is described in Table 1.

Rows describe the temporality and abstraction degree of information. Information at the upper row is relatively most abstract, future oriented and its effects are long-lasting. The lowest level contains information that updates fast, is concrete and is observable as immediate events. The column on the left contains cultural information described by Schein (1980 & 1992). The next column on the left contains actors´ internal information. Te next right contains information of expressed conclusions made by the actor. The column on the right describes information that comes from outside of an actor or is remarkably affected by the world outside the actor itself. Rough contents of the information categories are described, as well. This model describes the structure of indi-

Table 1. The high-level abstraction of human information handling ontology

Values, Competence	Internal facts	Conclusions	External facts
Basic assumptions Hidden assumptions that will guide the behaviour of an actor. The fundamental features of a culture.	**Mission, vision** A subjective and expressed impression of the end-state of the actor.	**Decision** A solution based on thinking and assessment.	**Task** Activities or work to be performed, activities originated by upper-level management or by the development of a situation.
Socially true values Assumptions that are mutually accepted in a certain group to be a basis of thinking and executing activities.	**Means** Activities or methods applied to reach an aim or fulfil a purpose.	**Alternatives to act** Description of realistically executable acting solutions.	**Foreseen end states** Future situations most certainly reached when activities are finished.
Physically true values Assumption about structures that can be accepted to be valid, e.g. organization, division of labour, competences.	**Resources** Available tangible resources such as people, financial resources, material, machinery and office space.	**Possibilities to act** Describes possible paths to the goal that the actor can choose and that provide something new to the actor. For example, strategy alternatives.	**Anticipated futures** Describes a thing, event or development that can be taught or is expected.
Social artefacts Structure of a social system, principles of interaction, description of nodes and their mutual positions, and observable behaviour.	**Action patterns** Describes how an actor can behave, e.g., process descriptions and instructions.	**Restrictions** Things that have to be considered before planning the use of resources and means in the context of anticipated futures.	**Environment** Describes an area or a space that affects an actor, e.g., activities of media, market trends, national trends, and global trends.
Physical artefacts Results of activity, like technical results of a group, written and spoken language, symbols, art.	**Features** Describes properties of objects such as the properties of an organization or equipment, e.g., infrastructure descriptions and properties of equipments.	**Event model** A description that enables the outlining of the pattern of a situation. For example, reports, documents, analyzed conclusions such as quality reports, statistics, pictures and maps.	**Events** Describes time-limited events caused by actors. For example, meetings and sales reports stock market prices.

vidual and shared information and sense-making. With the help of this ontology the complex information exchange activity can be simplified and emerging phenomena of inter-working network can be found.

Every layer of the model has a specialized task while handling the information for various purposes, such as situation follow-up, planning and decision-making. The layer that deals with event information produces an updated picture of events. On the next layer, restrictions are sorted out. The next two layers contain information about resources and means as internal facts. These facts as well as information about events and environment, and knowledge about the composition and the development of the situation and possible end-states are used as a basis of making conclusions. The possibilities to act and information about

alternate ways to operate are refined. The chain of deduction can be continued until the ultimate decision-making layer is reached. There, all output information from the lower layers shall be available in explicitly expressed form. Conclusions of a neighbor layer are relatively more meaningful than information on the other layers. The whole spectrum of tacit dimension shall be available for the decision-maker. The decision-maker must be able to know the action patterns, anticipate the change of the situation, foresee the end-state of the action and deeply understand the meaning of the mission as a part of the bigger continuum of action.

This ontology of human information handling structure is used to analyze various and different information sharing and information exploitation situations. Because it is universal, it can be used to analyze and develop knowledge discovery practices, too.

Methodology

Content analysis is used as methodology to find out information requirements abstractions in different working situations. Using Krippendorff (1980) criteria to define the context of content analysis results this research case as follows:

- Data of the content of various information exchange situations were analyzed. Analyzed data is described in the context of every studied case.
- Data was defined using expert evaluation criteria based on the ontology described in chapter 2.2. and illustrated in Table 1.
- Population of the data drawn is described in the context of each studied case, as well.
- Context relative to which data are analyzed is information exchange requirements of interacting actors in different situations.
- The target of generalization of data is to find out the patterns that may reveal the differences of information exchange profiles between various situations. (About) five of the most frequent categories described in Table 1 are **bolded** and (about) five next most frequent categories are underlined in the final analysis of each case to demonstrate the differences of information requirements between various situations. Quantification of analyzed and abstracted data is made by counting relative shares (%) of the analyzed data situated into each category. That makes final results comparable to each others.
- Boundaries of the analysis are defined by the limitations of the total amount of observed information exchange situations and ambiguity when sampling data into the nominated categories of the used ontological model.

Because of the boundaries of the analysis the method is not completely reliable. Only one observer was used to observe and analyze all studied cases. This observer categorized and counted manually key expressions and ideas of contents expressed in texts or speech. Categorization was done using Table 1 category definitions as reference. It is obvious that interpretation in this kind of situation is to some degree subjective. Because only one observer-analyst was used, the intra-rater reliability (stability) can be considered to be rather high, but the inter-rater reliability may be moderate. However, the reliability problem is not so severe that it sounds, because exact results are not searched. The aim of the content analysis in this research is to find out possible differences of information requirements in different using situations to demonstrate possible requirements to knowledge discovery techniques. Various cases were analyzed during the period beginning from August 2007 and ending to December 2007. A priori coding was used applying the ontology described in Table 1 as theory.

CASE STUDIES

Actor Profile Information

Twenty individual actors from military, governmental and non-governmental organizations taking part to cooperation experiment in December 2007 were surveyed to find out, what kind of information they would prefer to have from their potential networking partners. The actual question was: "When joining the network community, what types of information about your potential collaboration partners would you like to have?" The question did not concern general administrative information like contact information or technical information. Free word answers were analyzed like described in chapter 2.3. Results are shown in Table 2. All results in tables are converted into relative shares (%).

Table 2. Relative shares (%) of information needs for network partner choosing situations

Values, Competence	Internal facts	Conclusions	External facts
Basic assumptions 9	Mission, vision 21	Decision 0	Task 6
Socially true values 6	Means 6	Alternatives to act 0	Foreseen end states 0
Physically true values 3	Resources 9	Possibilities to act 0	Anticipated futures 0
Social artefacts	Action patterns 18	Restrictions 0	Environment 0
Physical artefacts 3	Features 18	Event model 0	Events 0

Table 3. Relative shares (%) of information categories that real organizations release about themselves

Values	Internal facts	Conclusions	External facts
Basic assumptions 6	Mission, vision 14	Decision 0	Task 6
Socially true values 6	Means 16	Alternatives to act 0	Foreseen end states 6
Physically true values 6	Resources 6	Possibilities to act 2	Anticipated futures 0
Social artefacts 0	Action patterns 14	Restrictions 0	Environment 4
Physical artefacts 4	Features 10	Event model 0	Events 0

In addition, web pages of five real organizations were analyzed using the Table 1 information categorization model and content analysis method. The categories that were found and their relative frequencies are shown in Table 3.

Those two tables look alike enough to be combined and mean value counted. As summarized and categorized and highlighted the result is as Table 4 describes.

It can be noticed that most important information in network foundation phase will concentrate to every actors internal facts added with values and competence information. In addition, after analysis of thirty crisis management professionals' experiences and somewhat comprehensive lessons learned report (Linder 2006) of crisis management practices on the field, one additional category raised up as a quite important one. (Kuusisto &

Kuusisto 2008) This category is "environment". Information about all working environment features and issues was found crucial to successfully work on the area. So, we need to know the basic features of our working environment in addition to the internal facts of organizations or individuals on the network.

Planning the Mission

Next, some findings based on the analysis of an inter-agency cooperation exercise are presented. Exercise was arranged in Finland on August 2007. Participants were professionals form several ministry- and agency level organizations. The nature of the exercise was to practice tactical management (i.e. optimizing the available resources to deal with ongoing situation to respond the

Table 4. Relative shares (%) of information requirement profile for network partner choosing situations

Values, Competence	Internal facts	Conclusions	External facts
Basic assumptions 8	**Mission, vision** 18	Decision 0	Task 6
Socially true values 6	**Means** 11	Alternatives to act 0	Foreseen end states 3
Physically true values 5	**Resources** 8	Possibilities to act 1	Anticipated futures 0
Social artefacts 0	**Action patterns** 16	Restrictions 0	Environment 2
Physical artefacts 4	**Features** 14	Event model 0	Events 0

Table 5. Relative shares (%) of unidirectional released information during briefings

Values, Competence	Internal facts	Conclusions	External facts
Basic assumptions 0	Mission, vision 0	Decision 9	Task 0
Socially true values 2	Means 20	Alternatives to act 3	Foreseen end states 0
Physically true values 1	Resources 18	Possibilities to act 3	Anticipated futures 1
Social artefacts 0	Action patterns 5	Restrictions 15	Environment 3
Physical artefacts 0	Features 3	Event model 3	Events 11

foreseeable near-term future). Observed activity phases concentrated to mission planning prior to mission execution. Three different information exchange situations were observed. First, a total of four general briefings were followed. Second, one decision discussion were observed. Finally, the information content that was released by all participants into the collaboration support system database, were analyzed at the title-level.

In briefing situations, mainly all information was shared in a unidirectional way by the briefer. About 10% of the information items were discussed. Discussion dealt merely with means, resources, alternatives to act, possibilities to act and restrictions (See Table 5 and Table 6).

The decision and planning discussion information exchange profiles concerning released and discussed information are described in Table 7

and Table 8. Now, because it was question of experts´ contribution to support decision making, about 50% of the released information was also discussed. Almost every other item was discussed expect the situation facts and final decisions. Information released and discussed situated mainly in the middle of the information exchange model. One deviation compared to discussions during briefings exists. More information about futures development was both released and especially discussed during decision-making situations than during briefings.

Table 9 shows the distribution of the information types of the generally published information. The classification criterion was the content of the title of released publication. As a whole, same kind of information types were released in general publication process than in unidirectional

Table 6. Relative shares (%) of discussed information during briefings

Values, Competence	Internal facts	Conclusions	External facts
Basic assumptions 0	Mission, vision 0	Decision 0	Task 0
Socially true values 0	Means 17	Alternatives to act 17	Foreseen end states 0
Physically true values 0	Resources 17	Possibilities to act 17	Anticipated futures 0
Social artefacts 0	Action patterns 0	Restrictions 29	Environment 0
Physical artefacts 0	Features 0	Event model 0	Events 0

Table 7. Relative shares (%) of released information during decision discussion

Values, Competence	Internal facts	Conclusions	External facts
Basic assumptions 0	Mission, vision 0	Decision 17	Task 7
Socially true values 0	Means 21	Alternatives to act 2	Foreseen end states 2
Physically true values 0	Resources 10	Possibilities to act 5	Anticipated futures 2
Social artefacts 0	Action patterns 2	Restrictions 5	Environment 2
Physical artefacts 0	Features 0	Event model 2	Events 21

phases during briefings and decision discussions.

Mean values of both released and discussed information were counted to get an idea, what kind of information exchange profiles exist while releasing and discussing about mission planning and if differences can be found between these two information using situations. Results are demonstrated in Table 10 and Table 11. Differences were observed, indeed. Information profiles while releasing information in briefings and discussing about further actions seem to be different.

Some brief conclusions can be made on behalf of those results presented above. In tactical planning situation, information in the middle of the model comes important in addition to situation follow-up and decision information releasing. During briefings, where lots of representatives of various organizations were present, discussions raised up mainly about available means and re-sources and about possibilities and alternatives to act, as well mutual restrictions for activities. In the case of small group decision-making discussion, the general information releasing profile was quite equal to the one with briefings. What comes into the discussed information categories, still the means and resources items were found to be important, but discussion about alternatives to act moved towards to anticipate the future and to evaluate the possible end-states of overall activity. Discussing about mutual future orients parties to work together more longer periods than to only deal with the emerging issues.

Executing Task

Barents Rescue 2007 (BR) search and rescue exercise tactical management execution activities was analyzed (http://www.pelastusopisto.fi/

Table 8. Relative shares (%) of discussed information during decision discussion

Values, Competence	Internal facts	Conclusions	External facts
Basic assumptions 0	Mission, vision 0	Decision 0	Task 0
Socially true values 0	Means 38	Alternatives to act 6	Foreseen end states 6
Physically true values 0	Resources 19	Possibilities to act 13	Anticipated futures 6
Social artefacts 0	Action patterns 0	Restrictions 6	Environment 6
Physical artefacts 0	Features 0	Event model 0	Events 0

Table 9. Relative shares (%) of collaboration support system database published information

Values, Competence	Internal facts	Conclusions	External facts
Basic assumptions 0	Mission, vision 0	Decision 4	Task 0
Socially true values 0	Means 24	Alternatives to act 1	Foreseen end states 1
Physically true values 0	Resources 15	Possibilities to act 5	Anticipated futures 6
Social artefacts 0	Action patterns 6	Restrictions 6	Environment 1
Physical artefacts 0	Features 4	Event model 6	Events 19

Table 10. Relative shares (%) of unidirectional released information during mission planning

Values, Competence	Internal facts	Conclusions	External facts
Basic assumptions 0	Mission, vision 0	**Decision** **10**	Task 2
Socially true values 1	**Means** **22**	Alternatives to act 2	Foreseen end states 1
Physically true values 0	**Resources** **14**	Possibilities to act 4	Anticipated futures 3
Social artefacts 0	Action patterns 4	**Restrictions** **10**	Environment 2
Physical artefacts 0	Features 2	Event model 4	**Events** **17**

pelastus/cmc/home.nsf/wLatestEng/ 0BF38AD-DB817B1E1C225726E003022B4, visited December 08, 2008). The nature of Barents Rescue was operational. Various authorities and volunteer organizations from four countries executed an airliner accident search and rescue operation in Finnish Lapland.

A collaboration support system was established to support the actors to release and use relevant planning and mission execution information. In-

Table 11. Relative shares (%) of discussed information during mission planning

Values, Competence	Internal facts	Conclusions	External facts
Basic assumptions 0	Mission, vision 0	Decision 0	Task 0
Socially true values 0	**Means** **28**	**Alternatives to act** **12**	<u>Foreseen end states</u> <u>3</u>
Physically true values 0	**Resources** **18**	**Possibilities to act** **15**	<u>Anticipated futures</u> <u>3</u>
Social artefacts 0	Action patterns 0	**Restrictions** **18**	<u>Environment</u> <u>3</u>
Physical artefacts 0	Features 0	Event model 0	Events 0

Table 12. Relative shares (%) of published information categories on collaboration support system in BR mission execution

Values, Competence	Internal facts	Conclusions	External facts
Basic assumptions 0	Mission, vision 0	**Decision** **10**	<u>Task</u> <u>6</u>
Socially true values 0	<u>Means</u> <u>3</u>	Alternatives to act 0	Foreseen end states 0
Physically true values 0	**Resources** **20**	Possibilities to act 0	Anticipated futures 0
Social artefacts 0	**Action patterns** **14**	Restrictions 0	<u>Environment</u> 6
Physical artefacts 0	**Features** **14**	<u>Event model</u> <u>3</u>	**Events** **23**

formation that was published on the collaboration support system was analyzed to get an idea about the pattern of the information exchange profile in the mission execution phase.

In the first phase information publishing was more concentrated to features - events layer, and when the rescue execution started the publishing contained decisions. It can be noticed that value and mission information was not released at all. That is because the mission was clear to all. Another interesting feature is that information about futures development and conclusions (expect decisions) was not released, as well (Table 12). This tells that various organizations did not have to make collaborative planning. This can have two explanations. Either the division of tasks was totally clear to everyone or the organizations did not see added value of on-line collaboration during mission execution phase.

Conclusive Findings

As a conclusion it can be argued that improvement of acting in networks would need a concept that provides as good a system as possible to improve the potential of focusing to relevant types of information of the knowledge discovery systems.

IT can be postulate that different kind of situations requires different kind of emphasis concerning the type of the required information. So, it can be concluded that the hypothesis set for this study, will be considered as truthful. Further on, we can postulate that different phases of activity require differently focused knowledge discovery.

Knowledge discovery practices shall be such that they guide the user to find and also release relevant type of information compared to this nominated activity phase. This is consistent with Habermas's theory of communication act (1984, 1989). He claims that to start communication, at least one common item must exist between interacting parties. Interaction and its development are based on this common item. The implication is that to conduct interaction between two or more actors, one or multiple common categories of information must be present. To gain mutual understanding, interacting parties require common information flows. Knowledge discovery practices shall be developed to enable these information flows to support users to both release and find relevant types of information related to ongoing or becoming situation.

Information using profiles differ in the cases of evaluating the network-partner potentiality for cooperation, preliminary planning work, the decision-making itself, as well as managing various networking situations. To re-iterate from above, at least one information category must be common between those functions. In general this means that organizations should understand what types of information are important for the activities between organizations. This can be used to produce and develop knowledge discovery practices. Those practices should support information exchange procedures across organizational boundaries to assure the information flow priorities, and to take into account the temporal demands of information exchange.

Information exchange profiles for networking shall be determined to optimize interactivity. Those organizations or parts of organizations that are working with the same kinds of issues should have common information exchange profiles. Networking can be enhanced when information content priorities and time frames of updating content are consistent across various, inter-organizational actors. It can be concluded that to develop inter-organizational working processes, it

is essential to identify, develop and exploit inter-working information exchange profiles. Finding and determining those profiles will give a good thrust to develop suitable knowledge discovery algorithms.

CONSEQUENCES FOR KNOWLEDGE DISCOVERY

Technological solutions have potential to increase organizations capability to perform its task. To increase capability even more the practices, processes and ways to act shall be renewed or adjusted to meet those demands that the holistic working environment causes. Further on, organizational culture shall be adjusted if success will be gained in longer period. If knowledge discovery solutions support required processes and practices with working phase dependant information discovery, the overall capability of the organization will increase. If information type requirements are well known, it will be easier to develop more situation precise knowledge discovery solutions for organizations needs in networked environment. This differs from the content based knowledge discovery that aims at finding certain defined information, not information requirements to deal with certain situation.

Table 13 combines four different cases of information exchange needs of organization that is acting in different networking situations described in chapter 3. Table 13 demonstrates rather clearly that information needs will vary from working phase to another. It is assumable that this happens despite the purpose of the organization. However, some more research shall be done to get comparative material from e.g. business organizations. Table 13 also shows that some information categories are emphasized in several phases of activity. Those categories are the ones that carry the networking activity from phase to another. Moving from partner finding and network establishing phase to start common

Table 13. The importance of information categories compared to activity phases

	Partnerizing	Planning published	Planning discussed	Execution
Basic assumptions	**8**	0	0	0
Socially true values	<u>6</u>	1	0	0
Physically true values	<u>5</u>	0	0	0
Social artefacts	0	0	0	0
Physical artefacts	<u>4</u>	0	0	0
Mission, vision	**18**	0	0	0
Means	**11**	**22**	**28**	<u>3</u>
Resources	**8**	**14**	**18**	**20**
Action patterns	**16**	<u>4</u>	0	**14**
Features	**14**	2	0	**14**
Decision	0	**10**	0	**10**
Alternatives to act	0	2	**12**	0
Possibilities to act	1	<u>4</u>	**15**	0
Restrictions	0	**10**	**18**	0
Event model	0	<u>4</u>	0	<u>3</u>
Task	<u>6</u>	2	0	<u>6</u>
Foreseen end states	3	1	<u>3</u>	0
Anticipated futures	0	<u>3</u>	<u>3</u>	0
Environment	2	2	<u>3</u>	<u>6</u>
Events	0	**17**	0	**23**

activity with planning the information about organizations' means, resources and action patterns acts as a bridge to proceed towards next phase. Moving from planning to execution information about resources and events are crucial to enable smooth glide forward. This means that knowledge discovery practices shall support not only in-phase mining but also in-between mining. This set flexibility requirements for knowledge discovery systems.

In addition to the type requirements of the information the time domain is important, as well. When searching for partners the required information shall be available for long periods of time. To publish this information is not very time critical. Its only criteria are that it is up-to-date, accurate and available for possible partners. This information typically changes rather slowly, as well.

Information released on briefings prior to activity planning and discussions shall be available early enough to guarantee sufficient amount of time for all networking partners to complete their planning before common activity execution. However, that information shall not be available for too long period, because its reliability will expire inevitably during time. When actively discussing about planning, execution principles, and possibilities of common activity the information shall be available on-line throughout the discussion. Same kinds of information availability requirement are valid during activity execution phase. This time criticality sets requirements for knowledge discovery systems, as well. Knowledge discovery systems shall be able to both support releasing relevant type of information and discover right kind of information profile of partners to answer quickly and reliably to the demands of the ongoing working phase. It is rather clearly noticeable that different situations set quite divergent requirements for knowledge discovery practices in both quality and type of information and in time domain.

Table 13 illustrates rather clearly that there are some key types of information that seem to be important in spite of which situation the networking parties are. Those categories are means and resources, as well as environment. Other frequently occurring categories are action patterns, decisions, restrictions, events, alternatives and possibilities to act, as well as futures information. However the emphases of those information categories vary from using phase to another. This has consequences especially how the discovered information will be expressed to the user. The user interface shall be such that it supports the user to find more quickly and accurately such information that is relevant for that nominated networking phase. This will support the user to take account right kind of information and make more reliable and accurate choices thus limiting the need for both time and bandwidth.

Knowledge discovery algorithms shall support to find information that is not only user content specific. Also such terminology and symbolic expressions that are specific for different networking situations shall be supported by knowledge discovery systems. Determining networking situation specific ontology that focuses on the networking situation phenomena itself may be challenging to construct. One example of that was introduced in Table 1. The ontology shall support the knowledge discovery algorithms to find such contents of the published information of very various networking parties that support to find relevant partners and doing collaboration in ever evolving technologically supported network. This means that there shall be both an ontology that focuses networking in different phases of activity and an ontology that focuses subjective content. In this kind of case, knowledge discovery algorithms use

both of these to dig both the activity phase relevant and content relevant information. This kind of knowledge discovery system supports the user by offering a platform that both guides the user to release situation relevant information and offers such content information that is relevant for the situation. Its power is in finding such knowledge that defines the comprehensive working situation.

REFERENCES

Ball, P. (2004). *Critical Mass: how one thing leads to another*. London: Arrow Books.

Bergson, H. (1983). Creative Evolution. Lanham, MD: University Press of America™, Inc.

Damasio, A. (1999). *The Feeling of What Happens: Body and Emotion in the Making of Consciousness*. London: Heinemann.

Habermas, J. (1984). The Theory of Communicative Action: *Vol. 1. Reason and the Rationalization of Society, (Trans. T. McCarthy)*. Boston: Beacon Press.

Habermas, J. (1989). The Theory of Communicative Action: *Vol. 2. Lifeworld and System: A Critique of Functionalist Reason, (trans. T. McCarthy)*. Boston: Beacon Press.

Hofstede, G. (1984). *Culture's Consequences: International Differences in Work-Related Values*. Beverly Hills, CA: Sage Publications.

Holland, J. H. (1996). *Hidden Order: How Adaptation Builds Complexity*. Cambridge, MA: Perseus Books.

Kauffman, S. (1995). *At Home in the Universe: The Search for the Laws of Self-Organization and Complexity*. New York: Oxford University Press.

Krippendorff, K. (1980). *Content Analysis: An Introduction to Its Methodology*. Newbury Park, CA: Sage.

Kuusisto, R. (2006). Flowing of Information in Decision Systems, *Proceedings of the Thirty-Ninth Annual Hawaii International Conference on System Sciences, (HICSS-39),* Hawaii, USA. Retrieved from http://csdl2.computer.org/comp/proceedings/ hicss/2006/2507/07/250770148b.pdf

Kuusisto, R. (2008). *SHIFT" Theoretically-Practically Motivated Framework. Information Exchange viewpoint on developing collaboration support system (Series 3, No 1/2008).* Helsinki, Finland: Edita Prima Oy, Finnish Defence University, Department of Tactics and Operations Art.

Kuusisto, R. (2008). Analyzing the Command and Control Maturity levels of Collaborating Organizations. In *proc of 13th International Command and Control Research and Technology Symposium (13th ICCRTS),* June 2008.

Kuusisto, R., & Kuusisto, T. (2008). Information Security Culture as a Social System: Some Notes of Information Availability and Sharing. In Gupta, M., & Sharman, R. (Eds.), *Social and Human Elements of Information Security: Emerging Trends and Countermeasures* (pp. 77–97). Hershey, PA: Information Science Reference.

Kuusisto, T., Kuusisto, R., & Nissen, M. (2008). Information Flow Aspects of Inter-organizational Crisis Management. *Journal of Information Warfare, 6*(2), 39–51.

Linder, R. (2006). *Wikis, Webs, and Networks: Creating Connections for Conflict-prone Settings,* CSIS (The Center of Strategic and International Studies) Report. Retrieved February 15, 2006, from http://www.csis.org/media/csis/pubs/061018_pcr_creatingconnections.pdf

Luhmann, N. (1999). *Ökologishe Kommunikation, 3. Auflage. Opladen.* Wiesbaden, Germany: Westdeutcher Verlag.

Maier, R. (2002). *Knowledge Management Systems. Information and Communication Technologies for Knowledge Management.* Berlin: Springler-Verlag.

Marakas, G. M. (2003). *Decision Support Systems In the 21st Century.* Upper Saddle River, NJ: Prentice Hall.

Merleau-Ponty, M. (1968). *The Visible and Invisible.* Evanston, IL: Northwest University Press.

Nonaka, I., & Takeuchi, H. (1995). *The Knowledge-Creating Company.* New York: Oxford University Press.

Pardo, T. A., Cresswell, A. M., Dewes, S. S., & Burke, G. B. (2004). Modeling the Social & Technical Processes of interorganizational Information Integration. In *Proc. of the Thirty-Seventh Annual Hawaii International Conference on System Sciences, (HICSS-37),* Hawaii, USA.

Parsons, T. (1951). *The Social System.* Glencoe, IL: Free Press.

Polanyi, M. (1966). *The Tacit Dimension.* London: Cox & Wyman Ltd.

Schein, E. H. (1980). *Organizational Psychology* (3rd ed.). Englewood Cliffs, NJ: Prentice-Hall.

Schein, E. H. (1992). *Organizational Culture and Leadership* (2nd ed.). San Francisco, CA: Jossey-Bass.

Turban, E., Aronson, J. E., & Liang, T.-P. (2005). *Decision Support Systems and Intelligence Systems.* Upper Saddle River, NJ: Pearson Education, Inc.

Wang, E. T. G., & Wei, H.-L. (2007). Interorganizational Governance Value Creation: Coordinating for Information Visibility and Flexibility in Supply Chains. *Decision Sciences, 38*(4), 647–674.

KEY TERMS AND DEFINITIONS

Information: Knowledge derived from study, experience, or instruction; Knowledge of specific events or situations that has been gathered or received by communication; intelligence or news; A collection of facts or data; The act of informing or the condition of being informed.

Knowledge: Knowledge is part of the hierarchy made up of data, information and knowledge. Data are raw facts. Information is data with context and perspective. Knowledge is information with guidance for action based upon insight and experience.

Knowledge Discovery: Knowledge Discovery and Data Mining (KDD) is an interdisciplinary area focusing upon methodologies for extracting useful knowledge from data.

Network: An interconnected system of things or people.

Networking Activity: The act of meeting new people in a business or social context by using computer networks as enablers.

Networked Environment: The social-technical system, where networking activity takes place.

Complex Adaptive System: A complex, nonlinear, interactive system which has the ability to adapt to a changing environment. Such systems are characterized by the potential for self-organization, existing in a non-equilibrium environment. CASs evolve by random mutation, self-organization, the transformation of their internal models of the environment, and natural selection.

Compilation of References

Aaltonen, J. (2007). Service oriented extension of roles-linkage model for travel business networks. In Saloheimo, M. (Ed.), *Operative Network Integration: working papers from research project, University of Lapland, Department of Research Methodology Reports, Essays and Working Papers 10* (pp. 166–181). Rovaniemi, Finland: University of Lapland Press.

Aaltonen, J., Krone, O., & Mustonen, P. (2008). Towards Information Security Ontology in Business Networka. In Y. Kiyoki & T. Tokuda (Eds.), *Proceedings of the 18th European-Japanese Conference on Information Modeling and Knowledge Bases (EJC 2008)*, (pp. 373-379). Kanagawa, Japan: EJC 2008 Program Committee.

Aaltonen, J., Rinne, J., & Tuikkala, I. (2006). A Multidisciplinary Framework for Concept Evolution: A Research Tool for Business Models. In Maula, M., Hannula, M., Seppä, M., & Tommila, J. (Eds.), *ICEB + eBRF 2006 Frontiers of e-Business Research 2006* (pp. 526–532). Tampere, Finland: Tampere University of Technology and University of Tampere.

Aaltonen, J., Tuikkala, I., & Saloheimo, M. (2007). Concept Modeling in Multidisciplinary Research Environment. In H. Jaakkola, Y. Kiyoki & T. Tokuda (Eds.), *Proceedings of the 17th European-Japanese Conference on Information Modeling and Knowledge Bases (EJC 2007)* (pp. 143-160). Pori, Finland: Tampere University of Technology.

Aaltonen, J., Tuikkala, I., & Saloheimo, M. (2007). Towards Semantic Resource Classification in Organizational Environment. In L. Uden, E. Damiani & G. Passiante (Eds.), *Proceedings of the 2nd International Conference on Knowledge Management in Organization (KMO): New trends in Knowledge management* (pp. 183-187). Lecce, Italy: Knowledge Management in Organizations 2007.

Abernethy, M., & Wyatt, A. (2003). *Study on the measurement of intangible assets and associated reporting practices*. Prepared for the European Communities Enterprise Directorate General.

Abramson, B., & Finizza, A. (1991). Using belief networks to forecast oil prices. *International Journal of Forecasting, 7*(3), 299–315. doi:10.1016/0169-2070(91)90004-F

Abramson, B., & Finizza, A. (1995). Probabilistic forecasts from probabilistic models: a case study in the oil market. *International Journal of Forecasting, 11*(1), 63–72. doi:10.1016/0169-2070(94)02004-9

Abul, O., Atzori, M., Bonchi, F., & Giannotti, F. (2007). Hiding Sequences. In *IEEE International Conference on Data Engineering Workshop* (pp. 147-156), Istanbul, Turkey.

Abul, O., Atzori, M., Bonchi, F., & Giannotti, F. (2007). Hiding Sensitive Trajectory Patterns. In *IEEE International Conference on Data Mining Workshops* (pp. 693-698), Omaha, NE.

Abul, O., Bonchi, F., & Nanni, M. (2008). Never Walk Alone: Uncertainty for Anonymity in Moving Objects Databases. In *International Conference on Data Engineering* (pp. 376-385), Cancun, Mexico.

Ackof, R. L. (1989). From Data to Wisdom. *Journal of Applies Systems Analysis, 16*, 3–9.

Adler, P. S., & Borys, B. (1996). Two Types of Bureaucracy: Enabling and Coercive. *Administrative Science Quarterly, 41*(1), 61–89. doi:10.2307/2393986

Adobe. (2009). *Adobe Flash Microphone Settings.* Retrieved May 25, 2009 from http://www.macromedia.com/support/documentation/en/flashplayer/help/settings_manager02.html

Adrangi, B., Chatrath, A., Dhanda, K. K., & Raffiee, K. (2001). Chaos in oil prices? Evidence from futures markets. *Energy Economics, 23*, 405–425. doi:10.1016/S0140-9883(00)00079-7

Aggarwal, C. C., & Yu, P. S. (Eds.). (2008). *Privacy Preserving Data Mining: Models and Algorithms.* New York: Springer-Verlag.

Agosta, L. (2000). *The Essential Guide to Data Warehousing.* Upper Saddle River, NJ: Prentice Hall.

Agrawal, R., & Srikant, R. (1994). Fast Algorithms for Mining Association Rules in Large Databases. In *International Conference on Very Large Data Bases* (pp.487-499), San Francisco, CA.

Agrawal, R., & Srikant, R. (2000). Privacy Preserving Data Mining. In *ACM SIGMOD Conference on Management of Data,* (pp. 439-450), Dallas, TX.

Agrawal, R., Imielinski, T., & Swami, A. (1993). Mining Association Rules between Sets of Items in Large Databases. In *ACM SIGMOD International Conference on Management of Data* (pp. 207-216), Washington, DC.

Al Faris, A. (1991). The determinants of crude oil price adjustment in the world petroleum market. *OPEC Review, 15*.

Alavi, M., & Leidner, D. (2001). Review: Knowledge Management and Knowledge Management Systems: Conceptual Foundations and Research Issues. *Management Information Systems Quarterly, 25*(1), 107–136. doi:10.2307/3250961

Aldendefrer, M., & Blasfield, R. (1984). *Cluster Analysis.* London: SAGE.

Aleksander, I., & Morton, H. (1995). *An introduction to neural computing.* New York: International Thompson Computer Press.

Allen, S. G. (1983). How much does absenteeism cost? *The Journal of Human Resources, 18*(3), 379–393. doi:10.2307/145207

Anderson, B., Ryan, V., & Goudy, W. (1984). Consistency in subjective evaluations of community attributes. Social Indicators Research, 14(2), 165–175. doi:10.1007/BF00293408doi:10.1007/BF00293408

Anderson, E. W., Fornell, C., & Rust, R. T. (1997). Consumer satisfaction, productivity, and profitability: differences between goods and services. *Marketing Science, 16*(2), 311–329. doi:10.1287/mksc.16.2.129

Andrews, R., Boyne, G. A., & Walker, R. M. (2006). Strategy Content and Organizational Performance: An Empirical Analysis. *Public Administration Review,* 66(1): 52–63. doi:10.1111/j.1540-6210.2006.00555.x

Andrews, R., Boyne, G. A., Law, J., & Walker, R. M. (2009). Strategy Formulation, Strategy Content and Performance: An Empirical Analysis. *Public Management Review, 11*(1), 1–22. doi:10.1080/14719030802489989

Annola, V. (2003). Sopimuksen dynaamisuus. Talousoikeudellinen rakennetutkimus sopimuksen täydentymisestä ja täydentymisen ohjaamisesta. Turku, Finland: Turun yliopisto.

Appelbaum, S., Adam, J., Javeri, N., Lessard, M., Lion, J. P., Simard, M., & Sorbo, S. (2005). A case study analysis of the impact of satisfaction and organizational citizenship on productivity. *Management Research News, 28*(5), 1–26. doi:10.1108/01409170510629023

Aracil, J., & Gordillo, F. (Eds.). (2000). *Stability Issues in Fuzzy Control.* Heidelberg, Germany: Physica-Verlag.

Arsham, H. (1994). *Time-Critical Decision Making for Business Administration.* (Web site checked on February 2nd, 2009) http://home.ubalt.edu/ntsbarsh/stat-data/Forecast.htm

Asbjorn, R. (1995). *Performance Management.* Boca Raton, FL: Chapman & Hall.

Atallah, M., Bertino, E., Elmagarmid, A. K., Ibrahim, M., & Verykios, V. S. (1999). Disclosure Limitation of Sensitive Rules. In *IEEE Workshop on Knowledge and Data Engineering Exchange* (pp. 45-52), Chicago, IL.

Atiyah, P. S. (1979). *The Rise and Fall of Freedom of Contract.* Oxford, UK: Clarendon Press.

Atiyah, P. S. (1981). *Promises, Morals and Law.* Oxford, UK: Clarendon Press.

Auslander, G., Dobrof, J., & Epstein, I. (2001). Comparing social work's role in renal dialysis in Israel and the United States: The practice-based research potential of available clinical information. *Social Work in Health Care, 33*(3/4), 129–152.

Ayre, L. B. (2006). *Data Mining For Information Professionals.* Retrieved May 6, 2008, from http://techessence.info/files/Ayre_DataMiningForInformationProfessionals_June2006.pdf.

Baard, E. (2002). Buying Trouble: Your Grocery List Could Spark a Terror Probe. *Village Voice.* Retrieved January, 2009, from http://www.villagevoice.com/2002-07-23/news/buying-trouble/

Bacon, R. (1991). Modelling the price of oil. *Oxford Review of Economic Policy, 7*(2), 17–34. doi:10.1093/oxrep/7.2.17

Bala, P. K. (2008). A technique for mining generalized quantitative associated rules for retail inventory management. *International Journal of Business Strategy, 8*(2), 114–127.

Ball, P. (2004). *Critical Mass: how one thing leads to another.* London: Arrow Books.

Balloch, S., & Taylor, M. (2001). Partnership working: Introduction. In Balloch, S., & Taylor, M. (Eds.), *Partnership working: Policy and practice* (pp. 1–14). Bristol, UK: The Policy Press.

Barandela, R., Rangel, E., Sánchez, J. S., & Ferri, F. J. (2003). *Restricted Decontamination for the Imbalanced Training Sample Problem,* (. *LNCS, 2905,* 424–431.

Barber, P., Graves, A., Hall, M., Sheath, D., & Tomkins, C. (2000). Quality failure costs in civil engineering projects. *International Journal of Quality & Reliability Management, 17*(4/5), 479–492. doi:10.1108/02656710010298544

Barnes, B. (1995). *The Elements of Social Theory.* Princeton, NJ: Princeton University Press.

Barney, J. (1991). Firm resources and sustained competitive advantage. *Journal of Management, 17,* 99–120. doi:10.1177/014920639101700108

Barone-Adesi, G., Bourgoin, F., & Giannopoulos, K. (1998). Don't look back. *Risk (Concord, NH),* (August): 100–107.

Beaulieu, A. (2005). Learning SQL. Sebastopol, CA: O'Reilly Inc.

Bellatreche, L., Karlapalem, K., & Mohania, M. (1999). OLAP query processing for partitioned data warehouses. In *DANTE '99: Proceedings of the 1999 International Symposium on Database Applications in Non-Traditional Environments,* (pp. 35). Washington, DC: IEEE Computer Society.

Benitez, J. M., Castro, J. L., & Requena, I. (1997, September). Are artificial neural networks black boxes? *IEEE Transactions on Neural Networks, 8*(5), 1156–1164. doi:10.1109/72.623216

Berger, P. L., & Luckmann, T. (1999). *Die gesellschaftliche Konstruktion der Wirklichkeit. Frankfurt/Main.* Germany: Fischer.

Bergson, H. (1983). Creative Evolution. Lanham, MD: University Press of America™, Inc.

Berka, P., & Bruha, I. (1998). *Principles of Data Mining and Knowledge Discover, Nantes, France*. Berlin: Springer.

Berne, R. (1992). *The relationship between financial reporting and the measurement of financial condition*. Government Accounting Standard Board, Research Report, (18), Nolwalk, CT.

Berry, J. A., & Linoff, G. (1997). *Data mining Techniques For Marketing, Sales and Customer Support*. New York: John Wiley & Sons Inc.

Berry, J. A., & Linoff, G. (2000). *Mastering data mining*. New York: John Wiley &Sons, Inc.

Berry, J. A., & Linoff, G. (2003). *Mining the web*. New York: John Wiley &Sons Inc.

Beynon, M. J. (2005). A Novel Technique of Object Ranking and Classification under Ignorance: An Application to the Corporate Failure Risk Problem. *European Journal of Operational Research*, *167*, 493–517. doi:10.1016/j.ejor.2004.03.016

Beynon, M. J. (2005). A Novel Approach to the Credit Rating Problem: Object Classification Under Ignorance. *International Journal of Intelligent Systems in Accounting Finance & Management*, *13*, 113–130. doi:10.1002/isaf.260

Beynon, M. J., Buchanan, K., & Tang, Y.-C. (2004). The Application of a Fuzzy Rule Based System in an Exposition of the Antecedents of Sedge Warbler Song Flight. *Expert Systems: International Journal of Knowledge Engineering and Neural Networks*, *21*(1), 1–10. doi:10.1111/j.1468-0394.2004.00258.x

Beynon, M.J., Peel, M.J., & Tang, Y.-C. (2004). The Application of Fuzzy Decision Tree Analysis in an Exposition of the Antecedents of Audit Fees. *OMEGA - International Journal of Management Science*, *32*(2), 231-244.

Beynon-Davies, P. (2002). *Information Systems: An Introduction to Informatics in Organisations*. Basingstoke, UK: Palgrave Macmillan.

Biggs, D., Ville, B., & Suen, E. (1991). A method of choosing multiway partitions for classification and decision trees. *Journal of Applied Statistics*, *18*(1), 49–62. doi:10.1080/02664769100000005

Blackwell, B., & Ravda, S. (n.d.). Oracle's Technology for Bioinformatics and Future Directions. In Y.-P. Chen, (ed.), *First Asia – Pacific Bioinformatics Conference, Adelaide, Australia. Conferences in Research and Practice in Information Technology*.

Blumenfield, S., & Epstein, I. (2001). Introduction: Promoting and maintaining a reflective professional staff in a hospital-based social work department. *Social Work in Health Care*, *33*(3/4), 1–14.

Böckerman, P., & Ilmakunnas, P. (2008). Interaction of working conditions, job satisfaction, and sickness absences: evidence from a representative sample of employees. *Social Science & Medicine*, *67*(4), 520–528. doi:10.1016/j.socscimed.2008.04.008

Bonneau, J., Anderson, J., Anderson, R., & Stajano, F. (2009) Eight Friends Are Enough: Social Graph Approximation via Public Listings. In *Second ACM Workshop on Social Network Systems*, Nuremburg, Germany.

Bouckaert, G. (1992). Productivity analysis in the public sector: the case of fire service. *International review of Administrative Sciences*, *58*(2), 175-200.

Bouckaert, G. (1993). Efficiency measurement from a management perspective: a case of the civil registry office in Flanders. *International review of Administrative Sciences*, *59*(1), 11-27.

Bouckaert, G., & Auwers, T. (1999). Prestaties meten in de overhead. Brugge, Belgium: Die Keure.

Boullé, M. (2006). MODL: a Bayes optimal discretization method for continuous attributes. *Machine Learning*, *65*(1), 131–165. doi:10.1007/s10994-006-8364-x

Boullé, M. (2007). Compression-based averaging of selective naive Bayes classifiers. [JMLR]. *Journal of Machine Learning Research*, *8*, 1659–1685.

Boullé, M. (2008). Khiops: outil de préparation et modélisation des données pour la fouille des grandes bases de données. In Extraction et gestion des connaissances (EGC), (pp. 229-230).

Bourgeois, L. (1980). Performance and Consensus. *Strategic Management Journal, 1,* 227–248. doi:10.1002/smj.4250010304

Bourgeois, L. J. III. (1985). Strategic goals, perceived uncertainty, and economic performance in volatile environments. *Academy of Management Journal, 28*(3), 548–573. doi:10.2307/256113

Bowman, C., & Amrosini, V. (1997). Perceptions of strategic priorities, consensus and firm performance. *Journal of Management Studies, 34,* 241–258. doi:10.1111/1467-6486.00050

Boyne, G. A., & Walker, R. M. (2004). Strategy content and public service organizations. *Journal of Public Administration: Research and Theory, 14*(2), 231–252. doi:10.1093/jopart/muh015

Bozeman, B. (1987). *All organizations are public.* San Francisco, CA: Jossey-Bass.

Brand, R. (2002). Microdata Protection Through Noise Addition. In *Inference Control in Statistical Databases* []. New York: Springer-Verlag.]. *Theory into Practice, 2316,* 97–116.

Brandt, A. (2006). Privacy watch: Phishers put their lures on cell phones. *PC World,* (November 20), 1-2.

Brans, M., Giesbers, S., & Meijer, A. (2008). Alle ogen op de ziekenhuizen gericht? De effecten van openbaarheid van prestatiegegevens. Bestuurswetenschappen, 62(2), 32–52.

Breiman, L. (2001). Random forest. *Machine Learning, 45.* Retrieved from www.berkeley.edu/users/breiman/Breiman.

Breiman, L., Friedman, J. H., Olshen, R. A., & Stone, C. J. (1984). *Classification and Regression Trees.* Belmont, CA: Wadsforth International Group.

Brennan, J. J., & Seiford, L. M. (1987). *Linear programming and l1 regression: A geometric interpretation.* Computational Statistics & Data Analysis.

Bridges, D. (2003). *Fiction written under Oath? Essays in Philosophy and Educational Research.* Dordrecht, The Netherlands: Kluwer Academic Publishers.

Brito, P., & Malerba, D. (2003). Mining official data. Intelligent Data Analysis, 7, 497–500.

Brown, S., & Sessions, J. G. (1996). The economics of absence: theory and evidence. *Journal of Economic Surveys, 10*(1), 23–53. doi:10.1111/j.1467-6419.1996.tb00002.x

Bryson, J. M. (2004). *Strategic Planning for Public and Nonprofit Organizations* (3rd ed.). San Francisco: Jossey-Bass.

Burrell, G., & Morgan, G. (1979). *Sociological Paradigms and Organizational Analysis.* London: Heinemann.

Bush, I., Epstein, I., & Saines, A. (1997). Social work utilization of social sciences literature: A content analysis of practice journal citations. *Social Work Research, 21,* 45–56.

Callens, M. (2007). *Efficiëntie en effectiviteit in de publieke sector.* Unpublished paper. Brussels: Studiedienst van de Vlaamse Regering.

Campo, K., Gijsbrechts, E., & Nisol, P. (2000). Towards understanding consumer response to stock-outs. *Journal of Retailing, 76*(2), 65–78. doi:10.1016/S0022-4359(00)00026-9

Canongia Lopes, J. N. (2004). On the classification and representation of ternary phase diagrams: The yin and yang of a T–x approach. *Physical Chemistry Chemical Physics, 6,* 2314–2319. doi:10.1039/b315799g

Cao, H., Mamoulis, N., & Cheung, D. W. (2006). Discovery of Collocation Episodes in Spatiotemporal Data. In *International Conference on Data Mining* (pp. 823-827), Hong Kong, China.

Capurro, R. (2008). Information Technology as an Ethical Challenge.19-28. *Journal of Information Ethics, 5* (2). Retrieved 09.08.2009 from http://www.acm.org/ubiquity/volume_9/v9i22_capurro.html

Castells, M. (2000). *The Rise of the Network Society* (*Vol. 1*). Oxford, UK: Blackwell Publisher.

Castells, M., Fernandez-Ardevol, M., Qiu, J. L., & Sey, A. (2007). *Mobile Communication and Society: A Global Perspective* (p. 77). Cambridge, MA: The MIT Press.

Chambers, M. J., & Bailey, R. J. (1996). A theory of commodity price fluctuations. *The Journal of Political Economy, 104*(5), 924–957. doi:10.1086/262047

Chan, W. (2007). *A clinical data-mining study of the psycho-social status of Chinese cancer patients in palliative care.* Doctoral dissertation, University of Hong Kong, Hong Kong.

Chan, W., Epstein, I., & Chen, C. (2008). (submitted to). Family predictors of psychosocial outcomes among Hong Kong Chinese cancer patients in palliative care: living and dying with the "support paradox". [Palliative Medicine.]. *Paper.*

Chang, L., & Moskowitz, I. S. (1998). Parsimonious Downgrading and Decision Trees Applied to the Inference Problem. In *Workshop on New Security Paradigms* (pp. 82-89), Charlottesville, VA.

Chang, R. L. P., & Pavlidis, T. (1977). Fuzzy decision tree algorithms. *IEEE Transactions on Systems, Man, and Cybernetics, 7*(1), 28–35. doi:10.1109/TSMC.1977.4309586

Chaudhuri, S., & Dayal, U. (1997). An Overview of Data warehousing and OLAP Technology. *SIGMOD Record, 26*(1), 65–74. doi:10.1145/248603.248616

Chawla, N. V., Bowyer, K. W., Hall, L. O., & Kegelmeyer, W. P. (2002). SMOTE: Synthetic Minority Over-sampling Technique. *Journal of Artificial Intelligence Research, 16*, 321–357.

Chawla, N. V., Japkowicz, N., & Kolcz, A. (2004). Editorial: special issue on learning from imbalanced data sets. *ACM SIGKDD Explorations Newsletter, 6*(1), 1–6. doi:10.1145/1007730.1007733

Chen, K., & Liu, L. (2005). Privacy Preserving Data Classification with Rotation Perturbation. In *IEEE International Conference on Data Mining* (pp. 589-592), Houston, TX.

Chen, Z. (2001). Data Mining and Uncertain Reasoning: An Integrated Approach. New York: John Wiley & Sons, US.

Chesney, T., & Penny, K. (2009). Data mining trauma injury data using C5.0 and logistic regression to determine factors associated with death. *International Journal of Healthcare Technology and Management, 10*(1/2), 16–26. doi:10.1504/IJHTM.2009.023725

Choi, S., & Stahl, D. (1997). *The Economics of Electronic Commerce.* Indiana: Macmillan Technical Publishing.

Choi, T., Dooley, K., & Rungtusanahan, M. (2001). Supply networks and complex adaptive systems. *Journal of Operations Management, 19*(3), 351–366. doi:10.1016/S0272-6963(00)00068-1

Choudat, D. (2003). Risque, fraction étiologique et probabilité de causalité en cas d'expositions multiples, i: l'approche théorique. *Archives des Maladies Professionnelles et de l'Environnement, 64*(3), 129–140.

Chow, A. (2005). *The bereavement experience of Chinese persons in Hong Kong.* Doctoral dissertation, University of Hong Kong, Hong Kong.

Ciro, D., & Nembhard, M. (2005). Collaborative data-mining in an adolescent mental health service: Clinicians speak of their experience. In K. Peake, I. Epstein & D. Medeiros, (Eds.), Clinical and research uses of an adolescent intake questionnaire: What kids need to talk about (pp. 305-318). Binghampton, NY: Haworth Press.

Clark, T. (1990). *Monitoring Local Governments.* Dubuque, IA: Kendal Hunt Publishing.

Clark, T. (1994). Municipal Fiscal Strain: Indicator and Causes. *Government Finance Review, 10*(3), 27–29.

Cleland, D. I and Ireland, L. R. (2006). Project management: strategic design and implementation, (5th Ed.). Clarksville, TN: McGraw-Hill.

Clementine, S. P. S. S. (2009). Retrieved from http://www.spss.com/clementine/

Clifton, C. (2000). Using Sample Size to Limit Exposure to Data Mining. *International Journal of Computer Security, 8*(4), 281–307.

Clifton, C., Kantarcioglou, M., Lin, X., & Zhu, M. (2002). Tools for Privacy Preserving Distributed Data Mining. *ACM SIGKDD Explorations, 4*(2), 28–34. doi:10.1145/772862.772867

Cloward, R., & Epstein, I. (1965). Private social welfare's disengagement from the poor: The case of family adjustment agencies. In *Proceedings of the annual social work day conference.* University of Buffalo. Reprinted in Brager, G., & Purcell, P. (Eds.), (1967). *Community action against poverty.* New Haven, CT: College & University Press (pp. 40-63).

Cohen, W. (1995). Fast effective rule induction. In *Proceedings of the 12th international conference on machine learning,* (pp. 115–123). Los Altos, CA: Morgan Kaufmann.

Collins, M., Schwartz, I., & Epstein, I. (2001). Risk factors for adult imprisonment in a sample of youth released from residential child care. *Children and Youth Services Review, 23,* 203–226. doi:10.1016/S0190-7409(01)00133-5

Commission of European Contract Law. (1999). *The Principles of European Contract Law.* Retrieved 17.10.2008 from <http://frontpage.cbs.dk/law/commission_on_european_contract_law/PECL%20engelsk/engelsk_partI_og_II.htm>

Cooke-Davies, T. (2002). The "real" success factors on projects. *International Journal of Project Management, 20,* 185–190. doi:10.1016/S0263-7863(01)00067-9

Copeland, R. E., & Ingram, R. (1983). *Municipal Financial Reporting and Disclosure Quality.* Reading, MA: Addison-Wesley.

Cordero, A. (2000). *When reunification works: A family strengths perspective.* Doctoral dissertation, Graduate Faculty in Social Welfare, The City University of New York, New York.

Cordero, A. (2004). When family reunification works: Data-mining foster care records. *Families in Society, 85*(4), 571–580.

Cordero, A., & Epstein, I. (2005). Refining the practice of reunification: "Mining" successful foster care case records of substance abusing families. In Mallon, G. P., & Hess, P. M. (Eds.), *Child Welfare for the Twenty-First Century: A Handbook of Practices, Policies and Programs.* New York: Columbia University Press.

CRA. (2003). *Four Grand Challenges In Trustworthy Computing.* Available at http://www.cra.org/reports/trustworthy.computing.pdf, last accessed on May 26, 2009.

Crisp, S., Eiken, S., Gerst, K., & Justice, D. (September 2003). *Money Follows the Person and Balancing Long-Term Care Systems: State examples.* A report for the US Department of Health and Human Services, Centers for Medicare and Medicaid Services, Disabled and Elderly Health Programs Division. Washington, DC: Medstat. http://www.cms.hhs.gov/promisingpractices/mfp92903.pdf

CRISP-DM. (2009). Retrieved from http://www.crisp-dm.org/

Crossman, G. (2008). Nothing to hide, nothing to fear? International Review of Law Computers & Technology, 22(1/2), 115–118. doi:10.1080/13600860801925003doi:10.1080/13600860801925003

Curtin, J., Kauffman, R. J., & Riggins, F. J. (2007). Making the 'MOST' out of RFID technology: A research agenda for the study of the adoption, usage and impact of RFID. *Information Technology and Management, 8*(92), 100.

Curtis, B., Krasner, H., & Iscoe, N. (1988). A field study of the software Design process for large Systems. *Communications of the ACM, 31*(11), 1268–1287. doi:10.1145/50087.50089

Czarniawska, B. (2001). Narrative, Interviews, and Organizations. In Gubrium, J. F., & Holstein, J. A. (Eds.), *Handbook of Interview Research; Context & Method* (pp. 733–749). London, New Delhi: Sage Publications.

Czarniawska-Joerges, B. (1998). *A narrative Approach to organizations Studies*. London: Sage Publications.

Czerniawska, F., & Potter, G. (1998). *Business in a Virtual World. Exploiting Information for Competitive Advantage*. Houndmills, UK: Palgrave MacMillan.

D'Adderio, L. (2002). Configuring Software, reconfiguring memories: the influence of integrated systems on knowledge storage, retrieval and reuse. In *Proceedings of the 2002 ACM symposium on Applied computing*, (pp. 726–731), Madrid, Spain.

Dale, C., & Zyren, J. (1997). Petroleum futures markets: volatile prices, controversial functions, stagnant volumes. In Petroleum 1996: Issues and Trends, (pp. 92-100). Washington, DC: DOE/EIA-0615.

Damasio, A. (1999). *The Feeling of What Happens: Body and Emotion in the Making of Consciousness*. London: Heinemann.

Dasseni, E., Verykios, V. S., Elmagarmid, A. K., & Bertino, E. (2001). Hiding Association Rules by Using Confidence and Support. In *International Workshop on Information Hiding* (pp. 369-383), Pittsburgh, PA.

DATAllegro. (2008). *Datallegro solves telecom data warehouse challenges*. Retrieved May, 2009, from http://www.datallegro.com/data_warehouse_solutions/telecommunications.asp

Datta, R. P. (2008). Data Mining Applications and Infrastructural Issues: An Indian Perspective. *ICFAI Journal of Infrastructure, 6*(3), 42–50.

Davis, W. (2009). *FTC's Leibowitz Opts For BT Opt-In*. Available at http://www.mediapost.com/publications/?fa=Articles.showArticle&art_aid=105954, last accessed on May 26, 2009.

Day, R., & Rogers, E. (2006). Enhancing NASA's Performance as a Learning Organization. *NASA Ask Magazine, 22*, 36–39.

De Bruijn, H. (2002). Prestatiemeting in de publieke sector. Strategieën om perverse effecten te neutraliseren. Bestuurswetenschappen, 56(2), 39–159.

De Bruijn, H. (2006). Prestatiemeting in de publieke sector. Tussen professie en verantwoording (2e druk). Den Haag, The Netherlands: Lemma.

De Mantores, R. L. (1990). *Approximate Reasoning Models*. Chichester, UK: Ellis Horwood.

De Peuter, B., De Smedt, J., & Van Dooren, W. (2007). Handleiding beleidsevaluatie. Deel 2: monitoring van beleid. Brussels: Steunpunt Beleidsrelevant Onderzoek – Bestuurlijke Organisatie Vlaanderen.

De Smedt, J., Conings, V., & Verhoest, K. (2004). De integratie van de beleids-, contract- en financiële cyclus. Het agentschapsperspectief: De managementsrapportage in de beheersovereenkomst in het kader van de koppeling van de cycli. Onderzoeksrapport, Beter Bestuurlijk Beleid. Brussels: Steunpunt Beleidsrelevant Onderzoek – Bestuurlijke Organisatie Vlaanderen.

Deaton, A., & Larque, G. (1992). On the behavior of commodity prices. *The Review of Economic Studies, 59*(198), 1–23. doi:10.2307/2297923

Defays, D., & Nanopoulos, P. (1993). Panels of Enterprises and Confidentiality: The Small Aggregates Method. In *Symposium on Design and Analysis of Longitudinal Surveys* (pp. 195-204). Ottawa, Canada: Statistics Canada.

Delaney, J., & Huselid, M. (1996). The impact of human resource management practices on perceptions of organizational performance. *Academy of Management Journal, 39*(4), 949–969. doi:10.2307/256718

Dembczyński, K., Kotłowski, W., & Słowiński, R. (2007). Ordinal Classification with Decision Rules. *Mining Complex Data – ECML/PKDD Third International Workshop, MCD 2007*, Warsaw, Poland, September 17-21, *Revised Selected Papers* (LNCS 4944). Berlin: Springer.

Dempster, A. P. (1967). Upper and lower probabilities induced by a multiple valued mapping. *Annals of Mathematical Statistics, 38*, 325–339. doi:10.1214/aoms/1177698950

Dempster, A. P. (2008). The Dempster-Shafer Calculus for Statisticians. *International Journal of Approximate Reasoning, 48*, 365–377. doi:10.1016/j.ijar.2007.03.004

Demšar, J., Zupan, B., & Leban, G. (2004). *Orange: From Experimental Machine Learning to Interactive Data Mining*. White Paper (www.ailab.si/orange), Faculty of Computer and Information Science, University of Ljubljana, Slovenia.

Denne, S. (2007). After being over-hyped, RFID starts to deliver. *The Wall Street Journal*, (November 7), B5F.

Dennis, A. R., Valacich, J. S., Speier, C., & Morris, M. G. (1998). Beyond Media Richness: An Empirical Test for Media Synchronicity Theory. In *Proceedings of the 31st Hawaii International Conference on Systems Sciences (HICSS '98)*", Los Alamitos, CA: IEEE Computer Society.

DeRosa, M. (2004). *Data Mining and Data Analysis for Counterterrorism*. Washington, DC: Center for Strategic & International Studies.

Dess, G. G. (1987). Consensus on strategy formulation and organizational performance: competitors in a fragmented industry. *Strategic Management Journal, 8*(3), 259–277. doi:10.1002/smj.4250080305

Dess, G. G., & Origer, N. K. (1987). Environment, structure, and consensus in strategy formulation: a conceptual integration. *Academy of Management Review, 12*(2), 313–330. doi:10.2307/258538

Dess, G. G., & Shaw, J. D. (2001). Voluntary turnover, social capital and organizational performance. *Academy of Management Review, 26*(3), 446–456. doi:10.2307/259187

DeTienne, K. B., DeTienne, D. H., & Joshi, S. A. (2003). Neural networks as statistical tools for business researchers. *Organizational Research Methods, 6*, 236–265. doi:10.1177/1094428103251907

Diagne, G. (2006). *Sélection de variables et méthodes d'interprétation des résultats obtenus par un modèle boite noire*. Unpublished master's thesis, UVSQ-TRIED.

Diesner, J., & Carley, K. (2005) Exploration of communication networks from the Enron email corpus. In *Workshop on Link Analysis, Counterterrorism and Security*.

Dillon, M. (2008). Underwriting Security. *Security Dialogue, 39*(2-3), 309–332. doi:10.1177/0967010608088780

Dills, A. K. (2005). Does cream-skimming curdle the milk? A study of peer effects. *Economics of Education Review, 24*, 19–28. doi:10.1016/j.econedurev.2004.01.002

Directorate General for Financial Coordination with Local Authorities, Spanish Ministry of Economy and Finance, *(1992-1999)*.

Dobrof, J., Dolinko, A., Lichtiger, E., Uribarri, J., & Epstein, I. (2000). The complexity of social work practice with dialysis patients: Risk and resiliency factors, interventions and health-related outcomes. *Journal of Nephrology Social Work, 20*, 21–36.

Dobrof, J., Dolinko, A., Lichtiger, E., Uribarri, J., & Epstein, I. (2001). Dialysis patient characteristics and outcomes: The complexity of social work practice with end stage renal disease. *Social Work in Health Care, 33*(3/4), 105–128.

Dobrof, J., Ebenstein, H., Dodd, S., & Epstein, I. (2006). Caregivers and professional partnership caregiver resource center: Assessing a hospital support program for family caregivers. *Journal of Palliative Medicine, 9*(1), 196–205. doi:10.1089/jpm.2006.9.196

Dollery, B., Crase, L., & Byrnes, J. (2006, September). Local Government Failure: Why Does Australian Local Government Experience Permanent Financial Austerity? *Australian Journal of Political Science, 41*(3), 339–353. doi:10.1080/10361140600848952

Dombi, J., & Gera, Z. (2005). The approximation of piecewise linear membership functions and Łukasiewicz operators. *Fuzzy Sets and Systems, 154*, 275–286. doi:10.1016/j.fss.2005.02.016

Domingo-Ferrer, J., & Mateo-Sanz, J. M. (2002). Practical Data-Oriented Microaggregation for Statistical Disclosure Control. *IEEE Transactions on Knowledge and Data Engineering, 14*(1), 189–201. doi:10.1109/69.979982

Domingo-Ferrer, J., & Torra, V. (2005). Ordinal, Continuous and Heterogeneous K-anonymity Through Microaggregation. *Data Mining and Knowledge Discovery, 11*(2), 195–212. doi:10.1007/s10618-005-0007-5

Dornier, P.-P., Ernst, R., Fender, M., & Kouvelis, P. (1998). *Global Operations and Logistics Text and Cases.* Chichester, UK: Wiley & Sons.

Downs, A. (1967). *Inside bureaucracy.* Boston: Little Brown.

Dresner, H. (2008). *Performance management revolution.* New York: John Wiley & Sons Inc.

Dutton, J. E., Fahey, L., & Narayanan, V. K. (1983). Toward understanding strategic issue diagnosis. *Strategic Management Journal, 4*(4), 307–323. doi:10.1002/smj.4250040403

Eagle, N., & Pentland, A. (2006). Reality mining: Sensing complex social systems. *Personal and Ubiquitous Computing, 10*(4), 255–268. doi:10.1007/s00779-005-0046-3

Earl, M. (2001). Knowledge Management Strategies: Toward a Taxonomy. *Journal of Management Inquiry, 18*(1), 215–233.

Edwards, M., & Clough, R. (2005). *Corporate Governance and Performance: An Exploration of the Connection in a Public Sector Context.* Issues paper 1. Retrieved October 1, 2008, from http://www.canberra.edu.au/corpgov-aps/pub/IssuesPaperNo.1_GovernancePerformance Issues.pdf

Eggen, D. (2006). Justice department database stirs privacy fears. *Washington Post,* (December 26), 2-3.

Eggink, E., & Blank, J. L. (2002). Efficiëntie in de publieke sector. Beleidswetenschap, 16(2), 144–161.

Eisenhardt, K. M. (1989). Agency Theory: An Assessment and Review. *Academy of Management Review, 14*(1), 57–74. doi:10.2307/258191

Eisenhardt, K. M. (1989). Building Theories from Case Study Research. *Academy of Management Review, 14*(4), 532–550. doi:10.2307/258557

Elizalde, F. (2006). *EU data retention directive: An onerous burden on service providers.* Retrieved January, 2009, from http://www.frost.com/prod/servlet/market-insight-top.pag?docid=83098430

Emmelhainz, M., Emmelhainz, L., & Stock, J. (1991). Consumer responses to retail Stock-outs. *Journal of Retailing, 67*(2), 32–49.

Emory, C. W. (1985). *Business research methods* (3rd ed.). Homewood, Illinois: Irvin.

Epstein, I. (1987). Pedagogy of the perturbed: Teaching research to the reluctant. *Journal of Teaching in Social Work, 1,* 71–89. doi:10.1300/J067v01n01_06

Epstein, I. (1992). Changing models of practice in research utilization. In Grasso, A. J., & Epstein, I. (Eds.), *Research utilization in the social services: Innovations for practice and administration* (pp. 7–10). Binghampton, NY: Haworth.

Epstein, I. (1995). Promoting reflective social work practice: Research strategies and consulting principles. In Hess, P., & Mullens, E. (Eds.), *Practitioner-researcher partnerships: Building knowledge from, in and for practice* (pp. 83–102). Washington, DC: NASW Press.

Epstein, I. (1996). In quest of a research-based model for clinical practice: Or, why can't a social worker be more like a researcher? *Social Work Research, 20,* 97–100.

Epstein, I. (2001). Using available clinical information in practice-based research: Mining for silver while dreaming of gold. In I. Epstein & S. Blumenfield (eds.), Clinical data-mining in practice-based research: Social work in hospital settings (pp. 15-32). Binghamton, NY: Haworth Press.

Epstein, I. (2005). Following in the footnotes of giants: Citation analysis and its discontents. *Social Work in Health Care, 41*(3/4), 93–101. doi:10.1300/J010v41n03_04

Epstein, I. (2007). From evaluation methodologist to clinical data-miner: Finding treasure through practice-based research. In Rehr, H., & Rosenberg, G. (Eds.), *The Social Work–Medicine Relationship: 100 Years at Mount Sinai* (pp. 107–111). Binghamton, NY: Haworth Press.

Epstein, I. (2008). *Clinical Data-Mining: Integrating Practice and Research.* Oxford, UK: Oxford University Press.

Epstein, I. (2009). Promoting harmony where there is commonly conflict: Evidence-informed practice as an integrative strategy. *Social Work in Health Care, 48*(3), 216–231. doi:10.1080/00981380802589845

Epstein, I. (2010). *Clinical data-mining: Integrating practice and research*. New York, N.Y.: Oxford University Press.

Epstein, I., & Grasso, A. J. (1990). Using agency-based available information to further practice innovation. In Weissman, H. (Ed.), *Serious play: Creativity and innovation in social work*. New York: NASW Press.

Epstein, I., & Hench, C. (1979). Behavior modification in the classroom: Education or social control? *Journal of Sociology and Social Welfare*, (September): 223–229.

Epstein, I., & Tripodi, T. (1978). *Research techniques for program planning, monitoring and evaluation*. New York: Columbia University Press.

Epstein, I., Grellong, B., & Kohn, A. (1992). Models of university-agency collaboration in research. *Research on Social Work Practice, 2*, 350–357.

Epstein, I., Zilberfein, F., & Snyder, S. (1997). Using available information in practice-based outcomes research: A case study of psycho-social risk factors and liver transplant outcomes. In E. J. Mullen, & J.L. Magnabosco, (eds.), Outcomes measurement in the human services: Cross-cutting issues and methods (pp. 224-233). New York: NASW Press.

European Parliament. (2007). *EU data retention directive 2006/24/e*. Retrieved January, 2009, from http://eur-lex.europa.eu/LexUriServ/site/en/oj/2006/l_105/l_10520060413en00540063.pdf

Express Scripts. (2009). Available at http://www.esisupports.com/, last accessed on May 29, 2009.

Fan, H.-Y., & Lampinen, J. (2003). A Trigonometric Mutation Operation to Differential Evolution. *Journal of Global Optimization, 27*, 105–129. doi:10.1023/A:1024653025686

Fan, Y., Liang, Q., & Wei, Y. M. (2008). A generalized pattern matching approach for multi-step prediction of crude oil price. *Energy Economics, 30*, 889–904. doi:10.1016/j.eneco.2006.10.012

Fan, Z.-P., Feng, B., Sun, Y.-H., & Ou, W. (2009). Evaluating knowledge management capability of organizations: a fuzzy linguistic method. *Expert Systems with Applications, 36*, 3346–3354. doi:10.1016/j.eswa.2008.01.052

Farrell, D., & Stamm, C. L. (1988). Meta-analysis of the correlates of employee absence. *Human Relations, 41*(3), 211–227. doi:10.1177/001872678804100302

Farrell, M. B. (2009). *Cellphone tracking services: Friendfinder or Big Brother?* Available at http://features.csmonitor.com/innovation/2009/05/01/cellphone-tracking-services-friend-finder-or-big-brother/, last accessed on May 26, 2009.

Faucett, A., & Kleiner, B. H. (1994). New developments in performance measures of public programmes. *International Journal of Public Sector Management, 7*(3), 63–70. doi:10.1108/09513559410061768

Faulkner, M. (2003). *Customer management excellence*. New York: John Wiley &Sons Inc.

Fawcett, T. (2003). *Roc graphs: Notes and practical considerations for data mining researchers*. Technical Report HPL-2003-4, HP Labs, 2003. Retrieved from citeseer.ist.psu.edu/fawcett03roc.html

Fayyad, U., Piatetsky-Shapiro, G., & Smyth, P. (1996). From Data Mining to Knowledge Discovery: An Overview. In Fayyad, U. M., Piatetsky-Shapiro, G., Smyth, P., & Uthurusamy, R. (Eds.), *Advances in Knowledge Discovery and Data Mining* (pp. 1–34). Menlo Park, CA: AAAI Press/The MIT Press.

Féraud, R., & Clérot, F. (2002). A methodology to explain neural network classification. *Neural Networks, 15*(2), 237–246. doi:10.1016/S0893-6080(01)00127-7

Féraud, R., Boullé, M., Clérot, F., & Fessant, F. (2008). Vers l'exploitation de grandes masses de données. In *Extraction et gestion des connaissances* (pp. 241–252). EGC.

Fern, X. Z., & Brodley, C. (2003). Boosting lazy decision trees. In *International conference on machine learning* (pp. 178–185). ICML.

Fiss, P. C. (2007). A Set-Theoretic Approach to Organizational Configurations. *Academy of Management Review*, *32*(4), 1160–1198. doi:10.2307/20159362

Floyd, C. (1992). Human Questions in Computer Science. In Floyd, C., Züllighoven, R., Budde, R., & Keil-Slawik, R. (Eds.), *Software Development and Reality Construction* (pp. 15–27). Berlin: Springer.

Floyd, C. (1992). Software Development and Reality Construction. In Floyd, C., Züllighoven, R., Budde, R., & Keil-Slawik, R. (Eds.), *Software Development and Reality Construction* (pp. 86–100). Berlin: Springer.

Framling, K. (1996). *Modélisation et apprentissage des préférences par réseaux de neurones pour l'aide à la décision multicritère.* Unpublished doctoral dissertation, Institut National des Sciences Appliquées de Lyon, France.

Frank, E., & Hall, M. (2001). A simple approach to ordinal classification. In *12th European Conference on Machine Learning,* Freiburg, Germany, September 5–7, (LNCS 2167). Berlin: Springer.

Freedman, C., Joubert, L., & Russell, N. (2005). Practitioner evaluation of a brief intervention approach in emergency services: The Sunshine Hospital Quick Response Team. *Social Work Research and Evaluation*, *6*(2), 207–216.

Freund, Y., Iyer, R., Schapire, R., & Singer, Y. (2003). An efficient boosting algorithm for combining preferences. *Journal of Machine Learning Research*, *4*, 933–969. doi:10.1162/jmlr.2003.4.6.933

Galguera, L., Luna, D., & Mendez, M. P. (2006). Predictive segmentation in action: using Chaid to segment loyalty card holders. *International Journal of Market Research*, *48*(4), 459–479.

Gambrill, E. (2006). Evidence-based practice and policy: Choices ahead. *Research on Social Work Practice*, *16*(3), 338–357. doi:10.1177/1049731505284205

Garcia, V., Sánchez, J. S., Mollineda, R. A., Alejo, R. & Sotoca, J. M. (2007). The class imbalance problem in pattern classification and learning. *CEDI 2007.*

Garnet, J., Marlowe, J., & Pandey, S. (2008). Penetrating the Performance Predicament: Communication as a Mediator or Moderator of Organizational Culture's Impact on Public Organizational Performance. Public Administration Review, 68(2), 266–281. doi: 10.1111/j.1540-6210.2007.00861.xdoi:10.1111/j.1540-6210.2007.00861.x

GASB. (1987). Concepts Statement N° 1 of Governmental Accounting Standards Board: Objectives of Financial Reporting, Norwalk, CT.

Ghoshal, S., & Moran, P. (1996). Bad for Practice: A critique of the Transaction Cost Theory. *Academy of Management Review*, *21*(1), 13–47. doi:10.2307/258627

Giannotti, F., & Pedreschi, D. (Eds.). (2008). *Mobility, Data Mining and Privacy: Geographic Knowledge Discovery.* New York: Springer-Verlag. doi:10.1007/978-3-540-75177-9

Giannotti, F., Nanni, M., & Pedreschi, D. (2006). Efficient Mining of Temporally Annotated Sequences. In *SIAM International Conference on Data Mining*, Bethesda, MD, (pp. 346-357).

Giannotti, F., Nanni, M., Pinelli, F., & Pedreschi, D. (2007). Trajectory Pattern Mining. In *ACM SIGKDD International Conference on Knowledge Discovery and Data Mining* (pp. 330-339), San Jose, CA.

Gibbs, L., & Gambrill, E. (2002). Evidence-based practice: Counter arguments and objections. *Research on Social Work Practice*, *12*, 452–476. doi:10.1177/1049731502012003007

Gibson, J. L., Ivancevich, J. M., Donnelly, J. H., & Konopaske, R. (2003). *Organizations: Behavior Structure Processes.* New York: McGraw-Hill Irwin.

Gilbert, N. (2007). Dilemmas of privacy and surveillance: Challenges of technological change. *The Royal Academy of Engineering*, March.

Giudici, P. (2003). *Applied Data Mining: Statistical Methods for Business and Industry.* New York: John Wiley &Sons Inc.

Giudici, P. (2004). *Applied data mining: statistical methods for business and industry.* Chichester, UK: John Wiley & Sons.

Gkoulalas-Divanis, A., & Verykios, V. S. (2006). An Integer Programming Approach for Frequent Itemset Hiding. In *ACM Conference on Information and Knowledge Management* (pp. 748-756), Arlington, VA.

Gkoulalas-Divanis, A., & Verykios, V. S. (2008). Exact Knowledge Hiding Through Database Extension. In IEEE Transactions on Knowledge and Data Engineering.

Gkoulalas-Divanis, A., & Verykios, V. S. (2009). Hiding Sensitive Knowledge without Side Effects. In Knowledge and Information Systems.

Goadrich, M., Oliphant, L., & Shavlik, J. (2006). Creating Ensembles of First-Order Clauses to Improve Recall-Precision Curves. *Machine Learning, 64*(1-3). doi:10.1007/s10994-006-8958-3

Goldstein, A. (2007). *"A place of my own" Homeless families in the New York City shelter system: The long-term stayers.* Doctoral dissertation, Graduate Faculty in Social Welfare, The City University of New York, New York.

Gomes, L. (2009). *The Hidden Cost of Privacy.* Available at http://www.forbes.com/forbes/2009/0608/034-privacy-research-hidden-cost-of-privacy.html, last accessed on May 26, 2009.

Gonzalez, A., Correa, A., & Acosta, M. (2002). Factores determinantes de la rentabilidad financiera de las pymes. *Revista Española de Financiación y Contabilidad, 31*(112), 395–429.

Goodman, L. A. (1979). Simple models for the analysis of association in cross-classifications having ordered categories. *Journal of the American Statistical Association, 74*, 537–552. doi:10.2307/2286971

Gramatikov, M. (2003). *Data Mining Techniques and the Decision Making Process in the Bulgarian Public Administration.* Paper presented at the NISPACee Conference, 10-12 April 2003, Bucharest, Romania.

Grant, R. M. (1996). Prospering in Dynamically-competitive Environments: Organizational Capability as Knowledge Integration. *Organization Science, 7*(4), 375–387. doi:10.1287/orsc.7.4.375

Grant, R.M. (1996). Toward a Knowledge-based Theory of the firm. *Strategic Management Journal,* (Winter Special Issue), 109– 122.

Grasso, A. J., & Epstein, I. (Eds.). (1992). *Research utilization in the social services: Innovations for practice and administration.* Binghampton, NY: Haworth Press.

Grasso, A. J., & Epstein, I. (Eds.). (1993). *Information systems in child, youth and family agencies: Planning, implementation and service enhancement.* Binghampton, NY: Haworth Press.

Gratzer, M., & Winiwarter, W. (2003). The role of the internet in the SME hotel sector in Austria. In C. Chung, C. Kim, W. Kim, T. W. Ling & K. H. Song (Eds.), *Human Society @ Internet Conference 2003,* (pp. 85-95). Seoul, South Korea: Springer-Verlag.

Greenberg, J., & Hillier, D. (1995). *Indicators of Financial Condition for Governments.* Paper presented at the 5th Conference of Comparative International Governmental Accounting Research, Paris-Amy, France.

Grobler, B. R., Bisschoff, T. C., & Moloi, K. C. (2002). The CHAID-technique and the relationship between school effectiveness and various independent variables. *International Studies in Educational Administration, 30*(3), 44–56.

Grönroos, C. (1984). A service quality model and its marketing implications. *European Journal of Marketing, 18*(4), 36–44. doi:10.1108/EUM0000000004784

Grönroos, C., & Ojasalo, K. (2004). Service productivity: towards a conceptualization of the transformation of inputs into economic results in services. *Journal of Business Research*, *57*(4), 414–423. doi:10.1016/S0148-2963(02)00275-8

Grossman, L. (2007). Tag, you are it: They are cheap, they are tiny, and they are everywhere. But are RFID chips good for humanity? *Time*, (October 29), 57.

Groves, M., Godsey, W., & Shulman, M. (2003). *Evaluating Financial Condition: A handbook of Local Government* (3rd ed.). Washington, DC: The International City/County Management Association.

Gruen, T. W., Corsten, D., & Bharadwaj, S. (2002). *Retail Out-of-Stocks: A Worldwide Examination of Causes, Rates, and Consumer Responses*. Washington, DC: Grocery Manufacturers of America.

Gulen, S. G. (1998). Efficiency in the crude oil futures markets. *Journal of Energy Finance & Development*, *3*(1), 13–21. doi:10.1016/S1085-7443(99)80065-9

Guyon, I. (2005). *Feature extraction, foundations and applications*. New York: Elsevier.

Guyon, I., Constantin Aliferis, C., & Elisseeff, A. (2007). In Liu, H., & Motoda, H. (Eds.), *Computational methods of feature selection* (pp. 63–86). Boca Raton, FL: Chapman and Hall/CRC.

Guyon, I., Saffari, A., Dror, G., & Bumann, J. (2007). Report on preliminary experiments with data grid models in the agnostic learning vs. prior knowledge challenge. In *International Joint Conference on Neural Networks (IJCNN)*.

Guzman, J., Moreno, P., & Tejada, P. (2008). The tourism SMEs in the global value chains - the case of andalusia. *Service Business*, *2*, 187–202. doi:10.1007/s11628-008-0034-6

Habermas, J. (1984). The Theory of Communicative Action: *Vol. 1. Reason and the Rationalization of Society*, *(Trans. T. McCarthy)*. Boston: Beacon Press.

Habermas, J. (1989). The Theory of Communicative Action: *Vol. 2. Lifeworld and System: A Critique of Functionalist Reason*, *(trans. T. McCarthy)*. Boston: Beacon Press.

Håkansson, H., & Johanson, J. (1992). A model of industrial networks. Indiustrial Networks. A New View of Reality, 1, (pp. 28-34).

Hakolahti, T., & Kokkonen, P. (2006). Business webs in the tourism industry. In Hitz, M., Sigala, M., & Murphy, J. (Eds.), *Information and communication technologies in tourism* (pp. 453–462). Vienna, Austria: Springer. doi:10.1007/3-211-32710-X_58

Hall, R. (1992). The strategic analysis of intangible resources. *Strategic Management Journal*, *13*(2), 135–144. doi:10.1002/smj.4250130205

Hamblen, M. (2007). Privacy concerns dog information technology (IT) efforts to implement RFID: Employees often rebel against plans to include chips in corporate identification (ID) badges. *Computerworld*, October 15, 26.

Hampel, R., Wagenknecht, M., & Chaker, N. (Eds.). (2000). *Fuzzy Control: Theory and Practice*. Heidelberg, Germany: Physica-Verlag.

Han, J., & Kamber, M. (2006). *Data mining: concepts and techniques*. San Francisco: Morgan Kaufmann.

Hand, D., & Yu, K. (2001). Idiot's Bayes - not so stupid after all? *International Statistical Review*, *69*(3), 385–399.

Hand, D., Mannila, P., & Smyth, P. (2001). *Principles of Data Mining*. Cambridge, MA: MIT Press.

Hanssen, D. (2003). *Looking inside the black box of intensive family preservation services*. Doctoral dissertation, Graduate faculty in Social Welfare, The City University of New York, New York.

Hanssen, D., & Epstein, I. (2006). A "black box" study of intensive family preservation services: Utilization of clinical data-mining. *Family Preservation*, *9*, 7–22.

Hanssen, D., & Epstein, I. (2007). Learning what works: Demonstrating practice effectiveness with children and families through retrospective investigation. *Family Preservation, 10*, 24–41.

HarrisInteractive. (2008). *Majority Uncomfortable with Websites Customizing Content Based Visitors Personal Profiles*. Available at http://www.harrisinteractive.com/harris_poll/index.asp?PID=894, last accessed on May 26, 2009.

Hart, S., & Banbury, C. (1994). How Strategy-making Processes can make a Difference. *Strategic Management Journal, 15*(3), 251–269. doi:10.1002/smj.4250150402

Hatch, M. J., & Cunliffe, A. L. (2006). *Organization Theory modern, Symbolic and Postmodern Perspectives*. Oxford, UK: University Press.

Hatry, H., Gerhart, C., & Marshall, M. (1994). Eleven Ways to Make Performance Management More Useful to Public Managers. International City/County Management Association [Washington, DC]. Public Management, (September): 15–18.

Hayes, M., & Pidd, M. (2005). *Public Announcement of Performance Ratings: implications for Trust Relationships*. Retrieved August, 15, 2008, from http://www.lancs.ac.uk/staff/smamp/working%20paper%20on%20trust.pdf

He, Y.-Q., Chan, L.-K., & Wu, M.-L. (2007). Balancing productivity and consumer satisfaction for profitability: statistical and fuzzy regression analysis. *European Journal of Operational Research, 176*(1), 252–263. doi:10.1016/j.ejor.2005.06.050

Hensher, D. A., & Jones, S. (2007). Forecasting Corporate Bankruptcy: Optimizing the Performance of the Mixed Logit Model. *Abacus, 43*(3), 241–264. doi:10.1111/j.1467-6281.2007.00228.x

Herbrich, R., Graepel, T., & Obermayer, K. (1999). *Regression models for ordinal data: A machine learning approach. Technical Report*. Germany: TU Berlin.

Herrera, F., Herrera-Viedma, E., & Martinez, L. (2000). A fusion approach for managing multi-granularity linguistic term sets in decision making. *Fuzzy Sets and Systems, 114*(1), 43–58. doi:10.1016/S0165-0114(98)00093-1

Hewlett-Packard. (2007). *Dragon, data retention and guardian online*. Retrieved May, 2009, from http://h20247.www2.hp.com/enterprise/cache/490843-0-0-82-150.html

Hicks, R. C., Dattero, R., & Galup, S. D. (2006). The five-tier knowledge management hierarchy. *Journal of Knowledge Management, 10*(1), 19–31. doi:10.1108/13673270610650076

Hicks, R. C., Galup, S. D., & Dattero, R. (2007). The Transformations In The Five Tier Knowledge Management Transformation Matrix. *Journal of Knowledge Management, 8*, 1.

Hinds, P. J., & Pfeffer, J. (2003). Why Organizations Don't "Know What They Know": Cognitive and Motivational Factors Affecting the Transfer of Expertise. In Ackerman, M., Pipek, V., & Wulf, V. (Eds.), *Sharing Expertise Beyond Knowledge Management* (pp. 3–26). Cambridge, MA: The MIT Press.

Hines, M. (2007). Black hat exposes RFID security risk. *InfoWorld*, (March): 5, 9–10.

Hiraki, T. (2007). *Factors affecting the "performance" of performance measurement systems: an analysis of the Japanese Practice*. Paper presented at the EGPA conference, EGPA Study Group on productivity and quality in the public sector, Madrid, Spain.

Hodgkinson, A. (1999). Productivity measurement and enterprise bargaining – the local government perspective. *International Journal of Public Sector Management, 12*(6), 470–481. doi:10.1108/09513559910301342

Hofstede, G. (1984). *Culture's Consequences: International Differences in Work-Related Values*. Beverly Hills, CA: Sage Publications.

Hoh, B., & Gruteser, M. (2005). Protecting Location Privacy through Path Confusion. In *International Conference on Security and Privacy for Emerging Areas in Communications Networks* (pp. 194-205), Athens, Greece.

Hoh, B., Gruteser, M., Xiong, H., & Alrabady, A. (2007). Preserving Privacy in GPS Traces via Uncertainty-Aware Path Cloaking. In *ACM Conference on Computer and Communications Security* (pp. 161-171), Alexandria, VA.

Holland, J. H. (1996). *Hidden Order: How Adaptation Builds Complexity*. Cambridge, MA: Perseus Books.

Holmstrom, B., & Tirole, J. (1989). The Theory of the Firm. In R. Schmalensee & R. Willig (Eds.), Handbook of Industrial Organization, (pp. 63–131). North-Holland: Elsevier Science Pub Co.

Hom, P. W., & Kinicki, A. J. (2001). Toward a greater understanding of how dissatisfaction drives employee turnover. *Academy of Management Journal*, *44*(5), 975–987. doi:10.2307/3069441

Homburg, C., Krohmer, H., & Workman, J. P. Jr. (1999). Strategic consensus and performance: the role of strategy type and market-related dynamism. *Strategic Management Journal*, *20*(4), 339–357. doi:10.1002/(SICI)1097-0266(199904)20:4<339::AID-SMJ29>3.0.CO;2-T

Hood, C. (1996). Exploring variations in public management reform of the 1980's. In H. Bekke, J. Perry, & T. Toonen (Eds.), Civil service systems in comparative perspective (pp. 268–287). Bloomington, IN: Indiana University Press.

Hood, C. (1998). *The Art of State*. Oxford, UK: Oxford University Press.

Hood, C., & Peters, G. (2004). The Middle Aging of New Public Management: Into the Age of Paradox? *Journal of Public Administration: Research and Theory*, *14*(3), 267–282. doi:10.1093/jopart/muh019

Hoopes, D. G., & Postrel, S. (1999). Shared Knowledge, "Glitches" and Product Development Performance. *Strategic Management Journal*, *20*(9), 837–865. doi:10.1002/(SICI)1097-0266(199909)20:9<837::AID-SMJ54>3.0.CO;2-I

Hopp, W., & Spearman, M. (2000). *Factory Physics* (International edition). New York: McGraw Hill.

Hubbard, D. (2009). *The Failure of Risk Management: Why It's Broken and How to Fix It*. Hoboken, New Jersey: John Wiley & Sons.

Huff, L., Fornell, C., & Anderson, E. W. (1996). Quality and productivity: contradictory and complementary. *Quality Management Journal*, *4*(1), 22–39.

Hughes, D. C., Leung, P., & Naus, M. J. (2008). Using a single-system analysis to assess the effectiveness of an exercise intervention on quality of life for Hispanic breast cancer survivors: A pilot study. *Social Work in Health Care*, *47*(1), 73–91. doi:10.1080/00981380801970871

Hughes, D., Elkin, C., & Epstein, I. (2004). Long-term Counseling: A feasibility study. of extended follow-up services with high-risk EAP clients. *Journal of Workplace Behavioral Health*, *22*(2/3), 27–41.

Hunt, E. B., Marin, J., & Stone, P. J. (1966). *Experiments in Induction*. New York: Academic Press.

Huntington, H. G. (1994). Oil price forecasting in the 1980s: what went wrong? *The Energy Journal (Cambridge, Mass.)*, *15*(2), 1–22.

Hurley, R. F., & Estelami, H. (2007). An exploratory study of employee turnover indicators as predictors of customer satisfaction. *Journal of Services Marketing*, *21*(3), 186–199. doi:10.1108/08876040710746543

Hutson, C., & Lichtiger, E. (2001). Mining clinical information in the utilization of social services: Practitioners inform themselves. *Social Work in Health Care*, *33*(3/4), 153–162.

Huysman, M., & de Wit, D. (2003). A Critical Evaluation of Knowledge Management Practices. In Ackerman, M., Pipek, V., & Wulf, V. (Eds.), *Sharing Expertise Beyond Knowledge Management* (pp. 27–55). Cambridge, MA: The MIT Press.

Ichihashi, H., Shirai, T., Nagasaka, K., & Miyoshi, T. (1996). Neuro-fuzzy ID3: a method of inducing fuzzy decision trees with linear programming for maximising entropy and an algebraic method for incremental learning. *Fuzzy Sets and Systems, 81*, 157–167. doi:10.1016/0165-0114(95)00247-2

Immon, W. H. (2002). *Building the data warehouse*. New York: John Wiley & Sons, Inc.

Inan, A., & Saygin, Y. (2006). Privacy-Preserving Spatiotemporal Clustering on Horizontally Partitioned Data. In *International Conference on Data Warehousing and Knowledge Discovery* (pp. 459-468), Krakow, Poland.

Inan, A., Kaya, S. V., Saygin, Y., Savas, E., Hintoglu, A., & Levi, A. (2006). Privacy Preserving Clustering on Horizontally Partitioned Data. *Data & Knowledge Engineering, 63*(3), 646–666. doi:10.1016/j.datak.2007.03.015

Iranmanesh, S. H., & Mokhtari, Z. (2008, August). Application of Data Mining Tools to Predicate Completion Time of a Project. In Proceedings of World Academy of Science (Vol. 32, pp. 234–239). Engineering and Technology.

Isomäki, H. (2002). *The Prevailing Conceptions of the Human Being in Information Systems Development: Systems Designer's Reflections*. Tampere, Finland: Tampere University Press.

ITRC. (2009). *Data Breach Total Soars*. Available at http://www.idtheftcenter.org/artman2/publish/m_press/2008_Data_Breach_Totals_Soar.shtml, last accessed May 26, 2009.

Jagannathan, G., & Wright, R. (2005). Privacy Preserving Distributed K-Means Clustering over Arbitrarily Partitioned Data. In *ACM SIGKDD Conference on Knowledge Discovery in Data Mining* (pp. 593-599), Chicago, IL.

Jagannathan, G., Pillaipakkamnatt, K., & Wright, R. (2006). A New Privacy Preserving Distributed K-Clustering Algorithm. In *SIAM International Conference on Data Mining*, Bethesda, MD.

Järvensivu, T., & Möller, K. (2008). *Metatheory of network management - a contingency perspective*. Upsala, Sweden: Helsinki Scool of Economics, Working papers.

Jensen, J., Rattingan, M., & Blau, H. (2003). Information Awareness: a prospective technical assessment. In *Proceedings of the ninth ACM SIGKDD international conference on Knowledge discovery and data mining*.

Jiang, W., & Clifton, C. (2005). Privacy Preserving Distributed K-anonymity. In *IFIP 11.3 Working Conference on Data and Applications Security,* (pp. 166-177), Storrs, CT.

Johnsten, T., & Raghavan, V. V. (2000). Impact of Decision-Region Based Classification Mining Algorithms on Database Security. In *IFIP TC13 WG11.3 International Conference on Database Security* (pp. 177-191), Deventer, Netherlands.

Johnston, R., & Jones, P. (2004). Service productivity. towards understanding the relationship between operational and customer productivity. *International Journal of Productivity and Performance Management, 53*(3), 201–213. doi:10.1108/17410400410523756

Jonas, J., & Harper, J. (2006). *Effective Counterterrorism and the limited role of predictive data mining*. Washington, DC: Cato Institute. Retrieved January 2009, from http://www.cato.org/ pub_display.php?pub_id=6784

Jones, M. (1995). Organisational Learning: Collective Mind or Cognitive Metaphor? *Accounting. Management and Information Technology, 5*(1), 61–77. doi:10.1016/0959-8022(95)90014-4

Jones, S., Statham, H., & Solomou, W. (2006). When expectant mothers know their baby has a fetal abnormality: Exploring a crisis of motherhood through qualitative data-mining. *Journal of Social Work Research and Evaluation, 6*(2), 195–206.

Jorgenson, T. (2006). Value consciousness and public management. *International journal of organiszation theory and behavior, 9*(4), 510-536.

Joubert, L. (2006). Academic-practice partnerships in practice research: A cultural shift for health social workers. *Social Work in Health Care, 43*(2/3), 151–161. doi:10.1300/J010v43n02_10

Joubert, L., & Epstein, I. (Eds.). (2005). Special Issue. Multi-disciplinary data-mining in allied health practice: Another perspective on Australian research and evaluation [Special Issue]. *Journal of Social Work Research and Evaluation, 6*(2).

Joubert, L., & Power, R. (2006). Using data-mining to explore the outcomes of an integrated care program: Looking for meaning behing key outcome indicators. *Social Work Research and Evaluation, 6*(2), 185–194.

Kabillo, R. (2005). *Family functioning and adolescent psychopathology: A comparison of content and process scoring indices on the McMaster Family Assessment Device in terms of association with adolescent clinical indicators of depression, self-esteem and behavior.* Doctoral dissertation, School of Psychological Science, Faculty of Science, Technology and Engineering, La Trobe University, Bundoora, Victoria, Australia.

Kaboudan, M. A. (2001). Compumetric forecasting of crude oil prices. In *The Proceedings of IEEE Congress on Evolutionary Computation*, (pp. 283–287).

Kafner, K. (2009). *Texting May Be Taking a Toll*. Available at http://www.nytimes.com/2009/05/26/health/26teen.html?scp=1&sq=texting&st=cse, last accessed on May 26, 2009.

Kallinikos, J. (2004). Deconstructing information packages: Organizational and behavioural implications of ERP systems. *Information Technology & People, 17*(1), 8–30. doi:10.1108/09593840410522152

Kamaja, I. (2009). DIT – IT:n uusi tiedekäsitys. DIT:n peruspiirteet ja ominaisuudet. Rovaniemi, Finland: Lapin yliopisto, Menetelmätieteiden laitos.

Kantarcioglu, M., & Clifton, C. (2004). Privacy Preserving Distributed Mining of Association Rules on Horizontally Partitioned Data. *IEEE Transactions on Knowledge and Data Engineering, 16*(9), 1026–1037. doi:10.1109/TKDE.2004.45

Kantarcioglu, M., & Vaidya, J. (2003). Privacy Preserving Naïve Bayes Classification for Horizontally Partitioned Data. In *IEEE International Conference on Data Mining Workshop on Privacy Preserving Data Mining* (pp. 3-9), Melbourne, FL.

Kapp, S., Schwartz, I., & Epstein, I. (1994). Adult imprisonment of males released from residential childcare: A longitudinal study. *Residential Treatment for Children & Youth, 12*, 19–36. doi:10.1300/J007v12n02_03

Käpylä, J., Jääskeläinen, A., Seppänen, S., Vuolle, M., & Lönnqvist, A. (2008). *Tuottavuuden kehittäminen Suomessa: haasteet ja tutkimustarpeet.* Helsinki, Finland: Finnish Work Environment Fund. (In Finnish)

Karalić, A. (1991). *Regression tree inductive system – Retis.* Ljubljana, Slovenia: Faculty of Computer and Information Science.

Kasanen, E., Lukka, K., & Siitonen, A. (1993). Constructive approach in management accounting. *Journal of Management Accounting Research, 5*, 243–264.

Kass, G. V. (1980). An exploratory technique for investigating large quantities of categorical data. *Applied Statistics, 29*, 119–127. doi:10.2307/2986296

Katsarou, A., Gkoulalas-Divanis, A., & Verykios, V. S. (2009). Reconstruction-Based Classification Rule Hiding through Controlled Data Modification. In *IFIP Conference on Artificial Intelligence Applications & Innovations*, Thessaloniki, Greece.

Kauffman, S. (1995). *At Home in the Universe: The Search for the Laws of Self-Organization and Complexity.* New York: Oxford University Press.

Kaydos, W. (1999). *Operational performance measurement: increasing total productivity.* Delray Beach, FL: St. Lucie Press.

Keating, B. (2008). Data Mining: What is it and how is it used? *The Journal of Business Forecasting, Fall*, 33-35.

Kecman, V. (2001). *Learning and Soft Computing: Support Vector Machines, Neural Networks, and Fuzzy Logic*. London: MIT Press.

Kellermanns, F. W., Walter, J., Lechner, C., & Floyd, S. W. (2005). The Lack of Consensus about Strategic Consensus: Advancing Theory and Research. *Journal of Management, 31*, 719–737. doi:10.1177/0149206305279114

Kim, D. (1999). Normalization methods for input and output vectors in backpropogation neural networks. *International Journal of Computer Mathematics, 71*(2), 161–171. doi:10.1080/00207169908804800

Kimball, R. (1996). *The data warehouse toolkit: practical techniques for building dimensional data warehouses*. New York: John Wiley & Sons Inc.

Kitchener, M., Beynon, M., & Harrington, C. (2004). Explaining the Diffusion of Medicaid Home Care Waiver Programs Using VPRS Decision Rules. *Health Care Management Science, 7*(3), 237–244. doi:10.1023/B:HCMS.0000039386.59886.dd

Klepac, G., & Mršić, L. (2006). *Poslovna inteligencija kroz poslovne slučajeve*. Zagreb, Croatia: Liderpress.

Klepac, G., & Panian, Ž. (2003). *Poslovna inteligencija*. Zagreb, Croatia: Masmedia.

Kloha, P., Weissert, C. S., & Kleine, R. (2005). Developing and testing a composite model to predict local fiscal distress. *Public Administration Review, 65*(3), 313–323. doi:10.1111/j.1540-6210.2005.00456.x

Kochkine, V. (2006). *Depressive symptoms and academic achievement in immigrant and American-born adolescents of diverse ethno-cultural backgrounds: A cultural data-mining exploration*. Doctoral dissertation, Graduate faculty in Social Welfare, The City University of New York, New York.

Kogan, G. (in progress). *A conceptual and empirical data-mining study of bullying and social power*. Doctoral dissertation, Graduate faculty in Social Welfare, The City University of New York, New York.

Kohonen, T. (2001). *Self-organizing maps*. Berlin: Springer.

Kohtamäki, M. (2005). *Strategisen verkoston ohjaus* [Governance of Strategic Network]. Vaasa, Finland: University of Vaasa.

Konsynski, B., & Tiwana, A. (2004). The improvisation-efficiency paradox in inter-firm electronic networks. *Journal of Information Technology, 19*, 234–243. doi:10.1057/palgrave.jit.2000029

Kostoff, R., & Geisler, E. (1999). Strategic Management and Implementation of Textueal Data Mining in Government Organizations. Technology Analysis and Strategic Management, 11(4), 493–525. doi:10.1080/095373299107302doi:10.1080/095373299107302

Kotler, P., Haider, D., & Rein, I. (1993). *Marketing places*. New York: The Free Press.

Kotzanikolaou, P. (2008). *Data Retention and Privacy in Electronic Communications*. IEEE Security and Privacy.

Kovalerchuk, B., & Vityaev, E. (2000). *Data Mining in Finance: Advances in Relational and Hybrid Methods*. Amsterdam: Kluwer Academic Publishers.

Kramer, M. S., Leventhal, J. M., Hutchinson, T. A., & Feinstein, A. R. (1979). An algorithm for the operational assessment of adverse drug reactions. i. background, description, and instructions for use. *Journal of the American Medical Association, 242*(7), 623–632. doi:10.1001/jama.242.7.623

Kramer, S., Widmer, G., Pfahringer, B., & DeGroeve, M. (2001). *Prediction of ordinal classes using regression trees*. Fundamenta Informaticae.

Kransdorff, A. (1995). Exit interviews as an induction tool. *Management Development Review, 8*(2), 37–40. doi:10.1108/09622519510084260

Krebs, B. (2008). *Spear Phishing Scam Targets LinkedIn Users*. Available at http://voices.washingtonpost.com/securityfix/2008/10/spear_phishing_attacks_against.html?nav=rss_blog, last accessed on May 26, 2009

Krippendorff, K. (1980). *Content Analysis: An Introduction to Its Methodology.* Newbury Park, CA: Sage.

Krone, O. (2007). *The Interaction of Organisational Structure and Humans in Knowledge Integration.* Rovaniemi, Finland: University of Lapland, Lapland University Press.

Kudyba, S., & Hoptroff, R. (2001). *Data mining and business intelligence: a guide to productivity.* Hershey, PA: Idea Group Publishing.

Kuhn, T. S. (1996). *The Structure of Scientific Revolutions.* Chicago: Chicago University Press.

Kuhry, B. (Ed.). (2004). Prestaties van de publieke sector. Den Haag, The Netherlands: SCP Nederland.

Kuusisto, R. (2006). Flowing of Information in Decision Systems, *Proceedings of the Thirty-Ninth Annual Hawaii International Conference on System Sciences, (HICSS-39),* Hawaii, USA. Retrieved from http://csdl2.computer.org/comp/proceedings/hicss/2006/2507/07/250770148b.pdf

Kuusisto, R. (2008). Analyzing the Command and Control Maturity levels of Collaborating Organizations. In *proc of 13th International Command and Control Research and Technology Symposium (13th ICCRTS),* June 2008.

Kuusisto, R., & Kuusisto, T. (2008). Information Security Culture as a Social System: Some Notes of Information Availability and Sharing. In Gupta, M., & Sharman, R. (Eds.), *Social and Human Elements of Information Security: Emerging Trends and Countermeasures* (pp. 77–97). Hershey, PA: Information Science Reference.

Kuusisto, T., Kuusisto, R., & Nissen, M. (2008). Information Flow Aspects of Inter-organizational Crisis Management. *Journal of Information Warfare, 6*(2), 39–51.

Kvale, S. (1995). The Social Construction of Validity. *Qualitative Inquiry, 1*(1), 19–40. doi:10.1177/107780049500100103

Lamberton, D. M. (1998). Information Economics Research: Points of Departure. *Information Economics and Policy, 10,* 325–330. doi:10.1016/S0167-6245(98)00002-X

Lambsdorff, J. G. (2003). How corruption affects productivity. *Kyklos, 56*(4), 457–474. doi:10.1046/j.0023-5962.2003.00233.x

Lanza, A., Manera, M., & Giovannini, M. (2005). Modeling and forecasting cointegrated relationships among heavy oil and product prices. *Energy Economics, 27,* 831–848. doi:10.1016/j.eneco.2005.07.001

Larose, D. T. (2005). *Discovering Knowledge in Data: An Introduction to Data Mining.* New York: John Wiley &Sons Inc.

Larose, D. T. (2006). *Data mining methods and models.* New York: John Wiley &Sons Inc.

Laszlo, M., & Mukherjee, S. (2005). Minimum Spanning Tree Partitioning Algorithm for Microaggregation. *IEEE Transactions on Knowledge and Data Engineering, 17*(7), 902–911. doi:10.1109/TKDE.2005.112

Lauriala, J. (2001). *Kontrolli, riski ja informaatio: tutkimus kasvuyrityksen rahoittamiseen ja transaktioihin liittyvistä juridisista ja liiketoimintariskeistä sekä niiden hallitsemisesta velvoite- ja yhtiöoikeudellisin keinoin modernin varallisuusoikeuden ympäristössä.* Saarijärvi, Finland: Kauppakaari.

Lawler, J., & Molluzzo, J. C. (2006). A study of data mining and information ethics in information systems curricula. *Information Systems Journal, 4*(34).

Leban, G., Zupan, B., Vidmar, G., & Bratko, I. (2006). VizRank: data visualization guided by machine learning. *Data Mining and Knowledge Discovery, 13*(2), 119–136. doi:10.1007/s10618-005-0031-5

Lee, C. C., & Yang, J. (2000). Knowledge value chain. *Journal of Management Development, 19*(9), 783–793. doi:10.1108/02621710010378228

Lehesvirta, T. (2004). Learning processes in a work organization: From individual to collective and/or vice versa? *Journal of Workplace Learning, 16*(1, 2), 92–100.

Lehtonen, V.-M. (2007). Henkilöstöjohtamisen tehosta-minen valtionhallinnossa henkilöstötilinpäätösinformaa-tion avulla – empiirinen tutkimus Suomen valtionhal-linnossa tuotettavan henkilöstötilinpäätösinformaation arvosta johtamisessa. Helsinki, Finland: Svenska handelshögskolan. (In Finnish)

Lemaire, V. Féraud, R., & Voisine, N. (2006, October). Contact personalization using a score understanding method. In *International Joint Conference on Neural Networks (IJCNN),* Hong-Kong.

Lemaire, V., & Féraud, R. (2008). Driven forward fea-tures selection: a comparative study on neural networks. In *International Joint Conference on Neural Network (IJCNN).*

Leonard-Barton, D. (1995). *Wellsprings of Knowledge Building and Sustaining the sources of Innovation.* Boston: Harvard Business School Press.

Leray, P., & Gallinari, P. (1998). *Variable selection.* Tech. Rep. No. ENV4-CT96-0314, University Paris 6, France.

Li, M.-T., Zhao, F., & Chow, L.-F. (2006). Assignment of Seasonal Factor Categories to Urban Coverage Count Stations Using a Fuzzy Decision Tree. *Journal of Trans-portation Engineering, 132*(8), 654–662. doi:10.1061/(ASCE)0733-947X(2006)132:8(654)

Lichtenstein, S., & Hunter, A. (2005). *Receiver Influences on Knowledge Sharing.* Retrieved 09.07.2009 from http://is.lse.ac.uk/asp/aspecis/20050103.pdf

Lichtsteiner, S., & Schibler, U. (1989). *A glycosylated liver-specific transcription factor stimulates transcrip-tion of the albumin gene.* CELL.

Lin, H. T., & Li, L. (2007). Ordinal regression by extended binary classifications. *Advances in Neural Information Processing Systems, 19,* 865–872.

Lindell, Y., & Pinkas, B. (2000). Privacy Preserving Data Mining. *Journal of Cryptology, 15*(3), 36–54.

Linder, R. (2006). *Wikis, Webs, and Networks: Creat-ing Connections for Conflict-prone Settings,* CSIS (The Center of Strategic and International Studies) Report. Retrieved February 15, 2006, from http://www.csis.org/media/csis/pubs/061018_pcr_creatingconnections.pdf

Lo, H. (in process). *A clinical data-mining study of symp-tom presentation of depression, anxiety and Cognitive Behavioral Therapy outcomes in a community–based mental health program.* Doctoral dissertation, University of Hong Kong.

Lönnqvist, A. (2004). *Measurement of intangible success factors: case studies on the design, implementation and use of measures.* Tampere, Finland: Tampere University of Technology.

Løwendahl, B. (1997). Strategic Management of Profes-sional Service Firms. Copenhagen: Handelshøjskolens forlag.

Luan, J. (2002). *Data Mining and Knowledge Manage-ment in Higher Education – Potential Applications; Presentation at AIR Forum, Toronto Canada.* Retrieved 09.05.2009 from www.cabrillo.edu/services/pro/oir_re-ports/DM_KM2002AIR.pdf

Luft, A. L. (1994). Zur begrifflichen Unterscheidung von 'Wissen', 'Information' und 'Daten'. R. Wille & M. Zickwolff (eds.), Begriffliche Wissensverarbeitung / Grundfragen und Aufgaben, (pp. 61–79). Mannheim, Germany: BI Wissenschaftsverlag.

Luhmann, N. (1999). *Ökologishe Kommunikation, 3. Auflage. Opladen.* Wiesbaden, Germany: Westdeutcher Verlag.

Lum, L., Kervin, J., Clark, K., Reid, F., & Sirola, W. (1998). Explaining nurse turnover intent: job satisfac-tion, pay satisfaction or organizational commitment? *Journal of Organizational Behavior, 19*(3), 305–320. doi:10.1002/(SICI)1099-1379(199805)19:3<305::AID-JOB843>3.0.CO;2-N

Lundquist, E. (2007). The next killer application?: It will be in the mobile segment, if CTIA Is Any Indication. *eWeek,* April 2/9, 6.

Lundquist, E. (2007). The view from Europe: United States lags in some areas, but hiring woes are similar. *eWeek*, (March 19), 9.

Luts, M., Van Dooren, W., & Bouckaert, G. (2008). Internationale rangschikkingen gerangschikt. Een meta-analyse van rangschikkingen van publieke sectoren. Leuven, Belgium: Steunpunt beleidrelevant onderzoek-bestuurlijke organisatie Vlaanderen.

M: Metrics Inc. (2006). *United States Mobile Subscriber: Monthly Consumption of Content and Applications. M:Metrics Inc., Benchmark Survey*, April, 16.

Macdonald, E. M., Carroll, A., Albiston, D., & Epstein, I. (2006). Social relationships in early psychosis: Clinical data-mining for practice-based evidence. *Journal of Social Work Research and Evaluation, 6*(2), 155–166.

Magidson, J. (1993). The use of the new ordinal algorithm in CHAID to target profitable segments. *The Journal of Database Marketing, 1*, 29–48.

Maier, R. (2002). *Knowledge Management Systems. Information and Communication Technologies for Knowledge Management*. Berlin: Springler-Verlag.

Mannila, H., & Hand, D. (2001). *Principles of Data Mining*. Cambridge, MA: The MIT press.

Mannila, H., & Toivonen, H. (1997). Levelwise Search and Borders of Theories in Knowledge Discovery. *Data Mining and Knowledge Discovery, 1*(3), 241–258. doi:10.1023/A:1009796218281

Marakas, G. M. (2003). *Decision Support Systems In the 21st Century*. Upper Saddle River, NJ: Prentice Hall.

March, J. G., & Simon, H. A. (1958). *Organizations*. New York: Wiley & Sons.

Margineantu, D., & Dietterich, T. (2001). Improved class probability estimates from decision tree models. In Nonlinear Estimation and Classification, (pp. 169–184).

Markoff, J. (2006). Taking spying to higher level, Agencies look for more ways to mine data. *New York Times,* February 25th. Technology, 1-4.

Markus, M. L. (1983). Power, Politics, and MIS Implementation. Association for Computing Machinery. *Communications of the ACM, 26*(6), 430–445. doi:10.1145/358141.358148

Markus, M. L. (2001). Toward a Theory of Knowledge Reuse: Types of Knowledge Reuse Situations and Factors in Reuse Success. *Journal of Management Information Systems, 18*(1), 57–93.

Martin, C. R., Horne, D. A., & Chan, W. S. (2001). A perspective on client productivity in business-to-business consulting services. *International Journal of Service Industry Management, 12*(2), 137–157.

Mason, J., Edlow, M., Lear, M., Scopetta, S., Walther, V., Epstein, I., & Guaccero, S. (2001). Screening for psycho-social risk in an urban prenatal clinic population: A retrospective, practice-based research study. *Social Work in Health Care, 33*(3/4), 33–52.

Matignon, R. (2005). *Neural Network Modeling Using SAS Enterprise Miner*. Bloomington, IN: AuthorHouse.

McCracken, S., & Marsh, J. C. (2008). Practitioner expertise in evidence- based practice decision-making. *Research on Social Work Practice, 18*(4), 301–310. doi:10.1177/1049731507308143

McLaughlin, C. P., & Coffey, S. (1990). Measuring productivity in services. *International Journal of Service Industry Management, 1*(1), 46–64. doi:10.1108/09564239010002847

Meier, K. J., O'Toole, L. J. Jr, Boyne, G. A., & Walker, R. M. (2007). Strategic management and the performance of public organizations: testing venerable ideas against recent theories. *Journal of Public Administration: Research and Theory, 17*(3), 357–377. doi:10.1093/jopart/mul017

Meilich, O. (2006). Bivariate models of fit in contingency theory: Critique and a polynomial regression alternative. *Organizational Research Methods, 9*, 161–193. doi:10.1177/1094428105284915

Memon, N., Hicks, D. L., & Larson, H. L. (2007). *How Investigative Data Mining Can Help Intelligence Agencies to Discover Dependence of Nodes in Terrorist Networks* (*Vol. 4632*). LNCS.

Menon, S., Sarkar, S., & Mukherjee, S. (2005). Maximizing Accuracy of Shared Databases when Concealing Sensitive Patterns. *Information Systems Research, 16*(3), 256–270. doi:10.1287/isre.1050.0056

Merleau-Ponty, M. (1968). *The Visible and Invisible.* Evanston, IL: Northwest University Press.

Meyer, A. D., Tsui, A. S., & Hinings, C. R. (1993). Configurational approaches to organizational analysis. *Academy of Management Journal, 36*(6), 1175–1195. doi:10.2307/256809

Michaelides, A., & Ng, S. (2000). Estimating the rational expectations model of speculative storage: a Monte Carlo comparison of three simulation estimators. *Journal of Econometrics, 96*(2), 231–266. doi:10.1016/S0304-4076(99)00058-5

Miles, R. E., & Snow, C. (1978). *Organizational strategy, structure and process.* New York: McGraw-Hill.

Miles, R., & Snow, C. (1978). *Organizational Strategy, Structure and Process.* London: McGraw Hill.

Miller, D. (1986). Configurations of Strategy and Structure: Towards a Synthesis. *Strategic Management Journal, 7*(3), 233–249. doi:10.1002/smj.4250070305

Miller, D. M. (1984). Profitability = productivity + price recovery. *Harvard Business Review, 62*(3), 145–153.

Miller, R. T., Murnane, R. J., & Willett, J. B. (2008). Do worker absences affect productivity? The case of teachers. *International Labour Review, 147*(1), 71–89. doi:10.1111/j.1564-913X.2008.00024.x

Ministry of International affairs of the Republic of Slovenia (1996-1999). *Annual reports of Administrative statistics*, Slovenia.

Mintzberg, H. (1978). *The structuring of Organizations.* Englewood Cliffs, NJ: Prentice Hall.

Mirabito, D. (2000). *Keeping the door open or keeping the door shut: How and why adolescents terminate from mental health treatment?* Doctoral dissertation, Graduate faculty in Social Welfare, The City University of New York, New York.

Mirabito, D. (2001). Mining treatment termination data in an adolescent mental health service: A quantitative study. *Social Work in Health Care, 33*(3/4), 71–90.

Miranda, M. J., & Glauber, J. W. (1993). Estimation of dynamic nonlinear rational expectations models of primary commodity markets with private and government stockholding. *The Review of Economics and Statistics, 75*(3), 463–470. doi:10.2307/2109460

Mirmirani, S., & Li, H. C. (2004). A comparison of VAR and neural networks with genetic algorithm in forecasting price of oil. *Advances in Econometrics, 19*, 203–223. doi:10.1016/S0731-9053(04)19008-7

Mitchell, T. M. (1997). *Machine Learning.* Boston: McGraw-Hill.

Mitra, S., Konwar, K. M., & Pal, S. K. (2002). Fuzzy Decision Tree, Linguistic Rules and Fuzzy Knowledge-Based Network: Generation and Evaluation. *IEEE Transactions on Systems, Man and Cybernetics. Part C, Applications and Reviews, 32*(4), 328–339. doi:10.1109/TSMCC.2002.806060

Modell, S. (2004). Performance measurement myths in the public sector: a research note. *Financial Accountability & Management, 20*(1), 39–55. doi:10.1111/j.1468-0408.2004.00185.xdoi:10.1111/j.1468-0408.2004.00185.x

Molluzzo, J., & Lawler, J. (2007). Integrating issues of location-based privacy with mobile Computing into international information systems curricula. *Information Systems Education Journal, 6*(32).

Monk, E., & Wagner, B. (2005). *Concepts in Enterprise Resource Planning* (2nd ed.). Boston: Thomson Course Technology.

Mooney, R. J., Melville, P., Shavlik, J., De Castro Dutra, I., & Santos Costa, V. (2002). Relational data mining with inductive logic programming for link discovery. In *Proceedings of the National Science Foundation Workshop on Next Generation Data Mining*.

Moore, M. H. (1995). *Creating public value: strategic management in government*. Cambridge, MA: Harvard University Press.

Morana, C. (2001). A semiparametric approach to short-term oil price forecasting. *Energy Economics, 23*(3), 325–338. doi:10.1016/S0140-9883(00)00075-X

Moskowitz, I., & Chang, L. (2000). A Decision Theoretic System for Information Downgrading. In *Joint Conference on Information Sciences*.

Motorola. (2007). *Mobile Device Security: Securing the Handheld, Securing the Enterprise*, Motorola Technology Group.

Mouritzen, P. (1992). *Managing cities in austerity*. London: Sage.

Moustakides, G. V., & Verykios, V. S. (2006). A Max-Min Approach for Hiding Frequent Itemsets. In *IEEE International Conference on Data Mining Workshops* (pp. 502-506), Hong Kong.

Možina, M., Demšar, J., Kattan, M., & Zupan, B. (2004). Nomograms for visualization of naive Bayesian classifier. In *Proceedings of the 8th european conference on principles and practice of knowledge discovery in databases (PAKDD)*, (pp. 337–348). New York: Springer-Verlag, Inc.

Mozina, M., Demsar, J., Zabkar, J., & Bratko, I. (2006). Why is rule learning optimistic and how to correct it. *Lecture Notes in Compututer Sc. (ECML'06)*, pp. 330-340. Berlin: Springer.

Muggleton, S. (1995). Inverse Entailment and {P}rogol. *New Generation Computing, 13*.

Mulder, I. (2004). *Understanding Designers Designing for Understanding*, (Telematica Instituut Fundamental Research Series, vol. 010). Enschede, the Netherlands. Retrieved 30/12/2008 from https://doc.telin.nl/dsweb/Get/File-41827/mulder4.0.pdf

Mullen, E. J., & Bacon, W. (2004). A survey of practitioner adoption and implementation of practice guidelines and evidenced-based treatments. In Roberts, A. R., & Yeager, K. (Eds.), *Evidence-based practice manual: Research and outcome measures in health and human services* (pp. 193–199). New York: Oxford University Press.

Murphy, C. K. (2000). Combining belief functions when evidence conflicts. *Decision Support Systems, 29*, 1–9. doi:10.1016/S0167-9236(99)00084-6

Nagadevara, V., Srinivasan, V., & Valk, R. (2008). Establishing a link between employee turnover and withdrawal behaviours: Application of data mining techniques. *Research and Practice in Human Resource Management, 16*(2), 81–99.

Nakache, J., & Confais, J. (2003). *Statistique explicative appliquée*. TECHNIP.

Namid, R. N., & Christopher, D. B. (Eds.). (2004). *Organizational Data Mining: Leveraging Enterprise Data Resources for Optimal Performance*. Hershey, PA: Idea Group.

National Research Council. (2008). Committee on Technical and Privacy Dimensions of Information for Terrorism Prevention and Other National Goals, National Research Council, Protecting Individual Privacy in the Struggle Against Terrorists: A Framework for Assessment.

Natwichai, J., Li, X., & Orlowska, M. (2005). Hiding Classification Rules for Data Sharing with Privacy Preservation. In *International Conference on Data Warehousing and Knowledge Discovery* (pp. 468-477), Copenhagen, Denmark.

Natwichai, J., Li, X., & Orlowska, M. (2006). A Reconstruction-Based Algorithm for Classification Rules Hiding. In *Australasian Database Conference* (pp. 49-58), Hobart, Australia.

Nayak, R., & Qiu, T. (2004). Data Mining Application in a Software Project Management Process. In *proceedings of Australian Data Mining Conference*, Cairns, Australia.

Nelson, R. R., & Winter, S. R. (1982). *An Evolutionary Theory of Economic Change.* Cambridge, MA: Belknap Harvard.

Nelson, Y. S., Stoner, G., & Gemis, H. D. (1994). *Nix: Results of Delphi VIII survey of oil price forecasts.* Energy Report, California Energy Commission.

Nemati, H. R., & Barko, C. D. (2002). Enhancing Enterprise Decisions Through Organizational Data Mining. *Journal of Computer Information Systems,* (Summer): 21–28.

Nergiz, M. E., Atzori, M., & Yucel, S. (2008). Towards Trajectory Anonymization: a Generalization-Based Approach. In *ACM GIS Workshop on Security and Privacy in GIS and LBS,* Irvine, CA.

Nilsson, D. (2001). Psycho-social problems faced by "frequent flyers" in a pediatric diabetes unit. *Social Work in Health Care, 33*(3/4), 53–70.

Nissen, M. E. (2000). An extended model of knowledge-flow dynamics. *Communications of the Association for Information Systems, 8,* 251–266.

Noaman, A., & Barker, K. (1999) A horizontal fragmentation algorithm for the fact relation in a distributed data warehouse. In *CIKM '99: Proceedings of the eighth international conference on Information and knowledge management,* (pp. 154–161). New York: ACM Press.

Nonaka, I., & Takeuchi, H. (1995). *The Knowledge creating Company How Japanese Companies create the Dynamics of Innovation.* New York: Oxford University Press.

Nowotny, H., Scott, P., & Gibbons, M. (2004). *Re-Thinking Science Knowledge and the Public in an Age of Uncertainty.* Cambridge, UK: Polity Press.

Nutt, P., & Backoff, R. (1995). Strategy for Public and Third Sector Organizations. *Journal of Public Administration: Research and Theory, 5,* 189–211.

Nysten-Haarala, S. (1998). *The Long-Term Contract. Contract Law and Contracting.* Jyväskylä, Finland: Gummerus Kirjapaino Oy.

O'Callaghan, C. (2001). *Music therapy's relevance in a cancer hospital researched through a constructionist's lens.* Doctoral dissertation, University of Melbourne, Melbourne.

O'Callaghan, C. (2005). Qualitative data-mining through reflexive journal analysis: Implications for music therapy practice development. *Journal of Social Work Research and Evaluation, 6*(2), 217–229.

O'Callaghan, C. (2008). Lullament: Lullaby and lament-therapeutic qualitaties actualized through music therapy. *American Journal of Hospice and Palliative Medicine, 25*(2), 93–99. doi:10.1177/1049909107310139

O'Sullivan, P. (2000). What you don't know won't hurt me: Impression management functions of communication channels in relationships. *Human Communication Research, 26,* 403–431. doi:10.1093/hcr/26.3.403

OASIS (2006). *Reference Model for Service Oriented Architecture.* (SOA Reference Model Technical Committee). 01.08.2006: OASIS

OECD. (2007). *OECD project on Management in Government: Comparative Country Data. Issues in Output Measurement for "Government at a Glance".* OECD GOV Technical Paper 2 (Second Draft).

Ohsawa, Y., & Yada, K. (2009). *Data Mining for Design and Marketing.* Boca Raton, FL: Chapman & Hall/Crc Data Mining and Knowledge Discovery.

Ojasalo, K. (2003). Customer influence on service productivity. *S.A.M. Advanced Management Journal, 68*(3), 14–19.

Olaru, C., & Wehenkel, L. (2003). A complete fuzzy decision tree technique. *Fuzzy Sets and Systems, 138,* 221–254. doi:10.1016/S0165-0114(03)00089-7

Oliveira, S. R. M., & Zaiane, O. R. (2003). Protecting Sensitive Knowledge by Data Sanitization. In *IEEE International Conference on Data Mining* (pp. 211-218), Melbourne, FL.

Oracle (2008). *Oracle Database Concepts 11g Release (11.1) B28318-05.* Retrieved 09.01.2009 from http://download.oracle.com/docs/cd/B28359_01/server.111/b28318.pdf

Oracle Sql Developer. (2009). Retrieved from Web site (checked on March 4, 2009): http://www.oracle.com//technology/products/database/sql_developer/index.html

Oracle Warehouse Builder. (2009). Retrieved from http://www.oracle.com/technology/products/warehouse/index.html

Orlikowski, W. J., & Gash, D. C. (1994). Technological frames: Making Sense of Information Technology in Organzations. *ACM Transactions on Information Systems, 12*(2), 174–207. doi:10.1145/196734.196745

Osbourne, D., & Gaebler, T. (1993). Reinventing Government. How the Entrepreneurial Spirit is Transforming the Public Sector. Harmondsworth, UK: Penguin Books.

Osmond, J., & O'Connor, I. (2004). Formalizing the unformalized: Practitioners' communication of knowledge in practice. *British Journal of Social Work, 34*(5), 677–692. doi:10.1093/bjsw/bch084

Pal, N. R., & Chakraborty, S. (2001). Fuzzy Rule Extraction From ID3-Type Decision Trees for Real Data. *IEEE Transactions on Systems, Man, and Cybernetics Part B, 31*(5), 745–754. doi:10.1109/3477.956036

Palace, B. (1996). Data Mining: What is Data Mining? *Anderson Graduate School of Management at UCLA.* Retrieved November 20, 2008, from http://www.anderson.ucla.edu/faculty/jason.frand/teacher/technologies/palace/datamining.htm

Panas, E., & Ninni, V. (2000). Are oil markets chaotic? A non-linear dynamic analysis. *Energy Economics, 22,* 549–568. doi:10.1016/S0140-9883(00)00049-9

Papakiriakopoulos, D., Pramatari, K., & Doukidis, G. (2009). A decision support system for detecting products missing from the shelf based on heuristic rules. *Decision Support Systems, 46*(3), 685–694. doi:10.1016/j.dss.2008.11.004

Parasuraman, A. (2002). Service quality and productivity: a synergistic perspective. *Managing Service Quality, 12*(1), 6–9. doi:10.1108/096045202104

Pardo, T. A., Cresswell, A. M., Dewes, S. S., & Burke, G. B. (2004). Modeling the Social & Technical Processes of interorganizational Information Integration. In *Proc. of the Thirty-Seventh Annual Hawaii International Conference on System Sciences, (HICSS-37),* Hawaii, USA.

Parolini, C. (1999). *The value net: A tool for competitive strategy.* New York: Wiley.

Parsons, T. (1951). *The Social System.* Glencoe, IL: Free Press.

Parsons, V. S. (2007). Searching for "Unknown Unknowns.". *Engineering Management Journal, 19*(1), 43–46.

Pathak, N., Mane, S., & Srivastava, J. (2006). Who thinks who knows who? Socio-cognitive analysis of email networks. In *ICDM '06: Proceedings of the Sixth International Conference on Data Mining,* (pp. 466–477). Washington, DC: IEEE Computer Society.

Pawson, R., & Tilley, N. (1997). Realistic Evaluation. London: Sage.

Payton, G. (1970). Webster's Dictionary of Proper Names. Springfield, MA: G & C Merriam, C O.

Peake, K., Epstein, I., & Medeiros, D. (Eds.). (2005). *Clinical and research uses of an adolescent intake questionnaire: What kids need to talk about.* Binghampton, NY: Haworth Press.

Peake, K., Mirabito, D., Epstein, I., & Giannone, V. (2005). Creating and sustaining a practice-based research group in an urban adolescent mental health program. *Social Work in Mental Health, 3*(1/2), 39–54. doi:10.1300/J200v03n01_03

Pearson, R. (2005). *Mining imperfect data: dealing with contamination and incomplete records.* SIAM.

Pečar, Z. (2002). *A model of Assessing the Efficiency of Work Processes in Public Administration Using Some Methods of Artificial Intelligence*. PhD thesis, Kranj, Faculty of Management Sc.

Pechenizkiya, M., Puuronenb, S., & Tsymbalc, A. (2008). Towards more relevance-oriented data mining research. *Intelligent Data Analysis, 12*, 237–249.

Pedrycz, W., & Gomide, F. (1998). *An Introduction to Fuzzy Sets: Analysis and Design of Complex Adaptive Systems*. Cambridge, MA: MIT Press.

Pennings, P. (2003). Beyond dichotomous explanations: Explaining constitutional control of the executive with fuzzy-sets. *European Journal of Political Research, 42*, 541–567. doi:10.1111/1475-6765.00095

Penrose, E. (1995). *The theory of the growth of the firm*. Oxford, UK: Oxford University Press. doi:10.1093/0198289774.001.0001

Pensa, R. G., Monreale, A., Pinelli, F., & Pedreschi, D. (2008). Pattern-Preserving K-Anonymization of Sequences and its Application to Mobility Data Mining. In *International Workshop on Privacy in Location Based Applications*, Malaga, Spain.

Perry, W. J. (2008). *Protecting Individual Privacy in the Struggle against Terrorists: A Framework for Assessment*. New York: National Academies Press.

Petronio, S. (2002). *Boundaries of Privacy: Dialectics of Disclosure*. Albany, NY: State University of New York Press.

Pfeffer, J., & Sutton, R. I. (2000). *The Knowing Doing Gap: how smarts companies turn knowledge into knowledge*. Boston: Harvard Business School Press.

Pidd, M. (2005). Perversity in Public Service Performance Measurement. International Journal of Productivity and Performance Management, 54(5/6), 482–493. doi:10.11 08/17410400510604601doi:10.1108/17410400510604601

Pinkas, B. (2002). Cryptographic Techniques for Privacy Preserving Data Mining. *ACM SIGKDD Explorations, 4*(2), 12–19. doi:10.1145/772862.772865

Pipek, V., Hinrichs, J., & Wulf, V. (2003). Sharing Expertise: Challenges for Technical Support. In Ackerman, M., Pipek, V., & Wulf, V. (Eds.), *Sharing Expertise Beyond Knowledge Management* (pp. 111–136). Cambridge, MA: The MIT Press.

Polanyi, M. (1966). *The Tacit Dimension*. London: Cox & Wyman Ltd.

Pollach, I. (2007, September). What's Wrong with Online Privacy Policies? *Communications of the ACM, 50*(9), 103–108. doi:10.1145/1284621.1284627

Pontikakis, E., Theodoridis, Y., Tsitsonis, A., Chang, L., & Verykios, V. S. (2004). A Quantitative and Qualitative Analysis of Blocking in Association Rule Hiding. In *ACM Workshop on Privacy in the Electronic Society* (pp. 29-30), Washington, DC.

Popper, K. R. (1972). *Objective Knowledge. An Evolutionary Approach*. Oxford, UK: Clarendon Press.

Posenelli, S., Joubert, L., Power, R., Vale, S., Lewis, A., & Elliot, R. (2005). Managerial collaboration through allied health data-mining: The St. Vincent's Health experience. *Journal of Social Work Research and Evaluation, 6*(2), 167–176.

Potharst, R., & Bioch, J. C. (2000). Decision trees for ordinal classification. *Intelligent Data Analysis, 4*(2), 97–112.

Pottick, K., Bilder, S., Vander Stoep, A., Warner, L., & Alvarez, M. (2007). US Patterns of mental health service utilization for transition-age youth and young adults. *The Journal of Behavioral Health Services & Research*, 1–16.

Poulin, B., Eisner, R., Szafron, D., Lu, P., Greiner, R., & Wishart, D. S. (2006). *Visual explanation of evidence with additive classifiers*. IAAI.

Pöyhönen, J. (1988). *Sopimusoikeuden järjestelmä ja sopimusten sovittelu*. Vammala, Finland: Vammalan Kirjapaino Oy.

Pratt, M. K. (2007). Your gadgets are springing leaks: Handheld electronics travel everywhere in your company, spilling data along the way. *Computerworld*, (March): 19, 34–36.

Priem, R. L. (1990). Top management team group factors, consensus, and firm performance. *Strategic Management Journal, 11*(6), 469–478. doi:10.1002/smj.4250110605

Pritchard, R. D. (1995). *Productivity measurement and improvement: organizational case studies*. Westport, CT: Praeger Publishers.

Proctor, E., & Rosen, A. (2008). From knowledge production to implementation: Research challenges and imperatives. *Research on Social Work Practice, 18*(4), 285–291. doi:10.1177/1049731507302263

Pyle, D. (1999). *Data preparation for Data Mining*. San Francisco: Morgan Kaufmann.

Pyle, D. (2003). Making the Case. *IBM Database Magazine, 8*(4). Retrieved November 20, 2008, from http://www.ibmdatabasemag.com/showArticle.jhtml?articleID=15300105

Quinlan, J. R. (1979). Discovering rules by induction from large collection of examples. In Michie, D. (Ed.), *Expert Systems in the Microelectronic Age* (pp. 168–201). Edinburgh, UK: Edinburgh University Press.

Quinlan, J. R. (1992). *C4.5 Programs for Machine Learning*. San Francisco: Morgan Kaufmann.

Quinlan, J. R. (1993). *C4.5: Programs for machine learning*. San Mateo, CA: Morgan Kaufmann.

Radhakrishnan, T., & Nandan, U. (2005). Milling force prediction using regression and neural networks. *Journal of Intelligent Manufacturing, 16*, 93–102. doi:10.1007/s10845-005-4826-4

Ragin, C. C., & Pennings, P. (2005). Fuzzy Sets and Social Research. *Sociological Methods & Research, 33*(4), 423–430. doi:10.1177/0049124105274499

Rai, A., Wareham, J., & Sambamurthy, V. (2005). Designing intelligent service supply networks. In Vervest, P., Preiss, K., van Heck, E., & Pau, L. (Eds.), *Smart business networks* (pp. 239–254). Berlin: Springer. doi:10.1007/3-540-26694-1_17

Ravetz, J. R. (1996). *Scientific Knowledge and Its Social Problems*. New Brunswick, NJ: Transaction Publishers.

Raymer, M. L., Doom, T. E., A., K. L. & Punch, W. L. (2003). Knowledge discovery in medical and biological datasets using a hybrid Bayes classifier/evolutionary algorithm. *IEEE Transactions on Systems, Man, and Cybernetics, Part B*.

Reeser, L., & Epstein, I. (1990). *Professionalization and activism in social work: The 60's, the 80's and the future*. New York: Columbia University Press.

Reihheld, F. F., & Sasser, W. E. (1990). Zero defections: quality comes to services. *Harvard Business Review, 68*(5), 105–111.

Reiss, S. P. (1984). Practical Data Swapping: The First Steps. *ACM Transactions on Database Systems, 9*, 20–37. doi:10.1145/348.349

Rennie, J., & Srebro, N. (2005). Loss functions for preference levels: Regression with discrete ordered labels. In *Proc. of the IJCAI Multidisciplinary Workshop on Advances in Preference Handling*.

Rennolls, K and AL-Shawabkeh, A. (2008). Formal structures for data mining, knowledge discovery and communication in a knowledge management environment. *Intelligent Data Analysis, 12*, 147–163.

Rexer, K., Gearan, P., & Allen, H.N. (2007). Surveying the field: Current data mining applications, analytic tools, and practical challenges. *Data Mining Survey Summary Report*, 1-7.

Ridgway, V. (1956). Dysfunctional Consequences of Performance Measurements. Administrative Science Quarterly, 1(2), 240–247. doi:10.2307/2390989doi:10.2307/2390989

Robey, D., Boudreau, M.-C., & Rose, G. M. (2000). Information technology and organizational learning: a review and assessment of research. *Accounting. Management and Information Technology, 10*(2), 125–155. doi:10.1016/S0959-8022(99)00017-X

Robnik-Sikonja, M. & Kononenko, I. (2008). *Explaining classifications for individual instances*, (to appear in IEEE TKDE).

Robnik-Sikonja, M., Likas, A., Constantinopoulos, C., & Kononenko, I. (2009). *An efficient method for explaining the decisions of the probabilistic RBF classification network.* (currently under review, partially available as TR, http://lkm.fri.uni-lj.si/rmarko)

Rodriguez, L. (2008). *Exploring pathways to independence: A data-mining study to research predictors of long-term stay among homeless men in the New York City family shelter system.* Doctoral dissertation, Graduate faculty in Social Welfare, The City University of New York, New York.

Roesmer, C. (2000). Nonstandard Analysis and Dempster-Shafer Theory. *International Journal of Intelligent Systems, 15*, 117–127. doi:10.1002/(SICI)1098-111X(200002)15:2<117::AID-INT2>3.0.CO;2-2

Romano, N. C. Jr, & Fjermestad, J. (2007). Privacy and security in the age of electronic customer relationship management. *International Journal of Information Security and Privacy, 1*(1), 103.

Romesburg, C. (2004). *Cluster analysis for researchers.* Raleigh, NC: Lulu.

Ross, J., Walther, V., & Epstein, I. (2004). Screening risks for intimate partner violence in primary care settings: Implications for future abuse. *Social Work in Health Care, 38*(4), 1–24. doi:10.1300/J010v38n04_01

Routledge, B., Seppi, D., & Spatt, C. (2000). Equilibrium Forward Curves for Commodities. *The Journal of Finance, 55*(3), 1297–1338. doi:10.1111/0022-1082.00248

Roy, N., & McCallum, A. (2001). Toward optimal active learning through sampling estimation of error reduction. In *Proc. 18th international conf. on machine learning* (pp. 441-448). San Francisco, CA: Morgan Kaufmann.

Saariluoma, P. (1990). *Taitavan Ajattelun Psykologia* [Psychology of skilled thinking]. Helsinki, Finland: Otava.

Sadorsky, P. (2006). Modeling and forecasting petroleum futures volatility. *Energy Economics, 28*, 467–488. doi:10.1016/j.eneco.2006.04.005

Safranek, R. J., Gottschlich, S., & Kak, A. C. (1990). Evidence Accumulation Using Binary Frames of Discernment for Verification Vision. *IEEE Transactions on Robotics and Automation, 6*, 405–417. doi:10.1109/70.59366

Sahay, B. S. (2005). Multi-factor productivity measurement model for service organization. *International Journal of Productivity and Performance Measurement, 54*(1), 7–22. doi:10.1108/17410400510571419

Saif Ghouri, S. (2006). Assessment of the relationship between oil prices and US oil stocks. *Energy Policy, 34*(17), 3327–3333. doi:10.1016/j.enpol.2005.07.007

Sainz, A., & Epstein, I. (2001). Creating experimental analogs with available clinical information: Credible alternatives to 'gold standard' experiments? *Social Work in Health Care, 33*(3/4), 163–184.

Sales, E., Lichtenwalter, S., & Fevola, A. (2006). Secondary analysis in social work research education: Past, present and future promise. *Journal of Social Work Education, 42*(3), 543–558. doi:10.5175/JSWE.2006.200404136

Saloheimo, M., Soukka, A., Tuikkala, I., & Aaltonen, J. (2007). Towards ICT-enabled SME supply networks within the tourism industry in Lapland. In Kankaanpää, P., Ovaskainen, S., Pekkala, L., & Tennberg, M. (Eds.), *Knowledge and power in the arctic* (pp. 134–139). Rovaniemi, Finland: University of Lapland.

Samarati, P. (2001). Protecting Respondents' Identities in Microdata Release. *IEEE Transactions on Knowledge and Data Engineering, 13*(6), 1010–1027. doi:10.1109/69.971193

Samarati, P., & Sweeney, L. (1998). *Protecting Privacy when Disclosing Information: K-Anonymity and its Enforcement Through Generalization and Suppresion (Technical Report).* Menlo Park, CA: SRI International.

Sandberg, J. (2005). How do we justify Knowledge Produced within Interpretative Approaches. *Organizational Research Methods, 8*(1), 41–68. doi:10.1177/1094428104272000

Sande, G. (2002). Exact and Approximate Methods for Data Directed Microaggregation in One or More Dimensions. *International Journal of Uncertainty. Fuzziness and Knowledge-Based Systems, 10*(5), 459–476. doi:10.1142/S0218488502001582

Santín, D. (2006). La medición de la eficiencia de las escuelas: una revisión crítica. *Hacienda Pública Española / Revista de Economía Pública, 177*(2), 57-82.

Saracostti, M. (2008). *Social networking as a strategy to overcome poverty in Chile: A data-mining evaluation of the Chile Solidario System.* Doctoral dissertation, Graduate faculty in Social Welfare, The City University of New York, New York.

Sartipi, K., Yarmand, M. H., & Down, D. G. (2007). Mined-knowledge and Decision Support Services in Electronic Health. In *IEEE International Workshop on Systems Development in SOA Environments (SDSOA'07).* Retrieved 09.08.2009 from http://portal.acm.org/citation.cfm?id=1270307

Saunders, C., Wu, Y., Li, Y., & Weisfeld, S. (2004). Interorganizational Trust in B2B Relationships. In M. Janssen, H. G. Sol & R. W. Wagenaar (Eds.), *Proceedings of the 6th International Conference on Electronic Commerce,* (pp. 272-279) (ICEC 2004). New York: ACM.

Saygin, Y., Verykios, V. S., & Clifton, C. (2001). Using Unknowns to Prevent Discovery of Association Rules. *SIGMOD Record, 30*(4), 45–51. doi:10.1145/604264.604271

Saygin, Y., Verykios, V. S., & Elmagarmid, A. K. (2002). Privacy Preserving Association Rule Mining. In *International Workshop on Research Issues in Data Engineering: Engineering E-Commerce/E-Business Systems* (pp. 151-163), San Jose, CA.

Schein, E. H. (1980). *Organizational Psychology* (3rd ed.). Englewood Cliffs, NJ: Prentice-Hall.

Schein, E. H. (1992). *Organizational Culture and Leadership* (2nd ed.). San Francisco, CA: Jossey-Bass.

Schubert, J. (1994). Cluster-based specification techniques in Dempster-Shafer theory for an evidential intelligence analysis of multiple target tracks. Department of Numerical Analysis and Computer Science Royal Institute of technology, S-100 44 Stockholm, Sweden.

Schwartz, D., Kaufman, A. B., & Schwartz, I. M. (2004). Computational intelligence techniques for risk assessment and decision support. *Children and Youth Services Review, 26*(11), 1081–1095. doi:10.1016/j.childyouth.2004.08.007

Schwartz, E. (2007). *Effective privatization of a community mental health agency: Assessing and developing an agency's readiness to change.* Doctoral dissertation, Graduate faculty in Social Welfare, The City University of New York, New York.

Scott, N., Baggio, R., & Cooper, C. (2008). The network concept and tourism. In Scott, N., Baggio, R., & Cooper, C. (Eds.), *Network analysis and tourism* (pp. 15–26). Clevedon, UK: Channel View.

Scriven, M. (1995). The logic of evaluation and evaluation practice. In Fournier, (Ed.), Reasoning in evaluation: Inferential links and leaps (New Directions for Program Evaluation, No. 68, pp. 49-70). San Francisco. Jossey-Bass.

Searle, J. R. (1995). *The Construction of Social Reality.* New York: The Free Press.

Seifert, J. W. (2007). *Data Mining and Homeland Security.* Washington, DC: CRS Report for Congress.

Shafer, G. A. (1976). *Mathematical theory of Evidence.* Princeton, NJ: Princeton University Press.

Shafer, G., & Srivastava, R. (1990). The Bayesian and belief-function formalisms: A general perspective for auditing. In Shafer, G., & Pearl, J. (Eds.), *Readings in Uncertain Reasoning.* San Mateo, CA: Morgan Kaufman Publishers, Inc.

Shambora, W. E., & Rossiter, R. (2007). Are there exploitable inefficiencies in the futures market for oil? *Energy Economics, 29,* 18–27. doi:10.1016/j.eneco.2005.09.004

Shapiro, C., & Varian, H. R. (1999). *Information Rules. A Strategic Guide to the Network Economy*. Boston: Harward Business School Press.

Shaw, I. (2005). Practitioner research: Evidence or critique? *British Journal of Social Work*, 35(8), 1231–1248. doi:10.1093/bjsw/bch223

Shortell, S., & Zajac, E. (1990). Perceptual and archival measures of Miles and Snow's strategic types: A comprehensive assessment of reliability and validity. *Academy of Management Journal*, 33, 817–832. doi:10.2307/256292

Shyne, A. B. (1960). Use of available material. In N.A. Polansky (ed.), Social work research (pp. 106-124). Chicago: University of Chicago Press.

Sia, S. K., Tang, M., Soh, C., & Boh, W. F. (2002). Enterprise Resource Planning (ERP) Systems as a Technology of Power: Empowerment or Panoptic Control? *The Data Base for Advances in Information Systems*, 33(1), 23–37.

Siler, W., & Buckley, J. J. (2005). *Fuzzy expert systems and fuzzy reasoning*. New York: John Wiley &Sons, Inc.

Singh, A., Nowak, R., & Ramanathan, P. (2006). Active learning for adaptive mobile sensing networks. In *Proceedings of the fifth international conference on information processing in sensor networks* (IPSN), (p. 60-68). New York: ACM Press.

Sink, D. S. (1983). Much ado about productivity: where do we go from here. *Industrial Engineering (American Institute of Industrial Engineers)*, 15(10), 36–48.

Skans, O. N. (2008). How does the age structure affect regional productivity? *Applied Economics Letters*, 15(10), 787–790. doi:10.1080/13504850600749123

Smets, P. (1990). The Combination of Evidence in the Transferable belief Model. *IEEE Transactions on Pattern Analysis and Machine Intelligence*, 12(5), 447–458. doi:10.1109/34.55104

Smith, P. (1995). On the unintended consequences of publishing performance data in the public sector. International Journal of Public Administration, 18(2&3), 277–310. doi:10.1080/01900699508525011doi:10.1080/01900699508525011

Snow, C. C., & Hrebiniak, L. G. (1980). Strategy, Distinctive Competence, and Organizational Performance. *Administrative Science Quarterly*, 25(2), 317–336. doi:10.2307/2392457

Spanhove, J., & Verhoest, K. (2007). Corporate governance vs. Government governance: translation or adoption? Paper, EIASM, 4th workshop on corporate governance, Brussels, 15-16 November 2007.

SPSS. (2006). *AnswerTree algorithm summary*. Retrieved from http://www.spss.com/download, (login required)

Sraeel, H. (2007). In the United States, privacy is not always convenient or wanted. *Bank Technology News*, May, 8.

Sraeel, H. (2007). Protecting data on-line is a top priority for consumer. *Bank Technology News*, April, 8.

Srinivas and Harding. J. A. (2008). A data mining integrated architecture for shop floor control. In Proc. IMechE Part B: J. Engineering Manufacture, 222, 605-624.

Srivastava, R. P., & Liu, L. (2003). Applications of Belief Functions in Business Decisions: A Review. *Information Systems Frontiers*, 5(4), 359–378. doi:10.1023/B:ISFI.0000005651.93751.4b

Stacey, R. A. (2001). *Complex responsive processes in organizations: learning and knowledge creation*. New York: Routledge.

Stahl, B. C., & Brooke, C. (2008). The contribution of critical IS research. *Communications of the ACM*, 51(3), 51–55. doi:10.1145/1325555.1325566

Stahlknecht, P., & Hasenkamp, U. (2002). *Einführung in die Wirtschaftsinformatik*. Berlin: Springer.

Stampfel, G., Gansterer, W. N., & Ilger, M. (2008). *Data Retention - The EU Directive 2006/24/EC from a Technological Perspective*. Vienna, Austria: Medien und Recht Publishing.

Steel, R. P., & Rentsch, J. R. (1995). Influence of cumulation strategies on the long-range prediction of absenteeism. *Academy of Management Journal*, 38(6), 1616–1634. doi:10.2307/256846

Stipak, B. (1979). Are there sensible ways to analyse and use subjective indicators of urban service quality. Social Indicators Research, 6(4), 421–438. doi:10.1007/BF00289436doi:10.1007/BF00289436

Storn, R., & Price, K. (1997). Differential Evolution – A simple and Efficient Heuristic for Global Optimization over Continuous Spaces. *Journal of Global Optimization, 11*, 341–359. doi:10.1023/A:1008202821328

Strambi, O. & Karin-Anne, T. (1998). Trip generation modeling using CHAID, a criterion-based segmentation modeling tool. *Journal of the Transportation Research Board,* (1645), 24-31.

Stross, R. (2006). Cellphone as tracker: X marks your doubts. *The New York Times,* Business Section, Sunday, November 19, 3.

Sun Microsystems. (2007). *Sun Microsystems launches unique data management appliance for communication service providers.* Retrieved, May 2009, from http://www.sun.com/aboutsun/pr/2007-06/sunflash.20070607.1.xml

Sun, X., & Yu, P. S. (2005). A Border Based Approach for Hiding Sensitive Frequent Itemsets. In *IEEE International Conference on Data Mining* (pp. 426-433), Houston, TX.

Sutherland, J. (2002). Job-to-job turnover and job-to-non-employment movement – a case study investigation. *Personnel Review, 31*(6), 710–721. doi:10.1108/00483480210445980

Sutton, B. (2005). *Why Projects Fail – Mastering the Monster (Part 2), Examining the underlying reasons for project failure, and how to use that knowledge to get your projects back on track.* ArchItect, Bearpark Publishing Ltd. Retrieved November 19, 2008, from http://www.itarchitect.co.uk/articles/display.asp?id=224

Swanborn, P. G. (1999). Evalueren: het ontwerpen, begeleiden en evalueren van interventies: een methodische basis voor evaluatie-onderzoek. Amsterdam: Boom.

Taipale, K.A. (2004). Technology, Security and Privacy: The Fear of Frankenstein, the Mythology of Privacy and the Lessons of King Ludd. *Yale Journal of Law and Technology, 7.*

Talukder, A. K., & Yavagal, R. P. (2007). *Mobile Computing: Technology, Applications and Service Creation.* New York: McGraw Hill.

Tan, P.-N., Steinbach, M., & Kumar, V. (2006). *Introduction to Data Mining.* Reading, MA: Addison-Wesley.

Tapac. (2004). *Safeguarding Privacy in the Fight Against Terrorism.* Technology and Privacy Advisory Committee, Department of Defense, Washington, DC: DIANE Publishing.

Tavani, H. T. (2004). *Ethics and Technology: Ethical Issues in an Age of Information and Communication Technology.* Hoboken, NJ: John Wiley and Sons.

Taylor, C. (2007). As RFID tracking booms, privacy issues loom. *Business 2,* May 11, 1-3.

Taylor, F. W. (1911). *The Principles of Scientific Management.* New York: Harper. Digital version available on http://melbecon.unimelb.edu.au/het/taylor/sciman.htm (link checked on February 22nd, 2009).

Taylor, H. (2003). *Most People Are "Privacy Pragmatists" Who, While Concerned about Privacy, Will Sometimes Trade It Off for Other Benefits.* Available at http://www.harrisinteractive.com/harris_poll/index.asp?PID=365, last accessed June 24, 2007.

Teradata Corporation. (2006). *Flexible solution launched by teradata and capgemini to enable compliance with eu data retention directive.* Retrieved, May, 2009, from http://www.teradata.com/t/page/160330/index.html

Terrovitis, M., & Mamoulis, N. (2008). Privacy Preservation in the Publication of Trajectories. In *Intl. Conference on Mobile Data Management* (pp. 65-72), Beijing, China.

Thabtah, F., Cowling, P., & Hammoud, S. (2006). Improving rule sorting, predictive accuracy and training time in associative classification. *Expert Systems with Applications, 31*, 414–426. doi:10.1016/j.eswa.2005.09.039

Thompson-Klein, J. (1996). *Crossing Boundaries Knowledge, Disciplinarities, and Interdisciplinarities.* London: Virginia University Press.

Thrun, S. (1995). Extracting rules from artificial neural networks with distributed representations. In Tesauro, G., Touretzky, D., & Leen, T. (Eds.), *Advances in neural information processing systems (NIPS)* (*Vol. 7*). Cambridge, MA: M. Press.

Timothy, J. C., & Eunnyeong, H. (2000). Price and inventory dynamics in petroleum product markets. *Energy Economics, 22*(5), 527–548. doi:10.1016/S0140-9883(00)00056-6

Toulmin, S. (1990). *Cosmpolis the Hidden Agenda of Modernity.* Chicago: The University of Chicago Press.

Trent, R., Stout-Wiegand, N., & Furbee, P. (1984). The nature of the connection between life course and satisfaction with community services. Social Indicators Research, 15(4), 417–429. doi:10.1007/BF00351447doi:10.1007/BF00351447

Tripodi, T., & Epstein, I. (1978). Incorporating knowledge of research methodology into social work practice. *Journal of Social Service Research, 2,* 65–78. doi:10.1300/J079v02n01_06

Tripodi, T., & Epstein, I. (1980). *Research techniques for clinical social workers.* New York: Columbia University.

Tripodi, T., Epstein, I., & MacMurray, C. (1970). Dilemmas of evaluation. *The American Journal of Orthopsychiatry, 40,* 850–857.

Tripodi, T., Fellin, P., & Epstein, I. (1978). *Differential social program evaluation.* Itasca, IL: F.E. Peacock.

Tsoukas, H., & Cummings, S. (1997). Marginalization and recovery: the emergence of Aristotelian themes in organizational studies. *Organization Studies.* http://findarticles.com/p/articles/mi_m4339/is_/ai_n27518846, last accessed 09.08. 2009

Tuomi, I. (1999). Data is More Than Knowledge: Implications of the Reversed Knowledge Hierarchy for Knowledge Management and Organizational Memory. *Journal of Management Information Systems, 16*(3), 103–118.

Turban, E., Aronson, J. E., & Liang, T.-P. (2005). *Decision Support Systems and Intelligence Systems.* Upper Saddle River, NJ: Pearson Education, Inc.

Turban, E., McLean, E., & Wetherbe, J. (2002). *Information technology for management: transforming the business in the digital economy.* New York: John Wiley & Sons, Inc.

Turner, K., & Zizzamia, F. (2008). Predicting Better Claims Management. *Risk Management, 55*(7), 52–55.

Turunen, A. (2005). *Innovations as Communication Processes. A Legal Architecture for Governing Ideas in Business.* Saarijärvi, Finland: Lapland University Press.

Vaidya, J., & Clifton, C. (2002). Privacy Preserving Association Rule Mining in Vertically Partitioned Databases. In *ACM SIGKDD International Conference on Knowledge Discovery and Data Mining* (pp. 639-644), Edmonton, AB.

Vaidya, J., & Clifton, C. (2003). Privacy Preserving K-Means Clustering over Vertically Partitioned Data. In *ACM SIGKDD International Conference on Knowledge Discovery and Data Mining,* (pp. 206-215), Washington, DC, USA.

Vaidya, J., & Clifton, C. (2004). Privacy Preserving Naïve Bayes Classifier for Vertically Partitioned Data. In *SIAM International Conference on Data Mining* (pp. 522-526), Lake Buena Vista, FL.

Väisänen, J., Kujansivu, P., & Lönnqvist, A. (2007). Effects of intellectual capital Investments on productivity and profitability. *International Journal of Learning and Intellectual Capital, 4*(4), 377–391. doi:10.1504/IJLIC.2007.016334

Van de Walle, S. (2006). The State of the World's Bureaucracies. Journal of Comparative Policy Analysis, 8(4), 439–450. doi:10.1080/13876980600971409doi:10.1080/13876980600971409

Van de Walle, S. (2008). Comparing the performance of national public sectors: Conceptual problems. International Journal of Productivity and Performance Management, 57(4), 329–338. doi:10.1108/17410400810 867535doi:10.1108/17410400810867535

Van de Walle, S., & Bouckaert, G. (2007). Perceptions of Productivity and Performance in Europe and The United. International Journal of Public Administration, 30(11), 1123–1140. doi:10.1080/01900690701225309doi :10.1080/01900690701225309

Van Dongen, W. (2004). *Kinderopvang als basisvoorziening in een democratische samenleving. Scenario's voor de toekomstige ontwikkeling van de dagopvang voor kinderen jonger dan drie jaar.* Brussel: Centrum voor Bevolkings - en Gezinsstudie.

Van Dooren, W. (2006). *Performance measurement in the Flemish public sector: A supply and demand approach.* Leuven: published doctoral dissertation, K.U. Leuven, Belgium.

Van Roosbroek, S. (2007). Rethinking governance indicators: What can quality management tell us about the debate on governance indicators? Paper EGPA annual conference. Study Group: Performance and Quality, Madrid, September 19-22, 2007.

Van Someren, M., & Urbancic, T. (2006). Applications of machine learning: matching problems to tasks and methods. *The Knowledge Engineering Review, 20*(4), 363–402. doi:10.1017/S0269888906000762

van Thiel, S., & Leeuw, F. (2003). De prestatieparadox in de publieke sector. Beleidswetenschap, 17(2), 123–144.

Vandewalle, S., Sterck, M., & Van Dooren, W. (2004). What you see is not necessarily what you get, een verkenning van de mogelijkheden en moeilijkheden van internationale vergelijkingen van publieke sectoren op basis van indicatoren. Leuven, Belgium: Instituut voor de Overheid.

Vandijck, E. & Despontin, M. (1998). Hoe komen we te weten wat we weten? Data mining. *VTOM, Vlaams tijdschrift voor overheidsmanagement, 3*(3), 21-25.

Vanhoof, K., Bloemer, J., & Pauwels, K. (1997). A case of loyalty and satisfaction research. In M. Van Someren, & G. Widmer (Eds.). *Proceedings 9th European Conference on Machine Learning, Prague, Czech Republic (ECML)* (pp. 290-297). Berlin: Springer.

Verhoest, K., & Spanhove, J. (2007). Inleiding tot het themanummer: Deugdelijk bestuur en government governance. [VTOM]. Vlaams Tijdschrift voor Overheidsmanagement, 4(1), 2–6.

Verlet, D. (2008) *Good governance, corporate governance, government governance: what's in a name? Een theoretische situering van Beter Bestuurlijk Beleid in Vlaanderen.* Brussel, Studiedienst van de Vlaamse Regering, SVR-nota 2008/4.

Verlet, D., Reynaert, H., & Devos, C. (2005). Burgers in Vlaamse grootsteden. Tevredenheid, vertrouwen, veiligheidsgevoel en participatie in Gent, Brugge en Antwerpen. Brugge, Belgium: Vanden Broele.

Verykios, V. S., Elmagarmid, A. K., Bertino, E., Saygin, Y., & Dasseni, E. (2004). Association Rule Hiding. *IEEE Transactions on Knowledge and Data Engineering, 16*(4), 434–447. doi:10.1109/TKDE.2004.1269668

Virtanen, P. (2001). Määräävän markkina-aseman kontrollointi. Oikeus ja taloustieteellinen vertaileva tutkimus Saksan, Suomen ja EU:n kilpailuoikeudesta. Helsinki, Finland: Suomalainen lakimiesyhdistys.

Von Krogh, G., Roos, J., & Slocum, K. (1994). An Essay on Corporate Epistemology. *Strategic Management Journal, 15*(1), 53–71.

Vonk, E., Tripodi, T., & Epstein, I. (2006). *Research techniques for clinical social workers* (2nd ed.). New York: Columbia University Press.

Vose, D. (2000). *Quantitative Risk Analysis.* New York: John Wiley & Sons Inc.

Wai, F. (2007). *Data-mining as a methodology for explaining written narratives: An application on understanding the breast cancer experience among Hong Kong Chinese women.* Doctoral dissertation, University of Hong Kong.

Walker, O., & Ruekert, R. (1987). Marketing's role in the implementation of business strategies: A critical review and conceptual framework. *Journal of Marketing, 51,* 15–33. doi:10.2307/1251645

Wang, E. T. G., & Wei, H.-L. (2007). Interorganizational Governance Value Creation: Coordinating for Information Visibility and Flexibility in Supply Chains. *Decision Sciences, 38*(4), 647–674.

Wang, K. (2007). Applying data mining to manufacturing: the nature and implications. *Journal of Intelligent Manufacturing, 18,* 487–495. doi:10.1007/s10845-007-0053-5

Wang, K., Fung, B. C. M., & Yu, P. S. (2005). Template-Based Privacy Preservation in Classification Problems. In *IEEE International Conference on Data Mining* (pp. 466-473), Houston, TX.

Wang, R. C., & Chuu, S. J. (2004). Group decision-making using a fuzzy linguistic approach for evaluating the flexibility in a manufacturing system. *European Journal of Operational Research, 154*(3), 563–572. doi:10.1016/S0377-2217(02)00729-4

Wang, S. L., & Jafari, A. (2005). Using Unknowns for Hiding Sensitive Predictive Association Rules. In *IEEE International Conference on Information Reuse and Integration* (pp. 223-228), New York.

Wang, X., Chen, B., Qian, G., & Ye, F. (2000). On the optimization of fuzzy decision trees. *Fuzzy Sets and Systems, 112*(1), 117–125. doi:10.1016/S0165-0114(97)00386-2

Wechsler, B., & Backoff, R. W. (1986). Policy making and administration in state agencies: Strategic management approaches. *Public Administration Review, 46,* 321–327. doi:10.2307/976305

Wehrle, P., Miquel, M., & Tchounikine, A. (2005). A model for distributing and querying a data warehouse on a computing grid. In *ICPADS '05: Proceedings of the 11th International Conference on Parallel and Distributed Systems,* (pp. 203–209).

Weiss, S. M., & Kulikowski, C. A. (1991). *Computer Systems that Learn.* San Francisco: Morgan Kaufmann.

Westin, A. F. (1996). *Harris-Equifax Consumer Privacy Survey.* Atlanta, GA: Equifax, Inc.

Westlund, A., & Löthgren, M. (2001). The interactions between quality, productivity and economic performance: the case of Swedish pharmacies. *Total Quality Management, 12*(3), 385–396. doi:10.1080/09544120120034528

Westphal, C., & Blaxton, T. (1998). *Data Mining Solutions: Methods and Tools for Solving real-World Problems.* New York: Wiley.

Willenborg, L., & DeWaal, T. (2001). *Elements of Statistical Disclosure Control.* New York: Springer-Verlag.

Williams-Gray, B. (in progress). *Accreditation as an intervention and a means for expanding organizational capacity: A data-mining study.* Doctoral dissertation, Graduate faculty in Social Welfare, The City University of New York, New York.

Williamson, O. E. (1991). Comparative Economic Organization: The Analysis of Discrete Structural Analysis. *Administrative Science Quarterly, 36*(2), 269–296. doi:10.2307/2393356

Wilson, T. D. (2002). The non-sense of 'knowledge management'. *Information Research, 8* (1). Retrieved 09.01.2009 from http://informationr.net/ir/8-1/paper144.html

Witten, I. H., & Frank, E. (2005). *Data Mining: practical machine learning tools and techniques.* San Francisco: Elsevier.

Wu, Y. H., Chiang, C. M., & Chen, L. P. (2007). Hiding Sensitive Association Rules with Limited Side Effects. *IEEE Transactions on Knowledge and Data Engineering, 19*(1), 29–42. doi:10.1109/TKDE.2007.250583

Xie, W., Yu, L., Xu, S. Y., & Wang, S. Y. (2006). *A new method for crude oil price forecasting based on support vector machines,* (. LNCS, 3994, 441–451.

Xu, K., Jayaram, J., & Xu, M. (2006). The effects of customer contact on conformance quality and productivity in Chinese service firms. *International Journal of Quality & Reliability Management, 23*(4), 367–389. doi:10.1108/02656710610657585

Yang, J.-B., Liu, J., Wang, J., Sii, H.-S., & Wong, H.-W. (2006). Belief Rule-Base Inference Methodology Using the Evidential Reasoning Approach—RIMER. *IEEE Transactions on Systems, Man, and Cybernetics. Part A, Systems and Humans, 36*(2), 266–285. doi:10.1109/TSMCA.2005.851270

Ye, M., Zyren, J., & Shore, J. (2002). Forecasting crude oil spot price using OECD petroleum inventory levels. *International Advances in Economic Research, 8*, 324–334. doi:10.1007/BF02295507

Ye, M., Zyren, J., & Shore, J. (2005). A monthly crude oil spot price forecasting model using relative inventories. *International Journal of Forecasting, 21*, 491–501. doi:10.1016/j.ijforecast.2005.01.001

Ye, M., Zyren, J., & Shore, J. (2006). Forecasting short-run crude oil price using high and low-inventory variables. *Energy Policy, 34*, 2736–2743. doi:10.1016/j.enpol.2005.03.017

Yin, X., & Yang, J. (2006). Efficient Classification across Multiple Database Relations: A CrossMine Approach. *IEEE Transactions on Knowledge and Data Engineering, 18*(6). doi:10.1109/TKDE.2006.94

Yu, C.-S., & Li, H.-L. (2001). Method for solving quasi-concave and non-cave fuzzy multi-objective programming problems. *Fuzzy Sets and Systems, 122*(2), 205–227. doi:10.1016/S0165-0114(99)00163-3

Yu, H., Vaidya, J., & Jiang, X. (2006). Privacy Preserving SVM Classification on Vertically Partitioned Data. In *Pacific-Asia Conference on Advances in Knowledge Discovery and Data Mining,* (pp. 647-656), Singapore.

Yu, L., Lai, K. K., Wang, S. Y., & He, K. J. (2007). *Oil price forecasting with an EMD-based multiscale neural network learning paradigm,* (. *LNCS, 4489*, 925–932.

Yu, L., Wang, S. Y., & Lai, K. K. (2005). A novel nonlinear ensemble forecasting model incorporating GLAR and ANN for foreign exchange rates. *Computers & Operations Research, 32*(10), 2523–2541. doi:10.1016/j.cor.2004.06.024

Yu, L., Wang, S. Y., & Lai, K. K. (2008). Forecasting crude oil price with an EMD-based neural network ensemble learning paradigm. *Energy Economics, 30*, 2623–2635. doi:10.1016/j.eneco.2008.05.003

Yuan, Y., & Shaw, M. J. (1995). Induction of fuzzy decision trees. *Fuzzy Sets and Systems, 69*(2), 125–139. doi:10.1016/0165-0114(94)00229-Z

Zadeh, L. A. (1975). Fuzzy Logic and Approximate Reasoning (In Memory of Grigore Moisel). *Synthese, 30*, 407–428. doi:10.1007/BF00485052

Zafra-Gómez, J. L. López-Hernandez, A.L. & Hernández-Bastida, A. (2009) Developing a Model to Measure Financial Condition in Local Government: Evaluating Service Quality and Minimizing the Effects of the Socioeconomic Environment: An Application to Spanish Municipalities. *The American Review of Public Administration.* Retrieved from http://arp.sagepub.com/cgi/rapidpdf/

Zafra-Gómez, J. L., López-Hernandez, A. M., & Hernández-Bastida, A. (2009, May). Developing an alert system for local governments in financial crisis. *Public Money & Management, 29*(3), 175–181.

Zafra-Gómez, J.L., López-Hernández, A.M., & Hernández-Bastida, A. (2009). Evaluating financial performance in local government. Maximising the benchmarking value. *International Review of Administrative Science, 75*(1), 151–167. doi:10.1177/0020852308099510

Zahra, S. A., & Pearce, J. A. (1990). Research evidence on the Miles-Snow typology. *Journal of Management, 16*, 751–768. doi:10.1177/014920639001600407

Zajac, E. J., & Shortell, S. M. (1989). Changing generic strategies: Likelihood, direction and performance implications. *Strategic Management Journal, 10*, 413–430. doi:10.1002/smj.4250100503

Zettinig, P. (2003). *Invisible Organisations: Inter-firm Organisational Formation and Form.* Turku, Finland: Turku School of Economics and Business Administration.

Zhang, X., Lai, K. K., & Wang, S. Y. (2008). A new approach for crude oil price analysis based on Empirical Mode Decomposition. *Energy Economics, 30*, 905–918. doi:10.1016/j.eneco.2007.02.012

Zhong, S., Yang, Z., & Wright, R. (2005). Privacy Enhancing K-anonymization of Customer Data. In ACM SIGMOD-SIGACT-SIGART Principles of Database Systems, (pp. 139-147), Baltimore, MD.

Zhou, S.-M., & Gan, J. Q. (2008). Low-level interpretability and high-level interpretability: a unified view data-driven interpretable fuzzy system modelling. *Fuzzy Sets and Systems, 159*, 3091–3131. doi:10.1016/j.fss.2008.05.016

Zhu, H. (2006). Role mechanisms in collaborative systems. *International Journal of Production Research, 44*(1), 181–193. doi:10.1080/00207540500247495

Zilberfein, F., Hutson, C., Snyder, S., & Epstein, I. (2001). Social work practice with pre- and post-liver transplant patients: A retrospective self-study. *Social Work in Health Care, 33*(3/4), 91–104.

Zondergeld-Hamer, A. (2007). Een kwestie van goed bestuur. Openbaar Bestuur, 17(10), 5–10.

About the Contributors

Antti Syväjärvi is professor of administrative science at the Lapland University in Finland and the Head of Research Methodology Department. Professor Syväjärvi's academic work is concentrated especially to the fields like public information management, leadership, human resource management, organizational information technology, electronic government and change in public administration. He is currently leading some academic research projects that are related to the abovementioned thematic areas. Professor Syväjärvi has numerous national and international academic publications in refereed science forums. In addition to Finnish Universities, Professor Syväjärvi has been teaching and doing research at the Aston University and at the Cardiff University. These Universities are in the United Kingdom.

Jari Stenvall is research professor at the University of Tampere in Finland. He has done, evaluated and conducted several assessments and research projects related to public administration reforms and applied information technology. His research has included topics like change management, trust, organizational reforms, service innovations, and the use of information technology in organizations. Professor Stenvall's scientific production contains more than one hundred national and international publications. Besides Finland, Professor Stenvall has also been teaching at the Kaunas University of Technology in Lithuania and the Queen's University in the United Kingdom.

***

Emanuel Camilleri occupies the post of Director General (Strategy & Operations Support) at the Ministry of Finance, Economy and Investment, Malta. Dr Camilleri has undertaken major government corporate projects, including the establishment of the Value Added Tax Department, Tax Compliance Unit and other major reforms in Tax Administration. He is also the Chairman, Accrual Accounting Task Force, responsible for the implementation of accrual accounting across government Ministries and their respective Departments. Dr Camilleri is a Visiting Senior Lecturer at the University of Malta, Faculty of Economics, Management and Accountancy, lecturing at Public Policy Department in Project Management, Information Management (Service Delivery in the Information Age) and Financial Management. He held senior posts with the Australian Public Service, Ministry of Defence Support related to Operations Research and Information Systems Development. He has extensive experience in management information systems development and has academic qualifications in information management, accountancy, engineering and business management.

John C. Molluzzo is a Professor and Chair of the New York Campus Information Technology Department in the Seidenberg School of Computer Science and Information Systems at Pace University. He has held positions at the City University of New York, and St. John's University. He is the author of six books in mathematics and computing, including C++ for Business Programmers, 2nd Edition. He has authored numerous articles in mathematics, computer science, and information systems. He has won awards for his teaching and scholarship. Currently professor Molluzzo is engaged in several research projects involving privacy issues in online advertising and in social networking Websites.

James P. Lawler is a Professor of Information Systems, in the Information Systems Department, of the Seidenberg School of Computer Science and Information Systems, at Pace University, in New York City, USA. His interests in research include competitive e-Commerce design methods, customer relationship management (CRM) marketing, sales and service systems, and privacy on mobile computing device systems and on social networking systems and technologies on the Web. He is the principal author of Service-Oriented Architecture (SOA): Strategy, Methodology, and Technology, a primer on the technology, and is an instructor in the topic. His recent interests in research include cloud computing and security. Professor Lawler is published in conference proceedings and journals in his interests in research in the United States, Europe, and northern Africa.

Pascale Vandepeutte is a Lecturer of Computer Science and e-Business, at the University of Mons-Hainaut, in Mons, Belgium. Her interests in research include e-Commerce methodologies and mobile computing systems and privacy and related technologies in the European Union. She is a co-author with Dr Lawler of An Exploratory Study of Apparel Dress Model Technology on European Web Sites, a paper in the Journal of Information, Information Technology, & Organizations, in Canada. Dr Vandepeutte's recent interests in research involve expanded surveying of the privacy practices of European Union students, especially in Belgium and France. She is a frequent collaborator with Dr Lawler and Dr Molluzzo at conference presentations and on published e-Commerce research in Europe and northern Africa.

Goran Klepac works as a Head of Strategic Development and Reporting Department in Credit Risk Management Division, Raiffeisen Bank Austria in Croatia. Dr Klepac has also worked on many data mining projects as a consultant in different domains like retail, finance, insurance, hospitality, telecommunication and production. He is an author/co-author of several books published in Croatian and English language in the domain of data mining. He achieved Ph.D. degree in temporal data mining at Faculty of Organization and Informatics, Varazdin, Croatia. He is an author of REFII model (which was also the subject of his Ph.D.), the model for temporal data mining.

Vincent Lemaire obtained his undergraduate degree from the University of Paris 12 in signal processing and was in the same period an electronic teacher. He obtained a PhD in Computer Science from the University of Paris 6, France. Thereafter he joined the R&D Division of France Télécom where he became a Senior Expert in data-mining. Dr Lemaire's research interests are the application of machine learning in various areas for telecommunication companies with an actual main application in data mining for business intelligence. He developed exploratory data analysis and classification interpretation tools. Active learning and data-space exploration are now his main research interests. Dr Lemaire obtained a HDR thesis ("Habilitation à diriger des recherches": French post-doctoral degree allowing its holder to supervise officially PhD students) in Computer Science from the University of Paris-Sud 11, Orsay).

Carine Hue has received the M.Sc. degree in mathematics and computer science and the PhD degree in signal and image processing from the University of Rennes 1, France. She has worked at INRA (French National Institute for Research in Agronomy) as full-time researcher on Bayesian statistical modelling for agronomy. During the last years she has worked with Orange Labs engineers, first as associated research engineer then as consultant hired by GFI Informatique. Dr Hue's research interests are statistical modelling and the application of data mining algorithms to various domains as signal and image processing, agronomy or data mining. More precisely, she proposed works on MCMC methods and on particle filtering. At the moment, Dr Hue works on the application of neural nets, decision trees and random forests for business intelligence.

Olivier Bernier has graduated from the "Ecole Polytechnique" and from the "Ecole Nationale Supérieure des Télécommunications". He thereafter joined the CNET, "Centre National d'Etude des Télécommunications", which became later the R&D Division of France Télécom. As a Senior Expert in computer vision, his main area of research are statistical learning, probabilistic modelling and computer vision, with a focus on applications of computer vision to advanced Human Computer Interfaces. He obtained a HDR thesis ("Habilitation à diriger des recherches": French post-doctoral degree allowing its holder to officially supervise PhD students) in Computer Science from the University Pierre et Marie Curie (Paris 6) in 2009.

Dries Verlet is an Advisor in Policy Evaluation at the Research Center of the Flemish Government and a Visiting Professor at the Faculty of Business Administration and Public Administration, Ghent University College. He is also former assistant professor at Department of Political Sciences of the Ghent University. Dr Verlet is an advisor on policy evaluation, within the team on quality of statistics, surveys, foresight studies and policy evaluation of the Research Centre of the Flemish Government. He's involved in a wide variety of policy evaluation programs and as an academic he's teaching methodology and statistics.

Carl Devos is a Professor at the department of political studies at Ghent University. He's president of the Ghent Institute for Political Studies (GhIPS) and editor-in-chief of Res Publica, the Flemish-Dutch scientific journal for political sciences. Carl Devos wrote a PhD on the impact of globalization on the power position of trade unions. He's head of the department section studying the Belgian internal politics. His main research topics are the Belgian political system, Belgian federalism, decision making and collective bargaining. Professor Devos has published on political parties, decision making, federalism, collective bargaining and the performance of public services.

Aki Jääskeläinen works as a Researcher on the Performance Management Team at Tampere University of Technology, Finland. He has written research articles on intellectual capital and performance measurement. He has also participated in many development projects related to performance management in Finnish organisations. His current research interests focus on productivity measurement of public services.

Paula Kujansivu works as a Senior Researcher at the Department of Industrial Management, Tampere University of Technology, Finland. Her research interests are the measurement and management of organisations' intellectual capital and business performance. Dr Kujansivu's research has been published in such journals as International Journal of Learning and Intellectual Capital, Journal of Knowledge Management Studies, Journal of Intellectual Capital, Measuring Business Excellence and Production Planning & Control. In addition, she has written books on those research topics. Dr Kujansivu also acts as the Managing Partner of Prodia Ltd.

Jaani Väisänen is working as a Researcher in Tampere University of Technology at the Department of Business Information Management and Logistics. His research interests include electronic commerce, service innovation, open source software, business intelligence, data mining and Internet marketing. The author is overseeing the usage of the SAS Enterprise Guide and Enterprise Miner software in his department as the manager for the faculty's SAS educational Analytical Suite program. He is currently finishing his doctoral dissertation which examines the usage of search engine marketing in Finnish small and medium-sized enterprises.

Malcolm J. Beynon is a Professor of Uncertain Reasoning in Business/Management in Cardiff Business Cardiff at Cardiff University (UK). He gained his BSc and PhD in pure mathematics and computational mathematics, respectively, at Cardiff University. His research areas include the theoretical and application of uncertain reasoning methodologies, including Dempster-Shafer theory, fuzzy set theory and rough set theory. Also the introduction and development of multi-criteria based decision making and classification techniques, including the Classification and Ranking Belief Simplex. Professor Beynon has published numerous research articles. He is a member of the International Rough Set Society, International Operations Research Society and the International Multi-Criteria Decision Making Society.

Rhys Andrews (PhD University of Wales) is a Senior Research Fellow in the Centre for Local and Regional Government Research at Cardiff Business School. Dr Andrews has ten years experience of researching public services in England and Wales, undertaking a variety of projects studying policy implementation, project delivery and service effectiveness in a range of public and voluntary sector bodies. His research interests focus on social capital, organizational environments and public service performance. His expertise in these areas has been recognised in the publication of over thirty sole and co-authored articles in academic journals, such as Journal of Public Administration Research and Theory, Public Administration Review, Urban Affairs Review and Urban Studies. He also currently serves as a member of the UK central government's Local Governance expert panel.

Jue Wang received the PhD degree in Applied Mathematics from Xidian University, Xi'an in 2005. She is currently an Assistant Research Fellow of Management Science at Academy of Mathematics and Systems Sciences of CAS. She has published 2 books and over 20 journal papers in journals including Soft Computing, Experts Systems with Applications. Dr Wang's current research interests include financial engineering, data mining, intelligent computing, economic forecasting and decision analysis.

Xun Zhang received the PhD degree in Management Sciences and Engineering from Institute of Systems Science, Academy of Mathematics and Systems Sciences, Chinese Academy of Sciences. She is currently an Assistant Researcher in Academy of Mathematics and Systems Science, Chinese Academy of Sciences. She published many papers in scientific journals including Energy Economics, International Journal of Information Technology & Decision Making, and Journal of Systems Science and Complexity. Dr Zhang's research interests are in the areas of decision support systems, knowledge management and prediction.

Wei Xu received the PhD degree in Management Sciences and Engineering from School of Management, Graduate University of Chinese Academy of Sciences, and Chinese Academy of Sciences. He is currently an Assistant Professor of School of Information, Renmin University of China. He has published various papers in journals including Fuzzy Sets and Systems, Computers & Mathematics with Applications, and Journal of Systems Science and Systems Engineering. Dr Xu's research interests include data mining, financial forecasting, intelligent detection, and decision support systems.

Yejing Bao received the PhD degree in Management Sciences and Engineering from Institute of Systems Science, Academy of Mathematics and Systems Sciences, Chinese Academy of Sciences. She is currently an Assistant Researcher in Beijing University of Technology. Dr Bao has published many papers in energy forecasting. Her research interests are in the areas of decision support systems and economic forecasting.

Ye Pang received the Master degree in Management Sciences and Engineering from Institute of Systems Science, Academy of Mathematics and Systems Sciences, Chinese Academy of Sciences. During the years at Chinese Academy of Sciences, she participated in projects such as export/import forecasting for Chinese Ministry of Commerce, Crude oil price forecasting for Sinopec and developing risk management system for People's Bank of China. From these projects, she gained valuable experience in macroeconomic and oil price analysis. She is currently a Risk Management Engineer in The People's Insurance Company (Group) of China and in charge of the risk management of the company and sub-company.

Shouyang Wang received the PhD degree in Operations Research from Institute of Systems Science, Chinese Academy of Sciences (CAS), Beijing in 1986. He is currently a Bairen Distinguished Professor of Management Science at Academy of Mathematics and Systems Sciences of CAS and a Lotus chair professor of Hunan University, Changsha. He is the editor-in-chief or a co-editor of 12 journals. He has published 18 books and numerous journal papers. Professor Wang's current research interests include financial engineering, e-auctions, knowledge management and decision analysis.

Mirco Nanni is a Researcher at the KDDLab of the ISTI institute of CNR, in Pisa, Italy. He holds a Laurea degree and a PhD in Computer Science, both from the University of Pisa. He has been a visiting fellow at UMCP (Maryland, USA), and recetly at MIT (Massachusetts, USA). Dr Nanni's research interests mainly focus on data mining and knowledge discovery, especially model and pattern extraction methods for spatio-temporal and mobility data. He collaborated in various roles to the organization of several international conferences and workshops in the field of data mining and databases. Dr Nanni is involved in several projects on mobility data analysis and applications (EU-GeoPKDD, the Italian Motus and MdM, the EU MOVE cost action). He served for several years as teacher and/or collaborator in courses on data mining and databases for graduate and undergraduate students.

Laura Spinsanti is a Senior Researcher in the Database Laboratory at Ecole Polytechnique Fédérale de Lausanne (Switzerland). Her current research interests include spatio-temporal conceptual modelling, geographic semantic enrichment and ontology application. She received her MS degree in Computer Science from University of Florence, Italy and her PhD in eLearning from Polytechnic University of Marche, Italy, respectively in 2002 and 2006. From 2006 to 2009 she was a scientific collaborator of KDD-Lab (Knowledge Discovery and Delivery Laboratory): a joint research group of ISTI (Institute of Italian National Research Council) and the Computer Science Department of University of Pisa. Dr Spinsanti has worked as group Coordinator, project supervisor and as a researcher on data base, data mining and applied ontology.

Irwin Epstein is the Rehr Professor of Applied Social Work Research (Health and Mental Health) at Hunter College School of Social Work of the City University of New York where he teaches in the PhD Program. An Adjunct Professor at the Mt. Sinai Medical Center, he has introduced the concept and methodology of "Clinical Data-mining" (CDM) into social work and allied health and has given CDM training workshops at universities, social agencies and hospitals in Australia, Britain, Finland, Hong Kong, Ireland, Israel, Singapore and the United States. Professor Epstein's current interest is in promoting practice-research integration by engaging professionals in research on their own practice by using routinely available clinical information for knowledge-generation. He is an author of several books and numerous articles on program evaluation, research utilization, practice-based research and CDM, his newest book is entitled Clinical Data-Mining: Integrating Practice and Research, and is published by Oxford University Press.

Lynette Joubert is an Associate Professor, trained as a Social Worker and Clinical Psychologist and has had experience as a clinician, teacher and researcher in mental health and health. She is a Senior Lecturer in Social Work, School of Health Sciences at the University of Melbourne, the Coordinator of the Health Practice Research Unit in the school, and a member of the Behavioural Research and Ethics Committee of the University of Melbourne. She has a research interest in the contribution of eco-systemic social and psychological factors to recovery and disease management with a particular focus on depression. Dr Joubert is the Principal Investigator on three Australian Research Council grants and works as a consultant in academic practice research collaboration with the Peter MacCallum Cancer Centre in Melbourne, Australia.

Aris Gkoulalas-Divanis received his BSc degree in computer science from the University of Ioannina (2003), the MS degree from the University of Minnesota (2005) and the PhD degree (with honors) from the University of Thessaly (2009). His doctoral dissertation received the Certificate of Recognition in the 2009 SIGKDD Dissertation Award. Currently, he is a Postdoctoral Research Fellow in the Department of Biomedical Informatics at Vanderbilt University. In the past he served as a research assistant in the University of Minnesota (2003-2005) and the University of Manchester (2006). His research interests are in the areas of databases, privacy preserving data mining, privacy and anonymity in trajectories and location-based services, and privacy in medical records. Dr Gkoulalas-Divanis is a member of ACM, IEEE, SIAM and UPE, a regular reviewer for DKE, KAIS and Computing Reviews, as well as he serves in the Editorial board of Crossroads and IJKBO.

Vassilios S. Verykios received the Diploma degree in computer engineering from the University of Patras in Greece (1992) and the MS and PhD degrees from Purdue University (1997 and 1999, respectively). In 1999, he joined the Faculty of Information Systems, College of Information Science and Technology, Drexel University, Philadelphia, Pennsylvania. Since 2005, he has been an Assistant Professor in the Department of Computer and Communication Engineering, University of Thessaly, Volos, Greece. He has also served on the faculty of Athens Information Technology Center, Hellenic Open University, and University of Patras. Dr Verykios has published more numerous papers in major referred journals and in the proceedings of international conferences and workshops. He has served in the program committees of several international scientific events. He is a member of the IEEE Computer Society, IEEE and UPE.

Konrad Stark is currently working a Research Assistant at the Institute of Knowledge and Business Engineering at the University of Vienna. He holds a master's degree in Computer Science from the University of Klagenfurt. Together with Wilfried Gansterer and Michael Illger he has been working on a technical report about the implications of the EU data retention directive. His main research interests include data warehousing, data mining, knowledge discovery, bioinformatics, statistics, data privacy and data security (k-anonymity), collaborative systems, and service-oriented architectures.

Michael Ilger currently lives and works as a Software Developer for a large international bank in Vancouver, BC. He holds master's degrees in Computer Science and Information Systems from the Vienna University of Technology and the University of Vienna. He has worked as a researcher at the University of Vienna for a number of years, studying the nature of spam and also doing research on process modelling and data exchange formats.

Wilfried Gansterer is currently an Associate Professor of Computer Science at the University of Vienna. He earned a masters degree in mathematics from Vienna University of Technology, an MSc in Scientific Computing/Computational Mathematics from Stanford University, and a PhD in Scientific Computing from Vienna University of Technology. He spent several years as post doctoral research associate at the Department of Computer Science at the University of Tennessee at Knoxville, and then joined the Department of Distributed and Multimedia Systems at the University of Vienna as assistant professor. Some years ago Dr Gansterer was promoted to associate professor and appointed head of the Research Lab Computational Technologies and Applications of the Faculty of Computer Science at the University of Vienna. His research interests include scientific computing and computational science, parallel and distributed computing, numerical and high performance computing, as well as internet security and data mining.

Jukka Aaltonen is a Researcher in the University of Lapland, Finland. His academic career includes mostly European based research projects that are multidisciplinary in their nature. He has done research in both University of Technology Helsinki and University of Lapland and in such fields as information technology, network management, cognitive sciences, philosophy of mind and performing arts (theatre). Current post-graduate studies, academic research and teaching focus on the cross-disciplinary conceptual analysis and information modelling supporting the operations and management of knowledge intensive IT-enabled business and public networks. Specifically Aaltonen has been interested in the fundamental nature of information and knowledge at the philosophically grounded metatheoretical level in the context of the semantization of information intensive web based environments.

Annamari Turunen has a PhD (law) degree and is momentarily working at the University of Lapland at the Department of Research Methodology. Dissertation thesis, discussing on intellectual property rights, was completed some year ago. The view was the mixed one of information law and property law and the aim was to question the plausibility of the system of intellectual property rights. Former posts of Turunen have been at the Faculty of Law at the University of Lapland: as an Assistant of Legal Informatics, an Assistant Professor, and as a Researcher in different research projects funded by the Academy of Finland. Dr Turunen has achieved practical experience by completing training on the chair in the District Court. The research of Dr Turunen has mainly been concentrating on finding new ways of seeing traditional legal areas, basically on property law and intellectual property rights.

Ilkka Kamaja is a Development Manager of the Faculty of Social Sciences at the University of Lapland. He has worked as a Lecturer in Information Technology (IT). The current sphere of responsibilities involves planning IT based research projects, and the development of cooperation between IT and other scientific fields. Additionally Kamaja has also been engaged in scientific research distinctly focusing on scientific theory. The objective of research has been to build a firm scientific philosophical and theoretical base for the scientific concept for IT, with the central goals of combining technological and social perspectives with the operating environments of modern information technology, and the development of epistemic communities through shared knowledge.

Oliver Krone has a master degree in Political Science with minors in Law and Education. Additionally he has a Master Degree in Business Administration (International Management). Dr Krone received a PhD in Public Administration in 2007 with the title "The Interaction of Organizational Structure and Humans in Knowledge Integration". His academic research areas are in the field of multiprofessional cooperation for product development (organizational innovation management) in a broad sense. He employs a framework entailing socio-psychological and knowledge difference as well as organizational structures. Dr Krone has published in peer-reviewed journals and he has contributed in many forums of knowledge and information systems. Dr Krone has also over ten year's practical experience in multiprofessional corporate work and seven years in depth project experiences of implementation and requirements engineering for ERP.

Martin Kitchener MBA PhD is Associate Dean at Cardiff Business School where he also serves as a Professor of Public Management and Policy, and Director of Cardiff Healthcare Organization and Policy Studies (CHOPS). His research and teaching concentrate on organization theory and public sector management and policy. Martin's research is published in journals including: Organization Studies, Organization, Health Services Research, Medical Care Research and Review, Health Affairs, Inquiry, and Journal of Health and Social Behavior. Professor Kitchener is also the co-author of two books: Managing Residential Children's Care: A Managed Service, and Major Works in Health Service Management.

Rauno Kuusisto is a Professor and Head of a Division at the Finnish Defence Force Technical Centre. He is also an Adjunct Professor of network enabled defence at Finnish National Defence University. Professor Kuusisto was granted as PhD at Helsinki University of Technology and on the area of corporate security and futures studies. Also he has general staff officer qualification. He has over 30 years experience mainly as a developer of heavy duty communication systems, intelligence systems and decision support systems as well as educating people up to doctoral programs. Professor Kuusisto has numerous scientific publications and research reports on the areas like network management, situation understanding, information and decision-making, and safety and security issues. He is an active member of several scientific advisory boards, and conference and journal reviewer.

José Luis Zafra-Gomez is an Associate Professor of Public Management at Granada University, Spain. He is a member of the Spanish Association of Accounting University Teachers, Spanish Association of Accounting and Management (AECA) and a member of the European Accounting Association. He teaches public sector management and control. His research interests are on management systems and financial information in central and local government. He has published in scientific journals such as The American Review of Public Administration, Public Money & Management and International Review of Administrative Science. Dr Zafra-Gomez is also the author of chapters in several science books.

Antonio Manuel Cortés-Romero is an Associate Professor of Financial Accounting at the Department of Accounting and Finance, University of Granada, Spain. Dr Cortés-Romero has studied economics and did his PhD at the University of Granada. His research interests are profitability analyses, investment projects, real options, ERP and data mining. Dr Cortés-Romero has numerous publication and science papers, while his current interests are on research projects like "Empirical Valuation of Real Options in Spanish Firms", "Entrepreneurial Stand", and "Financial Planning". These researches are funded by Spanish Ministries and Government.

Zdravko Pečar is an Associate Professor at Faculty of Public Administration at University of Ljubljana and a Chair for Management and Economics. He is also director of Institute for regional economics IREL. He received his undergraduate degree in economics from Brigham Young University, Provo (Utah), a master degree in business administration from Utah State University (Salt Lake City), and doctoral degree in organizational science from University of Maribor, Slovenia. His currently research interest is the field of public sector economics and management. Dr Pečar's recent projects include developing models for assessing quality in elementary, vocational and high school level within EU project Commenius (QiS – Quality in school), and developing quality assessment systems with TQM tools for higher education in Slovenia.

Ivan Bratko is a Professor of Computer Science at the Faculty of Computer and Information Science, Ljubljana University, Slovenia. He heads the AI laboratory at the University. Until 2002 he also directed the AI department of J. Stefan Institute. He has conducted research in machine learning, knowledge-based systems, qualitative modelling, intelligent robotics, heuristic programming and computer chess. Professor Bratko is the author of widely adopted text Prolog Programming for Artificial Intelligence (3rd edition) and numerous publications in scientific journals and conferences. Professor Bratko has been visiting professor at Edinburgh University, Strathclyde University, Glasgow University, Sydney University and University of New South Wales, etc.

Index

A

activity utility data 344
administrative districts 67, 68, 69, 70, 73, 74, 75, 76, 77, 78, 79, 80, 81, 82
administrative services 67, 68, 69, 70, 72, 79, 80, 82
administrative services, basic unit of 82
administrative services, work performance at 68
advertising campaigns 247, 248, 252, 262, 263
aggregation of findings 323
artificial neural networks (ANN) 184, 186, 187, 188, 189, 191, 203, 205
artificial neurons 203
assassins problem 270
asset turnover 22
asymmetric keys 155
Australia v, x, 316, 317, 325, 327, 328, 329, 333
autonomous government agencies 2

B

Bayesian theory 268
Belgium iv, vii, 106, 109
benchmarking 3
BI-Coop project 220, 242
binary-class classification 219
blocking techniques 126
body of evidence (BOE) 269, 270, 271, 272, 273, 274, 278, 279, 280, 281, 283
budgetary stability 21, 22
budgetary sustainability 21, 24, 28, 33, 40
budget authorities 69
budgets 21, 22, 23, 24, 28, 33, 39, 40

building blocks 360, 361
business cases 245, 246, 250, 251
business environment 245, 246
business intelligence (BI) 166, 220, 290
business networks 289, 290, 294, 297, 298, 299, 303, 307, 309, 310, 311, 312

C

C4.5 decision trees 24, 42
capital expenditure 21, 29, 30, 31, 32, 33, 35, 38, 40
CART decision trees 24, 25
certificate authority 155
CHAID (chi-squared automatic interaction detector) decision tree technique 21, 22, 24, 25, 28, 33, 40, 41, 42
child care 87
child day care services 83, 84, 87, 100
Children's Online Privacy Protection Act (COPPA) 108
churn 258, 264, 265
churn trends 245, 246, 247, 248, 249, 250, 258, 259, 260, 261, 262, 263, 264
classification 187, 203
classification and ranking belief simplex (CaRBS) 267, 268, 269, 271, 272, 273, 274, 275, 276, 277, 278, 279, 280, 281, 282, 283, 284, 285
classification model 204, 243
classification rule 243
classifier 205, 209, 212, 218
classifier, probabilistic 218
clinical data mining (CDM) 316, 317, 318, 319, 320, 321, 322, 323, 324, 325, 326, 327, 328, 329, 330, 336